Human Sexuality

IN HEALTH AND ILLNESS

Human Sexuality
IN HEALTH AND ILLNESS

Nancy Fugate Woods, R.N., Ph.D., F.A.A.N.

Professor
University of Washington
School of Nursing
Seattle, Washington

THIRD EDITION

Illustrated

THE C. V. MOSBY COMPANY

ST. LOUIS   TORONTO   1984

MOSBY

A TRADITION OF PUBLISHING EXCELLENCE

Editor: Julie Cardamon
Assistant editor: Bess Arends
Manuscript editor: Linda L. Duncan
Book design: Jeanne Bush
Cover design: Suzanne Oberholtzer
Production: Barbara Merritt

Cover photo: Lisa Suits

THIRD EDITION

The C.V. Mosby Company
11830 Westline Industrial Drive, St. Louis, Missouri 63146

Library of Congress Cataloging in Publication Data

Main entry under title:

Human sexuality in health and illness.

    Includes bibliographies and index.
    1. Sick—Sexual behavior. 2. Sex. 3. Sexual disorders.
4. Nursing. I. Woods, Nancy Fugate. [DNLM: 1. Sex
behavior. HQ 21 W896h]
RT87.S49H84   1984   612.6   83-8260
ISBN 0-8016-5628-1

GW/VH/VH 9 8 7 6 5 4 3 2 1   03/D/323

Contributors

PATRICIA BERKE, R.N., M.S.

Research Analyst, Family Medicine, University of Washington; formerly Research Assistant, University of Washington School of Nursing, Department of Psychosocial Nursing, Seattle, Washington

THOMAS DeMARIA, B.S., R.N.

Graduate Student, Health Services Administration, University of Washington, Seattle, Washington

GRETCHEN KRAMER DERY, R.N., M.S.

Associate Professor, Duke University School of Nursing, Durham, North Carolina

GORDON L. DICKMAN, M.A.

Sex Counselor and Educator; Co-Director, Seattle Sexual Health Center, Seattle, Washington

CATHERINE INGRAM FOGEL, R.N., M.S.

Associate Professor, University of North Carolina School of Nursing, Durham, North Carolina

CYNTHIA GATENS, R.N., M.N.

Clinical Nurse Specialist, Grant Hospital, Columbus, Ohio

JEANNE MINOR HERBERT, R.N., M.S.

Formerly Instructional Assistant, Duke University School of Nursing, Durham, North Carolina

ROSA M. JOHNSON, C.R.N., M.N.

Clinical Specialist, Northwest Hospital, Seattle, Washington

MARCIA KILLIEN, R.N., M.S.

> Associate Professor, University of Washington School of Nursing, Department of Parent and Child Nursing, Seattle, Washington

CANDACE KIRCHNER, R.N., M.N.

> Lecturer, University of Washington School of Nursing, Department of Physiological Nursing, Seattle, Washington

MARY BETH KNAPP, R.N., M.S.N.

> Formerly Assistant Professor, Department of Parent-Child Nursing, University of Washington School of Nursing, Seattle, Washington

CAROLYN A. LIVINGSTON, R.N., A.A., S.E.C.T., Ph.D.

> Certified Sex Therapist, Seattle Sexual Health Center, Seattle, Washington

CYNTHIA LUKE, R.N., M.S.

> Formerly Assistant Professor, Duke University School of Nursing, Durham, North Carolina

MARILYN C. McINTYRE, M.S.W.

> Co-Director, Seattle Institute for Sex Therapy, Education, and Research; Counselor, Educator, and Consultant in Private Practice, Seattle, Washington

CAROL L. STADE, R.N., M.S.N.

> Lecturer, Department of Parent-Child Nursing, University of Washington School of Nursing, Seattle, Washington

ANNE STAMER, R.N., M.S.P.H.

> Lecturer, Duke University School of Nursing, Durham, North Carolina

CONSTANCE VAUGHT, R.N., M.S.

> Formerly Instructor, Duke University School of Nursing, Durham, North Carolina

CARMEN GERMAINE WARNER, R.N., M.S.N., F.A.A.N.

> President and Publisher, Capistrano Press, Ltd., Garden Grove, California

MARILYN WHITLEY, R.N., M.S.

> Assistant Dean, Student Affairs, University of Portland School of Nursing, Portland, Oregon; formerly Lecturer, University of Washington School of Nursing, Department of Psychosocial Nursing, Seattle, Washington

JAMES S. WOODS, Ph.D., M.P.H.

> Health and Population Study Center, Battelle Human Affairs
> Research Centers, Seattle, Washington

NANCY FUGATE WOODS, R.N., Ph.D., F.A.A.N.

> Professor, Department of Physiological Nursing, University of
> Washington School of Nursing, Seattle, Washington

Preface

Human sexuality is a complex phenomenon, pervading every aspect of our being. It is a source of pleasure, even peak experiences. Sexuality can also be a source of great pain. It is vulnerable to the vicissitudes of stress and strain of daily living and illness.

Sexuality is multidimensional. Sexual health is reflected in the integration of biologic, intrapersonal, social, and cultural aspects of our being. Unit I examines human sexuality as a multidimensional phenomenon. Human sexual behavior, how it is influenced by social and biologic processes, variability in expression of sexual behavior, and the development of sexuality throughout the life span are considered. In Unit II sexual health and health care, including assessment of sexual health, sex education, counseling, and therapy, are discussed. In Unit III clinical aspects of human sexuality are examined.

This text views human sexuality in health and illness from a multidimensional perspective. Several life events influence sexuality. Pregnancy and lactation change a woman's biology, her image of herself, and her social relationships. Abortion, a crisis situation, may have some sequelae affecting a woman's sexuality and that of her partner. Sexual assault has the potential to negatively influence a woman's future sexual functioning, her concept of herself as a woman, and her social relationships. Fertility and infertility raise important sexual issues.

Hospitalization and illness warrant certain changes in life-style, one of which is altered sexual behavior patterns. Chronic illnesses such as diabetes, renal disease, cancer, arthritis, and heart disease; surgery that alters body image; spinal cord injury; stroke; and drug abuse or drug therapy are each capable of interfering with normal sexual functioning.

Sexually transmitted diseases are becoming increasingly prevalent in society. Their identification, treatment, and prevention constitute an important contemporary public health problem. Changes in the life patterns of individuals with developmental disabilities have brought sexual issues to the fore. Health professionals are asked to help the developmentally disabled embrace their sexuality at the same time that they are striving to become integrated in a world oriented to the nondisabled.

Throughout the book an attempt has been made to review current literature dealing with each topic; to examine the area in view of its biologic, psychologic, and social ramifications; and to suggest guidelines with which the health care practitioner can intervene with clients in certain life situations that threaten sexual integrity. Case examples are presented in review questions to help both students and practitioners apply the theories, principles, and research findings discussed in each chapter.

The guidelines for practice presented here are general in their orientation. Not every principle will be applicable in every situation or to each client. Practitioners will find it necessary to modify their approaches to their individual clients, to the context in which they practice, and to their own comfort and style of providing care.

Nancy Fugate Woods

Contents

Human Sexuality
IN HEALTH AND ILLNESS

I

Human sexuality: an overview

1

Human sexuality: a holistic perspective

Human sexuality is a highly complex phenomenon. Sexuality pervades human beings, influencing their self-images and feelings. It influences their relationships with others. In addition, sexuality involves the biologic basis for experiencing sexual pleasure, giving and receiving sensual pleasure, and is a powerful force in a person's ability to bond to another person. Sexuality is concerned with the biologic, psychologic, sociologic, spiritual, and cultural aspects of life.

The purposes of this chapter follow:
1. To review the physiologic components of the human sexual response cycle
2. To consider the psychologic components of the human sexual response
3. To discuss psychosocial and cultural factors influencing sexuality

Physiologic aspects of human sexual response

Little knowledge about the physiologic aspects of human sexual response existed until the publication of Masters and Johnson's classic volume in 1966.[17] Masters and Johnson sought to determine what physical phenomena developed as humans responded to sexual stimulation and what psychosocial factors influenced how they responded. Their method of study consisted of direct observation and measurement of the changes that occur during the sexual response.

In the monitoring of the human sexual response cycle Masters and Johnson[17] recorded two principal physiologic changes: vasoconstriction and myotonia. Vasoconstriction is defined as congestion of blood vessels, usually venous vessels, and is the primary physiologic response to sexual stimulation. Myotonia, increased muscular tension, is a secondary physiologic response to sexual stimulation. These two changes are responsible for the phenomena observed during the sexual response cycle.

Phases of the cycle. To facilitate description of their observations, Masters and Johnson arbitrarily chose to divide the cycle into four phases: excitement, plateau, orgasm, and resolution. The excitement phase develops from any source of bodily or psychic stimuli, and if adequate stimulation occurs, the intensity of excitement increases rapidly. This phase may be interrupted, prolonged, or ended by distracting stimuli.

The plateau phase is a consolidation period that follows excitement if adequate stimulation is maintained. Sexual tension becomes intensified to the level at which the person may experience orgasm. Like excitement, this phase may also be affected by distracting stimuli.

Orgasm, the involuntary climax of sexual tension increment, involves only a few seconds of the human sexual response cycle during which vasocongestion and myotonia are released. There appears to be greater variation of intensity and duration of orgasm among females than among males. Although the total body is involved, the sensual focus during orgasm is usually in the pelvic area.[17]

During the resolution phase the person undergoes involutional changes that restore the preexcitement state. Females may, if adequately stimulated, begin another sexual response cycle immediately before sexual excitement totally resolves. However, for males a refractory period during which they cannot be restimulated is superimposed on the resolution period. Unless orgasm has been overwhelming, sexual tension dissipates slowly. Usually the length of the resolution periods parallels the length of the excitement phase.

Masters and Johnson[17] described only one sexual response pattern for males, although it is highly unlikely that it is invariant. In this pattern, illustrated in Fig. 1-1, excitement proceeds rapidly, followed by a short plateau period, orgasm, and a resolution period. Although Masters and Johnson state that the variety of patterns for females is almost infinite, they described the three most prevalent patterns (Fig. 1-2). In pattern *A*, the female experiences multiple orgasms, with a fairly rapid resolution period. Pattern *B* depicts a nonorgasmic cycle in which several peaks are noted in the plateau phase and a longer resolution period occurs. Pattern *C* shows a cycle in which the female's excitement is first interrupted or distracted, an intense orgasm occurs, and resolution is very rapid.

A very important finding from the work of Masters and Johnson[17] is that human sexual response is a total body response rather than merely a pelvic phenomenon. Changes in

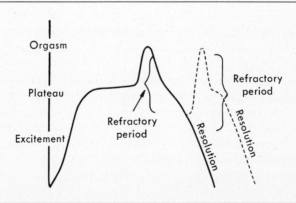

Fig. 1-1. Male sexual response cycle. (From Masters, W., and Johnson, V.: Human sexual response, Boston, 1966, Little, Brown & Co.)

the cardiovascular and respiratory function and reactions involving skin, muscle, breasts, and the rectal sphincter are observed during the sexual response cycle.

      Excitement phase. During the excitement phase of the human sexual response cycle the clitoral glans becomes tumescent, or enlarged, and the clitoral shaft increases in diameter and elongates. The appearance of vaginal lubrication, caused by vasocongestion and likened to a sweating process, occurs within 10 to 30 seconds after initiation of sexual stimulation. The vaginal barrel expands about 3.75 to 4.25 cm in transcervical width and lengthens 2.5 to 3.5 cm. In addition, the vaginal wall develops a purplish hue because of vasocongestion. Partial elevation of the uterus may occur if it lies in the anterior position. Irritation of the corpus uteri may also occur.

    In the nulliparous woman, flattening and separating of the labia majora occur as in an apparent effort to open the entrance to the vagina. In the multiparous woman the labia majora move slightly away from the introitus because of a vasocongestive increase in their diameter. The vaginal barrel is lengthened approximately 1 cm as a result of the thickening of the labia minora. No changes have been observed in Bartholin's glands during this phase.

    In the male there is rapid erection of the penis, which may be partially lost and regained during this phase. At this time there is also the possibility that distracting stimuli may interfere with erection.[17]

    Tensing and thickening of the scrotal skin occur with elevation of the scrotal sac. Both testes are partially elevated toward the perineum as the spermatic cords shorten.

    During this phase vasocongestion causes both penile erection and vaginal lubrication. Thickening of the scrotal skin, elevation of the scrotal sac, elevation and flattening of

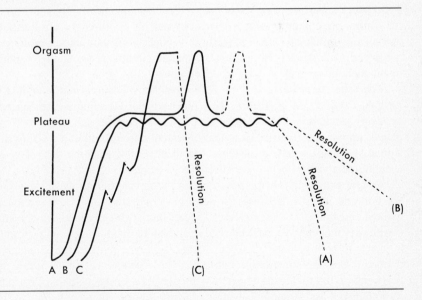

Fig. 1-2. Female sexual response cycle. (From Masters, W., and Johnson, V.: Human sexual response, Boston, 1966, Little, Brown & Co.)

the labia majora in the nulliparous woman, thickening of the labia majora in the multiparous woman, and extension of the labia minora are also vasocongestive reactions. As partial elevation of the testes occurs, the vasocongestive increase in their size begins. This reaction corresponds with the lengthening and broadening of the vagina.

During the excitement phase changes also occur in the extragenital organs. In the female, nipples may become erect, breast size increases, the areolae become engorged, and the venous pattern on the breast becomes more obvious. The "sex flush," a maculopapular rash, may appear over the epigastric area, spreading quickly over the breasts. Some involuntary muscle tensing may be evident, as in the tensing of intercostal and abdominal muscles. The heart rate and blood pressure also increase as sexual tension increases.

In some males, nipple erection occurs during this phase. There is also evidence of involuntary muscle tensing, such as tensing of the intercostal and abdominal muscles. The heart rate and blood pressure levels parallel sexual excitement.

Plateau phase. During the plateau phase the clitoris retracts against the anterior body of the symphysis pubis, underneath the clitoral hood. Vasocongestion of the outer third of the vagina and the labia minora causes an increase in size of this highly sensitive tissue, which is referred to as the orgasmic platform. Further increase in the depth and width of the vaginal barrel appears. The uterus becomes fully elevated, and as the cervix rises it produces a tenting effect in the inner part of the vagina. Irritability of the corpus uteri continues to intensify.

In both nulliparous and multiparous women the labia majora continue to become engorged, with this phenomenon being more pronounced in nulliparous women. The labia minora undergo a vivid color change from bright red to a deep wine-colored hue. This change in the "sex skin" is considered pathognomonic of impending orgasm. During the plateau phase a drop or two of mucoid material is secreted from Bartholin's glands; this secretion probably assists slightly in vaginal lubrication during prolonged coitus.

In the male there is an increase in penile circumference at the coronal ridge. An inconsistent deepening of color has been noted in this area.

The testes increase in size by 50% over their nonstimulated state and elevate to a position closer to the perineum. This full testicular elevation is pathognomonic of impending ejaculation. Two or three drops of mucoid material, secreted from Cowper's glands, appear at a time similar to that of secretion from Bartholin's glands in the female. Active spermatozoa have been observed in this fluid, negating the utility of coitus interruptus as a very effective contraceptive technique.

Several extragenital responses occur in the female during the plateau phase. Nipple erection and turgidity continue to develop, along with an increase in breast size and marked engorgement of the areolae. The sex flush, which began during excitement, may spread over the body. Facial, abdominal, and intercostal muscles contract; muscle tension is increased both voluntarily and involuntarily. Some females use voluntary rectal contraction to enhance stimulation during this phase. Hyperventilation occurs, along with a heart rate of 100 to 175 beats per minute, elevation of the systolic blood pressure of 20 to 60 mm Hg, and diastolic elevation of 10 to 20 mm Hg.

In the male, nipple erection and turgidity occur inconsistently. The sex flush, as described in the female, may appear late in this phase in some males. As in the female, a further increase in voluntary and involuntary muscle tension occurs. Again, there may be voluntary contraction of the rectal sphincter. Late in the plateau phase, hyperventilation appears. The elevation of heart rate is similar to that of the female, but the elevation of blood pressure is often greater for the male; the systolic rise may be 20 to 80 mm Hg and the diastolic 10 to 40 mm Hg.

Orgasm. During the orgasmic phase the primary response occurs in the female's orgasmic platform, as illustrated in Fig. 1-3. About five to twelve contractions occur in the orgasmic platform at 0.8-second intervals. After the first three to six contractions the interval between contractions increases, and the intensity diminishes.[17] The pelvic floor muscles that surround the lower third of the vagina contract against the engorged vessels, thus forcing out the blood trapped in them. It is thought that a stretch reflex mechanism is one factor responsible for orgasm.[27] Contractions of the uterus begin at the fundus and progress to the lower segment of the uterus. The contractile excursion of the uterus parallels the intensity of the orgasmic experience.

In the male there are expulsive contractions of the entire length of the penile urethra, as illustrated in Fig. 1-4. They start at 0.8-second intervals, as in the female. Again, the frequency of contraction is reduced after the first three or four contractions. The expulsive force of ejaculation is also reduced in the male after the initial forceful contractions. During orgasm there is also contraction of secondary organs such as the vasa efferentia of the testes (the epididymis, vas deferens, and seminal vesicles) and the prostate. At

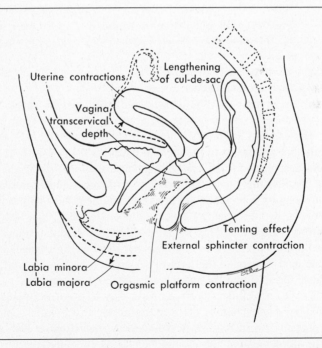

Fig. 1-3. Female pelvis: orgasmic phase. (From Masters, W., and Johnson, V.: Human sexual response, Boston, 1966, Little, Brown & Co.)

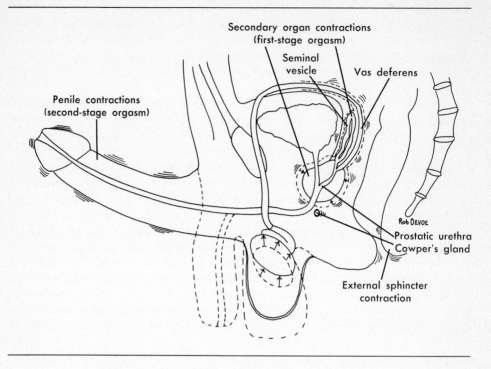

Fig. 1-4. Male pelvis: orgasmic phase. (From Masters, W., and Johnson, V.: Human sexual response, Boston, 1966, Little, Brown & Co.)

the onset of ejaculation the internal bladder sphincter closes or remains sealed, preventing retrograde ejaculation into the bladder.

The ejaculatory process may be divided into two separate stages. During stage I seminal fluid substrate is expelled from the accessory organs of reproduction, such as the seminal vesicles, into the prostatic urethra. During stage II the seminal fluid from the prostatic urethra progresses to the urethral meatus.

Extragenital responses for the female involve several organ systems during orgasm. The sex flush parallels the intensity of orgasmic experience and is present in about 75% of females. Involuntary contraction and spasm of muscle groups may be seen, including contractions of the rectal sphincter, which occur at the same intervals as those of the orgasmic platform. Respiratory rates as high as 40 breaths per minute have been recorded, along with pulse rates from 110 to 180 beats per minute. Fluctuations in the pulse and respiratory rate tend to parallel the level of sexual tension. The systolic blood pressure may be elevated 30 to 80 mm Hg and the diastolic 20 to 40 mm Hg.

In 25% of males a well-developed sex flush may be seen. Involuntary muscle contractions, including contraction of the rectal sphincter at 0.8-second intervals, are also seen during orgasm. An increase in respiratory and heart rates occurs, as seen in the female, but the blood pressure elevation in the male is more pronounced, with 40 to 100 mm Hg systolic elevation and 20 to 50 mm Hg diastolic.

Recent work has explored orgasmic expulsion of fluid occurring in some females and has compared it with the process of ejaculation. Although earlier studies of female sexuality[16,17] stressed that ejaculation was the only physiologic phenomenon in sexual response that was not homologous in males and females, there is a long history of literary and scientific reference to female ejaculation.[4] Females who experience orgasmic expulsions describe the experience as a gushing of fluids with orgasm. Often they have been diagnosed and treated for stress incontinence. Possible sources of the fluid expelled at orgasm might include Bartholin's gland, the vagina, the periurethral glands, or the urinary bladder.[4]

The orgasmic expulsions appear to be triggered by stimulation of the Gräfenberg spot, an anatomic site in the anterior vaginal wall corresponding to the site of Skene's glands. Stimulation of the Gräfenberg spot produces first an urge to urinate, followed by intense pleasure; the area increases in size with stimulation. Expulsions of fluid from the urethral meatus have been observed in response to stimulation of the Gräfenberg spot. Chemical analysis of specimens obtained from orgasmic expulsions in a single case study revealed that concentrations of prostatic acid phosphatase were higher in the orgasmic expulsions than in urine specimens obtained from the same subject, whereas urea and creatinine levels were significantly lower and glucose levels were similar. This would suggest that orgasmic expulsions are not urine but possibly glandular secretions. In this study it did not appear that orgasmic expulsions in females were followed by a refractory period.[1]

Resolution. During the resolution phase the female's clitoris returns to its normal position within 5 to 10 seconds after the contractions of the orgasmic platform cease. Vasocongestion and tumescence of the clitoris dissipate more slowly. Rapid detumescence, or loss of vasocongestion, of the orgasmic platform and relaxation of the walls of the vagina occur. The vaginal wall returns to its normal coloring in about 10 to 15 minutes. A gaping of the cervical os continues for 20 to 30 minutes after orgasm. The uterus returns to its unstimulated position in the true pelvis, and the cervix descends into the dorsal area of the vagina, termed the seminal basin. In the nulliparous woman the labia majora return to their preexcitement position, and in the multiparous woman the labial vasocongestion dissipates. The labia minora change from deep red to light pink, and they decrease in size as vasocongestion is lost.

Involution of nipple erection, a slow decrease in breast size, and rapid reversal of the sex flush are seen. Some myotonia may still be seen during resolution. The respiratory rate, pulse rate, and blood pressure return to normal levels. An involuntary widespread film of perspiration may appear.

In the male there is initially a rapid loss of vasocongestion until the penis is from one to one and one-half times as large as normal; this decrease in size is followed by a slower involution to preexcitement levels. There is a rapid loss of the congested appearance of the scrotum, with the reappearance of skin folds. The testes descend into the relaxed scrotum and return to their normal size. Rapid involution of nipple erection and reversal of the sex flush occur. As in the female, myotonia may persist for a few minutes. Vital signs return to normal. An involuntary sweating reaction of the palms of the hands and soles of the feet may appear.

In the male a refractory period, during which he cannot be restimulated, is superimposed on the resolution phase.[17] A questionnaire investigation of 78 males ranging from 15 to 68 years of age indicated that the refractory period is not as long as might be suspected. Comfort[7] asked these male volunteers to measure refractory periods in three trials. In 48 of the respondents the refractory period lasted no longer than 10 minutes in two out of three trials. Eleven others were able to be restimulated to erection in 30 minutes. Respondents who were 40, 54, 61, 66, and 68 years of age required 45 minutes or longer in two out of three trials, but only 9 subjects under 30 years required more than 10 minutes. However, 8 men between 50 and 60 years of age could secure another erection in 10 minutes. In general, refractory time did increase with age, but the imagined lengthy refraction time may be an illusion.

Sarrel[25] points out that a number of qualifications apply to the physiologic events outlined for each phase of the sexual response cycle. Not every individual will experience each response; for example, the sex flush or nipple erection in the male may not appear. The same individual may experience differing responses from cycle to cycle. The observations of physical accompaniments of sexual response appear regardless of the type of behavior: autoerotic, homosexual, or heterosexual. The sexual response has been observed in both sleeping and wakeful states.

Triphasic nature of sexual response. Although the four-stage sexual response cycle described by Masters and Johnson has been helpful in describing the sequential physiologic changes, Kaplan[14] suggests that the nature of human sexual response is actually triphasic. She delineates three phases that are related components of sexual response but are governed by separate neurophysiologic systems: desire, excitement, and orgasm. This notion is useful for understanding not only the physiology of sexual response but also the consequences of pathophysiology, the etiology of sexual dysfunction, and appropriate therapies.

The *desire phase* refers to the experiences of sexual appetite or drive produced by the activation of a neural system in the brain. Sexual desire is experienced as sensations that move the person to seek out sexual experience. Although the precise neural circuitry involved in sexual desire is unknown, it is believed to involve the limbic system and the preoptic nuclei of the hypothalamus. It is likely that the sexual centers of the brain have either neural or chemical connections with the pleasure and pain centers of the brain. The pleasure centers are stimulated when people have sex, accounting for the pleasurable quality of sexual behavior. The pain centers, on the other hand, can inhibit the sexual system. Some even suggest that the pleasure center is stimulated by release of endorphins in sexual behavior. If a sexual object or situation produces pain, then it will cease to evoke desire. Testosterone is important in mediating sexual desire in both males and females. Luteinizing hormone also may be important in mediating sexual desire. Two neurotransmitters, serotonin (5-HT) and dopamine, are also believed to be important. Serotonin seems to act as an inhibitor of and dopamine as a stimulant to the sexual centers of the brain. Bonding to another person and love are powerful stimuli to sexual desire. There seem to be many stimuli capable of evoking sexual desire, such as sight, smell, and other sensory cues, and some of these are conditioned by the culture. Fear and pain, however, are potent inhibitors. The connections between the sex centers and other parts of the brain also make it possible for people to "turn off" sexual desire when other stimuli are more important or when it is not to the individual's advantage to pursue sexual activity.[14]

The *excitement phase* of sexual response, similar to the excitement and plateau phases described by Masters and Johnson, is produced by reflex vasodilation of the genital blood vessels. Two centers in the spinal cord, S2 to S4 and T11 to L2, cause the arterioles to dilate. This vasodilation causes the genitals to swell and changes their shape to adapt to their reproductive function. The vasocongestion is primarily a parasympathetically mediated response, and the intense sympathetic response, such as that produced by fear and anxiety, can instantly lead to loss of erection. It is believed that erection is governed by two spinal reflex centers. The thoracolumbar center (psychogenic) appears to respond more to psychic stimuli, whereas the sacral center is stimulated from tactile input to the genitals. It is believed that the spinal reflex centers and the higher neural connections are analogous in males and females.

The *orgasm phase* of sexual response, corresponding to that described by Masters and Johnson, is also a genital reflex governed by spinal neural centers and consists of reflex contractions of certain genital muscles. Sensory influences that trigger orgasm enter the cord in the pudendal nerve at the sacral level, and the efferents are T11 to L2.

Subjective experience of sexual response

The people in the sample studied by Masters and Johnson[17] were polled with regard to the subjective experience associated with orgasm. Three distinct stages of the female orgasmic experience were found. Orgasm begins as a sensation of "stoppage" or "suspension." This instantaneous sensation is followed by an intense sensual awareness oriented to the clitoris. A loss of sensory acuity has been described during this period. Some women described a sense of bearing down occurring simultaneously with the clitoral-pelvic sensation. A feeling of receptive opening has also been expressed by parous women. This sensation has been compared to sensations felt during the second stage of labor.

The second stage of the female orgasmic response is described as a feeling of warmth that pervades the pelvis and then spreads throughout the body. The third stage of subjective experience is a feeling of involuntary contraction of the vagina, followed by a sensation of pelvic throbbing. However, the female experience is highly individual and varied.

Men reported two stages of the subjective orgasmic experience. The first stage is a feeling of ejaculatory inevitability that develops as seminal fluid collects in the prostatic urethra. Distention of the urethral bulb may also contribute to this sensation. The second stage of subjective experience involves two phases: the sensation of contractions of the urethral sphincter and the perception of the volume of seminal fluid as it is expelled through the penile urethra.

Since Masters and Johnson's studies, Singer and Singer[28] have found that females describe three different types of orgasms: the vulval, uterine, and blended types. The vulval orgasm involves involuntary contractions of the orgasmic platform, as described by Masters and Johnson. The uterine orgasm depends on deep stimulation of the cervix that displaces the uterus, thus stimulating the peritoneum. It is characterized by a gasping type of breathing, eventually culminating in an explosive type of exhalation. The blended orgasm combines features of both the vulval and uterine variety. Even in the presence of complete spinal cord transection, nocturnal emissions and orgasm are experienced. Cognitional eroticism thus persists independent of sensation in the genitals. The brain seems to be able to work independent of the genitals just as the genitals of persons with spinal cord injuries work reflexly and independent of the brain.

Factors affecting sexual response

Many factors are capable of affecting sexual response, and most of them involve the brain, not the genitals. People's thoughts and feelings can produce physiologic signs of arousal and are just as capable of inhibiting sexual response.

Feelings such as anxiety and guilt may interfere with progression of the sexual response cycle. In addition, fear of failure may have a profound effect on sexual performance and may become internalized to the point of becoming a self-fulfilling prophecy. Stimuli from the environment, if interpreted as threatening or inconsistent with sexual actvity, may inhibit the development of desire, arousal, or orgasm.

Bardwick[2] suggests that among women there is a learned pattern involved in the achievement of orgasm, and she defines distinct levels of orgasmic response on the basis of interviews with a female sample. These three patterns are shown in Fig. 1-5. The first pattern *(A)* involves several surges toward orgasm once the woman reaches the plateau level. The sensation may be characterized as tingly, or as what Bardwick terms a minor orgasm. After a slow resolution the woman has experienced a nice feeling without frustration. Bardwick theorizes that the primary source of gratification is the affection or love that these women achieve; sex as a physical gratification is secondary. Some women never leave this level of arousability.

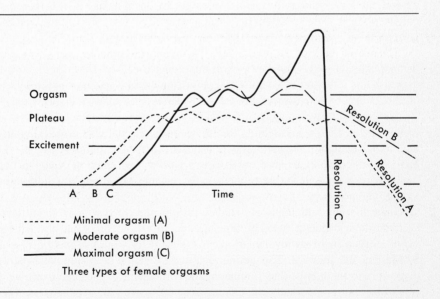

-------- Minimal orgasm (A)
— — — Moderate orgasm (B)
———— Maximal orgasm (C)
Three types of female orgasms

Fig. 1-5. Female sexual response patterns. (From Bardwick, J.: Psychology of women: a study of bio-cultural conflicts, New York, 1971, Harper & Row, Publishers, Inc.)

With sexual experience and experimentation, some women learn to maximize sensation, feelings, and pleasure in a trusting, stable relationship. Bardwick[2] believes that these women learn to deinhibit old inhibitions and forget the self. She hypothesizes that pattern *B* represents an intermediate level of arousability. In this pattern the woman achieves an orgasm but remains at the plateau level and can continue to have recurrent orgasms with some stimulation.

In pattern *C* the woman rapidly reaches plateau, achieves a maximal orgasm, and experiences a swift, total resolution. She requires 15 to 20 minutes of recovery time. Bardwick's model (pattern *C*) differs from that of Masters and Johnson in that, after this type of orgasm, the woman is actually at a level of sexual arousal lower than when sexual excitement was initiated. Some women reported being able to control their level of arousal to have several less intense orgasms before the explosive one that calls a halt to their immediate sexual excitement.

Pattern *C* was least frequently reported in Bardwick's sample.[2] She describes the excitement as desperate or imperative. Waves of pelvic sensation are felt. Bardwick theorizes that women who have achieved the pattern *C* orgasm are frustrated when it is not achieved on other occasions. Pelvic congestion and edema from the unrelieved high level of arousal and the expectation of the pattern *C* level of gratification contribute to their physical and psychologic discomfort.

Sherfey[27] proposes that a woman has an infinite capacity of orgasmic response if physical exhaustion does not intervene. This capacity she attributes to the presence of fulminating pelvic congestion and edema. During the last 14 days of the menstrual cycle parous women will be most likely to experience sexual insatiation because of the peculiar combination of progesterone levels and pelvic congestion. This is not to suggest that the woman is always unsatisfied at the conscious level but merely that she has a nearly infinite capacity to be orgasmic. Sherfey also develops interesting anthropologic theories related to the evolution of present-day female roles, which she postulates were largely based on the suppression of aggressive sex drives and woman's insatiation.

Psychosocial influences on sexual response patterns

Female patterns. There is some evidence that women's experience of orgasm depends more on their acceptance of their sexuality than is true for men. For many years authorities encouraged women to pretend orgasm, thus discouraging couples from communicating honestly about their sexual feelings. Changes in women's social situations, such as marriage, or demands made of them, such as parenting, can cause women to reevaluate or reorient their sexual behavior. For example, familiarity with and trust in a partner may make it possible for a woman to share her preferences about coital technique.

Masters and Johnson[17] found that variables relating to the woman's relationship influenced her subjective perception of sexual pleasure. Although self-pleasuring produced the most profound physiologic response to sexual stimuli, followed by partner manipulation and intercourse, the women in their study registered the most pleasurable feelings in response to intercourse.

Fisher,[10] in his study of female orgasm, found that certain psychosocial factors were correlated with orgasm consistency. Feelings of dependability with regard to the love object seemed to be the most influential variable in relation to orgasm consistency. Fisher theorized that fear of object loss, which is perhaps fostered by relations with an undependable father figure, may be subsequently revived as the woman experiences a blurring of perception during orgasm. This fear may have an inhibiting effect on orgasm attainment.

Male patterns. Masters and Johnson[17] state that the male's ejaculatory necessity has historically relieved him of psychosocial pressures that limit the female's orgasmic experience. His sexual behavior is much more acceptable to him and to others. It is interesting that fears of performance in American culture are primarily directed toward the male's erection rather than ejaculation, on the presumption that orgasm is not as problematic for the male as it is presumed to be for the female.

Guilt and anxiety. Guilt and anxiety about sexual performance are capable of interfering with the progression of the sexual response. Fear of failure may perpetuate failure and guilt may lead to sexual dysfunction. Since both guilt and anxiety are learned, they can be unlearned.

Perception and communication. Many people who are dissatisfied with their sexual experiences have problems communicating. One does not hesitate to tell another person how to scratch an itchy spot on his or her back: "A little more here, a little harder, now a little to the right." Unfortunately, many people are not nearly so candid or comfortable when communicating to a partner what is sexually pleasurable.

Sociocultural influences on sexual behavior. Sexual behavior is a product of both society and culture, as well as biologic structure and function. Cultural norms prescribe not only what types of behavior are acceptable but also who may perform them. Usually norms for males and females within a culture differ. To some extent, social structural variables such as class seem to influence sexual relationships.

What becomes most apparent in cross-cultural comparisons is the variety in forms of sexual expression. Indeed, a search for a definition of "normal" sexual behavior is likely to become a futile obsession. Comfort[8] asserts that the problem of defining "normal" sexual behavior is complicated by the many meanings of the word "normal," some of which follow:

1. Prevalent
2. Optimal function
3. Distributed in a statistical pattern
4. Fashionable
5. Socially acceptable

Comfort cautions clinicians not to define normal as what they, as counselors, find they are able to admit enjoying, although not necessarily what they actually enjoy or practice in private. He suggests that there are only three questions for clinicians to use as a guide when considering a particular behavior:

- What does the behavior mean to the individual?
- Does the behavior enrich or impoverish the sexual life of the individual and those persons with whom sexual relations are shared?
- Is the behavior tolerable to society?

With these considerations in mind, the wide variation in human sexual behavior can be appreciated rather than impugned (see Chapter 2 for a discussion of sexual variations).

Cultural variations. Davenport[9] suggests that in every society the culture of sex is linked not only to biologic inheritance but also to the internal logic and consistency of the total culture. The culture of a society defines the boundaries between what is sexual and what is not. Thus there are broad differences among and between cultures as to what might be considered ''sexual'' behavior. For example, in some cultures sharing food is considered a sexual act.

Some cultures view human sexuality as evil, and the Shakers of New England attempt to avoid heterosexual relations altogether. Others link sexual behavior to the state of health, believing that sexual activity causes weakness and poor health. Still others, such as some Polynesian societies, view sexuality in a very positive light, encouraging sexual activity.

The culture of every society provides for a variety of erotic actions, but in nearly all, sexual modesty is a concern. Incest taboos are common to most societies, but the definition of what constitutes the incestuous relationship varies from culture to culture and is in concert with the logic of the culture. Often the definition of incest is based on inheritance rights or relationships that might cause the family to incur obligations.

Each society has a jural system for regulating sexual behavior. Sexual intercourse may be restricted to marriage or to a similar relationship in some societies. In others there may be legitimized extramarital rights. For example, in some Eskimo groups a male visitor who was not accompanied by his wife was offered the wife of his host. Some societies permit or encourage nonmarital* sexual freedom. These societies are organized so that children born outside of a marital relationship are not stigmatized.

Ford and Beach[11] concluded that many aspects of sexual response are influenced by culture and subculture. The position for intercourse varies between cultures and within cultures. Although the female-supine, male-prone position is the most common in the United States and several other societies, intercourse in other cultures may most commonly occur in a squatting position, side to side, or with the female above the male. Although most mammals, except humans, copulate in the rear-entry position, this approach prevails in only a few societies. Usually the position assumed for intercourse reflects other aspects of the culture, such as privacy for sexual relations. In some cultures families may sleep in the same close quarters; often side-to-side positions are used to afford some privacy from children and other occupants of the one-room household.

Culture also dictates whether the female plays an active or passive role in sexual activity. In some societies females are expected and encouraged to initiate sex, in others to merely tolerate it.

The duration of the act of intercourse is modified by culture. Males are expected to achieve ejaculation in a few minutes in some societies, and in others the male's ability to prolong intromission by delaying ejaculation is valued.

A variety of sexual stimulation exists. Precopulatory stimulation may be brief or lengthy. Language may be used to convey symbols that enhance sexual excitement. Many mutual and reciprocal physical activities are also used as stimuli. Kissing is nearly ubiquitous in American culture, but in some societies it is believed to be unsanitary because of the possible exchange of saliva.

---

*We prefer to use the term *nonmarital* rather than *premarital*.

Grooming and delousing behavior are prevalent in certain societies before copulation. Stimulation of the female breasts is extremely common in humans but rare in other species. Women have reported experiencing orgasm solely from breast stimulation provided by a partner or as experienced while nursing infants. In some cultures breast stimulation may be the only form of coital play. Both manual and oral contact with the breasts was more common among college graduates than among less educated men in American society.[15] Often the woman's breasts are left uncovered, and nudity of the breasts is not inconsistent with feminine modesty in some cultures.

Manipulation of the female genitalia by the male is a common part of foreplay in several societies in addition to American society. Oral stimulation of the female genitals (cunnilingus) was practiced by nearly half of the well-educated Kinsey men[15] and has been found among other cultures. Many variations of this approach are described by Ford and Beach.[11]

The American female is perhaps less inclined to manually manipulate the male genitals than the male hers. Fellatio, or oral stimulation of the male's penis, was also much less common in American society. In fact, it was avoided in about 58% of cases in the Kinsey sample.[16]

Painful stimulation, such as biting, scratching, pinching, and poking, is common foreplay in some cultures. It may be that the sensations of pain actually enhance erotic arousal. In some societies techniques that involve pain during sex play are considered normal. Anticipation of pain along with sexual arousal becomes a desirable part of the sex act.

Circumstances for coitus do vary from culture to culture, but privacy is commonly sought. Sexual frequency may also be governed by norms. In some cultures sex is prohibited during the menses, lactation, or pregnancy, and abstention may be required before hunts or wars. In American culture the restrictions apply only to the menses and a short period of time before and after childbirth, and adherence to these is highly variable.

Although heterosexuality constitutes the most prevalent form of sexual expression among adults of known societies, it is rarely the only type of sexual behavior in which humans indulge. Homosexual behavior is found in most species of mammals; it is most common in humans among adolescents and males. Some cultures may even prescribe homosexuality for a variety of reasons.

Normal sexual response may be determined by cultural norms and physiologic, phylogenetic, legal, statistical, moral, and social standards. This, of course, makes hard-and-fast definitions of ''the normal state'' nearly impossible except from the individual's own perspective.

Sexual behavior in the United States

Historical perspectives. Kinsey's studies revealed a number of social variables influencing human sexual behavior. Although the data were obtained in the 1940s, the findings will be reviewed here because some of the social trends observed at that time still prevail in American society.

Petting. In discussing heterosexual petting and its social significance, Kinsey and colleagues[15,16] point out that the English-speaking culture teaches its youth that touching should be restrained, especially when two people of the opposite sex are involved. In later life both men and women are expected to forget the restraints placed on their natural urges and become "natural" and "unrestrained" after a marriage ceremony. The problem associated with socializing the child and adolescent to one set of norms, later to be instantaneously replaced with a new set, is obvious.

Sexual maladjustment was found to be a contributing factor in the failure of about three fourths of the upper-class marriages that ended in separation or divorce, as opposed to only a small percentage of the lower-class marriages that were dissolved. The sexual factors that seemed to cause the most difficulty in upper-class marriages were the failure of the husband to demonstrate skill in his sexual techniques and approaches and the failure of the wife to participate in an uninhibited fashion.[15,16] The Kinsey data showed that the incidence of marital coitus was much lower among more religiously inclined men and upper-class men than among those less religiously inclined and those at lower educational levels. The inhibitions of women in the upper social classes appeared even more extreme than those of men in the same social level.[15,16]

Petting, rather than any other source of sex information, including books, classes, religious instruction, or parents, provided most of the women in the Kinsey sample[16] with their first understanding of a heterosexual experience. Among women who had not petted to the point of orgasm before marriage, 35% never reached orgasm during the first year of marriage. More important than the experience with orgasm seemed to be the physical, psychologic, and sociologic problems that the woman was made aware of as she adjusted to intimacy with another individual.

Nonmarital intercourse. Nonmarital intercourse has been a cause for concern in many cultures. Proscriptive codes that condemned nonmarital intercourse were developed even in ancient civilizations (often to ensure that property rights were safeguarded). Despite modern social codes, most men have intercourse before marriage. Class differences account for variation in men's ages at first coitus. Among men in the Kinsey sample who had attended college, 67% had had coitus before marriage; for those who finished high school the percentage was 84%; and for those who did not progress beyond grade school, 98% had had premarital coitus. The sexual outlet for college-age men was a prostitute or companion in 21% of the cases, but for men of lower educational levels, 68% had experienced coitus with a prostitute or companion. Only a very small proportion of contacts were between upper-class men and prostitutes. By age 21, about 75% of the males in the Kinsey study had had coitus. In male sexual practices there was a major departure from the publicly held and overtly expressed attitudes toward nonmarital coitus.[16]

Even among women there was a surprising incidence of nonmarital coitus in the Kinsey sample. Nearly 50% of the women who were married by the age of 20 years had had nonmarital intercourse, but it occurred rarely during their early teens. Perhaps the reason is that there are severe legal penalties for men who have intercourse with young girls or that few young adolescent girls are sexually uninhibited. In the mid-1940s coitus as a source of nonmarital outlet accounted for 43% of sexual activity, but during the late 1940s this figure began to decline. For all groups of women masturbation provided the major nonmarital outlet.

Most social factors, such as level of education, had little effect on the pattern of nonmarital intercourse among women in the sample. Age seemed to be an important factor for women, rather than level of education, as in the male sample.

Among women of various social classes there was little difference in the incidence of nonmarital intercourse. However, the reason may be that the women from lower-class homes in this sample had married at an earlier age. By age 35, there was a much higher incidence of coitus among unmarried white-collar women. As was true for the men in the Kinsey sample, the women who rose from lower-class homes and moved into an upper educational level were more likely to be restrained sexually than those women who came from upper-class homes and remained in that class.

A greater percentage of women who considered themselves to be less active and devout religiously had experienced nonmarital coitus than those who considered themselves religiously active. This smaller percentage of sexually experienced women among the religiously active was not related to religious affiliation. Similar results were reported for men.[15,16] Perhaps the role of guilt feelings in those who were extremely devout led to a decrease in sexual satisfaction and, in turn, more limited experience.

Factors that restricted the incidence of nonmarital coitus for women included fear of venereal disease, lack of opportunity, fear of public opinion, fear of pregnancy, sexual unresponsiveness, and moral objections. Most of these factors contain common themes: fear of the consequences and the element of guilt. Lack of experience and the sexual unresponsiveness of many young females were also important.

Despite these variables, 69% of the still-unmarried women in the sample did not regret their experience, nor did 77% of the married women. Religious orthodoxy may have influenced the remainder of the sample, who expressed regret at having had nonmarital coitus.

Even though the data presented represent a select sample and were collected during the 1940s, some of the inferences made from this study may help explain sexual behavior today. Many of the youth in today's culture have been influenced by the morals and traditions of their parents, contemporaries of the Kinsey sample. Whether youth emulate or reject these patterns, it is of value to be conversant with them, since they help to lend perspective to behavior that may be otherwise unwittingly attributed to a "sexual revolution."

Sex during the seventies. A 1974 study of the sexual attitudes and behavior of 2026 persons in 24 cities and suburban areas indicated that Americans are engaging in a wider variety of sexual activities more frequently than they did when Kinsey surveyed American sexual behavior over 20 years ago.[13] An increased number of persons, especially those in younger age groups, are more accepting and tolerant of many forms of sexual behavior. To illustrate some of these changes, an overview of Hunt's findings about several sexual practices will be presented.

Nonmarital sexual activity is prevalent and accepted. A comparison of Kinsey's data and Hunt's data shows that the greatest increase in nonmarital sex has occurred among women. Hunt found that approximately 75% of single women in the study had had intercourse before the age of 25, although nonmarital sex among men has increased only slightly. Among noncollege males, about three fourths of the group had nonmarital coitus by age 17, and of males with some college education, more than half had nonmarital coitus by age 17.

Extramarital sexual activity has also increased more for women than for men. For those under 25 years of age, 24% of wives and 32% of husbands had had extramarital coitus.

Oral sex is practiced more widely than in the past, especially among younger men and women. Approximately 90% of married persons under 25 years of age had recently practiced cunnilingus or fellatio or both. Oral sex was also engaged in by over 80% of single men and women between 25 and 34.

Tavris and Sadd,[30] in a survey of female sexuality, found that the majority of women had experienced oral-genital sexual contact occasionally or frequently, and most enjoyed cunnilingus more than fellatio. Almost half of the women whom they studied had tried anal intercourse and thought it was acceptable with someone with whom they had a close, trusting relationship.

Heterosexual anal intercourse is also more commonly practiced today. However, it is only an occasional coital variation and engaged in most often by younger persons.

Variation in coital techniques and frequency of sexual intercourse have both increased. The increase in frequency is especially noteworthy in sexually active single women between 18 and 24, who have a median frequency of intercourse greater than once per week. This contrasts sharply with Kinsey's finding that sexually active single females between 16 and 20 had intercourse about once every 5 to 10 weeks.

Although most of the myths about masturbation are no longer as prevalent as they were in the past, many people remain embarrassed about their own current masturbatory experiences. Today masturbation begins at younger ages in males and females and continues for more years at a higher frequency than at the time of Kinsey's survey in the 1940s. The increase in masturbation is especially apparent in young married men and women. The Hunt survey found that seven out of ten husbands in their late twenties and early thirties masturbated. Almost as many wives in this age group masturbated, although they did so less frequently.

The double standard. With the advent of the women's liberation movement, the climate for freedom of expression of one's sexuality has changed. Admittedly the effect of altered roles for women has not yet totally pervaded Western society.

The "double standard" in this culture has meant that certain sexual behaviors, such as nonmarital intercourse, are acceptable for men but not for women. Reiss,[20] in a review of the concept, suggested that the double standard, if universally applied among women, would indeed be a single standard. If no women engaged in nonmarital intercourse, men would be unable to do so. In further developing the concept he suggests that the double standard encourages sexual relationships outside of the group in which one has an established identity. In an effort to maintain a "good" image the woman seeks partners outside her community, social class, racial group, or religious group. By the same token, men seek out "bad women." The potential for role and psychologic conflict is evident. The double standard also creates conflict in a man who may require virginity in his wife but who is encouraged to eliminate virginity in all his premarital partners.

This concept also defies justice: one person who participates in an act is praised, whereas the other person is blamed. That a double-standard approach to nonmarital intercourse may interfere with a mutually satisfying sexual adjustment during marriage is obvious. Both partners must unlearn inhibitions—for the woman some generalized attitudes about sexual intercourse and for the man some inhibitions with regard to specific sexual acts that he has come to associate with "bad girls" only.

It is true that double-standard behavior has been declining over the past decades. Indeed, trends in sexual attitudes of unmarried university students show that between 1968 and 1972 students reported more permissive attitudes toward nonmarital sexual behavior, a convergence in attitudes of women and men, and less adherence to the double standard.[5] The future of greater equality for women suggests that the trend toward a single standard for sexual behavior will evolve.

Marital status. Marital status is a more important determinant of sexual behavior for women than for men. Whereas the separated, divorced, or remarried man tends to continue the same type and frequency of sexual activity, the woman tends to be less sexually active, especially during the first year after widowhood or divorce. In general divorced women tend to be more sexually active than widows, probably because of the differences in age, previous sexual habits, religion, and their response to trauma. Remarriage is a common type of sexual adjustment following divorce or widowhood. Widowers have more sexual freedom than widows because of traditional sex roles and also because there are fewer widowers than widows. Whether the marital status is changed by separation, divorce, or widowhood, the effects of the dissolution crisis may leave one or both persons depressed and consequently sexually dysfunctional.[19]

Tavris and Sadd[30] found that married women had intercourse less frequently as the length of their marriage increased and that the decline after the first year was the most pronounced. Whereas 27% of newly married women had intercourse more than four times a week, only 7% of women married 5 to 7 years did so. Most women were satisfied with the frequency of marital intercourse, but 38% felt the frequency was not high enough. In this study 80% of the women had had intercourse before marriage, and 29% of the married women had had intercourse with a partner other than their spouse while they were married.

Race and class. Several studies of the relationship of race and social class with sexual behavior were conducted during the 1960s. Reiss[21] found that blacks and whites differed in permissiveness, and Broderick[10] found that black youths were less inhibited than whites with regard to sexual behavior. Both found differences between men and women in sexual permissiveness among both racial groups.

Reiss[22] found that characteristics that were assumed to reflect a liberal or conservative dimension influenced behavior. In a liberal attitudinal setting there was a positive relationship between social class and permissiveness, with more permissiveness in high social classes. In a conservative setting the opposite was seen. Upper-class permissiveness was influenced by a conservative or liberal setting to a greater degree than lower-class permissiveness. Within each class studied, whites were influenced more by the liberal or conservative dimension than were blacks.

Rainwater[18] explored aspects of lower-class sexual behavior in the context of marriage. Lower-class husbands and wives were less likely than middle-class couples to find sexual relations gratifying. Rainwater theorized that the lower value placed on sexual relations by lower-class wives, and also to a lesser extent by their husbands, may be an extension of the high degree of segregation in their marital role relationships in general. In other words, where a joint involvement and participation in each other's activities are already lacking, separateness may be extrapolated to the sexual relationship. If the marital parties have separately organized roles, perhaps the sexual relationship serves a different function in their marriage. The woman's great fear of pregnancy also contributed to lessened enjoyment.

In the middle class, and among those in the lower class whose marital relationships were more jointly organized, it appeared that the sexual relationship was an extension of an overall conjugal mutual involvement. Wives in lower-class, highly segregated marriages found that sexual relations provided psychophysiologic pleasure and relief only, whereas those in the lower-class, intermediately segregated marriages, as well as those in the middle class, found that a socioemotional closeness and exchange were provided. It is interesting to note that men's feelings paralleled women's in this study.

Recent literature dealing with class differences in sexual behavior suggests that there may be more similarities than differences between the classes.[23,26] Adolescents from the working class seem to have heterosexual experiences at earlier ages, are more limited in the variety of their sexual behavior, and have more restricted attitudes toward noncoital sex than middle-class youth. Sexuality may be a significant opportunity for the working-class male adolescent to achieve male identity. For the adolescent working-class female, the family is largely the opportunity for her identity, since the working world may be disappointing. Despite some of their differences, adolescents of both classes reveal a liberal romantic love ideology. Coital relationships before marriage are approved by both sexes. Love, fidelity, and partner or marriage orientation remain important values.[26]

Religion. A final variable influencing sexual behavior is religion. To attempt to summarize the teachings of the great religions in a few pages would do a severe injustice to the teachings of each.* Judaic teachings regard the sexual drive as a divine endowment to be exercised within controlled boundaries. However, the libidinal instincts are to be directed toward establishment of a family. The exclusiveness of matrimony is zealously guarded.[24] Protestant and Roman Catholic Christianity are struggling with issues of sexual ethics. Efforts to personalize the ethics of sexuality while maintaining the biblical image of humans is a major challenge to Catholicism. Because of these efforts, there are tensions between Rome and the faithful elsewhere.[29] The sexual ethics of Protestantism mainly concentrate on determining the value of human relationships.[31]

Changing sex roles: androgyny. During the 1970s a new concept, androgyny, began to influence sexuality and sexual behavior. Androgyny implies the presence of both male and female characteristics in both men and women. The androgynous individual is not hampered or limited by the traditional constraints of sex-stereotyped roles but rather enjoys the characteristics of both sexes. It has been suggested that rather than adhering to traditional stereotypes about how men and women should behave, individuals should allow themselves to experience the better characteristics traditionally experienced by the opposite sex. Indeed, it has been suggested that being androgynous is a much healthier state than adhering to narrow definitions of what men and women

---

*The reader is referred to the references at the end of this chapter for a more detailed discussion of each.

can do. Men can cry and women can be assertive without being labeled atypical or inappropriate. In the future, androgyny may be synonymous with mentally healthy sex role behavior and may free both men and women to be more human.

Summary

This chapter has explored the human sexual response cycle as described by Masters and Johnson and psychologic and sociologic variables influencing sexual response and sexual behavior. In addition, alternative modes of sexual expression were discussed.

Key considerations for practice include the following:

1. Physiologic aspects of the human sexual response cycle are similar for males and females and are dependent on myotonia and vasocongestion.
2. Biologic aspects of human sexual response may be influenced by psychologic and sociologic variables.
3. Some components of human sexual response may be learned or conditioned.
4. Aspects of sexual behavior other than orgasm may be pleasurable.
5. A number of alternative sexual response patterns exist.
6. Patterns of sexual behavior differ among and between cultural groups.
7. Sexual customs in the United States are changing. There is an increasing concern for the quality of human relationships. The double standard is disappearing, perhaps as a result of the technologic control of conception. Sexual behavior has become a matter of individual choice. This change is especially apparent for women, who are now subject to fewer social sanctions for their sexual activity than in the past.

Questions for review

1. Consider how you would describe human sexual response (the Masters and Johnson or Kaplan model) to the following audiences:

   • Your professional peers
   • A client of your same sex and age with a high school education
   • A client of the opposite sex who is 20 years older than you
   • A 10-year-old student in a health class

   How will your language differ? What concepts will you present? What background information would the person(s) need to know for your explanation to be effective?

2. Given the range of variability of sexual behavior, what is most likely to account for your own current sexual behavior? What factors have been important in your experience of sexual response?

References

1. Addiego, F., et al.: Female ejaculation: a case study, Journal of Sex Research **17**(1):13-21, 1981.
2. Bardwick, J.: The psychology of women, New York, 1971, Harper & Row, Publishers, Inc.
3. Beach, F.A., editor: Human sexuality in four perspectives, Baltimore, 1977, The Johns Hopkins University Press.
4. Belzer, E.: Orgasmic expulsions of women: a review and heuristic inquiry, Journal of Sex Research **17**(1):1-12, 1981.
5. Bem, S.: Probing the promise of androgyny. In Kaplan, A., and Bean, J., editors: Beyond sex role stereotyping: readings toward a psychology of androgyny, Boston, 1976, Little, Brown & Co.
6. Broderick, C.B.: Social heterosexual development among urban Negroes and Whites, Journal of Marriage and the Family **27**:200-203, 1965.
7. Comfort, A.: Refractory period after ejaculation, Lancet **1**:1075, 1972.
8. Comfort, A.: The normal in sexual behavior: an ethological view, Journal of Sex Education and Therapy **2**:1-7, 1975.
9. Davenport, W.: Sex in cross-cultural perspective. In Beach, F.A., editor: Human sexuality in four perspectives, Baltimore, 1977, The Johns Hopkins University Press.
10. Fisher, S.: The female orgasm, New York, 1973, Basic Books, Inc., Publishers.
11. Ford, C.S., and Beach, F.A.: Patterns of sexual behavior, New York, 1951, Harper & Row, Publishers, Inc.
12. Hite, S.: The Hite report: a nationwide study of female sexuality, New York, 1976, Dell Publishing Co., Inc.
13. Hunt, M.: Sexual behavior in the 1970s, New York, 1974, Playboy Press.
14. Kaplan, H.S.: Disorders of sexual desire and other new concepts and techniques in Sex therapy, New York, 1979, Simon & Schuster, Inc.
15. Kinsey, A.C., Pomeroy, W.B., and Martin, C.W.: Sexual behavior in the human male, Philadelphia, 1948, W.B. Saunders Co.
16. Kinsey, A.C., et al.: Sexual behavior in the human female, Philadelphia, 1953, W.B. Saunders Co.
17. Masters, W., and Johnson, V.: Human sexual response, Boston, 1966, Little, Brown & Co.
18. Rainwater, L.: Some aspects of lower-class sexual behavior, Journal of Social Issues **22**:96-108, 1966.
19. Reed, D.: Sexual behavior in the separated, divorced and widowed. In Sadock, B., Kaplan, H.S., and Freedman, A.: The sexual experience, Baltimore, 1976, The Williams & Wilkins Co.
20. Reiss, I.L.: The double standard in premarital sexual intercourse: a neglected concept, Social Forces **34**:224-230, 1956.
21. Reiss, I.L.: Premarital sexual permissiveness among Negroes and Whites, American Sociological Review **29**:688-698, 1964.
22. Reiss, I.L.: Social class and premarital sexual permissiveness: a reexamination, American Sociological Review **30**:747-756, 1965.
23. Reiss, I.: Changing sociosocial mores. In Money, J., and Musaph, H., editors: Handbook of sexology, New York, 1977, Excerpta Medica.

24. Rosenheim, E.: Sexual attitudes and regulations in Judaism. In Money, J., and Musaph, H., editors: Handbook of sexology, New York, 1977, Excerpta Medica.

25. Sarrel, P.: Sexual physiology and sexual functioning, Postgraduate Medicine **58**(1):67-72, 1975.

26. Schmidt, G.: Working-class and middle class adolescents. In Money, J., and Musaph, H., editors: Handbook of sexology, New York, 1977, Excerpta Medica.

27. Sherfey, M.J.: The nature and evolution of female sexuality, New York, 1966, Random House, Inc.

28. Singer, J., and Singer, J.: Types of female orgasm, Journal of Sex Research **8:**255-267, 1972.

29. Sporken, P.: Marriage and sexual ethics in the Catholic Church. In Money, J., and Musaph, H., editors: Handbook of sexology, New York, 1977, Excerpta Medica.

30. Tavris, C., and Sadd, S.: The Redbook report on female sexuality, New York, 1977, Delacorte Press.

31. Van Gennep, F.O.: Sexual ethics in Protestant churches. In Money, J., and Musaph, H., editors: Handbook of sexology, New York, 1977, Excerpta Medica.

Media

"The nurse and homosexuality," Concept Media Series on Human Sexuality and Nursing Practice, Concept Media, Inc., 1500 Adams Avenue, Costa Mesa, CA 92626.

"Physiological responses of the sexually stimulated female in the laboratory," "Physiological responses of the sexually stimulated male in the laboratory," and "Sexual intercourse," Focus International, Inc., 505 West End Ave., New York, NY 10024.

References for clients

Barbach, L.G.: For yourself the fulfillment of female sexuality—a guide to orgasmic response, New York, 1975, Doubleday & Co., Inc.

Brecher, R., and Brecher, E.: An analysis of human sexual response, New York, 1966, Bantam Books, Inc.

Comfort, A.: More joy—a lovemaking companion to the joy of sex, New York, 1973, Crown Publishers, Inc.

Comfort, A.: The joy of sex, New York, 1974, Simon & Schuster, Inc.

Heiman, J., LoPiccolo, L., and LoPiccolo, J.: Becoming orgasmic: a sexual growth program for women, Englewood Cliffs, N.J., 1976, Prentice-Hall, Inc.

Hite, S.: The Hite report: a nationwide study of female sexuality, New York, 1976, Dell Publishing Co., Inc.

Hunt, M.: Sexual behavior in the 1970s, New York, 1974, Playboy Press.

Katchadourian, H.A., and Lunde, D.T.: Fundamentals of human sexuality, New York, 1975, Holt, Rinehart & Winston.

Martin, D., and Lyon, P.: Lesbian woman, New York, 1972, Bantam Books, Inc.

McCarthy, B., Ryan, M., and Johnson, F.A.: Sexual awareness—a practical approach, Oakland, 1975, Scrimshaw Press.

McCary, J.L.: Human sexuality, New York, 1973, D. Van Nostrand Co.

Silverstein, C., and White, E.: Joy of gay sex, New York, 1977, Crown Publishers, Inc.

Sisley, E., and Harris, B.: Joy of lesbian sex, New York, 1977, Crown Publishers, Inc.

Tripp, C.A.: Homosexual matrix, New York, 1976, The New American Library, Inc.

Zilbergeld, B.: Male sexuality: a guide to sexual fulfillment, Boston, 1978, Little, Brown & Co.

2

Sexual variation

GORDON L. DICKMAN and CAROLYN A. LIVINGSTON

The purpose of this chapter is to assist health care providers in delivering health care to sexual minorities. The chapter encourages health care providers to examine their attitudes and beliefs about sexual variations so that they can serve their patients with compassion and understanding. Specific knowledge about sexual variations is included so that health care can be delivered with accuracy. As society moves into a time when the wide range of human sexual expression becomes more visible and asserted, the demand increases for accurate information about and bias-free attitudes toward sexuality and health care. The objectives for this chapter follow:

1. To describe varieties of human sexual expression
2. To clarify the most common conflicts of the health care provider in dealing with varieties in sexual expression
3. To describe the reality, health care concerns, and nursing implications of sexual minorities
4. To describe the problematic varieties of human sexual expression

A community provides its members with standards by which they can pattern their behavior and judge its appropriateness. Sexual standards have been typically the most clearly prescribed. Religious and ethnic groups, the media, and other groups overtly and covertly teach ''appropriate'' sexual behavior. Any other forms of sexual expression are more or less tolerated, depending on the specific community in which they occur.

Sexual expression that does not conform to the accepted standard usually remains hidden from view. Homosexual and bisexual life-styles are only now becoming more visible to the general public. Transsexualism appears as an infrequent curiosity in the media. Transvestism, sadomasochism, pedophilia, exhibitionism, and voyeurism conjure up exotic and sometimes frightening images for many people. All of these forms of human sexual expression and life-styles are present throughout society. The people who engage in them both work in and seek out health care systems.

Defining sexual variations

Labels, language, and listening. Human beings tend to view life from an either/or perspective. Labels for human sexual behavior can reinforce this either/

or thinking, particularly when the behavior is not understood. Since sexual variations are invisible to most people, the words used to describe the life-style or behavior become laden with stereotypes and myths.

The first lesson for the health care provider is to understand the loaded nature of sexual labels. Actual sexual behavior can become lost in the words used to describe it. In fact, sexual labels tend to have a life of their own, quite separate from the behavior they are supposed to describe. It is important when working with sexual minorities to keep this dual nature of sexual language in mind. The way sexual minorities describe themselves and the way society describes them involve the same words, yet the meaning and emotion they convey are different.

The second lesson for health care providers is to understand that human sexual behavior is not fixed throughout one's lifetime. Kinsey[20] described sexuality as being on a continuum along which some people move throughout their lifetime. Both in fantasy and in fact, people report a variety of sexual experiences in a lifetime. To capture this reality, Kinsey devised a scale ranging from 0 (exclusively heterosexual behavior) to 6 (exclusively homosexual behavior) with 3 as the midpoint. He found that most sexual behavior falls somewhere in between 0 and 6 and that it may change with time. Hunt's study[19] of the 1970s indicated that approximately 25% of males and 15% of females had had at least one same-sex experience.

The problem with understanding statistical studies of sexual behavior is that they can reflect past as well as present behavior. They can reflect fantasy as well as actual practice. The most compassionate thing health care providers can do when dealing with their patients' sexual concerns is listen to patients' sexual language and focus on their description of the sexual behavior. Both parties need to be on guard against emotionally charged and sometimes inaccurate sexual labels.

Homosexuality. Homosexuals describe themselves as having a clear erotic attraction to a person of the same sex.[17] The word is used for females and males. The attraction is the same kind that heterosexuals describe when they talk about their sexuality. Homosexuals view their biologic sex as congruous with their role as a female or a male. They see their genitals as appropriate. Females may use the word "lesbian" to describe themselves, and males may use the word "gay." In some communities and in the media "gay" may refer to both female and male homosexuals.

Bisexuality. Bisexuals describe themselves as relating sexually to both sexes. Heterosexuals and homosexuals have been quick to accuse the bisexual of riding the fence with respect to sexual orientation. This attitude of waiting for the other shoe to drop goes back to the desire to see life in either/or terms. Bisexuals often refer to themselves as being "bi."

The bisexual identity has been around for a number of years. These people fall in the middle range between 2 and 5 on the Kinsey scale. Recent popularity in bisexual behavior has increased awareness about it but not necessarily understanding of it. The special health care issues of bisexuals have not yet appeared in the literature. The articles available are descriptive and anecdotal in nature.[38] Bisexuality is on its way to becoming a clearly defined and separate sexual life-style. As more and more people come forth with their experiences, a clearer picture of their issues will be gained. Their health care concerns will then take their rightful place in health care texts such as this one.

Transsexuality. Transsexuals believe that they are in the body of the wrong biologic sex. They may describe themselves as female, trapped in the body of a male, or as male in a female's body. Their behavior must be viewed from their internal perspective of their sexuality and not from their biologic sex. Some transsexuals are heterosexual and seek out partners who are, for them, of the opposite sex. Other transsexuals are homosexual and seek out partners of the same sex. Cross-dressing for a transsexual is not for sexual gratification. Their dress is appropriate for their inner perspective of their sexuality.

Other sexual variations include transvestism, sadomasochism, pedophilia, exhibitionism, and voyeurism. Descriptions of these sexual behaviors and life-styles are presented in the last section of the chapter.

Conflicts of health care providers

Health care providers often find themselves in conflict when dealing with sexual minorities. On the one hand, they have received the same values training about sex as other members of their community. This training has historically viewed sexual variations as unnatural or abnormal. On the other hand, they feel committed to providing compassionate and accurate health care to their patients. They may, themselves, be members of a sexual minority. Talking about these conflicts increases the chances that the relationship between sexual minorities and health care providers will be supportive and mutually enhancing.

Purpose of sex. Sex in American culture is generally assumed to be penis-in-vagina intercourse between females and males. The assigned purpose for intercourse has been for procreation and/or communicating love within a marriage. This traditional view of sex is supported throughout society. Religious teaching leaves no doubt whatsoever about the importance of this point of view. As anyone who has read the advice columns in the newspapers already knows, sexual behavior does not strictly conform to the assigned purpose for it. However, society has been able to tolerate this sexual double standard as long as it is heterosexual.

What seems to be difficult for people to accept is sexual attraction and sexual behavior between people of the same sex. In this arena the heterosexual model is often described as "natural," whereas anything deviating from it becomes "perverse" or "unnatural." It is important to remember that other variations are "unnatural" from a heterosexual point of view. A lesbian perceives her loving a partner and her sexual expression with a partner as a most natural act. Sexual minorities use sex for all of the reasons that heterosexuals do. One of these purposes may include procreation, since the desire to be a parent is part of the human experience. Calderone[9] offers a truly humane description of the purpose of sex: sex should provide people with a sense of pleasure, communication, and well-being. How that happens and with whom remains a matter for each individual to decide.

Masculine-feminine. Gender role is the masculine or feminine role people learn in their community. Young girls and boys adopt attitudes and beliefs about their role in society that will shape their sexual behavior as adults. Perhaps no other profession has felt the sting of traditional attitudes toward gender role behavior more than the health care field. The feminist movement has helped dramatize the emotional price both women and men pay when they ignore their own inner sense of self in favor of what they believe society expects of them.

One of the price tags on "acceptable" male behavior in society is avoiding doing anything that might be considered "feminine," at least in public. Effeminate behavior by a male will quickly earn him the label of "fag" or "queer." Females, on the other hand, are able to adopt a much wider range of behaviors, including those considered "masculine."

Homophobia. Homophobia is characterized as an irrational intolerance or fear of attraction to or sexual behavior involving people of the same sex. This aversion to homosexuality seems to be strongest among males. Extreme forms of homophobia may result in physical assault on homosexuals. It has been suggested that homophobia stems from a fear of one's own same-sex tendencies. Homophobia seems to be strongest among those people who come from a rigid, authoritarian, and intolerant background.[27]

Health care bias. American health care usually reflects a heterosexual medical model. The fear and distrust that sexual minorities describe in dealing with a society generally intolerant of their sexual behavior may show up in the health care setting. Homosexuals and transsexuals have encountered ignorance of their specific health care needs and intolerance of their life-styles.[22,28,31]

Heterosexual bias shows up in a multitude of ways. Lesbians report that if they have children, the assumption is that the lesbians are heterosexual. Medical personnel usually do not understand how gays and lesbians transmit sexually transmitted diseases to one another. Partners of lesbians and gay patients often are not viewed as being as important to the patient as partners in a heterosexual relationship. Lesbians and gays overhear derogatory remarks and jokes about their sexuality.[22,28,31]

Ground rules for talking about sex. Sex is a loaded subject. Emotions can run high when discussion turns to sexual variations. Health care providers are no different from anyone else in their attitudes toward sexual minorities. These attitudes range from very accepting to very intolerant. There is no reason why compassionate and accurate health care cannot be delivered to sexual minorities when there is understanding and respect for the variety of human sexual expression. Both sexual minorities and health care providers have a responsibility to keep the dialogue going. Discussion about sex is enhanced when both parties keep a few basic affirmations in mind:

1. I am entitled to my own sexual values and beliefs.
2. I am the adult in charge of my sexuality.
3. I am aware that other people have sexual values and beliefs different from my own.

Both the health care profession and sexual minority communities have taken measures to end biased and stereotyped medical treatment of sexual minorities. It is important for members of sexual minorities who have "come out" publicly to help educate the health care professions about their life-styles. It is important for the medical profession to read about and, most important, listen to the health care needs of sexual minorities.

Homosexuality

Homosexuality is as old as humankind. It has existed at all times and in all places in history. In the Judeo-Christian heritage, in which heterosexuality is the approved "norm," homosexual behavior has been viewed as evil, perverted, and sick. Living with homosexuality means living with two realities. One reality consists of the myths, stereotypes, intolerance, and fears that surround it. The other reality consists of the lives of millions of American women and men who work in and seek out health care—and who are homosexual.

Health care providers operate in the context of this dual reality. They need to know the health care concerns of a group of people whose sexual life-style has been hidden from view. Health care providers need to be aware of how the myths, stereotypes, and fears prevent homosexuals from receiving caring and accurate health care. Fleeting glimpses of the more flamboyant fringes have only served to reinforce myths and stereotypes.

Incidence. Kinsey[20] was the first to offer a statistical model that expressed the full range of human sexual behavior. The results of his studies in the late 1940s and early 1950s challenged contemporary notions about sexual behavior. It became clear from Kinsey's research that sexual aim is not an either/or behavior. The Institute for Sex Research at Indiana University defines a homosexual as anyone who has had sex more than six times with partners of the same sex. The Institute suggests that 15% of all males and 5% of all females in the United States are homosexual.[27]

Etiology. Law and religion have addressed the nature of homosexuality, but they have not addressed its cause. Most religions have traditionally viewed it as evil and as such intolerable in the religious community. Some religious groups have changed their stand and now speak out only against homosexual acts. The law does not speak to homosexuality itself as being illegal, but it does define certain sexual acts as illegal. Like religion, the law has not concerned itself with why people may seek out partners of the same sex. That job has fallen to mental health and medical communities.

The operating model of the health care professions centers around incidence, etiology, and cure. Where homosexuality is viewed as a sickness by health care professionals, the attitude toward it is to discover, through research, a means of curing it.[10] This attitude also existed in the mental health field. Until the 1970s, homosexuality was on the American Psychiatric Association's list of diagnostic mental illness categories. The category was changed in 1973 to describe only those homosexuals who were in conflict with or wanted to change their sexual orientation.[18] The issue is far from resolved, however.

Both biologic and environmental factors have been identified as causes of homosexuality. It is still not clear if people are born with it or learn it. The one clear fact that emerges from all of the attempts to find a cause is that there is no clear, definitive cause.

Some researchers are suggesting that hormonal or other chemical imbalances cause homosexuality. There are studies showing that male homosexuals have less androgen than male heterosexuals.[27] Prenatal hormonal influences are being considered. However, there is still no clear evidence that endocrinology plays an important role in the development of homosexual behavior.[18] Genetics has also provided no clear-cut answers. Chromosomal studies of homosexuals do not show any significant differences from heterosexuals.

The search for social factors that might be a cause has focused on the family constellation. Most often, abnormal relationships with parents have been blamed. Bieber[5] found that of 106 male homosexuals who were psychotherapy patients, 73% had over-protective, domineering mothers and fathers who tended to be hostile, weak, or detached. These and other social learning theories still do not explain the homosexual behavior of those people who had "normal," happy childhoods.

Roles and relationships. Being homosexual means having to come to terms with a self-identity and incorporate that into relationships with other individuals and communities. As such, it is similar to the developmental tasks of any human being. The difference of course is the intolerance and ignorance that often greets the emerging homosexual life-style.

The process of becoming homosexual seems to involve three stages. First, there is a sense of being different sexually from other people, involving feelings of attraction to one's same sex. Next, there is the exploration of these feelings. Finally, there is the admitting to oneself and others that this difference is called homosexuality.[27]

The coming out process may happen very quickly or take several years. Males seem to have more difficulty than females in accepting a homosexual identity. Blumstein and Schwartz[6] relate it to males' conflict with their masculine role in society. Coming out has its risks. Homosexuals have lost family, friends, and jobs when they revealed their sexual identity. For many, however, this price is not as high as the price paid for not reconciling what they tell themselves they are with the life-style they lead.

Coming out is still usually reserved for homosexual cliques and communities invisible to the general public.[10] As gay activist groups and gays who have come out continue to inform and challenge the old stereotypes about homosexuality, the general public will get a more accurate and humane picture of gays and lesbians.

Female homosexuals are less studied as a group than male homosexuals. This may reflect the traditional bias toward male sexuality in general, or it may be a result of the fact that society is more tolerant of intimacy between women than between men. Lesbians are subject to the same traditional role expectations as heterosexual women. One of these expectations is that lesbian relationships will reflect monogamous, enduring, and emo-tionally close values. It is true that lesbians tend to be less promiscuous than gay men.[10] Also, the women's movement, with its emphasis on human potential and independence, is changing women's role expectations. Married lesbians or single-parent lesbians, how-ever, are still especially vulnerable to coming out, since they fear the loss of their right to parent their children.

Male homosexuals are a much more visible and studied group. They must come to terms with their own sense of masculinity, society's expectations of masculine behavior, and society's stereotyped picture of male homosexuals. The biggest stereotype issue centers around effeminate behavior. Although there are some gay men who act effeminate, the majority of gays are traditionally "masculine" in the way they dress and behave and in the jobs they choose.[10] Like lesbians, many gay men have been or are married and are parents.

Studies of homosexual social behavior, like studies of its etiology, can be of particular value to health care providers. They serve as an ongoing reality check of myth and fact. It is a myth that homosexuals are effeminate males or "butch" females who wish to be the opposite sex. It is a myth that they are promiscuous and incapable of forming long-term relationships. It is a myth that they recruit others and molest children. It is a myth that they could become heterosexual if they only chose to do so.[12] It is a fact that homosexuality has no definite characteristics, location, and boundaries.[27] It occurs in all social groups, classes, and situations. It is as varied as heterosexuality.

Health care concerns. Homosexuals seek out health care for all of the same reasons heterosexuals do. However, the health care system may not be familiar with those medical concerns that relate to lesbian and gay sexual behavior. The level of medical treatment they receive will be determined in part by the knowledge of both the health care provider and the homosexual about sexually transmitted diseases (STDs) (see Chapter 14) and sexual injuries. Health care professionals may have a limited understanding of sexual behavior in general and homosexual sexual behavior in particular. If penis-in-vagina sex is the only model they know or understand, it may be very difficult for them to imagine other forms of sexual behavior. They may not recognize or explore their patients' health complaints as possibly resulting from sexual behavior.

Lesbians and gays may perceive themselves as having different sexual health care needs. This stems in part from their sexual life-styles. Lesbians may view the health care system as male dominated and, as such, unsympathetic to and ignorant of their needs as lesbian women. Gay males tend to be sexually active with more different partners than do lesbians; thus they are at greater risk of contracting an STD.[28] What is important here is to understand how lesbians and gays contract STDs.

Sexual behavior involves more than just the genitals.* The whole body can be a source of giving and receiving during sex. The mouth, ears, nose, and throat can be penetrated and pleasured by a tongue or fingers. During oral-genital sex the mouth can kiss and lick genitals. Tongues can penetrate vaginas, and penises can penetrate mouths. The anus, rectum, and perineum are highly erotogenic for many people, and these people incorporate those areas into their lovemaking. Anuses can be licked with tongues or stroked with fingers. Rectums can be penetrated with fingers, penises, dildos, or hands. Penises and clitorises can be stroked and rubbed. Scrotums can be pulled and stretched, as can inner and outer labia. Vaginas can be massaged and penetrated. Any part of the body is therefore susceptible to an STD. Any soft part of the body can be irritated, torn, or bruised during sex.

The most common complaints for which lesbians seek medical help deal with vaginal infections.[28] It is a common complaint for all women. Fungal, bacterial, and trichomonal infections are transmitted between women by mixing vaginal secretions. This may happen in many ways. Infection can occur by pressing the genitals together. Sleeping together with legs intertwined can pass secretions from thigh to vagina. Vagina-to-finger or finger-to-vagina contact will spread infections. Even clothing or sex toys that have been used recently by an infected woman can transmit an infection. Bacteria from the anus can also trigger vaginal infections. Women must remember to wash their hands and clean under their nails after anal contact, particularly during lovemaking when there is anal and vaginal stimulation.

The vagina is also susceptible to injury during penetration. Fingernails that are ragged,

---

*The following discussion may apply to heterosexual sexual activity as well as homosexual sexual activity.

long, or dirty can tear and irritate the vaginal mucosa. Vibrators and dildos can pull and tear soft tissue when there is not sufficient lubrication. Sometimes putting a vibrator in the vagina first and then turning it on can cause tissue trauma.[18]

It should be remembered that the anus and rectum may represent a very important part of a patient's sexuality. As such, it should be considered as essential to that person's sex life as the genitals or any other erotogenic area. There are men who enjoy having their prostate massaged. There are women and men who enjoy anal stimulation and penetration. As such, these areas are susceptible to disease and injury. Hemorrhoids and constipation can significantly interfere with anal or rectal pleasuring.

Rectal gonorrhea is an acute infection of the mucous membranes of the rectum and is contracted through anal intercourse with an infected partner. It is often asymptomatic. Syphilis can be contracted anally. The first-stage chancre symptoms may remain hidden and undetected in the folds of the rectum. Anal warts, which are tiny, viral, pink swellings, can be spread to the anus nonsexually as well as sexually. Herpes can also infect the anal area.[29]

Intestinal infections can be spread sexually by oral contact with the anus, sometimes referred to as "rimming." Fingers or a penis that has been in or near the anus can transmit the disease to the mouth. *Amoeba, Giardia, Shigella,* and *Salmonella* infections thus contracted can be manifested with a variety of symptoms that range from vague abdominal discomfort to severe cramping, diarrhea, and nausea.[26] If the patient confuses the symptoms with the common "flu" and does not seek treatment, loss of body fluids and electrolyte imbalance could even lead to shock and death before help is sought.

Gay males with a large number of sexual contacts may have more than one rectal intestinal infection at the same time. Called the *gay bowel syndrome,*[26] it may be overlooked if the health care provider does not ask about the patient's sexual behavior or if the patient does not volunteer the information.

Fissures in the anal canal may result from stretching and thrusting a penis, dildo, or hand into the rectum during sexual activity. Some people like to have very large objects pushed up into their rectums. These objects can tear the sensitive rectal tissue or even become lodged there, requiring emergency care. Homosexuals who engage in these forms of sexual behavior should be warned of the significant danger of damage to the rectum and ensuing risk to life that they incur.

The mouth and throat in both lesbians and gay males are susceptible to STDs. Many of the diseases that fall into the STD category can flourish in and be transmitted by this part of the body. There is a slight possibility that lesbians could pass fungal infections to a partner's throat during oral-genital sex. Other vaginal infections will not thrive there.[28] Throat cultures and careful mouth and throat examinations for herpes, blisters, chancres, and gonorrhea should be part of the health care of lesbians and gay males who are sexually active with partners whose STD history they do not know.

Implications for the health care provider. Receiving medical treatment, including hospitalization, creates a relationship between the health care consumer and provider. The relationship can be one in which the consumer is viewed as the ill, powerless party seeking a cure and the provider the powerful party with knowledge about the cure. Or the relationship can be viewed as a mutually enhancing partnership in which both consumer and provider share the power. When homosexuals enter the health care system, the relationship takes on an added dimension. Both the health care provider and the homosexual are subject to intolerant attitudes and myths about homosexuality. Both may make assumptions about the other's attitudes and expectations. This can lead to an imbalance of power, resulting in feelings of helplessness and hopelessness on the part of the homosexual and feelings of anxiety or distaste on the part of the health care professional.[8]

There is evidence that intolerance and bias on the part of the health care provider does influence homosexual health care. Patients report that they hear snide remarks and snickers when they are identified as gay or lesbian. Nurses' touch may change when they know the patient's sexual preference. Back rubs may be forgotten and other caring gestures ignored.[31] Homosexual patients have been known to withhold important medical information about themselves because they feared a negative response from their health care provider.[31] In a sample of 1000 physicians surveyed in 1970 three fourths responded that knowing a male patient was homosexual would adversely affect their medical management.[30]

The first step for health care providers in dealing with their homosexual patients is self-awareness. They can begin by assessing their own attitudes and beliefs about homosexuality. Next, the attitudes on the part of other people working in the health care environment need to be examined. Finally, homosexual patients' attitudes about homosexuality and their expectations about how they will be treated need to be expressed. Out of such a dialogue will come a better understanding of some of the special concerns of the homosexual patient. Such concerns involve feeling helpless and at the mercy of more powerful people, being separated from a partner, and not knowing where to find alternative sources of health care.

Homosexuals need to know that they have the same rights as other patients. They need to know that if a nurse is not comfortable treating them that there are other people available who are. They need to know that the information they share about themselves as it relates to their health care will not be judged and is confidential. Confidentiality is particularly important. Family members seeking information about their family member may not know about the homosexuality. There is a very real threat to homosexuals' housing and employment if confidential information about their sexual orientation shared in the health care setting is also shared in their community.

Some gay and lesbian patients who have partners may face separation during health care treatment. Hospitalization can be a stressful and frightening experience. At the very time when homosexual patients need the touch and support of their loved one it may be denied them. Homosexual relationships differ from heterosexual relationships in one significant way: homosexual relationships do not have public sanction. They do not receive the societal support and recognition that heterosexual relationships do, even though the emotional content is exactly the same.[22] Partners do not have the same legal status as a spouse or family and can thus be denied access to patients. Even when they are visiting, they may not feel they can touch, hold hands, or hold one another in bed.

Sex education is not a common experience in American society. What little there is in the public sector usually involves reproduction and contraception as taught in schools. There is little reason to suspect that much more is taught within the family. Homosexuals, like heterosexuals, may not know about or understand their own sexual health care needs.

Nurses can provide a source of information and advice. Homosexuals need to know about clinics and agencies that deal with their specific needs. Addresses, phone numbers, and brochures of gay and lesbian agencies and support groups need to be available to homosexual patients.

Both health care providers and homosexual patients have a role in accurate and nonjudgmental health care delivery. Both parties can provide one another with positive leadership, guidance, and support. Homosexual nurses and physicians[24] also have a leadership role to play in overcoming prejudicial myths and stereotypes about homosexuality.

Transsexuality

One of the tasks for the very young is to learn a gender role identity that matches up with their biologic sex. When this process is complete, there is congruity between what they see in the mirror and what they feel about themselves as girls or boys. This process goes awry for transsexuals. They feel themselves to be, and want to be, the opposite sex from their biologic sex.[32] Thus a biologic male would see himself as a female locked in a male's body. A female would see herself as a male in a female's body. Most often this awareness comes early in life and starts a long and often agonizing search to end the identity crisis and lead a life in which body and identity are congruous.[15]

Some transsexuals simply endure their emotional pain and lead "normal" lives. They behave according to the way society views their biologic sex. They may marry and have children. Others seek out endocrine therapy and surgical reassignment of their sex organs.[7]

It is important not to confuse transsexuality with transvestism or homosexuality. Homosexuals like their genitals and see their biologic sex and sexual feelings as congruous. Transvestites dress like the opposite sex, but they do not want to be the opposite sex. Transsexuals want to change their bodies to fit their feelings of maleness or femaleness. They believe that their dress and behavior, although incongruous with their biologic sex, reflects their true sexual identity.

Incidence. It has been estimated that from 1:20,000 to 1:40,000 males in the United States are transsexuals. There are no reliable statistics for females, although Pomeroy[32] estimates the male/female ratio to be 4:1.

Etiology. It is not any easier to find a cause for transsexuality than it is to find out why females and males are heterosexual or homosexual. The answer most likely involves a number of factors: genetic, hormonal, identity, behavioral, and environmental. As each of these factors is investigated, one gets a clearer picture of the causative forces. Green and Money[16] suggest that there is an identity confusion at an early age in a transsexual's life, between 18 and 36 months. The subsequent behavior becomes imprinted on the central nervous system. Benjamin[3] theorizes a prenatal neuroendocrine abnormality as a primary cause for a majority of transsexuals. He believes that it would be inaccurate to state that transsexuals are made, not born. Studies of the family constellations of transsexuals describe fathers as ineffectual and absent and mothers as strong and protective.[36] The difficulty with considering such environmental factors is that transsexuals also come from families in which there was shared and effective parenting.

Health care concerns. Transsexuals are not interested in changing their inner identity. They seem to have one all-consuming desire: to change their bodies.[10] Male transsexuals, for example, describe their penises as a source of shame and anxiety rather than a source of pleasure. They seldom masturbate because by touching their genitals, they are reminded of their maleness.[16] Their goal is usually hormone therapy and reassignment surgery so that their bodies appear female. Women seek hormone therapy to acquire male body characteristics. In some cases they also elect genital reassignment surgery.

The Harry Benjamin International Gender Dysphoria Association has developed standards of care that are meant as minimal requirements for sex reassignment treatment. The following statements from the standards of care document are worth reprinting here because they clarify and standardize terms[4]:

> *Hormonal sex reassignment:* Hormonal sex reassignment refers to the administration of androgen to genotypic females, and the administration of estrogens and/or progesterone to genotypic and phenotypic males for the purpose of effecting somatic changes in order for the patient to more closely approximate the physical appearance of the genotypically other sex.

> *Surgical sex reassignment:* Surgical sex reassignment refers to surgery of the genitalia and/or breasts performed for the purpose of altering the morphology in order to approximate the physical appearance of the genetically other sex.

Surgery is only the final step in the process of sex reassignment. The candidate has already passed through a screening process and life-style change regimen that may have lasted for several years. During this time the candidate may have been a member of a gender identity group, dressed and lived the desired sex role, and received hormone therapy. Under ideal conditions the support team will have included counselors, surgeons, endocrinologists, nurses, family, and friends.

Male-to-female surgery. There is no technique available at this time for transplanting sex organs. Current surgical practice involves the removal of existing sex structures and the recombining of tissue flaps to simulate natural sex organs. Markland[23] describes the process of constructing an artificial vagina as creating a cavity between the prostate and the rectum that is lined with scrotal and penile tissue. Testicles, the spongy tissue inside the penis, and most of the urethra are removed. The procedure has several variations, all of which involve creating labia and a vaginal barrel out of penile and scrotal tissues. The potential to be orgasmic may remain. The patient is now sterile and requires ongoing hormone therapy to maintain the feminized body.

Immediate postoperative care focuses on maintaining the shape of the healing vagina, preventing infection, and managing pain. The health care provider can provide clear and frequently repeated instructions as the patient learns to manage her own genital care. A vaginal splint or mold must be worn for several weeks following surgery. Initially, rotating and removing the splint may be very painful and require pain management. Following the initial period of healing, the patient learns to dilate her own vagina manually or with a mold. Taking warm sitz baths before genital care eases the stretching and discomfort.[11,13] It is essential that she follow her surgeon's instructions so that scar tissue does not distort her vagina. She will need assistance in learning how to prevent contamination of the wound by urine or stool. Artificially lubricating and stretching her vagina, together with new genital hygiene, will be initially strange and unfamiliar tasks for her.[18]

Postoperative complications are not usual; however, the health care provider should look for vaginal stricture or stenosis, rectovaginal fistula, and urethral stenosis.[3] Assuming an uneventful recovery, healing is well advanced in 6 to 8 weeks. The vagina is usually able to tolerate sexual activity in 2 to 3 months. Further vaginal surgery may be necessary if the vaginal barrel proves to be too short.[18]

In addition to vaginal construction, there are other surgeries available to the trans-sexual. Some patients have their Adam's apple reduced. Plastic surgery can refine the nose and other facial features. Surgical implants can shape and increase the size of breasts. Electrolysis removes hair and defines hairlines.[3]

Female-to-male surgery. The usual method of sex reassignment for biologic females emphasizes hormone therapy. Removal of the ovaries and uterus, together with the hormone therapy, promotes the development of male secondary sex character-istics. Hormone therapy will be a part of the patient's ongoing health care. Breast tissue can be surgically removed, leaving a barely discernible scar and a masculine-appearing chest.[3]

Construction of a penis is not as common as construction of a vagina in transsexual surgery. Surgery for creating an artificial penis is long and complicated and thus not often recommended. The surgeon uses a flap of lower abdominal tissue to surround an artificial urethra, sometimes using a segment of small intestine for the conduit. Since an artificial urethra is not self-cleansing, there is always the risk of infection. To avoid the compli-cations involved in creating an artificial urethra, the original urethral opening is sometimes incorporated into the base of the new penis. The penis is not capable of erection and penetration. Some sort of support or insert is necessary for penetration.[3] The clitoris, reduced in size by the hormone therapy, is incorporated into the base of the penis and may leave the orgasmic response intact.

Implications for the health care provider. The health care provider in the surgical setting sees only a portion of a transsexual's treatment program. It is a vital portion, and the professionals involved have an opportunity to make a significant contribution to the rehabilitation process. Postoperative health care information is only one of these contributions. Of equal importance are the support, morale boosting, and compassionate acceptance of another human being in a stressful situation.

A first step in this support process is for the nurses and physicians involved to prepare themselves for the patient. It is not unusual for people who have had little or no contact with transsexuals to respond to them with great curiosity or disapproval.[21] It can be an unnerving experience the first time a nurse sees a clearly female or male patient with the genitals of the opposite sex. Some professionals may even challenge a hospital's decision to perform the surgery. It is helpful to provide the health care team with debriefing sessions in which each team member has an opportunity to talk about all of the feelings surrounding transsexualism. Ventilating gut-level feelings in a supportive environment reduces the chances that the transsexual will overhear jokes and snide remarks in the hallways. The opportunity to leave the patient care assignment needs to be built in for those team members who feel they cannot provide supportive care.[21]

All of the non–health care concerns of the transsexual will be brought into the hospital along with the overnight bag. Some of these concerns may have been dealt with in a gender identity group or therapeutic setting. Health care providers may find that their supportive, nonjudgmental attitude will invite questions and concerns from their patients. Transsexuals are concerned about money and the expense of the surgery. They need to change school records and social security numbers, deal with family reactions, and perhaps change jobs.[11] They may be anxious about their appearance and dress and behave in exaggerated feminine ways while on the unit.

The health care professional can provide a helpful role model in all of these situations.[37] It is important to keep in mind that the most supportive posture is to view the transsexual not as sick but as being in a rehabilitation process. The majority of them will feel a vast sense of relief to finally have the opportunity to get on with a congruous and productive life.

Other sexual variations

The sexual variations described in this section express themselves in ways that range from the banal to the exotic and from the harmless to the illegal. It would be easy to think of the people who participate in them as demented social outcasts haunting darkened stairways. This is a popular public stereotype, but it is not true. Transvestism, sado-masochism, pedophilia, exhibitionism, and voyeurism are practiced by women and men throughout society. This is an important fact to remember, since they are consumers in the health care system.

These variations have as their driving force the same sexual energy that drives all other sexual behavior. The desire to be sexual is a combination of mental, physiologic, and environmental factors.[27] People become aroused through the interplay of thoughts, images, genital lubrication and swelling, and environmental cues that have been learned as sexual. These feelings have been described variously as a general warmth, tension, or even exhilaration. For some people the release of this sexual energy happens in ways that appear strange or are clearly inappropriate. When the behavior is compulsive, it may be beyond the ability of the person to control it. When the behavior is harmless, it may find some degree of tolerance in a private or semipublic arena. When the behavior involves unconsenting victims and is clearly a nuisance or harmful to society, then it becomes a concern of the protective and legal system.

Transvestism. Transvestism is another word for cross-dressing. People who cross-dress fall into several different categories. There are those who do it for sexual gratification and those who do it for fun. It is, for the most part, a male phenomenon.[34] Women do not seem interested in doing it. Women have always enjoyed a far greater range of dress behavior than men; thus cross-dressing is practiced by more men than women throughout society.

The majority of cross-dressers are married heterosexual men. They often have the acknowledgment, if not consent and support, of their partners. Wearing women's garments brings them sexual relief and gratification, generally leading to intercourse or orgasm. They may wear a single garment, several garments, or whole outfits, including makeup.[25]

A flamboyant version of transvestism is the ''drag'' scene that occurs among some heterosexual and homosexual men. The cross-dressing usually involves outrageously flamboyant wigs, makeup, and clothing. It most often does not have a sexual component. Cross-dressers may do it to "camp it up" for fun, for professional reasons (entertainers), or for the attention they get from its shock effect.[35]

Sadomasochism. Sadism is the desire to hurt or humiliate a partner sexually, and masochism is the desire to be sexually humiliated or hurt. Sadomasochism (S & M) refers to both attitudes, since they most often occur together. It may seem abhorrent at first to think that anyone would want to inflict pain or experience pain during sex, yet it is not an uncommon experience. Hitting, scratching, pinching, biting, or being tied up is reported among heterosexuals and homosexuals.

Sadomasochism is a more extreme form of this phenomenon. It can involve S & M games, which entail the use of elaborate black leather garments and sexual paraphernalia. Participants who become injured during sadomasochistic sex may lie about the cause of their injuries during treatment to avoid real or assumed negative reactions from health care providers.

Problematic sexual variations. The next group of sexual variations are clearly inappropriate and illegal because they involve unsuspecting and unwilling partners: pedophilia, exhibitionism, and voyeurism. At their most harmless the behaviors are a public nuisance. At their worst they violate innocent peoples' dignity and rights and as such are clearly intolerable in society.

Pedophilia. Pedophiles are adults who are not able to form sexual relationships with adults and thus seek out young children as sex partners. Most often they are heterosexual adult men who are gentle and moralistic. The children more often than not know the adult as their neighbor, relative, or family friend. A study by Gebhard et al.[14] found that the average age of heterosexuals who sought out girls under 12 years of age for sex was 35 years. About one third were married. The average age of men who sought out boys was 31 years. About 16% of these men were married. Men who seek out young boys as sex partners are referred to as pederasts.

Exhibitionism. Exhibitionism is the exposure of the sex organs where it is socially inappropriate. It is done for the exposer's own sexual arousal or gratification. The exposer's behavior usually surprises, disgusts, and frightens those who see it. Exposers are almost always male, averaging 30 years in age. Less than one third are married. About two thirds could be described as disturbed.[10] They almost always expose themselves to strangers. Generally quiet, submissive men, they rarely attack. If uninterrupted, they may masturbate while exposing.

Voyeurism. Haeberle[17] describes voyeurism as the compulsive observing of nudity or sexual behaviors. Again, voyeurs are almost always men in their late twenties or early thirties. They seem to be attracted by the danger and risk of seeing what they have no right to see.[34] Their victims are usually unaware that they are being watched. The act of "peeping" and the masturbation that may accompany it brings some sexual relief and gratification.

Implications for the health care provider. There are several different ways in which the health care provider may find out about patients' variant sexual behavior. Some patients will bring up the subject if they are feeling troubled and sense that the nurse is sympathetic and understanding. Nurses can ask about it if they suspect that a sexual issue is interfering with health care. A patient may act out sexually in the hospital or clinic. The issue for the health care provider remains the same as for any other patient: provide caring, accurate health care in an atmosphere that does not judge or condemn. This does not mean that the nurse should overlook sexual behavior that is disruptive.

Transvestites may wish to bring their garments with them to a hospital setting, particularly if doing so relieves sexual tension. An aware health care team can work together in ensuring the patient the same sexual privacy as any other patient. Patients who expose themselves or who "peep" at other patients need very clear limits set on their behavior. If the behavior is truly compulsive, the unreleased tension will still be there for the patient. Nurses are not therapists and are not expected to treat their patients' sexual tension. They can assist their patients in dealing with tension by listening, asking for assistance from other hospital personnel, and enlisting patients' help in setting realistic limits for their sexual behavior.

Summary

Health care providers can promote effective health care for females and males who lead variant sexual life-styles in two significant ways. They can work toward creating a bias-free and nonjudgmental attitude toward human sexual behavior. They can seek out accurate and up-to-date information about the specific health care needs of these people.

1. Human sexual behavior ranges along a continuum from heterosexual to homosexual. It may change over a lifetime.
2. Labels, such as homosexual and transvestite, have two realities: the historic stereotype and the actual human behavior.
3. A patient's sexual behavior and the health care provider's own beliefs and values about sex may create a conflict for the health care provider.
4. Homosexuality occurs in all levels of society. Fear and ignorance on the part of both the nurse and homosexual can interfere with effective health care delivery.
5. Homosexuals have specific health care needs with respect to STDs. Their emotional needs in the health care setting may be overlooked because their relationships are not sanctioned by society.
6. Transsexuals challenge society's most basic beliefs about masculine and feminine roles. Their medical treatment for sex reassignment must be viewed as positive rehabilitation.
7. Other variations of sexual behavior may appear in the health care setting, particularly if the behavior is compulsive. Nurses can learn to work with these patients in dealing with their sexual tension by listening, providing privacy, and setting limits.

Questions for review

List in the left column of the page at least 15 different types of sexual behavior of which you are aware. Think about which of these are acceptable to you in relation to *both* yourself and others. For those behaviors that you find unacceptable, try to identify what *specific* aspect "turns you off" or bothers you. What criteria do you seem to be using? For example, phylogenetic normalcy, social sanctions, legal sanctions, and religious doctrine may all be used as criteria for determining what sexual behaviors are acceptable.

Behavior	Acceptable to me in self	Acceptable to me in others	Unacceptable
1.			
2.			
3.			
4.			
5.			
6.			
7.			
8.			
9.			
10.			
11.			
12.			
13.			
14.			
15.			

After you have completed this exercise, write a short statement that describes any prevailing *themes* personally and/or in others. Decide which aspects of this exercise you would like to share with your colleagues.

•   •   •

The following statements represent some commonly (and uncommonly) encountered situations in nursing practice. Please think about each of these situations, and locate where you stand on the values barometer to the right of the item.

	TOTALLY UNACCEPTABLE				TOTALLY ACCEPTABLE
	1	2	3	4	5
1. A homosexual visits his lover in the hospital.	1	2	3	4	5
2. A lesbian wants to be the support person for her lover who is in labor	1	2	3	4	5
3. An older male patient has an erection while you are bathing him.	1	2	3	4	5

	TOTALLY UNACCEPTABLE				TOTALLY ACCEPTABLE
4. A young man confides that he has fantasies of "doing it with a dog."	1	2	3	4	5
5. A young woman says she really enjoys being tied up before having sex.	1	2	3	4	5
6. A male patient brings into the hospital his overnight bag with women's nightgowns and underwear.	1	2	3	4	5
7. You overhear snide remarks being made about your sex reassignment patient.	1	2	3	4	5

In your journal jot down any new insights you have about your sexual value system. In particular note those areas that seem to be especially unacceptable to you. How can you cope with these situations when they arise in clinical practice?

References

1. Bell, A., and Weinberg, M.: Homosexualities, New York, 1978, Simon & Schuster, Inc.
2. Benjamin, H.: The transsexual phenomenon, New York, 1966, Julian Press.
3. Benjamin, H., and Ihlenfeld, C.: Transsexualism, American Journal of Nursing **73**(3):457-461, 1973.
4. Berger, J., et al.: Standards of care—the hormonal and surgical sex reassignment of gender dysphoric persons, Galveston, Tex., 1979, University of Texas Medical Branch (Janus Information Facility, distributor).
5. Bieber, I.: Homosexuality, New York, 1962, Basic Books, Inc., Publishers.
6. Blumstein, P., and Schwartz, P.: Bisexuality: some social psychological issues, Journal of Social Issues **33**(2):30-45, 1977.
7. Bradshaw, P.L.: Gender surgery: aspects of its nursing care and management, Nursing Times, **77**(37):1595-1597, 1981.
8. Brossart, J.: The gay patient: what you should be doing, R.N. **42**:50-52, April 1979.
9. Calderone, M.S.: The family book about sexuality, New York, 1981, Harper & Row, Publishers, Inc.
10. DeLora, J., and Warren, C.A.: Understanding sexual interaction, Boston, 1977, Houghton Mifflin Co.
11. Erickson Educational Foundation: Guidelines for transsexuals, ed. 1, Baton Rouge, 1974, The Foundation.
12. Evans, R.B.: Homosexuality and the role of the family physician, Medical Aspects of Human Sexuality **13**:10-31, Sept. 1979.
13. Faber, H.: Specifics of physical care, American Journal of Nursing **73**(3):463, 1973.
14. Gebhard, P.H., and others: Sex offenders, New York, 1965, Harper & Row, Publishers, Inc.

15. Green, R.: Children called "sissy" and "tomboy," adolescents who cross-dress, and adults who want to change sex. In Green, R. editor: Human sexuality—a health practitioner's text, Baltimore, 1979, The Williams & Wilkins Co.
16. Green, R., and Money, J., editors: Transsexualism and sex reassignment, Baltimore, 1969, The Johns Hopkins University Press.
17. Haeberle, E.J.: The sex atlas, New York, 1978, The Seabury Press.
18. Hogan, R.: Human sexuality: a nursing perspective, New York, 1980, Appleton-Century-Crofts.
19. Hunt, M.: Sexual behavior in the 1970's, Chicago, 1974, Playboy Press.
20. Kinsey, A.C., et al.: Sexual behavior in the human female, Philadelphia, 1953, W.B. Saunders Co.
21. Lark, C.: Nurses' reactions to transsexual surgery, A.O.R.N. Journal **22**(5):743-749, 1975.
22. Lawrence, J.: Homosexuals, hospitalization and the nurse, Nursing Forum **14**(3):305-317, 1975.
23. Markland, C.: Transsexual surgery. In Wynn, R., editor: Obstetrics and gynecology annual, Englewood Cliffs, N.J., 1975, Prentice-Hall, Inc.
24. Messer, H.D.: The homosexual as physician. In Green, R., editor: Human sexuality—a health practitioner's text. Baltimore, 1979, The Williams & Wilkins Co.
25. Mims, F.H., and Swenson, M.: Sexuality: a nursing perspective, New York, 1980, McGraw-Hill, Inc.
26. Morin, J.: Anal pleasure and health, Burlingame, Calif. 1981, Down There Press.
27. Nass, G., et al.: Sexual choices, Belmont, Calif. 1981, Wadsworth, Inc.
28. O'Donnell, M., et al.: Lesbian health matters, Santa Cruz, 1979, Santa Cruz Women's Health Collective.
29. Ostrow, D., and Sandholzer, T.A.: Homosexuality and sexually transmitted diseases, New York, 1980, The Haworth Press.
30. Pauly, I., and Goldstein, S.: Physicians attitudes in treating homosexuals, Medical Aspects of Human Sexuality **4**(12):26-45, 1970.
31. Pogoncheff, E.: The gay patient: what not to do, R.N. **42**:46-49, April 1979.
32. Pomeroy, W.: The diagnosis and treatment of transvestites and transsexuals, Journal of Sex and Marital Therapy **1**(3):215-225, 1975.
33. Sadoff, R.: Other sexual deviations. In Sadock, B., Kaplan, H., and Freedman, A., editors: The sexual experience, Baltimore, 1976, The Williams & Wilkins Co.
34. Sagarin, E.: Power to the peephole, Sexual Behavior **3**:2-7, 1973.
35. Stoller, R.: The term transvestism, Archives of General Psychiatry **24**:230-237, 1971.
36. Stoller, R.: Gender identity. In Sadock, B., Kaplan, H., and Freedman, A., editors: The sexual experience, Baltimore, 1976, The Williams and Wilkins Co.
37. Strait, J.: The transsexual patient after surgery, American Journal of Nursing **73**(3):462-463, 1973.
38. Thomas, S.P.: Bisexuality: a sexual orientation of great diversity, Journal of Psychiatric Nursing and Mental Health Services, **18**(4):19-27, 1980.

References for clients

Bell, A., and Weinberg, M.: Homosexualities, New York, 1978, Simon & Schuster, Inc.

Benjamin, J.: The transsexual phenomenon, New York, 1966, Julian Press.

Clark, D.: Loving someone gay, Millbrae, Calif. 1977, Celestial Arts.

Fenwick, R.D.: The advocate guide to gay health, New York, 1978, E.P. Dutton.

Martin, D., and Lyon, P.: Lesbian woman, New York, 1972, Bantam Books, Inc.

Morin, J.: Anal pleasure and health, Burlingame, Calif., 1981, Down There Press.

O'Donnell, M., et al.: Lesbian health matters, Santa Cruz, Calif., 1979, Santa Cruz Women's Health Collective.

Ostrow, D., and Sandholzer, T.A.: Homosexuality and sexually transmitted diseases, New York, 1980, The Haworth Press.

Silverstein, C., and White, E.: Joy of gay sex, New York, 1977, Crown Publishers, Inc.

Sisley, E., and Harris, B.: Joy of lesbian sex, New York, 1977, Crown Publishers, Inc.

Tripp, B.: Homosexual matrix, New York, 1976, The New American Library, Inc.

3

Sexuality throughout the life cycle: prenatal life through adolescence

NANCY FUGATE WOODS and ANNE F. MANDETTA

From its earliest moments the human organism is indeed sexual. At conception, when sex is genetically determined, individuals are guided toward a specific and sex-related concept of themselves and fulfillment of certain socially approved roles.

Much of the literature about sexuality deals largely with adult sexuality or problems of sexuality specific to the older population, as if to ignore the sexual nature of infants and children. It is important to recall that the beginning of life is also shaped by sexuality; long before birth, characteristics of sex are evident. During the first moments after birth it is customary for the parents to inquire first about the sex and then about the health of their child.

The purpose of this chapter is to examine the changes in sexual functioning throughout the early part of the life cycle: the prenatal period, infancy, childhood, and adolescence. To maintain a holistic approach to sexual development, it is useful to view changes in sexuality from a biologic, psychologic, and social perspective. Although sexual development will be viewed from these different perspectives, it is useful to remember that these influences interact to determine how an individual develops sexually, especially in terms of the differentiation of gender identity, that is, the sense one has of being male or female.

The prenatal period and infancy

Biologic beginnings. Chromosomal sex is determined at the moment of fertilization when the sperm contributes either an X or Y chromosome to pair with the X chromosome of the female ovum. Barring any idiosyncrasies during cell division, the outcome of this pairing is either an XX (female) or XY (male) combination.[24] The combination of XX or XY chromosomes sets in motion a very complex process analogous to a relay race. In early fetal development the embryo is undifferentiated. The external and internal structures initially are identical.

At about 5 to 6 weeks of fetal life an XX or XY chromosomal combination determines whether the undifferentiated fetal gonads become ovaries or testes. After this point in sexual differentiation the sex chromosomes appear to have no more direct influence.

Further sexual differentiation occurs under the influence of the hormonal secretions of the fetal gonads (Fig. 3-1). It is actually the secretions of the male testis, the fetal androgens, that influence further differentiation between the seventh and the twelfth

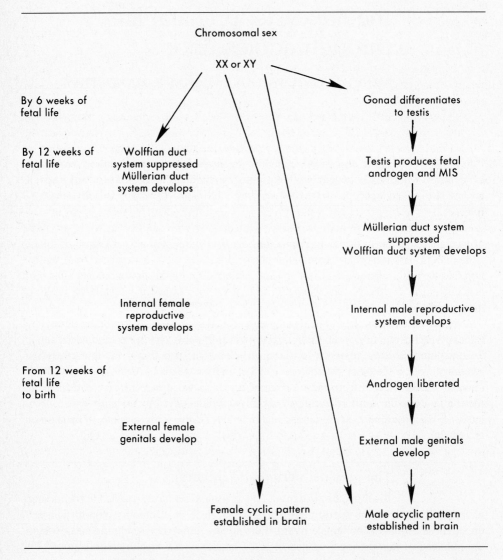

Fig. 3-1. Fetal sexual development. (Modified from Money, J., and Ehrhardt, A.A.: Man and woman, boy and girl: the differentiation and dimorphism of gender identity from conception to maturity, Baltimore, 1972, The Johns Hopkins University Press.)

prenatal weeks. For a male fetus to develop, male hormones must be added. If androgens are not present in appropriate amounts at critical times, male structures will not develop from the wolffian ducts. Another substance, the müllerian-inhibiting substance, which has not yet been isolated, is thought to prevent further development of the müllerian or female duct system. In rare cases the müllerian-inhibiting substance does not act, and a genetic male will be born with fallopian tubes and a uterus, as well as male internal organs. In the absence of fetal gonadal hormones female reproductive structures will begin to develop from the müllerian ducts regardless of whether the fetus is a chromosomal male or female. At this stage estrogen does not seem to be essential for female development. Although hormonal influence can still alter the genital appearance, biologic sex is fairly well established by the twelfth week of fetal life.[24] During the third or fourth month of pregnancy androgens convert the undifferentiated external genitals to the male pattern.

Although estrogens are probably not essential for the continued feminization of the reproductive tract, they are released in the genetically female embryo. If the gonads are removed before the seventh week of prenatal life, the fetus will continue to develop as a female, regardless of chromosomal sex. There does not appear to be an ovarian inductor substance elaborated in the female, as is necessary for the male. However, estrogens are required for full development of the female genital pattern. Hormonal induction enables the male embryo to offset the influence of his mother's hormones with his own testosterone. It is believed that there is a critical stage, just before or soon after birth, at which another set of sexual controls is introduced. Testosterone may influence the hypothalamus, in a process referred to as sex-typing of the brain. The brain that is influenced by testosterone will develop the male, or acyclic, pattern for the release of pituitary hormones, the gonadotropins. In the female-typed brain a cyclic pattern of gonadotropin release is established.

There appear to be two critical points in fetal sexual development: the prenatal point at which development of the internal and external genitals is induced in the male embryo by testosterone and the point during prenatal life or early childhood (some time before 3 years of age) when the brain becomes appropriately sex typed. Both chromosomal and hormonal factors influence the development of reproduction and bodily appearance. The infant's appearance at birth sets in motion a complex social process leading to differentiation of gender identity. Gender identity is the sense one has of maleness or femaleness, and gender role is the social expression of that gender identity. Parents and others in the infant's immediate environment play an important role in the differentiation of the child's gender identity. From the moment that they know "It's a girl" or "It's a boy," parents and significant others relate to the child in a way that confirms masculinity or femininity. Gender assignment, rearing the child as a male or female, has a powerful influence on the development of gender identity, which is usually well established by age 3 to 4 years.[24] As the infant develops, he or she also receives cues about gender identity from his or her bodily appearance.

Several rare conditions can cause the development of ambiguous genitals or genitals that are incongruous with genetic sex. Two such conditions are androgen-insensitivity syndrome and adrenogenital syndrome. With androgen-insensitivity syndrome, also called testicular feminization syndrome, a genetic male is born with incompletely masculinized genitals that may appear to be normal female external genitals. This occurs because the cells of the body are unable to respond to androgen even if it is produced by the testes in normal amounts. Incomplete masculine internal development prevents internal female development.

Elevated androgen levels that occur with the adrenogenital syndrome can produce an enlarged clitoris or normal-looking penis and scrotal sac in the genetic female. If not treated, this syndrome also causes severe virilization of females. Infants with both androgen-insensitivity syndrome and adrenogenital syndrome may have their sex reannounced or reassigned when their conditions are diagnosed. In such cases medical treatment and counseling are usually required.

The child who is born with ambiguous genitals becomes the object of parental confusion unless definitive counseling is obtained early. Although successful sex reassignment may occur at age 3, Money and Ehrhardt[24] believe that 18 months is an age ceiling for sex reassignment in the majority of cases. By this age, gender identity is advanced in its differentiation, and behavior patterns of those who are significant in the child's rearing are well established.

The transsexual is an individual who believes that he or she is trapped in the body of the wrong sex. The etiology of transsexualism, like homosexuality, is unknown. Various investigators have attributed the transsexual's plight to fetal, metabolic, hormonal, neural, familial, or social factors.[24] The external genitals of the human contribute to the formation of gender identity inasmuch as they are used in ascribing the sex of the infant at birth, in subsequent rearing, and in eliciting response from the parents based on their preferences for a son or daughter. Although parental preference may lead to inappropriate child-rearing patterns, these patterns alone do not appear to be responsible for the problems faced by the transsexual. It is probable that a biologic error in the differentiation of gender may occur either in infancy or during early childhood.[1,22,23]

Because tissues in the infant develop at differing rates, it is possible that there may be a mechanism by which the transsexual develops normal external genitals before birth but does not acquire the same sex typing at the critical period of brain differentiation. Because there are more male than female transsexuals, it is believed that the hormonal-induction mechanism is probably responsible for this disorder of gender. The male transsexual, as a fetus, probably receives adequate hormonal stimulation to develop normal internal and external genitals but during the second critical period, either shortly before or after birth, does not receive adequate stimulus to cause neural differentiation.[23,24] As a result, the discrepancy between biologic gender and perceived gender identity develops.

Infant sexuality. A major developmental task of infancy is development of trust, achieved through predictable relationships with primary caretakers. At the same time infants are learning to differentiate the "self" from others and are developing a sense of their bodies as good or bad. Infants experience sensations from being touched and from nursing. Feelings of pleasure, warmth, and satisfaction attained through touch and nursing are important early sensual experiences. Without touch, infants develop miasma or even die, and with early weaning from nursing they may develop oral deprivation.

Female infants have the potential for lubrication and orgasm, and males can have erections. Sometimes these evidences of infant sexuality are disturbing to parents who worry about the "normalcy" of these responses.

Gender differences. Recently investigators have explored the nature of behavioral differences between male and female infants and have proposed a number of theories to account for them. In a review of a number of studies of sexual differences among children during the first year of life, Bardwick[1] points out that even at birth there are significant differences between male and female infants. Males tend to be larger, have more muscle mass, and be more active. Females tend to be more passive in their motor responses and more sensitive to tactile stimuli and pain. At 6 months the female infant has a longer attention span for visual stimuli, has a better fixation response to a human face, and is more responsive to social stimuli. She prefers complex stimuli, such as jazz music, whereas the male infant has a better fixation response to a helix of light and is more attentive to an intermittent tone.

By 13 months there are additional sex differences. The male makes a maximal response to verbal stimuli that are high in meaning and low in inflection and the female to stimuli that are high in both meaning and inflection. The male prefers low-complexity stimuli and the female highly complex stimuli. Usually the female has already demonstrated earlier language development than the male and seems to be more aware of contextual relationships.[1]

Bardwick[1] hypothesizes that the sex typing of the brain causes the infant's personality to have qualities that are either rewarded or punished by parents according to their definition of sex-appropriate behavior. For example, the female as an infant and child tends to exhibit less physical activity, less aggressiveness, more pain sensitivity, lower sexual impulses, and less masturbation. She pays more attention to a wide variety of stimuli and is aware of contextual influence. Even the very young female is more aware of social demands, can better assess parental wishes, and is more likely to be rewarded for being good. She is conditioned to be more dependent on others for her self-esteem, which is based on being loved.[1]

Because of differences in their behavior patterns, there is less parental cultural stress exerted on girls than on boys. According to Bardwick,[1] girls' behavior tends to be less troublesome than that of boys of comparable ages. This lack of stress, however, leads to dependency, and the girl develops less impulse control, since she has fewer unacceptable impulses to control. On the other hand, the boy is pushed to conform. When he finds that he cannot adopt all the standards of his parents, he develops his own self-regard system. In general, most parents respond to the infantile quality of the male child until he is about 2 to 2½ years, and then sex-role discrimination becomes more enhanced.

That sex differences exist by the age of 13 months was borne out by studies of Goldberg and Lewis.[10] A free-play situation was used to observe sex differences in the infant's behavior toward the mother, toys, and a frustration situation in a group of 64 subjects (half boys and half girls). Girls spent a significantly shorter time away from their mothers than boys and returned significantly more frequently to their mothers. Girls also spent significantly more time touching their mothers than the boys. Girls also spent significantly more time looking at their mothers, in proximity to their mothers, and vocalizing to them. When a barrier was placed in a room separating the infants from their mothers, the girls were more frustrated than the boys. Boys made more attempts to get around the barrier, whereas girls tended to stand in the middle of the room and cry.

Toys that offered the most varied possibilities for manipulation seemed to get the more attention from the infants. There were no significant sex differences in the choice of toys, but girls preferred toys with faces and those that required more motor coordination. Boys spent more time playing with nontoys in the room. In general, boys were more active and vigorous. A comparison of the infant's behavior with data obtained about the mother-child relationship when the infants were only 6 months old revealed that mothers of the girls touched their infants more than the mothers of boys; girls were also more likely to be breast-fed than the males, and their mothers vocalized more to them.[10]

The investigators suggest that the girls were more dependent and less exploratory because of the differential behavior of the mother. It is possible that parents reinforce the behaviors they consider sex-role appropriate even while the infant is very young. As a result, the infant learns a sex role much like any other response to the parent. Parental cues and behavior are important influences on the child's developing gender role.[10]

The discomfort experienced by transsexuals may also be a result of the constraining effects of sex roles. If expectations of men and women were similar, perhaps the need to change gender might be perceived as less acute.

Differences in behavior can be explained by a number of factors. Biologists attribute gender differences in behavior to the effect of hormones on sex typing and the hemispheric specialization of the brain. Social scientists attribute gender differences to the way in which the child is socialized to behave.

Childhood

Childhood encompasses several stages of development, including the toddler, preschool, and school-age years (those years between infancy and preadolescence) and puberty. During this period several changes are seen in the rapidly growing and maturing individual. Physical growth occurs rapidly in nearly every system except the reproductive system. The genital organs remain quiescent, although the uterus regains its birth size by the time the girl is 10 or 11 years old. No major changes are seen in the ovaries, testes, or breasts until puberty.

The toddler years. As discussed earlier, gender identity is well developed in toddlers. They are usually well aware of gender differences and are able to tell others that they are a "girl" or "boy."

Neuromuscular control contributes to toddlers' ability to be mobile and become toilet trained. It also begins to provide them with the means to explore their environment and interact with peers of both sexes. As children grow, they also become more independent and are able to meet more of their own basic needs. Soon they discover that by self-stimulation they are able to experience sexual pleasure.

Finally, throughout this period the ability of children to communicate becomes more refined. As their vocabulary grows, they become able to express ideas and convey questions about their own sexuality to both parents and peers. They develop vocabulary relating to their genitals and elimination; the nature of their vocabulary may make it difficult for them to discuss these functions in later years. Between the ages of 2 and 3 years children become more interested in excretory functions. This period is usually characterized by some ambivalence toward the caretakers and is often termed the *pregenital* or *anal* period. Usually these years coincide with toilet training and are characterized by an increased awareness by children of their genitals.

During the transition period from infant to toddler, core gender identity is solidified. Children can look at a picture and clearly differentiate sexual differences. They can distinguish between male and female by means of the differences in hair and clothing. Children continue to be able to identify body parts, especially areas responsible for excretion. They also develop distinct pride and pleasure in their own bodies, sometimes specifically in the genital area. Pleasurable genital self-stimulation also enhances this self-satisfaction. At about 21 months, children can refer to themselves by their own names, an event pivotal in the emergence of identity. By 2 years of age, children are able to categorize people by gender and have some awareness of the anatomic differences if they have had an opportunity to view them.[16]

During the third year and after that time children continue to develop verbal categorizations, which become more precise for the sexes. At the middle of the third year they become aware of and interested in the parental relationship, including their roles, sleeping arrangements, and bathing. During the last part of the third year children continue to refine the meanings of gender terms and the roles associated with them. Often the father is emerging as a special love object for the female child as is the mother for the male.[16]

As their muscles mature, children are able to hold on and let go. It is during the period of life that Freud would term *anal* that children must cope with developing a sense of autonomy instead of shame and doubt. At this stage they require some parental limits and some guidance in autonomy. Children are particularly vulnerable to shaming experiences and may be purposefully shamed for acting out sexually in inappropriate places. If they are given an opportunity to develop self-control without losing self-esteem, they will probably achieve a sense of autonomy instead of shame and self-doubt.[8]

The preschool years. During the preschool years the child learns much about sex roles, especially appropriate behavior for boys and girls. The preschooler identifies with the parent of the same sex and simultaneously forms attachments to the parent of the opposite sex.

It is not uncommon for children of this age to engage in sexual play involving exploration of their own bodies and those of their friends. Self-pleasuring activities (masturbation) are also common.

During the preschool years gender identity disorders become evident. The history of the male-to-female transsexual typically dates the onset of cross-gender behavior back to early childhood. Often the transsexual recalls wanting to be a female or to wear female clothing. Parents comment that the child verbalizes wanting to be a girl, is preoccupied with feminine toys, tends to take on female roles in play, has feminine gestures, and is artistically inclined.[11] These characteristics engender great conflict in parents, who are fearful of frustrating their son. Many say they waited for the boy to outgrow the unacceptable behavior.[11] It is also quite possible that given less constraining notions about sex roles, the child could demonstrate those characteristics previously associated with only men or women without arousing parental anxiety.

Some authors implicate the family in the transsexual's etiology, but there does not appear to be consistent evidence for this conclusion. Others hypothesize that the disturbance is related to temperament of the child, with the child's temperament leading the parent to treat the child as an infant of the opposite sex.[22]

In either event several attempts have been made to objectively document childhood behavior that is inconsistent with sexual norms. Although authors suggest that such tests be used in conjunction with other tools to diagnose gender problems, it should be kept in mind that norms for these tests are based on what is traditionally viewed as ''normal male'' or ''normal female'' behavior rather than what is viewed as ''normal human'' behavior.

The school-age years. During the early school years children usually exhibit curiosity about sex. Most of their friends are of the same sex, but physical and emotional aspects of sexual development are commonly shared concerns. During these years children explore language about sex and may use terms for their shock value. Although Freud described this developmental period as a ''latency period,'' children's obvious interest in their sexuality attests to its importance. When children to do not receive the information they need, they may become fearful or develop negative feelings about their sexuality. Misinformation gleaned from their peers may confuse or frighten them. School-age children need to know which sexual behaviors are socially acceptable and in what contexts they may practice them.

As children enter school, a number of sex differences in intellectual functioning become apparent. First, there is a tendency for girls to test higher on intelligence tests during the preschool years and for boys to test higher during high school. In preschool and early school years girls show a decided advantage in verbal ability. Girls say their first words sooner, articulate better and earlier, and use longer sentences. By the beginning of grade school, however, vocabularies are similar. Girls learn to read sooner, but by the age of 10 years, boys catch up. Girls appear better at grammar, spelling, and word fluency.[19]

Usually girls learn to count earlier, but boys tend to outperform girls on tests of arithmetic reasoning. Boys appear to be more proficient at spatial and analytic abilities, but girls are able to pay more attention to detail. Boys are more apt to break set, that is, pick details that require divergence from the context. Finally, girls obtain better grades than boys during school, but men tend to be more achievement oriented than women during later life.[18]

Although some suggest that these gender differences are biologically determined, others claim that differential socialization of boys and girls is responsible.[18] Some implicate educational systems in the maintenance, if not the exaggeration, of gender differences in intellectual functioning.[1]

A childhood experience that can lead to future problems is sexual abuse, which includes a wide variety of sexual activities that an adult engages in with a child, with or without the child's willingness or consent. Sexual abuse of children may be the least reported but most common crime committed against children. Leaman[17] states that the intervention goal during this situational crisis is to return family functioning to normal quickly by resolving feelings about the abusive event. She divides early management of the family into the following 12 steps:

1. Interviewing the child and the parents separately to learn about the sexual abuse
2. Thoroughly explaining all procedures and examinations to the child and parents
3. Informing the parents that the medical examination may not prove or disprove sexual abuse
4. Explaining significant findings to the parents
5. Assuring the parents that the child will almost certainly not be emotionally or physically damaged for life by the abusive experience, if their reaction to the event is calm and reasonable
6. Informing the parents that their reaction will greatly influence the reaction of their child
7. Helping prevent further problems for the child by helping parents to resume their usual home life
8. Explaining to the parents that the child will probably be influenced more by their reaction than by the event
9. Knowing and informing the parents of the role of law enforcement authorities
10. Facilitating ventilation of the parents' feelings about the event
11. Helping the parents gain needed support from other sources such as relatives and other professionals
12. Documenting the results of interviews and examinations

Care should be taken not to further frighten or upset the child during the interview and medical examination. The families that often need the most help are the ones in which the offender is a relative or close friend. Details about these situations, especially incest, are less likely to be disclosed to health professionals. Cases involving incest often require further exploration and follow-up counseling.

In many schools children are now being taught sexual assault prevention tools. These include knowledge of parts of their bodies considered private, awareness of who may touch these body parts, discrimination between "good touching" and "bad touching," and the assertiveness to tell a responsible adult if sexual abuse is threatened or occurs.

Indications of sexual assault are varied but may include personality change, transition from outgoing to "clingy" behavior, changes in toilet training habits, being uncomfortable with someone previously trusted, withdrawal, discussion of sexual acts about which the child has had no instruction, or unusual interest in her or his own or others' genitals. In addition, many other behavior changes, such as sudden unfounded fears or changed eating or sleeping habits, may be signals.

Parents or others who suspect that a child has been sexually abused can receive help from child protective services, child abuse agencies, rape counseling centers, and sexual assault centers. The National Child Abuse Hotline Referral Service (1-800-423-5805) may also be helpful.

Adolescence

Adolescence refers to the period of transition from childhood to adulthood. It is marked by the onset of puberty, the second major period of physiologic and anatomic sexual development. There is perhaps no period in the life cycle during which changes in sexual anatomy and physiology are as profound as during adolescence. Immediately before and coincident with puberty, the genital organs develop rapidly, finally reaching their adult maturity.

Among the complex biologic changes seen during puberty are the budding of the breasts in girls and the beginning growth of pubic hair. These events occur at about age 10 to 11 years (but may occur between the ages of 8 and 13 years) and usually predate menstruation, which usually begins between the ages of 11 and 13 years. In boys the comparable events of testicular enlargement and growth of pubic hair occur between the ages of 12 and 16 years. Ejaculation and enlargement of the penis tend to occur later between the ages of 13 and 17 years.[14]

Hormonal influences responsible for secondary sex characteristics trigger changes in both the contour and the function of the body that challenge the adolescent's coping mechanisms. Responses to the altered body may be problematic or may reflect the adolescent's pleasure with his or her "adult" body. Usually the physical transitions proceed fairly gradually, and timetables for certain aspects of development are predictable (Fig. 3-2). For example, once the vellus type of hair appears on the inner aspects of the girl's labia majora, it darkens and spreads in a predictable sequence from an upright triangular

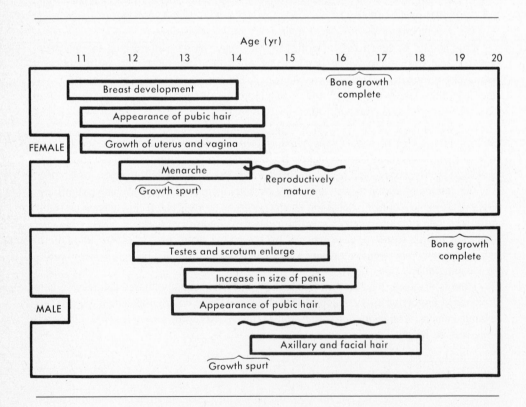

Fig. 3-2. Physical changes of adolescence by age and sex. (From Phipps, W.J., Long, B.C., and Woods, N.F.: Medical-surgical nursing, ed. 2, St. Louis, 1983, The C.V. Mosby Co.)

shape to the inverted triangle of the adult female escutcheon. About midway in this transition, menarche usually occurs. Breast development can also be predicted in a similar fashion.[24]

For the male, physical development is especially important. The common belief that one's virility and potency can be equated with the size of the testicles and penis probably contributes to his concern. Boys are also often concerned about other changes they experience. Nocturnal emissions, or "wet dreams," may worry some boys, especially if they have not been prepared for this event before it happens. If boys are provided with some basic information, such as that the discharge of semen during sleep is a natural occurrence that periodically relieves the pressure of fluid in the seminal vesicles, it will usually allay their anxiety. Another source of concern in boys at puberty is swollen, femalelike breasts. Adolescent gynecomastia is so common that it is viewed as a normal developmental variation for a small amount of glandular growth of the breasts to occur. The boy's concern is usually decreased if he is informed that this common condition does not indicate the development of other female characteristics and usually disappears without treatment. Similar preoccupations may be found among girls. Their concerns tend to be breast development and menstruation. The cultural emphasis placed on breasts as a symbol of femininity probably intensifies the young woman's worries about her changing body contours. In addition, the irregular menstrual pattern characteristic of the first year after menarche may cause her to be preoccupied with her physiology, particularly if her developmental timetable differs from that of her peers.[5,14]

Other aspects of growth such as height, weight, or transient skin problems (e.g., acne) may create anxiety. Changes in physiology, which are commonly reflected in reactions such as sweating or fatigue, also serve to heighten adolescents' preoccupation with their bodies.[13]

In general, the anatomic and physiologic changes seen during adolescence generate anxieties about maturation. For most adolescents, changes in sexual physiology are translated into new feelings and drives that demand new methods of coping.

A major task for the adolescent is the establishment of identity in the face of role confusion. The newly experienced sexual maturity activates not only questions about maleness or femaleness but also concerns about who one is within the peer group. For this reason the adolescent attempts to band together with others sharing similar characteristics and to fall in love. Both of these activities may be considered means of testing a definition of one's identity.[8] Within the present social climate of roles in transition, establishing identity may be a different and less limiting process.

The incredible change in the adolescent's appearance necessitates a change in the earlier concept of the body. Perceptions related to an increased awareness of sexual feelings must also be integrated into an acceptable view of the self. It is unfortunate that events, such as slow breast development, that vary from the prevailing stereotypes cause the adolescent to experience anxiety about development. Fantasies about sexual function or anatomy may interfere with evolution of a positive image of the self.[14] However, it currently seems that adolescents are becoming more accepting of less-than-perfect bodies and more concerned with aspects of human relationships.

Another change the adolescent must cope with is an excess of physical energy. Physical activity and impulsive behavior may be constructive ways of coping with tension and anxiety associated with the rapidly changing body.[14] Sexual impulses push the need for personal controls to the forefront.

Adolescents are faced with a new status in society, have new demands made on them, and are subject to moral proscriptions that are in conflict with changes in their physiology. Society attributes new status to adolescents: at 16 years of age they may obtain a driver's license, and at age 18 they are allowed to vote. Although adolescents are physiologically mature and experience intense sexual drives, society does not sanction adolescent non-marital sexual behavior. Sexual privilege does not necessarily derive from rites of passage.

Certain universal tasks are defined for adolescents as they develop: learning to be a productive member of society and developing a relationship with a member of the opposite sex. Cultures vary with regard to demands on adolescents and also in their ability to facilitate development of adult maturity. Middle-class American adolescents have a special status: they are members of a large, influential group. The peer group provides strong support.

However, even in light of their special status, adolescents are in somewhat of a bind: although they are sexually mature, they do not have full adult privileges. Middle-class morality still dictates the value of virginity in some sectors, but even within this class some groups advocate sexual freedom. The social conflicts over sexual morality only serve to intensify the confusion experienced by adolescents as they attempt to cope with intense sexual feelings. The dilemma adolescents face is strong repression of sexuality versus rebellion against sexual mores.

Sexual problems and concerns. Many sexual issues can generate concerns or problems for adolescents. Their rapidly changing bodies may be a source of anxiety. It is not uncommon for them to have a poor body image and believe that any difference between them and their peers is a mark of inadequacy. Any negative experience with their bodies, such as acne or divergence from the typical developmental timetable, may be the cause of a poor self-image. Inadequate knowledge is often responsible for sexual concerns. Providing adolescents with adequate information about sexual development can alleviate some of the anxiety about pubertal changes.

A girl's experience with menstruation serves as an example. Social customs such as terming the menstrual period "the curse" only abet fantasies of injury and undermine the concept of womanhood.[5] Fortunately, today fewer girls are told that menstruation is an illness during which they should refrain from activities such as bathing and engaging in sports. Even though the adolescent female may not view menstruation as an illness, she may be troubled about certain aspects of her "period." Providing adequate information about the normal range of age of onset of menstruation, length of cycles, and days of menstrual flow is useful. Some menstrual problems should be investigated medically if they persist over a period of months. These include amenorrhea (absence of menses), menorrhagia (abnormally heavy menstrual flow), secondary amenorrhea (irregularity or absence of periods that have previously been regular), scanty menstrual flow (except for users of contraceptive pills), and dysmenorrhea. Onset of the menses and development of secondary sex characteristics can be problematic if the rapidly developing or slowly developing girl perceives herself as radically different from her peers.

A boy may have anxiety about masturbation even though it is a normal aspect of sexual development. At this age he is probably much more aware of the pleasurable stimuli from his sexual organs than is a girl, and this is probably a result of the differences in socialization of boys and girls. However, both may experience guilt and shame in conjunction with masturbation, especially if parents have conveyed that masturbation is abnormal or immoral. First ejaculations may also be anxiety provoking if they have not been preceded by education.

A girl's experience with masturbation differs from a boy's in that she may be less aware of her external genitals. Although self-pleasuring is a normal component of sexual maturation, it frequently leads to guilt or shame, and some females consider masturbation a perversion or at least not a topic for conversation. Self-pleasuring or sexual fantasies, when used as an escape from real problems, may have negative consequences for the adolescent's development.

Despite publicity about sexually active adolescents, there is a large proportion who do not have their first heterosexual intercourse until their twenties. These adolescents may have worries about the normalcy of their virginity. For those who become sexually active during adolescence, there may be awkwardness in their early sexual encounters.

Nonmarital sex can produce guilt and fear of pregnancy or sexually transmitted disease (see Chapter 14). Some adolescents associate sex with guilt and shame rather than view it as positive and pleasurable. These feelings can provide the foundation for later sexual dysfunction.

Unwanted pregnancy among adolescents is increasing in the United States. Hundreds of thousands of teenagers are having children each year. The problem is much greater than the numbers of births alone reflect because pregnant teenagers are high risks medically, socially, and educationally. Early childbearing is associated with high rates of toxemia, fetal and neonatal mortality, and prematurity.[26] In addition to several social problems, pregnant adolescents often face a triple crisis of establishing their identity, adjusting to pregnancy and parenthood (or abortion or adoption if they select one of those options), and coping with a rapidly arranged marriage. Frequently they do not complete high school or vocational training. This often leads to a self-destructive cycle of failures— failure to finish school, failure to establish a stable family life, failure to be self-supporting, and failure to prevent repeated unwanted pregnancies.[27] Many interdisciplinary programs are working with pregnant adolescents to help them capitalize on their strengths and minimize the health, psychosocial, and educational problems that they face.

Preventing unwanted adolescent pregnancy is often a concern of professionals working with sexually active teenagers. The values as well as the knowledge of professionals about adolescent sexual behavior may influence their approach. Some focus on encouraging the unmarried adolescent to abstain from sexual intercourse. Others try to provide contraceptive information and services for adolescents to prevent unwanted pregnancy. The American Academy of Pediatrics supports this latter approach and has recommended that medical consultation and effective contraceptive advice and methods consistent with girls' physical and emotional needs should be available to teenage girls whose sexual behavior exposes them to the risk of pregnancy.[20] Helping sexually active adolescents use contraception effectively is a challenge. Often this group lacks adequate knowledge about conception and contraception. Although important, providing accurate information about these topics is usually not enough to facilitate effective contraceptive practice. Several other factors that influence whether or not a young woman will use a contraceptive need to be considered. These factors include the influence of significant others, especially parents, peers, and her sexual partner; her own values and attitudes about sexuality, children, contraceptives, and sex roles; her self-esteem, degree of assertiveness, and ability to communicate with her partner; and the health care delivery system's ability to provide contraceptive services that are accessible, available, and acceptable.[19] The adolescent's acceptance or nonacceptance of her sexual behavior is one of the most important determinants of contraceptive behavior. If a young woman accepts her sexual behaviors as positive, she is more likely to use a contraceptive than a young woman who believes her sexual behavior is wrong and bad. An adolescent with the latter view and the guilt that accompanies it will often say to herself and others, "I am never going to engage in sexual intercourse again and therefore do not need to use contraception." This denial can be so strong that a teenager who has intercourse each weekend for months will swear each Monday that she will never do so again until she is married. The adolescent who accepts her sexual relations and relationships can plan ahead and take responsible contraceptive action.[19]

Development of a sexual value system is an important task for adolescents. Their values will influence the kinds of relationships they develop, sexual activities they engage in, and sexual life-styles they choose. Adolescents who have no parental limits probably have difficulty clarifying their values about sexuality. On the other hand, those who are exposed to very rigid limitations are not encouraged to clarify their own values and may not learn self-control. If they have established a pattern of trust and communication, adolescents can discuss their feelings openly with their parents or another significant adult in their lives. This opportunity for discussion enhances the adolescent's ability to explore a range of values and their consequences.

Adolescence is also a time for validation of one's sexual orientation. It is a time of learning a repertoire of sexual behaviors, sex roles, and life-styles characteristic of the majority of society. For homosexuals the tasks are complicated by society's response to their sexual orientation. Homosexual adolescents face not only the challenges that typify all adolescents' sexual development but also those that are particular to their sexual orientation. Often they lack access to information because of the lack of understanding of homosexuality that pervades society.

During adolescence nearly all homosexually oriented girls and some heterosexually oriented girls have homosexual experiences of one form or another. Usually these involve visual inspection, caressing of the genitals, or mutual masturbation. Experiences of males are similar, with homosexual and heterosexual boys engaging in mutual masturbation, fellatio, or the rubbing of bodies together to experience orgasm.[3] Heterosexuals who engage in sexual activity with others of the same sex may be confused about their sexual orientation. Transient homosexual experiences in adolescence need to be considered in context as a part of a maturational process that is not incompatible with adult heterosexuality.

For homosexual adolescents, conflict may exist about whether, with whom, and how to share information about their sexual orientation. They may risk parental and peer rejection, live in fear of being discovered, or defer acting on their sexual feelings. Little is known about how to foster healthy development in the homosexual adolescent.

Autonomy in sexual relationships is another problem area for the adolescent. Since sexuality is represented to youth as a fringe benefit of adult status, it seems only natural that adolescents should seek it. However, Western society seems more concerned with parameters of sexual behavior than aspects of reproduction: even with contraceptive technology it does not permit adolescents the adult privilege of intercourse. Sex is simultaneously presented as good and bad, and procreation ability and adult sexual responsibility appear to develop out of phase with one another.

Gadpaille[9] lists a number of options for resolving adolescent sexual conflict. The first option is compliance with prohibitions that appear to be parentally derived rather than self-determined standards. Adolescents may defy authority or adult ownership of sex and openly refuse to wait for adult status. They may refuse to pretend to wait, openly challenging cultural definition. Open refusal to accept the social consequences of overt sexuality, such as ostracism for behavior, is yet another option. Mocking the authority position can be another strategy: adolescents act on ideals rarely practiced, such as "make love, not war." Finally, adolescents can repudiate authority or adult ownership of sex by redefining sexual traditions; for example, the female adolescent may demand sexual freedom, and the male adolescent may accept a nondominant role.

Adolescents who sexually act out sometimes reflect the sexual problems of their parents. Acting out is often precipitated by parental conflicts that result in disturbed family communication.[30]

A final problem of adolescent sexuality is inadequate health services. Again, the "hiatus" status of adolescents is responsible for difficulties they encounter: although sexually active and mature, in many areas they cannot obtain contraception, treatment for sexually transmitted diseases, or problem pregnancy counseling without parental consent. Parental consent may deter adolescents from obtaining needed health care. In addition, judgmental health practitioners or those uncomfortable with their own sexuality may further discourage adolescents. Free clinics or teen clinics have evolved in many parts of the United States but are not available for many youth.

Summary

This chapter has focused on sexuality throughout the early portion of the life cycle: the prenatal period, infancy, childhood, and adolescence. Sexual problems common to each age group were explored. Key considerations for the health practitioner include the following:

1. Each individual is a sexual being from the moment of conception.
2. During infancy and early childhood, sexuality is influenced profoundly by socialization. Sex differences in the behavior of infants are the products of environment, as well as gender.
3. During early childhood, core gender identity is solidified.
4. Sexual problems encountered in childhood may include problems related to sexual myth or misconception, gender identity disturbances, an environment supportive of sexual confusion, and sexual abuse.
5. Adolescence is the period of the life cycle during which sexual maturation is biologically established by means of widespread anatomic and physiologic changes.
6. The adolescent is faced with establishing identity, accepting a

changed body image, coping with new energies, and resolving conflicts.

7. Adolescence is socially a "hiatus status": adolescents have a new set of sexual functions but are told that they must wait for adult status to enjoy them.
8. Sexual concerns arising in adolescence may include accepting altered physiology such as menstruation, engaging in early sexual experiences, achieving sexual autonomy, resolving conflicts about relationships, and obtaining sex-related health services.

Questions for review

1. Consider the complex processes involved in the evolution of gender identity. Discuss the relative influences of socialization and biology. In what ways might social constraints of sex role stereotypes explain disorders of gender identity?
2. Consider the sexuality of the toddler. In what ways might the parents of toddlers reinforce and validate their sexuality? How might the parents negate their children's sexuality?
3. Consider school-age children and their sexuality. What evidence is there that the "latency period" described by Freud is an inappropriate label for this developmental stage?
4. Adolescents, as a population, have many sexual concerns, yet there is evidence that health professionals are poorly equipped to deal with them. Devise an assessment guide for an adolescent health care clinic that will help you identify their concerns. What items should be included in a comprehensive assessment?

References

1. Bardwick, J.M.: Psychology of women: a study of bio-cultural conflicts, New York, 1971, Harper & Row, Publishers, Inc.
2. Bates, J.E., Bentler, P.M., and Thompson, S.K.: Measurement of deviant gender development in boys, Child Development **44:**591-598, 1973.
3. Bell, A., Weinberg, M., and Hammersmith, S.: Sexual preference: its development among men and women, Bloomington, Ind., 1981, Indiana University Press.
4. Braverman, S.: Homosexuality, American Journal of Nursing **73:**652-655, 1973.
5. Brown, F.: Sexual problems of the adolescent girl, Pediatric Clinics of North America **19:**759-764, 1972.
6. Canfield, E.: Toward a manifesto of rights and responsibilities for the sexual adolescent, Journal of Clinical Child Psychology **3**(3):Fall/Winter, 1974.
7. Douvan, E.: Sex differences in adolescent character processes. In Bardwick, J.M.: Readings on the psychology of women, New York, 1972, Harper & Row, Publishers, Inc.
8. Erikson, E.H.: Childhood and society, ed. 2, New York, 1963, W.W. Norton & Co., Inc.

9. Gadpaille, W.J.: Adolescent sexuality and the struggle over authority, Journal of School Health **40:**479-483, 1970.

10. Goldberg, S., and Lewis, M.: Play behavior in the year-old infant: early sex differences. In Bardwick, J.M.: Readings on the psychology of women, New York, 1972, Harper & Row, Publishers, Inc.

11. Green, R.: Diagnosis and treatment of gender identity disorders during childhood, Archives of Sexual Behavior **1:**167-173, 1971.

12. Green, R., and Fuller, M.: Family doll play and female identity in preadolescent males, American Journal of Orthopsychiatry **43:**123-127.

13. Group for the Advancement of Psychiatry: Sex and the college student, New York, 1965, Mental Health Materials Center, Inc.

14. Group for the Advancement of Psychiatry: Normal adolescence: its dynamics and impact, New York, 1968, Charles Scribner's Sons.

15. House, E.: Medical services for sexually active teenagers, American Journal of Public Health **63:**285-287, 1973.

16. Kleeman, J.A.: The establishment of core gender identity in normal girls. 1. (a) Introduction; (b) Development of the ego capacity to differentiate, Archives of Sexual Behavior **1:**103-116, 1971.

17. Leaman, K.: The sexually abused child, Nursing '77 **7:**68-72, 1977.

18. Maccoby, E.E.: Sex differences in intellectual functioning. In Bardwick, J.M.: Readings on the psychology of women, New York, 1972, Harper & Row, Publishers, Inc.

19. Mandetta, A.: Family planning at a school for pregnant girls: development of a conceptual framework for practice. In Hall, J., and Weaver, B., editors: Distributive nursing practice: a systems approach to community health, Philadelphia, 1977, J.B. Lippincott Co.

20. Marinoff, S.C.: Contraception in adolescents, Pediatric Clinics of North America **19**(3):811-819, 1972.

21. McCoy, K.: Adolescent sexuality: a national concern, Journal of Clinical Child Psychology **3**(3):Fall-Winter, 1974.

22. Money, J.: Sex reassignment therapy in gender identity disorders, International Psychiatry Clinics **8:**197-210, 1972.

23. Money, J., and Ehrhardt, A.A.: Fetal hormones and the brain: effect of sexual dimorphism on behavior—a review, Archives of Sexual Behavior **1:**241-262, 1971.

24. Money, J., and Ehrhardt, A.A.: Man and woman, boy and girl: the differentiation and dimorphism of gender identity from conception to maturity, Baltimore, 1972, The Johns Hopkins University Press.

25. Neumann, F., and Steinback, H.: Influence of sex hormones on the differentiation of neural centers, Archives of Sexual Behavior **2:**147-162, 1972.

26. Osofsky, H.J.: The pregnant teenager, Springfield, Ill., 1968, Charles C Thomas, Publisher.

27. Sarrel, P.: Caring for the pregnant teenager, The Family Planner **3**(4):Jan./ Feb. 1970.

28. Semmens, J.P., and Semmens, J.H.: Sex education of the adolescent female, Pediatric Clinics of North America **19:**765-778, 1972.

29. Sherfey, M.J.: The nature and evolution of female sexuality, New York, 1972, Random House, Inc.

30. Sonne, J.C.: Family therapy of sexually acting-out girls, International Psychiatry Clinics **8:**95-118, 1971.
31. Wilbur, C., and Aug, R.: Sex education, American Journal of Nursing **73:**88-91, 1973.

References for clients

Andry, A., and Schepp, S.: How babies are made, New York, 1968, Life Books, Inc.

Bernstein, A.: The flight of the stork, New York, 1978, Delacorte Press.

Boston Women's Health Book Collective: Our bodies, ourselves, New York, 1977, Simon & Schuster, Inc.

Dayee, F.: Private zone: a book teaching children sexual assault prevention tools, Edmonds, Wash., 1982, Charles Franklin Press.

Gordon, S.: Facts about sex for today's youth, New York, 1973, The John Day Co.

Hart, C., et al.: Free to be you and me, New York, 1974, McGraw-Hill, Inc.

Mayle, P.: Where did I come from? Seacaucus, N.J., 1973, Lyle Stuart, Inc.

Mayle, P.: What's happening to me? Seacaucus, N.J., 1975, Lyle Stuart, Inc.

Morris, J.: Conundrum, New York, 1974, Harcourt, Brace, Jovanovich, Inc.

Pogrebin, L.: Growing up free, New York, 1980, McGraw-Hill, Inc.

Stein, S.: Making babies, New York, 1974, Walker & Co.

4

Sexuality throughout the life cycle: young adulthood through aging

Sexuality during the adult years has the configuration of a diamond. Men and women seem most similar at the age of emancipation. During their twenties they differentiate with respect to sexual capacity, social roles, and their sense of themselves. The gap gets largest during the late thirties and early forties. During the fifties the differences begin to resolve in a way that makes them more alike.[45] In this chapter we will examine the changes in sexuality as people age and explore the similarities and differences in women's and men's experiences.

Young adulthood

Young adulthood has rather nonspecific boundaries, but its beginning is marked by the end of adolescence, and it usually ends at the time parenthood begins. The young adult is faced with a number of social demands: selecting a vocation, obtaining an education, and perhaps participating in military service. In addition, the young adult faces many intimacy issues: learning to give and receive love, choosing whether or not to marry, and choosing a marital or sexual partner(s).[13]

One of the tasks for the young adult is developing intimacy and solidarity rather than existing in isolation. Usually this closeness is developed mutually in marriage or a close relationship, and sexual intimacy is an important aspect. Unless young adults are able to achieve intimacy, they may maintain stereotyped and formalized relationships, lacking an exchange of emotional involvement.

Young adulthood is a period of maximal sexual self-consciousness. Young adults' sexual statuses become a part of their public statuses. Most make some kind of commitment to a relationship whether marital or nonmarital. As a result, they have increased chances for regular sexual activity. They experience, perhaps for the first time, social legitimization of their sexual experiences.

During the 1970s sex roles became less rigid. Women are increasingly entering the labor force and remaining in it during their childbearing years. Some men are finding that sharing in or performing traditionally ''female'' roles offers them new freedoms. The women's movement has fostered values of equal opportunity and self-actualization for women and men. For some young adults less rigid sex roles provide opportunities to explore new life-styles. For others this flexibility is confusing in contrast with comfortable stereotypes.

The physical changes seen in this age group are not as pronounced as those seen during adolescence. However, in this period there is frequently a concern about one's image, especially as related to body contour and size. Since acceptance of one's body image has a great influence on one's ability to relate to a sexual partner, self-consciousness and shame about one's body may interfere with the establishment of sexual relationships. This concern is especially crucial in Western society, where much value is placed on the "body beautiful."

Sexual concerns and problems. During the young adult years non-marital sexual activity is prevalent; some suggest it is virtually normal. The increased opportunity for sexual activity may evoke sexual concerns simply because there are more opportunities to experience them. For example, more regular opportunity may lead to a decline in activity. Young adult men may experience sexual dysfunctions, in particular, difficulty in attaining an erection (secondary impotence) and difficulty with ejaculatory control (premature ejaculation). They may have concerns about the adequacy of their bodies, such as genital size. Some may find it difficult to integrate their sexual behavior with romantic love. Still others may have difficulty in making a transition from autoerotic practices to sharing sexual pleasure with a partner. Women may experience painful intercourse and difficulty having orgasms. Like men, they may have a negative image of their bodies. They may also have difficulty in expressing their sexual needs and preferences to a partner. Both men and women often have concerns about family planning, the adequacy of contraceptive measures, and their effects on sexual relationships (see Chapter 11). Some men and women develop an awareness of the waxing and waning of their sexual desires, sometimes attributed by women to their menstrual cycles and by men to androgen cycles.

Anxiety, guilt, and lack of information may interfere with sexual activity. Individuals who are especially concerned about "performing" well may find that anxiety inhibits orgasm if not sexual arousal. Persons who feel guilty about their sexual behavior may be unable to adequately communicate their needs to a partner, may find that their anxiety leads to sexual dysfunction, or may enjoy sexual activity but later feel remorse. This is likely to be true for some women who have inhibited their sexual feelings for many years and subsequent to marriage have difficulty unlearning those inhibitions.

Lack of information about one's own body and its functions, the variety of forms of sexual expression, and the technology for separating procreative from recreative sex may lead to sexual concerns or problems and unplanned pregnancy. Many young adults have problems resulting from misinformation, myth, or lack of information. Often society expects them to assume total responsibility for sexual education of their children.

In the context of a relationship both partners are faced with an adjustment to individual needs and desires of the other. Some mutual decisions about what variations in sexual expression are acceptable must be encountered early in a relationship. Guilt, hostility, and shame may become interwoven with sex unless each partner is aware of and respects the other's concerns. Ability to discuss sexual issues with one another is essential for mutuality in the relationship. Early disappointments and frustrations may interfere with the continuing sexual relationship if avenues of communication are blocked.[13]

Young adults today frequently do not marry or may marry with a variety of assumptions about the relationship. They may live in a coupled but nonmarital relationship in which sexual exclusivity and permanence predominate. Others may live in a coupled relationship in which the individuals may seek other relationships. Some individuals choose not to be involved in a relationship and may live as celibates. With the high divorce rate, many young adults are separated or divorced and may establish a close relationship (or relationships). There is growing acceptance of the single adult who may or may not be involved in a sexual relationship(s).

Adulthood

Adulthood is that portion of the life cycle typically devoted to parenting and consolidation of the marital union or a relationship. The tasks specific to this phase of the family life cycle are too numerous to be mentioned here, but they usually involve the beginning of a new life cycle for children and usually end at the time the children leave home. Societal demands in the United States have changed rapidly in the last decade. Recognition of the need for population control measures and the trend toward earlier marriages and later parenting have provided many couples with a longer life span together, without children.[13] Recently some married couples have elected to be nonparents. In view of these new trends the adulthood portion of the life cycle may offer new challenges and sources of pleasure unknown to previous generations.

The task critical to this age is the achievement of a feeling of generativity rather than stagnation or self-absorption. It is at this point that one asks, "What have I accomplished? What have I done with my life?" The common interest is the establishment and guidance of the next generation.[14]

The capacity to give and receive gratification in a stable relationship will probably prevail as a social task even in attempts at communal living and alternative life-styles. A crucial component of the interpersonal relationship, whether marriage or an alternative, is the sexual relationship. It includes not only the physiologic aspects of sexuality discussed previously but also the partner's concept of self as a sexual being and his or her sex role.

There are a number of potential adult crises that are linked to alteration of the concept of a "sexual self." Disfiguring surgery or trauma, illness that interferes with sexual function, and pregnancy all have in common the capability to change the way in which one sees the body and body competency and the way in which one meets the societal demands for sex role performance.

The influence of legislation and social conscience that created new opportunities for women in the marketplace cannot help but have reverberations in the lives of men. Role conflicts may plague those women maintaining careers and mothering children simultaneously.[2] Men may find that their roles, as traditionally defined, are no longer reciprocated. As both sexes assume responsibilities previously labeled "male" or "female," there are strains and gains in sexual relationships.

The process of aging, gradually underway since young adulthood, proceeds throughout the thirties and forties with only minimal overt changes. Maximal height is usually attained between the ages of 20 and 30 years. The frame may become slim or portly during this stage. Usually some wrinkling of the skin and graying of the hair appears. These changes may produce fear and concern in the adult who values a youthful image in a youth-oriented society.

Sexual concerns and problems. There is probably no set of well-defined sexual problems common only to childbearing adults. However, a number of familial and social variables can influence the sexual relationship.

Pregnancy may be a source of stress in the sexual relationship, since it often imposes lengthy periods of sexual abstinence for both spouses and may alter the woman's body image. Sexual desire may decrease for both partners.[13] The birth of a child focuses the couple's attention on the infant and initially away from one another. The presence of children may greatly decrease privacy and consequently the opportunity for sexual grat-ification. However, mothers of school-age children are probably at the peak of their sexual capacity. (It has been suggested that women reach their peak sexual capacity between age 25 and 30, whereas men reach their peak sexual capacity during the young adult years.) Demands placed on adults by their careers may physically or emotionally interfere with their sexual interest and activity.[7]

Many of the sexual problems arising at this point in the life cycle have their roots in inability to communicate about and negotiate sexual needs. As a consequence, people experience sexual dysfunction, boredom, stereotypic behavior, and lack of satisfaction.

Middle years

During the middle years, approximately the period of time between the age of 50 years (or when the children leave home) and the age of retirement, people are faced with major changes in life-styles. There are a number of demands placed on persons during the middle years, including emancipating adolescent children, making a comfortable home, achieving a peak in one's career, maintaining relationships with aging parents, and developing satisfaction from use of leisure time, social responsibility, and friendship. In addition to these rather monumental tasks, men and women are faced with accepting and adjusting to the physiologic aspects of middle age and developing new satisfactions in their relationships with their spouses.

The critical task for this portion of the life cycle is resolving feelings of self-esteem versus feelings of despair.[14] The issue is accepting one's own life cycle, rather than feeling despairing, disappointed, and abandoned. Social pressures and expectations, feedback from significant others, and finally self-perception all influence how one evaluates the success of one's life.

Depression in middle-aged women has frequently been attributed to the onset of menopause alone. However, recent studies suggest that the melancholia of middle age may be rooted in the role loss associated with the period during which children leave the home. This loss seems particularly profound for women who have been highly or solely involved in mothering and maintaining a home and who consequently have limited access to self-esteem from other sources.[4]

Couples who have had children must return to a relationship involving two parties, probably something they have not experienced for the preceding 20 years. Since both persons have probably reached the peak of their respective life's work, they may need to adjust values and goals for the remainder of their lives. The unmarried individual may be faced with similar concerns.

Superimposed on the social and psychologic demands of this phase are the physiologic components of aging. A decrease in height, muscle mass, strength, and cardiac power may become noticeable during this phase. Frequently, people in their fifties and sixties gain weight, and often an increase in adipose tissue is seen in the hips and thighs. Changes in the digestive capacity may cause discomfort. The skin becomes thinner, and wrinkles become more pronounced.

Physiologic changes are seen in the sexual function of both men and women during the middle years, among them, the menopause. However, involution of some sexual structures cannot be equated with cessation of sexual function or diminution of its importance.

Menopause and the male climacteric. Both men and women experience changes in their bodies during the middle years. As estrogen levels decrease, women experience the transition to menopause, characterized by increasing intervals

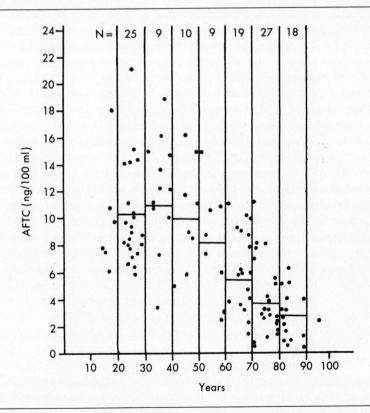

Fig. 4-1. Free testosterone concentration (AFTC) decreases with age. (Modified from Vermeulen, A.: Journal of Biosocial Science Suppl. **6:**5-18, 1979.)

between their menstrual cycles. The majority of women have their last menstrual period between age 50 and 52. Changes in estrogen-dependent tissues, including breast tissue and vaginal tissues, follow. Some women have hot flushes and vaginal irritation as a consequence of their diminishing estrogen levels. Some women also have a variety of emotional symptoms. The origin of menopausal symptoms is most likely multicausal, consisting of biologic changes coupled with the influence of the environment in which menopause occurs. With the current concern over the hazards of estrogen replacement therapy,[16,55] investigators may be encouraged to consider nonpharmacologic measures to treat menopausal symptoms.

Androgen levels in men also decrease during this part of the life cycle, but the rate at which androgen diminishes appears gradual (Fig. 4-1). In middle age, men may first notice changes in androgen-dependent tissues, such as the penis, and a decrease in the growth of sexual hair.

Sexual function in aging women. As women age, the intensity and duration of the physiologic aspects of the sexual response diminish gradually. (Fig. 4-2). Steroid changes produce changes in the genitals and breasts and may be responsible for some of the altered physiology. In middle-aged women a delay in the production of vaginal lubrication becomes evident. It is interesting to note that women who have been consistently sexually active throughout their lives do not appear to experience this lubrication difficulty.[31] There is a significant reduction in expansion of the vagina, both in length and width, with sexual arousal. Although estrogen replacement during the postmenopausal years may restore vaginal expansion in response to sexual stimulation, its use is now under close scrutiny because of evidence of an association between estrogen replacement therapy and endometrial cancer.[46,55] During the plateau phase the uterus does not elevate into the false pelvis to the extent that it does in younger women. The labia minora do not demonstrate the sex skin characteristic of younger women, and the labia majora do not elevate and flatten against the perineum as occurs in younger women. Clitoral size may decrease slightly but usually not until the woman reaches 60 to 70 years of age. The clitoral hood becomes less full, as does the fat pad over the mons. The orgasmic phase also becomes significantly shorter in middle years. In some women uterine contractions become spastic, causing abdominal pain. Finally, the resolution phase occurs much more rapidly. These changes are summarized in Table 4-1.

Despite a number of physiologic alterations in female sexual response, women do have the capacity to enjoy sexual arousal and orgasm far into later life. The presence of an interesting and interested sexual partner and reasonably good health are the only requisites.

Sexual function in aging men. As men age, many factors influence sexual responsiveness. Masters and Johnson[31] noted several recurrent themes in interviews about waning sexual responsiveness. Monotony in the sexual relationship or the feeling of being taken for granted was a common factor in loss of interest in sexual performance. Concerns with economic or career pursuits, mental or physical fatigue, physical and mental illness of the individual or his spouse, and overindulgence in food or drink also interfered with sexual activity. Finally, fear of failure caused many men to retreat from sexual activity rather than risk repeated embarrassment.

Physiologic changes in the middle-aged man's sexual response parallel those seen in

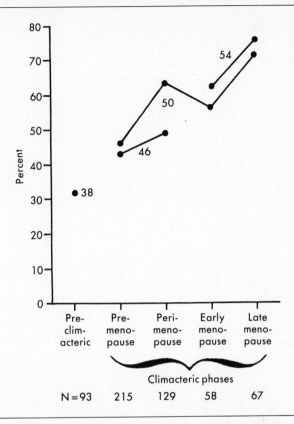

Fig. 4-2. Menopausal stage appears to have an effect on sexual interest despite woman's age. Interest decreases as woman proceeds through menopausal transition. (Modified from Hällström, T.: Journal of Biosocial Science Suppl. **6:**165-175, 1979.)

the woman. During these years the man may experience a significant delay in attaining an erection, and the erection may not be as full as that to which he is accustomed. There may be little testicular elevation, and the vasocongestive phenomena in the scrotum and testes are much less pronounced. Preejaculatory emission may diminish or cease. The plateau phase may be prolonged, and consequently control of ejaculatory demand is much better than in younger men.

The orgasmic experience encompasses a shorter time span. The feeling of ejaculatory inevitability may gradually disappear from the orgasmic phase, may be present but shortened, or may be prolonged if there is prostatic spasm. The expulsive force of ejaculation decreases, as does the volume of seminal fluid expelled. The resolution period proceeds more quickly, and the erection is lost rapidly. The refractory period is extended and may last several hours. These changes are summarized in Table 4-2.

As the man ages, his ejaculatory control actually improves, and simultaneously he experiences a reduced ejaculatory demand; that is, he may be satisfied to ejaculate during

Table 4-1. Phase-specific changes in selected organs in the sexual response cycle of the aging woman

| Target tissue | Phase of sexual response | | | |
	Excitement	Plateau	Orgasm	Resolution
Breast	Vasocongestive increase in size less pronounced, especially in more pendulous breasts	Engorgement of areolae less intense	—	Loss of nipple erection slowed
Clitoris		—	—	Retracts rapidly; tumescence lost rapidly
Labia majora	Flattening, separation, and elevation of major labia less evident or absent	—	—	
Labia minora	Vasocongestion reduced	Labial color change (sex skin) usually pathognomonic of orgasm less evident or absent	—	—
Vagina	Rate and amount of vaginal lubrication decreased; vaginal expansion in breadth and width decreases	Inner two thirds of vagina may still be expanding during this phase; vasocongestion of orgasmic platform reduced in intensity	Postmenopausal orgasmic platform contracts less frequently than in younger women	Rapid involution and loss of vasocongestion
Uterus	Uterine elevation and tenting of transcervical vagina develops more slowly and is less marked	Uterine elevation and tenting of transcervical vagina develops more slowly and is less marked	Some women report painful contractions with orgasm	—

Summarized from Masters, W., and Johnson, V.: Human sexual response, Boston, 1966, Little, Brown & Co., pp. 223-247.

Table 4-2. Phase-specific changes in selected organs in the sexual response cycle of the aging man

Target tissues	Phases of sexual response			
	Excitement	Plateau	Orgasm	Resolution
Penis	Erection may be less full; requires two to three times as much time as necessary for younger men; can be maintained for extended periods without ejaculation; if erection is lost without ejaculation, there may be a secondary refractory period (rare in men under 50 years)	Color changes at coronal ridge not observed in men over 60 years of age	Ejaculatory force is decreased (expulsion of semen 6 to 12 inches versus 12 to 14 inches in younger men); volume of semen decreases; fewer contractions with orgasm	Refractory period lasts for an extended period; rapid loss of erection
Scrotum	Decreased evidence of vasocongestion; less "tensing" of scrotal sac evident		—	Slow involution of vasocongestion
Testes	Testes do not elevate fully to the perineum; less contractile tone of cremasteric musculature observed; rare vasocongestive increase in size		—	Testicular descent extremely rapid

Summarized from Masters, W., and Johnson, V.: Human sexual response. Boston, 1966, Little, Brown & Co., pp. 248-270.

every second or third intercourse. There is evidence that the involuntary nocturnal erections during sleep persist well into the later years.[23,25] As men age, they can still enjoy a full and satisfying sexual relationship if they have an interested and interesting partner and are in reasonably good general health.

Sexual interest and activity. A study of 261 white men and 241 white women between the ages of 46 and 69 years from middle and upper socioeconomic levels revealed that although a decline in overall interest and activity occurred as age increased, sex continued to be a very important aspect of middle life. Men from each age group generally reported greater interest and activity than did women. Only 6% of the men and 33% of the women were no longer interested in sex; 12% of the men and 44% of the women were no longer sexually active. A decline in sexual interest and activity was most noticeable between the ages of 46 and 55 years. Women and men attributed responsibility for cessation of sexual relations to the men.[39]

Between the ages of 46 and 60 years, 44% to 70% of women in this sample described their sexual interest as moderate to strong, and 31% to 60% enjoyed intercourse at least once a week or more frequently. Among men between 46 and 60 years of age, 69% to 91% described their sexual interest as moderate to strong; 55% to 95% of the men enjoyed intercourse at least once or more each week. Interest exceeded activity for men.

A later study of the factors influencing sexual activity and interest during middle and old age revealed that for men the most important variables were past sexual experience, age, subjective and objective health factors, and social class. Marital status, age, and the enjoyment derived from sex during younger years influenced women's sexual activity and interest during middle and late years.[38] Sexual activity and interest in aging women depend on the availability of a socially approved and capable sexual partner. The theory is proposed that aging women adaptively inhibit their sexual strivings, since little opportunity for sexual fulfillment exists.[38] Little is known about the sexual adaptation made by widows.[36] The incidence and frequencies of sexual intercourse are shown for middle-aged and aging persons in Table 4-3. Although aging persons undoubtedly enjoy sexual experiences other than intercourse, few investigators have documented their frequency.

A recent study using longitudinal data on the sexual activity of 278 married men and women showed that levels of sexual activity remain remarkably stable over time. When the same individuals were observed for 6 years, both middle-aged men and women were much more likely to maintain the same level of activity rather than increase or decrease activity. Men were more active than women and the younger more than the older middle-aged persons. The only group who experienced a significant change over the 6 years were men aged 56 to 65 at entry to the study, and their levels of activity decreased.[19]

Hällström's study[20] of 800 middle-aged Swedish women (38 to 54 years of age) demonstrated a significant effect of the menopausal stage on declining sexual interest. As women passed from premenopause to postmenopause, their sexual interest declined. Declining sexual interest was not associated with total estrogen output in urine but instead with insufficient emotional support from the husband, negative development of marital relations, poor health of the husband, a high number of psychosocial stressors in the past year, unhappiness with work outside the home, and selected personality dimensions.

Table 4-3. Incidence and frequencies of sexual behaviors among research populations of well aging persons

Study	Population	Frequency of sexual behavior		
		Age	*Mean frequency/week*	*N*
Kinsey, Pomeroy, and Martin (1948)[25]	126 men (87 white, 39 black) 60 years and older	65	1.0	Not given
		75	0.3	
		80	0.1	
		Frequency of intercourse was noted for white men only 20% of men impotent at age 60 and 75% at age 80		
		Age	*Mean frequency/week*	*N*
Kinsey, et al. (1953)[26]	431 women ranging from 46 to 60 years of age	46-50	1.4	261
		51-55	1.2	120
		56-60	0.8	50
		Frequency of intercourse restricted to marital coitus		
		Age	*Mean frequency/year*	*N*
Finkle, et al. (1959)[16]	101 randomly selected male clinic patients, excluding those with genitourinary problems	55-59	29	16
		60-64	28	16
		65-69	12	19
		70-74	25	28
		75-79	11	17
		80+	5	10
		Age	*Sexually active (%)*	*N*
Newman and Nichols (1960)[34]	250 volunteer well aging persons	60-64	60	35
		65-69	64	36
		70-74	58	41
		75+	26	27
		Findings on 149 married couples		

Continued.

Table 4-3. Incidence and frequencies of sexual behaviors among research populations of well aging persons—cont'd

Study	Population	Frequency of sexual behavior
Freeman (1961)[17]	74 male respondents; population sampled included physician's patients; initial number to whom questionnaire was sent not known	Frequency of intercourse decreased with age

	N	Percent
Persistence of ability	41	55.4
Persistence of desire	56	75.6
Absence of spouse or illness influenced sexual activity		

Study	Population
Christenson and Gagnon (1965)[9]	241 white women 50 years and older from case history files of the Institute for Sex Research; data for marital sexual activities

Age	Median frequency/year	N
50	69.4	160
55	57.9	74
60	40.7	33
65	—	16
70	—	3

Study	Population	Frequency of sexual behavior
Rubin (1965)[42]	Questionnaire survey of aging men sent to 6000 men 65 and older listed in *Who's Who in America*; 832 replies	60% indicated satisfactory coitus. 30% were impotent. Incidence of satisfactory coitus decreased with age
Pfeiffer, Verwoerdt, and Wang (1969)[41]	39 survivors of cohort of 254 for whom data on sexual interest and activity were complete for all four studies (examination conducted at 3-year intervals)	Marital sexual activity in both men and women tended to decrease over time. Sexual activity and interest actually increased for some. Proportion of men continuing to demonstrate sexual interest over the 10-year period exceeded that for women
Pfeiffer, Verwoerdt, and Davis (1972)[39]	502 well aging persons 45 to 69 years of age (261 white men and 241 white women)	Frequency of intercourse (%)

Age	N	None	Monthly	Once a week+
Women				
46-50	43	14	26	60
51-55	41	20	41	39
56-60	48	42	27	31
61-65	44	61	29	10
66-71	55	73	16	11
TOTAL	231	44	27	28

Men				
46-50	43	0	5	95
51-55	41	5	29	66
56-60	61	7	38	55
61-65	54	20	43	37
66-71	62	24	48	28
TOTAL	261	12	34	54

Awareness of a decline in interest and activity occurred between 46 and 50 years of age

Primary reason for stopping intercourse attributed to men by both spouses

Christenson and Johnson (1973)[10] — 71 never married white women 50 years and over from case history files of the Institute for Sex Research

Age	Incidence (%)	N
45	32	71
50	25	71
55	15	34
60	8	14

Hällström (1979)[20] — 800 women ranging from 38 to 54 years of age

Age	Mean frequency/week	N
38	59	111
46	48	309
50	37	290
54	25	90

Garde and Lunde (1980)[18] — 225 Danish women 40 years of age

Approximately 80% engage in coitus at least once per week

Persson (1980)[37] — 266 women and 166 men 70 years of age in Sweden

	Persons having intercourse (%)
All	
men	46
women	16
Married	
men	52
women	36

Later years

Several social changes confront people during the last decades of their lives. Adjusting to retirement, establishing comfortable household routines and living accommodations, and maintaining relations with friends and relatives are only a few of the social demands facing the aging. In addition, aging persons may find it necessary to nurture one another in poor health, cope with bereavement and widowhood, and finally find new meanings in life.[13]

Role changes may be necessitated by the illness of a spouse. Loss of a peer group may be especially threatening for those who have spent a lifetime in an occupational setting. Loss of the husband may force a woman to develop a social identity of her own, since social systems linked to her husband's occupation and economic group may become closed to her. Assuming a dependent role may be necessitated by debilitating illness. Any or all of these events may assume crisis proportions for the aged individual.

Other tasks include acceptance of or resignation to old age and death. Unfortunately, social systems do not offer much preparatory support to the aging individual for either of these events.

Little preparation is provided for aging, much less changes in sexual function and relationships. The belief that elderly people cannot and do not enjoy sex may become a self-fulfilling prophecy or may cause elderly people to experience guilt and shame in conjunction with their sexual desires.

A number of observable changes occur throughout the later years: wrinkling of the skin, diminished visual acuity, diminution of hearing, joint changes, decrease in height, and diminution of muscle strength and muscle mass. Estrogen and androgen-dependent changes occurring in the genitals and other body tissues during the middle years become more pronounced. The physiologic changes that appear in the human sexual response cycle during middle age continue throughout the later years.

Sexual function and behavior. As early as 1960, published reports attested to the fact that people were sexually active in the seventh, eighth, and ninth decades. With good health and an available sex partner, older people were able to enjoy sexual relationships. Drives appeared to remain constant throughout life, and in one study blacks appeared more active than whites, men more than women, and those of lower socioeconomic status more than those from upper classes.[34]

Most studies show a decline in sexual activity and some a decline in interest. Two hundred and fifty-four community volunteers (131 females, 123 males) with an average age of 70.9 years, with a range of 60 to 94 years, were studied over a 9-year period. Although there was a decline in the frequency of sexual intercourse over time, this decline was not statistically significant. Among the subjects who were 60 to 71 years of age, 40% to 65% engaged in intercourse fairly frequently, whereas only 10% to 20% of those over 78 years of age were still active. A significant inverse correlation existed between age and sexual interest. In nearly all instances the cessation of sexual intercourse was attributed to the male partner. However, a significant portion of elderly subjects who were observed over a period of years actually showed rising patterns of sexual activity (13%) and interest (15%).[40]

Interest and activity levels in a group of biologically advantaged individuals (those who survived longest) were studied over a 10-year period. Men tended to maintain a high level of sexual interest throughout the decade, but sexual activity declined over time. Women showed less interest in sex, and a smaller proportion reported continued activity. An interest-activity gap became larger for men over the years but remained small for women.[41] The gender differences in the interest-activity gap may be a consequence of men feeling social pressure to express more sexual interest (the macho orientation) and women feeling social pressure not to express an interest in sex unless they had access to an acceptable partner. The findings about women may also be a function of the age cohort interviewed. These later studies also revealed no significant difference between blacks and whites in patterns of sexual interest or activity.

Ludeman's 1979 inquiry[29] about the sexuality of 15 formerly married women over 60 demonstrated that most of the women continued to be interested in sex and interpreted sex as more inclusive than intercourse. Most expressed an interest in the satisfaction they experienced in a male-female relationship or in touching. Their interest in sex and degree of pleasure remained constant throughout the life cycle. Although most of the women were not currently involved in a sexual relationship and did not see themselves as sexually appealing, those who continued to be interested in sex reported sexual fantasies and the channeling of their sexuality into nonsexual touching relationships with friends, children, or pets.

Persson's study[37] of 70-year-old Swedish men (166) and women (266) revealed gender differences in variables associated with sexual activity. For men, bereavement early in life, poorer mental health, weaker sex drives in early adult life, and negative attitudes toward sexuality and aging were associated with less sexual activity. For women, having an older husband, poorer mental and physical health, unhappy marriage, negative experiences of sexual intercourse, and negative attitudes toward sexuality among the aged were associated with less sexual activity.

The recent study by Starr and Weiner[49] of 800 men and women over 60 years of age from U.S. senior centers sought older people's perspectives on sexuality, as well as interest and activity levels. Most men and women indicated that a good sexual experience included intercourse or orgasm. Most felt sex was the same or better than when they were younger. Most liked sex. When asked how often they would like to have sex, most answered once a week or more often. Most thought sex had positive effects on health. Most rated orgasm as somewhat or very important, and the majority rated touching and cuddling in a similar way. Many found sexy pictures, books, and movies exciting. About half of the women and men masturbated, although the majority said this was an acceptable behavior. About half said that foreplay was the most exciting aspect of lovemaking. When asked what embarrassed them about sex, a small percentage of men and women included nudity, erection problems, and unconventional practices. Most said sex had not changed or become better since menopause. Although the majority of men and women said sexual experiences left them satisfied, some men and women reported that when they were not satisfied they masturbated, felt frustrated or angry, continued trying, or engaged in diversion.

Most reported that their sex activity took longer than it did when they were younger. When asked why they thought some older people did not have sexual relations as often as they would like, lack of a partner and poor health were mentioned most often. Most approved of older people who were not married having sex together, but when asked about how older women could cope with the excess of older women to men, most women recommended diversionary measures, and most men recommended finding a partner.

Most men and women said they could discuss sex with their partner, and most said they felt comfortable being nude with their partner. When asked what a couple could do when the man was unable to have an erection, half recommended using other stimulation, and one fourth recommended doing nothing; others said they would get professional help. Men were less accepting of women having younger lovers than were women of men having younger lovers. In addition, 30% of women versus 50% of men indicated an interest in trying new sexual experiences.

Thus there is evidence that sexual activity persists well into the last decades of life. Studies have shown that although the frequency of sexual intercourse and masturbation tends to decrease with age, sexual interest and activity remain fairly consistent throughout life. Cessation of intercourse is most often attributed to ill health or sexual dysfunction of the man.

Attitudes about sex. Aging persons' attitudes toward nontraditional sexual behavior, including premarital, extramarital, and homosexual sex, appear to be more conservative than are the attitudes of younger persons. However, a great range of differences in their attitudes suggests that aging individuals are not a homogeneous group.[29,48]

Summary

This chapter has considered biologic, psychologic, and sociologic aspects of the aging process and sexuality from young adulthood through the later years. Factors likely to interfere with sexual function throughout these stages of the life cycle were explored.

Key considerations for health care practice include the following:
1. Although there is a decline in both reported sexual interest and activity with age, there does not seem to be a single point in the life cycle at which sexual activity must cease.
2. Psychosocial demands placed on individuals throughout adult life have the capability of influencing sexual interest, activity, and function.
3. Aging is accompanied by changes in sexual anatomy and physiology for both men and women.
4. The young adult faces the task of establishing intimacy.
5. During adulthood, responsibilities of parenting and of maintaining a career can modify the nature of earlier sexual relationships.
6. During the middle years both men and women face the monumental task of adjusting to physiologic changes in sexual function at a time when they may also face a new phase in their relationship—the contracting family.
7. Sexual activity and interest persist well into old age, provided the individual is in relatively good health and has an interested and interesting partner.

Questions for review

1. Menopause is regarded as a biologic transition point in women's lives but occurs during a period of social transition for many women. How do these biologic and social transitions affect women's sexuality?
2. Men experience changing patterns in their sexuality throughout the life cycle. What factors seem most important in accounting for age-related changes in sexual function?
3. Choose one portion of the life cycle that is most relevant to your practice and/or your interests. Consider one *client* with whom you have been working. Describe the most significant aspects of sexuality for a person during this part of the life cycle. In what respects does your client differ from your expectations? What factors seem to contribute to these differences?
4. Reflect on your sexual development. How did you see your sexuality during childhood? What kinds of attitudes did your parents convey to you? What was your response to learning about menstruation? Nocturnal emissions (wet dreams)? Intercourse? How do you feel about yourself now? Your sexuality? Are your feelings about yourself changing as you age?
5. Consider the literature on sexuality and aging. Research examining sexual functioning in the elderly typically focuses on a very narrow set of behaviors. What questions do you think should be included in a survey of sexuality in the elderly?

References

1. Aletky, P.: Sexuality of the nursing home resident, Topics in Clinical Nursing **1:**53-60, 1980.
2. Bardwick, J.M.: Psychology of women: a study of biocultural conflicts, New York, 1971, Harper & Row, Publishers, Inc.
3. Bardwick, J.M.: A predictive study of psychological and psychosomatic responses to oral contraceptives. In Bardwick, J.M.: Readings on the psychology of women, New York, 1972, Harper & Row, Publishers, Inc.
4. Bart, P.: Depression in middle-aged women. In Bardwick, J.M.: Readings on the psychology of women, New York, 1972, Harper & Row, Publishers, Inc.
5. Braiman, A.: Psychosexual disorders of young adulthood, Clinical Obstetrics and Gynecology **13:**734-745, 1970.
6. Burnside, I., editor: Sexuality and aging, Los Angeles, 1975, Ethel Percy Andrus Gerontology Center.
7. Busse, E., and Eisdorfer, C.: Two thousand years of married life. In Palmore, Ed., editor: Normal aging: reports from the Duke longitudinal study, 1955-1969, Durham, N.C., 1970, Duke University Press.
8. Butler, R., and Lewis, M.I.: Sex after sixty: a guide for men and women for their later years, New York, 1966, Harper & Row, Publishers, Inc.
9. Christenson, C.V., and Gagnon, J.H.: Sexual behavior in a group of older women, Journal of Gerontology **20:**351-356, 1965.
10. Christenson, C.V., and Johnson, A.B.: Sexual patterns in a group of older never-married women, Journal of Geriatric Psychiatry **7**(1):88-98, 1973.
11. Comfort, A.: Drug therapy and sexual function in the older patient. In Comfort, A., editor: Sexual consequences of disability, Philadelphia, 1978, George F. Stickley Co.

12. Dickinson, P.A.: The fires of autumn: sexual activity in the middle and late years, New York, 1974, Drake Publishers, Inc.

13. Duvall, E.M.: Family development, ed. 4, Philadelphia, 1971, J.B. Lippincott Co.

14. Erikson, E.H.: Identity and the life cycle, Psychological Issues **1** (entire volume), 1959.

15. Finkle, A.L.: Urologic counseling in male sexual impotence, Geriatrics **27:**67-72, 1972.

16. Finkle, A., et al.: Sexual potency in aging males: frequency of coitus among clinic patients, Journal of the American Medical Association **170**(12):1391-1393, 1959.

17. Freeman, J.T.: Sexual capacities in the aging male, Geriatrics **16:**37-43, 1961.

18. Garde, K., and Lunde, I.: Female sexual behavior in a random sample of 40 year old women, Maturitas **2:**225-240, 1980.

19. George, L., and Weiler, S.: Sexuality in middle and late life, Archives of General Psychiatry **38:**919-923, 1981.

20. Hällström, T.: Sexuality of women in middle age: the Goteberg study, Journal of Biosocial Science Suppl. **6:**165-175, 1979.

21. Hunt, M.: Sexual behavior in the seventies, New York, 1974, Playboy Press.

22. Kahn, E., and Fisher, C.: REM sleep and sexuality in the aged, Journal of Geriatric Psychiatry **2:**181-199, 1969.

23. Kahn, E., and Fisher, C.: Some correlates of rapid eye movement sleep in the normal aged male, Journal of Nervous and Mental Diseases **148:**495-505, 1969.

24. Karacan, I., Hursch, C.J., and Williams, R.L.: Some characteristics of nocturnal penile tumescence in elderly males, Journal of Gerontology **27:**39-45, 1972.

25. Kinsey, A., Pomeroy, W., and Martin, C.: Sexual behavior in the human male, Philadelphia, 1948, W.B. Saunders Co.

26. Kinsey, A., et al.: Sexual behavior in the human female, Philadelphia, 1953, W.B. Saunders Co.

27. Lauritzen, D., and Müller, P.: Pathology and involution of the genitals in the aging female. In Money, J., and Musaph, H., editors: Handbook of sexology, New York, 1977, Excerpta Medica.

28. Lowenthal, M.F., and Chiriboga, D.: Transition to the empty nest: crisis, challenge, or relief, Archives of General Psychiatry **26:**8-14, 1972.

29. Ludeman, K.: The sexuality of the older person: review of the literature, Gerontologist **21**(2):203-208, 1981.

30. Martin, C.: Sexual activity and the aging male. In Money, J., and Musaph, H., editors: Handbook of sexology, New York, 1977, Excerpta Medica.

31. Masters, W., and Johnson, V.: Human sexual response, Boston, 1966, Little, Brown & Co.

32. Masters, W., and Johnson, V.: Human sexual inadequacy, Boston, 1970, Little, Brown & Co.

33. Neugarten, B., et al.: Women's attitudes toward the menopause, Vita Humana **6:**140-150, 1963.

34. Newman, G., and Nichols, C.R.: Sexual activities and attitudes in older persons, Journal of the American Medical Association **173:**33-35, 1960.

35. Offer, D., and Simon, W.: Sexual development. In Sadock, B., Kaplan, H., and Freedman, A., editors: The sexual experience, Baltimore, 1976, The Williams and Wilkins Co.

36. Parkes, C.M.: The first year of bereavement: a longitudinal study of the reaction of London widows to the death of their husbands. In Bardwick, J.M.: Readings on the psychology of women, New York, 1972, Harper & Row, Publishers, Inc.

37. Persson, G.: Sexuality in a 70-year-old urban population, Journal of Psychosomatic Research **24:**335-342, 1980.

38. Pfeiffer, E., and Davis, G.C.: Determinants of sexual behavior in middle and old age, Journal of the American Geriatrics Society **20:**151-158, 1972.

39. Pfeiffer, E., Verwoerdt, A., and Davis, G.C.: Sexual behavior in middle life, American Journal of Psychiatry **128:**1262-1267, 1972.

40. Pfeiffer, E., Verwoerdt, A., and Wang, H.S.: Sexual behavior in aged men and women, Archives of General Psychiatry **19:**753-758, 1968.

41. Pfeiffer, E., Verwoerdt, A., and Wang, H.S.: The natural history of sexual behavior in a biologically advantaged group of aged individuals, Journal of Gerontology **24:**193-198, 1969.

42. Rubin, I.: Sexual life after sixty, New York, 1965, Basic Books, Inc.

43. Scheingold, L., and Wagner, N.: Sound sex and the aging heart, New York, 1974, Human Sciences Press.

44. Selickman, M.A.: Medical care in a facility for the healthy aged, Geriatrics **26:**107-117, 1971.

45. Sheehy, G.: Passages: predictable crises of adult life, New York, 1976, E.P. Dutton Co., Inc.

46. Smith, D., et al.: Association of exogenous estrogen and endometrial carcinoma, New England Journal of Medicine **293:**1164-1167, 1975.

47. Sommer, B.: The effect of menstruation on cognitive and perceptual-motor behavior: a review, Psychosomatic Medicine **35:**515-534, 1973.

48. Snyder, E., and Spreitzer, E.: Attitudes of the aged toward non-traditional sexual behavior, Archives of Sexual Behavior **5**(3):249-254, 1976.

49. Starr, B., and Weiner, M.: The Starr-Weiner report on sex and sexuality in the mature years, New York, 1981, Stein & Day, Publishers.

50. Tucker, S.: The menopause: how much soma and much psyche? Journal of Gerontologic Nursing **6**(5):40-47, 1977.

51. Udry, J.R., and Morris, N.: The distribution of events in the human menstrual cycle, Journal of Reproductive Fertility **51:**419-425, 1977.

52. Van Keep, P., and Gregory, A.: Sexual relations in the aging female. In Money, J., and Musaph, H., editors: Handbook of sexology, New York, 1977, Excerpta Medica.

53. Vermeulen, A.: Decline in sexual activity in aging men: correlation with sex hormone levels and testicular changes, Journal of Biosocial Science Suppl. **6:**5-18, 1979.

54. Voigt, K., and Schmidt, H.: Sex and the involution of the genitals in the aging male. In Money, J., and Musaph, H., editors: Handbook of sexology, New York, 1977, Excerpta Medica.

55. Ziel, H., and Finkle, W.: Increased risk of endometrial carcinoma among users of conjugated estrogens, New England Journal of Medicine **293:**1167-1170, 1975.

Media

"Menopause and after: male and female, Part I. Changes in males and couples. Part II. Changes in females," Focus International, Inc., 505 West End Ave., New York, New York 10024.

References for clients

Boston Women's Health Book Collective: Our bodies, ourselves, New York, 1975, Simon & Schuster, Inc.

Dickinson, P.A.: The fires of autumn: sexual activity in the middle and late years, New York, 1974, Drake Publishers, Inc.

Scheingold, L., and Wagner, N.: Sound sex and the aging heart, New York, 1974, Human Sciences Press, Inc.

Troll, L., Israel, J., and Israel, K., editors: Looking ahead: a woman's guide to the problems and joys of growing older, Englewood Cliffs, N.J., 1977, Prentice-Hall, Inc.

Yates, M.: Coping: a survival manual for women alone, Englewood Cliffs, N.J., 1976, Prentice-Hall, Inc.

II

Sexual health and health care

5

Assessment of sexual health

Sexual health

Although a definition of sexual health seems essential to guide the professional in promoting or restoring sexual health, such a definition has not appeared in the literature until recently. To be sure, everyone has a notion of what is sexually healthy and unhealthy, but this alone is not a sufficient basis for providing sexual counseling or education. The World Health Organization (WHO)[18] has proposed that "sexual health is the integration of the somatic, emotional, intellectual, and social aspects of sexual being in ways that are positively enriching and that enhance personality, communication, and love."

The WHO definition implies that there are several components of sexual health. First, the capacity to enjoy and control sexual and reproductive behavior in accord with social and personal ethics is seen as important. Freedom from fear, shame, guilt, misconceptions, and other factors that inhibit sexual response and that can impair sexual relationships is another component of sexual health. Being free from organic disorders, diseases, and deficiencies that may interfere with either sexual or reproductive functions or both is yet another component of sexual health.[18]

Maddock[10] offers four components that may be evaluated in judging a person's sexual health. First is the conviction that the individual's personal and social behaviors are congruous with the individual's gender identity ("I am a man" or "I am a woman"). Maddock also suggests that comfort with a range of sex role behaviors is desirable, although it is unclear whether this component implies being androgynous. In any case it seems that behaving within a range that is acceptable for a male or a female is an important component of sexual health. The next component is the ability to engage in effective interpersonal relationships with both sexes and in relationships that might include the potential for love or long-term commitment. The third is the capacity to respond to erotic stimulation in a way that can make sexual activity both a positive and a pleasurable part of one's experience. The final component Maddock suggests is the ability to make mature judgments regarding one's sexual behavior that are congruous with one's values and beliefs. Maddock's list of components implies that sexually healthy persons have not only cognitive awareness of sexual phenomena but also personal awareness about their own values and attitudes about sex, value systems that influence sexual decisions, and comfort and emotional stability in relation to their sexual activities.

Both definitions explicitly state components of sexual health, including biologic, psychologic, sociocultural, and spiritual ones. Both imply that sexual behavior has the capacity to enhance the self and others. Both emphasize the necessity of sexual relationships. However, one needs to guard against too conservative an interpretation. The definitions are appropriate general guides for practitioners to use as tools rather than as yardsticks. As with definitions of general health, these must be applied liberally so that lack of a single component is not cause for labeling the client "unhealthy." It is important to keep in mind that sexual health is a relative matter; even the most disabled person can then be considered sexually healthy.

Subjective data: the sexual history

The definitions of sexual health provide a point of departure for the assessment of sexual health. This assessment, like that of other components of general health, includes both subjective and objective findings. To some extent, the scope of sexual assessment will be dictated by the professional's orientation to practice. Nurses are likely to be concerned with the client's sexual health from biologic, psychologic, sociocultural, and spiritual perspectives. Other professionals may restrict their attentions to one or more of these areas; thus their approach to assessment is likely to differ. In addition, the extensiveness of sexual assessment will be dictated by professionals' preparation and experience, as well as by clients' complaints or lack of them. Green[5] recommends that a sexual history be obtained for any male or female from puberty throughout the remainder of life. It is essential to obtain a sexual history from the client who initially has complaints of sexual dysfunction. It is also important to obtain a sexual history from clients whose illnesses or surgery may affect their sexual functioning, from those who have sexually transmitted diseases, infertility, or planned or problem pregnancies, and from clients who seek contraceptive or sexual counseling.

Health professionals usually do not hesitate to explore a client's bowel or urinary status, yet many have a great deal of discomfort at the thought of eliciting a sexual history. This response has no doubt been conditioned by the social prohibitions regarding the discussion of sexual matters. However, the consumer is becoming much more aware of sex and sexuality and frequently will present sexual concerns with a great deal of candor. This newfound openness creates the need for health professionals to be prepared to discuss sexual concerns and to educate and counsel clients.

Sexual assessment is a legitimate concern of the health professional and increasingly is integrated into general health assessments. The sexual history provides the professional with a data base on which to make diagnoses and to subsequently initiate a plan for education or counseling, or perhaps referral to another professional. Principles useful for obtaining a sexual history will be described next, followed by a discussion of several sexual assessment formats that can be applied to a number of clinical settings.

Principles. There is no single approach to taking a sexual history that is equally effective for all clients, nor is there an approach that is equally effective for all professionals. However, some general principles may be elaborated that will facilitate obtaining a sexual history with a fair degree of precision and with comfort for the client and professional as well. Provision of privacy is absolutely essential. This may imply not only physical privacy, such as closing the door of the office or conducting the history in a place where the professional and client will be uninterrupted, but also the assurance of trust between professional and client, such as that conveyed by a pledge of confidentiality.

Obtaining a sexual history early in the professional-client relationship conveys that sexual health is a legitimate and appropriate component of health. This probably facilitates reporting of sexual difficulties or concerns in later parts of the history or during subsequent contacts with the professional.

The sexual history is not merely a form of assessment but may also be therapeutic. During the process of collecting data the professional has the opportunity to provide permission for the client to discuss concerns, may provide limited information or suggestions to the client, and can validate that the client's concerns or practices are normal and acceptable (see Chapter 8). Avoidance of overreaction and underreaction is important, for it is unlikely that the client will respond honestly to a professional who is overtly shocked or to one whose boredom is evident.

Using language the client understands is also important in obtaining an adequate picture of client concerns. Both the client and the professional may need to define terms. Highly technical language may be ineffective if the client does not understand it, just as street language is ineffective for professionals who are unfamiliar with the terms. For example, a practitioner recounts asking a male client if he was having trouble getting an erection. He replied in the negative. However, later in the interview he revealed that he was having great difficulty with his "nature," a colloquialism for erection.

The technique of progressing from the less sensitive issues to the more sensitive issues is especially useful. The professional may find it wise to explore the client's childhood sexual development and education before exploring current sexual behavior and practices.

"Unloading" a question is a technique that implies that a wide variation of sexual behavior is acceptable. For example, one may determine the frequency of intercourse in the following way:

> • Some women have intercourse several times a week, some more often than that, some a few times a week, and still others not at all. On the average, how often do you have intercourse?

Referring to the ubiquity of sexual practices is yet another useful strategy. This approach requires that the professional ask clients "how" or "when" they began certain sexual practices. It can be readily seen that this approach is less threatening than the "Did you ever—" approach. Inquiries prefaced with statements such as "Many men experience—" convey that the individual's practices or experiences are not too unusual to relate. Although referring to the ubiquity of practices is a useful technique when obtaining a sexual history, the practitioner must guard against making assumptions about the client's sexual behavior. For example, the practitioner should not assume that the client is sexually active or heterosexual.

Using a life cycle chronology when taking a sexual history provides for a logical unfolding of events and often builds a progression from less to more threatening topics.

The sexual history can be terminated with an offer to respond to the client's questions or to discuss any other concerns of the client. This approach to termination of the interview conveys that the practitioner is willing to further explore sexual matters.

It is important to point out that attitudes may be communicated nonverbally during the interview. The client who senses that the clinician is acutely uncomfortable will probably not feel free to discuss a sexual problem. Frequently, values held by the client will be at variance with those of the counselor. If the client views the counselor as an authority, she or he may feel "abnormal" or unacceptable if any discomfort is conveyed. Reassurance that there is a wide range of "normal" may allay anxieties and guilt about sexual behavior.[5]

Privacy, warmth, and time are important aspects of the environment in which the sexual history is conducted. More than one interview may be necessary to complete the history.

Obtaining a sexual history affords the practitioner an opportunity to educate. Misconceptions can often be corrected and terminology clarified in the interview.

An awareness of a person's feelings, attitudes, and values about sex, coupled with a knowledge base related to the biologic and psychosocial aspects of sexuality, provides a substantial base for counseling. However, interpersonal skills that facilitate discussion of sexual problems and an awareness of the counseling process are essential to building a therapeutic relationship.

Approaches

A brief sexual history. A brief sexual history can be integrated with a health history such as that taken by a nurse or physician. The history presented here includes only three questions. The first addresses the person's sexual roles:

- Has anything (illness, pregnancy) interfered with your being a (mother, wife, father, husband)?

This question may be revised to specifically address life events, health problems, or hospitalization as the situation requires.

The second item deals with the way the person views himself or herself as a sexual being:

- Has anything (e.g., heart attack) changed the way you feel about yourself as a (man, woman)?

The third item addresses sexual function directly:

- Has anything (e.g., surgery, disease) changed your ability to function sexually (to engage in sexual activities)?

These brief items encourage clients to explore sexual concerns.* Often it is unnecessary for the practitioner to ask the second and third item. Many clients proceed to state their concerns about masculinity, femininity, and sexual functioning without further prompting. Examples of the application of the brief assessment are given on p. 89. Excerpt 1 illustrates how the sexual history unfolded after only the first question was asked. Excerpt 2 shows a history in which all three items were used.

---

*Similar items may be found in the format for the nursing history described by Mc-Phetridge.[13]

Excerpt 1

Practitioner	Client
"Has your heart disease interfered with your being a mother or wife?"	"No—I can't say that it has been much trouble because I don't need to pick up my children any more. That's because they're older. But I do have some trouble with my husband. I'd like to spend more time with him. . . ."
"More time?"	"Well, I only get to see him on the weekends because we both work and don't have much time during the week."
"So you don't have much time together during the week. . . ."	"No, and we feel pretty pushed on the weekends. That's really the only time my heart trouble bothers me."
"What's that like when your heart trouble bothers you?"	"Well, when we are together, in bed, I sometimes get chest pain."
"When you are together? Do you mean when you have sex?"	"Yes! It's kind of hard to talk about . . . but when we have sex, sometimes my chest pounds, and I have to stop."

Excerpt 2

Practitioner	Client
"Has your colostomy interfered with your being a husband or father?"	"No . . . I can't say it has been any trouble—as far as being a father and husband. I can still go to work."
"Has it [the colostomy] made any difference in how you think about yourself as a man?"	"Mostly I feel like a big baby. After all, what adult can't control his bowels?"
"Has it changed your ability to have sex?"	"Yes, in some ways I'm just too ashamed."
"You're ashamed?"	"Yes—of the bag and . . ."
"And anything else?"	"Yes—of the trouble I have sometimes—getting ready."
"Do you mean trouble having an erection?"	"Yes, sometimes I can't."

A sexual problem history. A sexual problem history can be used to supplement a brief history such as the one described in the excerpts or in the context of sexual counseling or therapy. Although the parameters explored in a sexual problem history will vary with the theoretical framework guiding the clinician's practice, there are commonalities to be explored regardless of the approach to therapy. The approach described here has been suggested by Annon.[2]

Excerpts from a sexual problem history

Practitioner	Client
"Hello, Ms. James. Please come in. I'm Ms. Forrest."	"Hi." [Nervously takes a seat.]
"Ms. Bradsher called me earlier this week to say that you would be coming to see me."	"Yes, I spoke to her when I had my Pap smear at the clinic. Did she tell you all about me?"
"No, but she did tell me that you had some sexual concerns."	"Oh good—I'm glad she said that."
"Would you like to tell me about your concerns?"	"Well, it's kind of hard to say some of it. . . . I'm not sure I even know the words."
"That's okay—I'll try to help. . . ."	"Well, I've been married almost 2 years now, and I just can't seem to enjoy sex."
"You don't enjoy sex?"	"Not really—I mean, I like to be with my husband, but he just goes so fast I can't keep up with him."
"Can you tell me more about that?"	"Well, before we were married it used to be pretty good. We could take a lot of time, and sometimes I would come to a climax four or five times."
"And things are different now?"	"Yes. It seems that we're just having sex now—and not really making love."
"So you are in a situation now where you don't spend as much time making love. Is that what you meant when you said your husband goes so fast?"	"Well, sort of. But it's more than that. I mean, he hardly gets inside me before he has come—and then it's all over for both of us."
"I see—and that leaves you feeling pretty bad?"	"Sure. I guess so. I try not to get upset at the time it happens—but later on it comes out."

Excerpts from a sexual problem history—cont'd

Practitioner	Client
"You mean you get angry later?"	"Yes—I sometimes shout at Bob."
"Can you tell me a bit about when this problem started?"	"It's hard to say exactly when—but, after my mother died my father came to live with us. We didn't have as much privacy—oh, he has his own room—but we didn't feel right about staying in bed so long anymore."
"Is that when your lovemaking started getting faster?"	"Yes—sometimes we would have to sneak it in."
"So since your father came to live with you, you and your husband have had this problem?"	"Yes."
"Did it ever get better, or has it gotten worse?"	"Well, shortly after [Dad] came, we went to San Francisco for a vacation. Things got better then."
"You mean you were able to come to climax then?"	"Yes—but we had a lot of time to ourselves."
"Have things improved since your trip?"	"No, they've only gotten worse because Bob still comes too fast."
"Have you had any other good times since your trip to San Francisco?"	"No, we even spent a week at the beach together, and nothing helped."
"What do you think is causing your problem?"	"Well, for a while I didn't think he loved me anymore, or maybe he was having an affair. Then I thought it might be my father being here. We never had that trouble when we were alone."
"Have you tried anything that you thought might help you with this problem?"	"Yes, I did try stimulating myself so I could get ready faster. But Bob could only last a few seconds, and that's still not enough. Then we tried not having sex for a while, and that made things worse."
"Things got worse?"	"Yes, then he came even quicker."
"That's likely to happen to men when they haven't ejaculated or come for a while."	"Oh—that's good to know."

Continued.

Excerpts from a sexual problem history—cont'd

Practitioner

Client

"Have you tried talking to someone about your concerns?"

"Only the nurse at the clinic, and she sent me here."

"I think I can help you and Bob talk about your concerns. Would you like that?"

"Yes, but I don't know if he will."

"Do you think you can ask him?"

"Sure, I'll ask anyway."

"I'd like to be able to see both of you together. Do you want to keep working on this problem?"

"Well, I did feel like giving up because of it. Is there anything that can be done for us?"

"I think that the two of you can help one another with this problem. What would you like us to work on together?"

"Well, first I'd like it if he could slow down a bit—like it was before. And maybe I could learn to hurry a little?"

"I think your choice of words is very good. Often we learn sexual habits just as we learn other habits. Of course, one can learn new ways of behaving, too."

"Does this mean things could get better?"

"I think so. I think you and Bob can learn ways of behaving that can give you both more pleasure."

"Good. I'd hate to think it was all over—should I make another appointment?"

"Yes. But you may want to phone me after you've talked to Bob."

"What if he won't come?"

"We'll face that when we know what his answer is."

"Okay. Could I come alone if he won't?"

"Yes—I think that would work, too."

"I'll see you next week."

The first component of a sexual problem history is a *description*, in the client's terms, of the current problem or concern. Next, the *onset and course* of the problem are elicited. The practitioner may wish to inquire about the age of the client at the time that the problem began and whether it had an insidious onset or occurred suddenly. The client is asked to identify any events that may have precipitated the problem initially or that cause it to persist. The course of the sexual problem can be described, including its fluctuations over time, and whether the problem has any functional relationships to phenomena such as medication, alcohol use, and so forth. The *client's concept of the cause and persistence of the problem* is extremely important. Past attempts at treatment and their results are explored next, including help from other health practitioners, as well as the self-help attempts that the client has made to cope with problems.

The last component of a sexual problem history includes an examination of the *client's current expectations and the goals* for treatment. It is important to explore the client's goals carefully, since she or he may want to achieve goals that the practitioner may not be able to facilitate or goals that would be best achieved in another therapeutic relationship. If expectations are not stated precisely, the practitioner may inappropriately treat or refer the client to a practitioner whose goals would be incongruous with those of the client. An example of a sexual problem history is given on preceding pp. 90-92.

Alternative approaches. Many other approaches for obtaining a sexual history exist. Masters and Johnson[12] describe the format for an intensive sexual history that includes exploration of the current problem, statistics of the current relationship, life cycle influences and events, self-perception, experience via the special senses, and environmental influences on sexual function. Kaplan[7] recommends the use of a "conflict-oriented history" designed to investigate psychodynamic phenomena. Lo Piccolo and Steger[9] and Annon[2] recommend paper-and-pencil measures to obtain data about the dyad and the individual who seeks help with sexual problems. Schiller's approach[16] focuses on the sexual relationship as a system.

Objective data: physical assessment

An essential sequel to identification of sexual concerns or problems is a thorough physical examination. Because the genitals have special significance for sexuality, the following discussion will focus on the breast examination, pelvic examination for women, and genital examination for men. Treating both men and women with dignity and conveying respect for their sexuality is important in any aspect of the physical examination. It is particularly important for breast and genital examination because most people have been socialized to consider their genitals private and sometimes even unacceptable.

Examination of women. Examination of women begins with inspection of the secondary sex characteristics, breast development, hair distribution, and the development of the external genitalia, including the mons, vulva, clitoris, labia minora and majora, and vaginal outlet. The female breasts are inspected to determine size and symmetry, contour, and appearance of the skin. Although there is often some difference in breast size (e.g., the left breast may be smaller than the right), the breasts usually are relatively symmetric. Variations in breast contour may include the presence of masses, dimpling, or flattening. The color of the skin of the breasts, presence of thickened areas, and abnormalities of the venous pattern may be indicative of pathologic processes. The nipples may be inverted, but this is usually not pathologic. However, the direction in which the nipples are pointing may provide clues to masses when there is asymmetry. Discharge from the nipples may indicate pathology or may merely vary in certain women with the hormonal fluctuation of the menstrual cycle. Ulcerated areas and other nipple lesions require further exploration.

Typically the professional makes body contact with the woman before the breast examination, such as in palpation of the cervical nodes or auscultation of the chest. Ideally, instruction in or a review of the breast self-examination can occur as the practitioner performs the breast examination. Women can be encouraged to examine their breasts on a monthly basis. The conclusion of their menstrual period or a few days thereafter is the best time for this, since premenstrual engorgement of the breasts may cause them to have a lumpy consistency or to be tender. Because of the cyclic changes in the consistency of breast tissue, it is recommended that the self-examination be performed at a consistent point in the menstrual cycle. The American Cancer Society provides instructional material for patients describing the technique to follow for breast examinations.[1]

The practitioner can inspect the external genitalia, including the labia majora, the mons, and the vulva, before the pelvic examination, noting inflammatory processes, ulcerations, congenital or surgical absence of structures, lesions, nodules, and discharge. It is customary for the examiner to inspect the labia minora, clitoris, urethral opening, and vaginal introitus before the pelvic examination.

It is general practice for the examiner to wear gloves on both hands during the genital examination. Although some women may safely practice self-examination without gloves, practitioners commonly wear gloves to prevent the transmission of infection to their clients. The practitioner can interpret the reason for wearing examination gloves to the woman so that she does not perceive the practice as an indication that she is abnormal or unclean.

Usually physical contact is made with the woman's knees before touching the thighs or genitals. The labia minora, clitoris, and urethral opening can be revealed by separating the labia majora. Evidences of pathologic processes cited earlier are noted. While the labia are separated with the examiner's middle and index fingers, the woman can be requested to strain down, allowing the examiner to note any bulging of the vaginal walls or gaping of the introitus. The former may be indicative of cystocele and rectocele, the latter of injury to the pubococcygeus muscle surrounding the vaginal outlet. Presence of surgical scarring, such as at an episiotomy site, may also be noted at this time. This part of the examination affords the practitioner the opportunity to teach the woman Kegel's exercises[8] in the event that she does not already know how to do them. A set of instructions for exercises of the pubococcygeus muscle is given on p. 95.

A pelvic examination is customarily performed as part of a total health assessment for women. It consists of two primary components: the speculum examination of the cervix and vagina and the manual palpation of the uterus and ovaries. Because this is described in detail in physical assessment texts, only those aspects of the examination that are not widely discussed and are related to the woman's sexuality will be addressed here.

The pelvic examination can be an educational experience for the woman, as well as an experience that validates her sexuality. It is recommended that the practitioner avoid assumptions about whether the woman is sexually active and with whom, as well as assumptions about her desire for fertility control. The examination should be begun with the woman in a sitting position, rather than greeting the examiner from the lithotomy position (usually this causes poor, if any, eye contact and a feeling of being vulnerable). The examiner can offer the woman the choice of whether or not she would like a drape. Some women prefer to see what the examiner is doing. Some women prefer not to use a drape because this reinforces that their bodies and the procedure are something shameful. Other women believe the drape adds to their dignity. Asking whether the woman would like a drape while offering it to show that it is available allows the client to choose what is most comfortable. The examiner can also ask the woman whether she would like a

Exercises for the pubococcygeus muscle

Sit on a toilet seat with your knees as far apart as possible. Start and stop the flow of urine. This will enable you to feel the pubococcygeus muscle.

Begin exercising this muscle gradually at intervals throughout the day. The following exercises can be done each day:

1. Contracting the pubococcygeus muscle and holding for 3 seconds (this feels the same as it did when you stopped the flow of urine)
2. Contracting the pubococcygeus muscle rapidly
3. Breathing deeply and tightening the pubococcygeus muscle as you inhale
4. Bearing down, then relaxing, and as you relax, tightening the pubococcygeus muscle

Ten to twenty-five contractions each day are usually sufficient to maintain good muscle tone.

---

mirror. This often enables the woman to see her cervix for the first time. Indeed, it may enable some women to see their genitals for the first time. Many examiners use a lighted speculum to facilitate the woman's viewing of her own anatomy.

By explaining what is happening, the examiner can validate the woman's sexuality and health. For example, the examiner might say "I'm going to look at your labia and clitoris now. They look very healthy." As the examiner gets ready to insert the speculum, she or he can advise the woman of any noise the speculum might make (plastic speculums are especially noisy) and also advise her of what will be done: for example, "Now I'm going to put two fingers in your vagina. I'm going to put the speculum into your vagina, and I'll open it up so you can see your cervix. Your vagina looks very healthy. Can you see your cervix?" Insertion of the speculum can be facilitated by using warm tap water as a lubricant. Some practitioners advocate inserting the speculum blades at only a slight oblique angle, whereas others advocate inserting the blades horizontally. The primary concern is avoiding pressure on the urethra, which causes pain. When removing the speculum, the blades are closed after the cervix is cleared, otherwise the cervix may become pinched between the speculum blades.

During the bimanual examination the woman can also be included. For example, she may wish to palpate her ovaries. This orientation to the pelvic examination affords many opportunities for teaching and modeling that sexuality is a wholesome, positive phenomenon.

Examination of men. Inspection of the penis, scrotum, and testicles is usually integrated with the physical examination. As these structures are examined, the practitioner also notes the hair distribution pattern over the axillary and pelvic area, as in the examination of the woman. Abnormalities of the male breast may also be noted, including the presence of gynecomastia, an enlargement of breast tissue that often occurs during normal puberty and at other times during the life cycle. The male breast may be inspected for deviations in contour, symmetry, abnormalities in the skin of the breast, and irregularities of the nipple. Men do develop breast cancers, so caution is in order if abnormal discharges or lesions are found.

Inspection of the penis includes observations of the skin for ulcers or lesions. The shaft is observed for deviations in shape and size or symmetry. The foreskin may be present in uncircumcised men, and the client may be asked to retract it to facilitate inspection of the glans area for the presence of lesions. Abnormalities of the glans and urethral meatus may also be noted, including deviations in the location of the urethra, ulcerations of the glans, and discharge from the urethral meatus.

The scrotal skin is usually inspected next for the presence of nodules or inflammation and to check contour. Usually the left testicle is somewhat lower in the scrotal sac than the right. Absence or atrophy of the testicles may also be identified by inspection. Palpation may be used to examine the penis, scrotal sac and contents, prostate gland, and rectum. Usually the genitalia are examined with a gloved hand. Inspection and palpation of the external genitalia can be accomplished with the client lying on the examination table. As with female clients, a drape may be offered. Inspection of the perineum and scrotum and palpation of the seminal vesicles and prostate can be easily accomplished by asking the client to turn on his left side with his legs flexed, a somewhat less vulnerable position than the spread-eagle stance advocated by some.

Approaches such as the explanations provided to women can be used when examining men. Some men may elect to use a mirror to see their own genitals. Instruction in testicular self-examination can be integrated with this portion of the physical examination.

Other useful data. To fully evaluate the cause of clients' sexual difficulties, relevant historical and laboratory data are obtained. Clients are queried about their cardiovascular, respiratory, gastrointestinal, genitourinary, central nervous system, and endocrine functions, as well as the presence of intercurrent illnesses, their use of prescription and nonprescription drugs, and habits such as alcohol use. Problems in other body systems, use of medications affecting sexual performance, and habits interfering with sexual appreciation or function may be corrected with appropriate medical therapy, and, in turn, the sexual problems are often corrected.

Laboratory data useful in the determination of the cause of sexual dysfunction include blood work, such as complete blood counts, thyroid fnction tests, glucose tolerance tests, and chemistry determinations. Vaginal cytology, endocrine workups, electrocardiograms, and chest x-ray films may reveal underlying conditions responsible for sexual problems.

Sexual assessment in the context of counseling and therapy

Sexual assessment constitutes an important component of therapy or counseling. In the event that the practitioner is not a nurse or physician, it is strongly recommended that clients seeking sexual counseling or therapy have a complete physical examination to identify organic causes of sexual problems.

Some practitioners integrate sexual assessment into the therapy format. For example, Masters and Johnson include extensive physical examinations in the early part of their therapy format.[2] Whatever form the physical examination takes, it can be a positive experience. Clients have an opportunity for learning about themselves and for validation of their sexuality.

One of the challenges of sexual assessment is identifying whether the sexual complaint is the problem or a symptom of another problem. In some instances the sexual complaint is the symptom of a relationship problem and in others the symptom of an intrapersonal problem, such as depression. Thus difficulty with erection might be treated as a problem, as a symptom of interpersonal difficulties, or as an indicator of depression.[6]

Identification of sexual problems

Etiology. Just as most diseases once viewed from a monoetiologic framework are now recognized to be determined by a multiplicity of factors, so it is also recognized that sexual problems have multiple etiologies. Three classes of etiologic variables are explored here, including biologic, behavioral, and socioenvironmental determinants.

Biologic determinants. Biologic determinants of sexual problems may relate to illness, use of pharmacologic agents, and the aging process. Although these variables may negatively influence an individual's sexual function, it should be kept in mind that even given optimal health, sexual response is vulnerable to interference from behavioral and socioenvironmental factors. Kaplan[7] estimates that the number of sexually dysfunctional patients who have organic problems ranges from 3% to 20%.

Interferences with vasocongestion and myotonia may be a direct result of diseases affecting the nervous system or circulatory system, as well as pharmacologic agents that act in a similar fashion. Pathologic or pharmacologically induced processes that reduce the individual's androgen level can interfere with libido in both sexes and impair male erection. Any entity causing painful sensations in response to sexual stimulation or intercourse can interfere with sexual function. Although biologic aspects of aging may lead to concerns about sexual response, aging does not of necessity lead to cessation of interest or activity.[12,15]

Behavioral determinants. There are a number of theories explaining the psychologic origins of sexual dysfunction. There is general agreement that most sexual difficulties are attributable to experiential factors. Psychoanalytic theorists believe that unconscious conflicts resulting from childhood experiences are the roots of sexual problems, whereas systems theorists attribute sexual dysfunction to unhealthy transactions between sexual partners. Learning and behavioral theorists attribute sexual problems to conditioning of unhealthy responses.[7] Guilt, anxiety, and other emotions can interfere with sexual response (see Chapter 8).

Socioenvironmental determinants. Several schools of sex therapy focus primarily on interpersonal components of sexual problems, and their proponents treat both partners or the relationship as the client. This approach is based on the assumption that neither partner is uninvolved in the cause and treatment of the dysfunction. A dyadic approach to therapy implies recognition of the power of social stimuli to create and maintain a sexually dysfunctional relationship.[12]

Environmental stimuli may lead to sexual problems or inability to express oneself sexually; these may include the presence of stimuli that compete with sexual sensation, the absence of a partner, or obstacles to interacting sexually with a partner. An example of the first is competing environmental noises and the last, institutionalization. Although sexual concerns and problems may result from any one of these, it is likely that a combination of these contributes to the problems of any individual client.

Clients at risk. Many clients will identify their sexual concerns and problems, but in some instances practitioners need to initiate discussion of issues of potential concern to clients. Many clients who seek health services are "at risk" of experiencing sexual concerns or problems. Potential threats to sexual health include structural alterations, changes in one's physiology, distortion of body image, environmentally induced problems, and behavioral problems. Life events and changes throughout the life cycle may also cause clients to be at risk of sexual dysfunction.

Table 5-1. Structural alterations and their hypothesized interferences with sexual health*

System	Hypothesized mechanism of interference
Central and peripheral nervous systems	
Spinal cord injury	
Spinal cord tumors	
Herniated disk	Disrupts integrity of peripheral nerves and spinal cord reflexes involved in sexual response, for example, erection
Multiple sclerosis	
Spina bifida	
Amyotrophic lateral sclerosis	
Tumors of the frontal or temporal lobes	
Cerebrovascular accident	May interfere with function of centers controlling sexual drive
Trauma to the frontal or temporal lobes	
Cardiovascular system	
Thrombus formation in vessels of the penis	
Leriche syndrome	
Sickle cell disorders	May interfere with the blood supply to the penis, thus interfering with erection
Leukemia	
Trauma to vasculature supplying sexual organs	
Genital system	
Radical perineal prostatectomy	May destroy nerve supply, interfering with sensory and motor aspects of sexual response
Abdominal perineal resections	
Lumbar sympathectomy	May result in disturbed ejaculation
Rhizotomies	May result in impotence as well as disturbed ejaculation
Absence of the penis or penile injury	
Imperforate hymen	Precludes or discourages intromission
Congenital absence of the vagina	
Obstetric trauma or poor episiotomy	Leaves gaping vaginal opening or painful scarring, discouraging intercourse
Damage to pubococcygeus	

*From Phipps, W., Long, B., and Woods, N.F.: Medical surgical nursing; concepts and clinical practice, ed. 2, St. Louis, 1983, The C.V. Mosby Co.

Table 5-2. Physiologic alterations and sexual health*

Interferences	Hypothesized mechanism of action
Systemic diseases Pulmonary disease Renal disease Malignancies Infections Degenerative diseases Some cardiovascular diseases	Debility, pain, and depression probably interfere with sexual libido as well as expression
Metabolic disruptions Cirrhosis Mononucleosis Hepatitis	Hepatic problems in the male result in estrogen buildup due to inability of the liver to conjugate estrogens; similar processes occur in the female along with general debility
Hypothyroidism Addison's disease Hypogonadism Hypopituitarism Acromegaly Feminizing tumors Cushing's disease Diabetes mellitus	By depression of CNS function, general debilitation and depression libido may be decreased, and impaired arousal in the female and impaired erectile abilities in the male may result With diabetes there is a hypothesized relationship between neuropathic and vascular damage and impotence or impaired sexual response in women
Diseases of the genitals Priapism Peyronie's disease Balanitis Phimosis Genital herpes Trauma to the penis Vaginal infections Senile vaginitis Vulvitis Leukoplakia Bartholin cyst Allergic response to vaginal sprays, deodorants Vaginitis following radiation therapy Pelvic inflammatory disease Fibroadenomas Endometriosis Uterine prolapse Anal fissures, hemorrhoids Pelvic masses Ovarian cysts	Each of these problems involves damage to the genital organs, which may result in painful intercourse
Prostatitis Urethritis	Local irritability, damage to genitals, and consequent interference with reflex mechanisms involved in erection and ejaculation
Medical or surgical castration Orchiectomy Radiation therapy Ovariectomy, adrenalectomy	Lowered androgen levels depress libido and lead to impotence, retarded ejaculation, and/or impaired sexual responsiveness

*From Phipps, W., Long, B., and Woods, N.F.: Medical surgical nursing; concepts and clinical practice, ed. 2, St. Louis, 1983, The C.V. Mosby Co.

Table 5-3. Some health problems resulting in changes in body image and self-concept*

Surgically induced	Traumatically induced	Others
Mastectomy	Burns	Dermatologic disorders
Ostomy	Lacerations, scarring	Obesity
Hysterectomy	Amputations	Congenital anomalies of the sexual
Amputation of limb(s)		organs, such as absence of penis, hypospadias
		Unusual breast size, including immaturity or hypertrophy

*From Phipps, W., Long, B., and Woods, N.F.: Medical surgical nursing: concepts and clinical practice, ed. 2, St. Louis, 1983, The C.V. Mosby Co.

Structural changes are probably best exemplified by the person with a spinal cord injury who has sustained irreversible damage to neural pathways and consequently has some degree of interference with his or her usual method of functioning sexually. *Physiologic alterations,* such as those associated with diabetes and circulatory insufficiency, probably alter the individual's ability to respond to sexual stimuli by interfering with the processes of vasocongestion and sensory-motor conduction essential to sexual response. Being chronically ill or fatigued may also interfere with sexual function. *Pharmacologic* agents are capable of inducing sexual problems, especially if they interfere with neurologic and circulatory mechanisms. *Body image distortion* and *change in self-concept* may follow surgery or traumatic injury and affect the person's ability to relate to a sexual partner. *Environmental restrictions,* such as those experienced in a nursing home or hospital, may minimize sexual opportunity or limit accessibility of a partner. *Life events,* such as pregnancy, although not pathologic entities, require adaptation to changes in biology, as well as feeling. Certain parts of the *life cycle* bring sexual issues to the forefront, especially adolescence and menopause. Finally, *behavioral problems,* such as inability to form a relationship with another person, may result in inappropriate sexual expression or thwart the client's attempts. A summary of structural and physiologic alterations and their hypothesized interferences with sexual health is given in Tables 5-1 and 5-2. Some health problems resulting in body image changes that may raise sexual concerns are given in Table 5-3.

Summary

This chapter included several definitions of sexual health. Approaches to assessment of sexual health including sexual histories and the physical examination were discussed. The etiologies of sexual problems were reviewed, and a variety of populations at risk of sexual difficulties was enumerated.

Key considerations to guide the assessment of sexual health follow:
1. Sexual health is a multidimensional phenomenon.
2. Both objective and subjective data are important for the assessment of sexual health.

3. Several formats are available for taking a sexual history.
4. Principles for obtaining a sexual history are designed to facilitate comfort on the part of both client and practitioner.
5. Most sexual problems do not have an organic cause.
6. Populations at risk of having sexual concerns or problems can be identified.

Questions for review

Before taking a sexual history from a patient, think about your own sexual history. Try to respond to the following questions about your own sexual development as honestly as possible. If some of the questions do not apply to your experience, just skip to the next question.

1. How old were you when you first discovered the differences between female and male anatomy?
2. How did you find out about these differences?
3. How did you feel about your discovery?
4. What were your parents' attitudes about sex?
5. How were these attitudes communicated?
6. What were your peers' attitudes about sex?
7. What was your response to your first menstruation (ejaculation)?
8. How did you learn about it?
9. Do you remember when you first stimulated yourself or pleasured yourself in a sexual way (masturbation)?
10. Do you remember the first time you had intercourse?
11. What was it like?
12. How do you feel about your body now?
13. How do you feel about your role as a woman (man)?
14. How do you feel about your sexual relationship?
15. Are you satisfied with your current sexual options? How would you change them?
16. How does your partner feel?
17. Can you describe a peak sexual experience?

Consider what behaviors by a nurse would enhance your comfort in discussing your sexual history. What behaviors would cause you to feel uncomfortable?

References

1. American Cancer Society, Inc.: Close-up standard breast examination, CA **24:**291-293, 1974.
2. Annon, J.: The behavioral treatment of sexual problems, Honolulu, 1974, Enabling Systems, Inc.
3. Friedl, E.: Women and men: an anthropologist's view, New York, 1975, Holt, Rinehart & Winston.
4. Fordney-Settlage, D.: Pelvic examination of women: genitorectal examination of men. In Green, R., editor: Human sexuality: a health practitioner's text, Baltimore, 1979, The Williams & Wilkins Co.

5. Green, R.: Taking a sexual history. In Green, R., editor: Human sexuality: a health practitioner's text, Baltimore, 1975, The Williams & Wilkins Co.

6. Group for the Advancement of Psychiatry: Assessment of sexual function: a guide to interviewing, New York, 1973, The Group for the Advancement of Psychiatry.

7. Kaplan, H.S.: The new sex therapy, New York, 1974, Brunner/Mazel, Inc.

8. Kegel, A.H.: Sexual functions of the pubococcygeus muscle, Western Journal of Obstetrics and Gynecology **60:**521-524, 1952.

9. Lo Piccolo, J., and Steger, J.: The sexual interaction inventory: a new instrument for assessment of sexual dysfunction, Archives of Sexual Behavior **3:**585-593, 1974.

10. Maddock, J.: Sexual health and health care, Postgraduate Medicine **58**(1):52-58, 1975.

11. Magee, J.: The pelvic examination: a view from the other end of the table, Annals of Internal Medicine **83**(4):563-564, 1975.

12. Masters, W., and Johnson, V.: Human sexual inadequacy, Boston, 1970, Little, Brown & Co.

13. McPhetridge, L.M.: Nursing history: one means to personalize care, American Journal of Nursing **68:**68-75, Jan. 1968.

14. Money, J., and Ehrhardt, A.: Man, woman, boy, girl, Baltimore, 1972, The Johns Hopkins University Press.

15. Pfeiffer, E., Verwoerdt, A., and Davis, G.C.: Sexual behavior in middle life, American Journal of Psychiatry **128:**1262-1267, 1972.

16. Schiller, P.: Creative approach to sex education and counseling, New York, 1977, Association Press.

17. Whitley, M., and Willingham, D.: Adding a sexual assessment to the health interview, Journal of Psychiatric Nursing and Mental Health Services **16:**17-22 + , April 1978.

18. World Health Organization: Education and treatment in human sexuality: the training of health professionals, Report of a WHO Meeting, Technical Report Series no. 572, Geneva, 1975, WHO.

6

Sex education

NANCY FUGATE WOODS and ANNE STAMER

During the 1960s and 1970s the media bombarded people with sex and sexuality. Although some found this more open approach to sexuality controversial, others have found it helpful in accepting their own sexuality. This newfound openness about sex has created a different climate for health care. Expectations of the health consumer reflect an ever-growing curiosity about sexual behavior in health and illness. No longer is the discussion of sexual matters restricted to the family planning clinic or the gynecologist's office. Practitioners in a variety of settings are being confronted with requests for information about sex. In addition to responding to requests for information, health care practitioners in a wide variety of settings have the opportunity and responsibility to promote sexual health. The variety of ways in which this can be done is discussed in Chapter 7 in the section on roles of health care practitioners in the delivery of sexual health services. Several of these roles, including provider of anticipatory guidance, validator of normalcy, and educator, are primarily educational ones.

Unfortunately, until recently, most nurses and other health professionals did not acquire the knowledge and skills during their formal education that would enable them to provide sexual education and other sexual health services. In 1974 Jacobson[13] stated that nursing was still in the Dark Ages when it came to sexual aspects of patient care. She went on to state that both nurses and physicians had failed to provide patients with information about how their sexuality might be affected by illness, drugs, and procedures. She urged nurse educators, administrators, and practitioners to ''free themselves from the shackles of rigidity, ignorance, submissiveness, and prudity and concern themselves with the sexual rights of humans, including their own.''[13] In the same year Lief,[19] a pioneer in the area of sex education for medical students, reported that this group lacked knowledge and had generally conservative sexual attitudes.

Fortunately health professionals are beginning to move out of the Dark Ages. Human sexuality has become an accepted component of total health care. The number of courses on sexuality in medical schools is increasing,[4] more attention is being given to this topic in nursing school curricula, and during the past few years there has been an increase in articles about sexuality in journals for health professionals. More will be said about preparation of the health professional in a later section.

Scope of sex education

Health care practitioners' involvement in the sex education process may vary from answering simple questions to planning, presenting, and evaluating formalized courses of instruction for clients, professionals, students, or peers. Because of the individual's varying needs for information about sexuality throughout the life cycle, practitioners deal with a wide variety of issues and may practice on a variety of levels.

Need. The American Association of Sex Educators, and Counselors and Therapists (AASECT)[1] defined several target areas for sex educators. The entire area of human reproduction is a basic concern to people throughout the life cycle. To children, concern about the birth of a sibling may spark interest in the entire reproductive process. Preadolescents need information about menstruation, conception, and pregnancy. To be able to accept the responsibility for sexual encounters, young adults need an understanding of contraception, as well as an awareness of their own attitudes and values about sexuality and contraception. The couple experiencing fertility problems may require information about physiologic aspects of sexual function. The childbearing family may have special questions about issues such as sex determination, fetal development, and safe sexual practices during the prenatal and postpartum periods. Roesel[34] states that the prenatal period is an appropriate time to begin discussions with parents about rearing their children in ways that influence positive sexual health. It is useful for parents to be aware that their verbal and nonverbal interaction with the child affects the child's sexual self-perception, sex role, and attitudes and values toward many aspects of sexuality.

As the human grows and develops, sexual components of the physical, mental, and emotional self change. These alterations give rise to questions about sexuality that, if unanswered, may create anxieties about one's "normalcy." As children grow they become more curious about their bodies and also about their new feelings of sexual responsiveness. Phenomena such as nocturnal emissions, sexual fantasies, homosexual attraction, and masturbation may be anxiety provoking unless youth can put them in perspective as fairly common aspects of sexual development. Myths and fallacies may plague those without access to accurate information. It is crucial that health professionals be able to give clients accurate information about the human sexual response, but perhaps of equal importance are the knowledge of sexual inadequacy and the availability of therapy.

Although factual information is essential for a healthy sexuality, an awareness of attitudes and clarification of personal values are also important. These factors are usually more important than knowledge in determining sexual behavior and positive sexual adjustment or lack of it. Values governing sexual behavior become an integral determinant of the person's response to sexual phenomena. The role of culture and mores, religious dogmas, and familial beliefs cannot be ignored, since they strongly influence the development of sexual attitudes and values.

In the era of the women's liberation movement youth are faced with models of sex roles reflecting both traditional stereotypes and the blurred role relationships characterized by a sharing of tasks previously labeled "masculine" or "feminine." Parents eloquently convey models of gender roles through their behavior. It is essential that both children and adults have information to help them differentiate biologic sex, or gender, and gender identity from gender roles. Understanding of male and female sex characteristics is important. However, knowledge that a young boy's desire for a doll is compatible with being a "normal" male may alleviate anxiety in both parent and child and therefore may be of equal importance.

Sexual adjustment in marriage is perhaps the least emphasized aspect of wedding preparations. The couple is seldom prepared for the necessary compromises and new intimacies of marriage. Sexual practices in emerging types of relationships, such as communal living, also need to be considered. Finally, the alternative approaches to marital sex, such as mate swapping and group sex, are not generally well understood. Clinicians may be confronted with questions about all these issues.

It is essential that individuals of any age have knowledge about healthy sexuality appropriate to their level of understanding. Presenting this knowledge is an important aspect of preventive health care. It is also important that individuals who are ill be informed about the effects of disease and related treatment and drug therapy on their sexual functioning. Mythology about mental illness resulting from sexual practices may cause great concern to healthy individuals; knowledge about sexuality may prevent anxiety. Finally, sexually transmitted diseases can be combated only by individuals who are well informed about the causes and cures of these illnesses.

Dealing with the various aspects of sex and sexuality is important for the individual and society because the client's achievement of a well-integrated, positive well-being at all levels of living can result in a more fulfilled individual, a more peaceful family life, and a more productive and peaceful society.[2]

Objectives. The objectives of sex education programs vary widely according to many factors, such as goals of the program, age of students, type of group, length of course, and values of the persons planning the program. Although the objectives of many programs focus only on providing knowledge, some programs also include objectives that deal with clarifying personal attitudes and values, becoming more accepting of personal sexual values and behavior as well as those of others, and helping students increase their ability to comfortably communicate about sexual topics. Sex education is still viewed by some as a threat to religious teachings, political beliefs, and the family's function as a teacher. Unfortunately, the majority of Western civilization has not accepted sex education as a tool to broaden children's knowledge about sexuality and make them aware of a variety of sexual phenomena so that they have a basis for an intelligent choice.[9] A common argument against sex education in the public schools is that if students, particularly adolescents, are given information about sexual topics, they will also be given "ideas" that will encourage them to become more active sexually. Research has not shown this to be true. In fact it seems that participation of adolescents in sex education programs that present information about conception and contraception and also facilitate open discussion of attitudes and values about sexual intercourse, caring relationships, love and sex, and possible emotional and physical consequences of sexual intercourse increases the likelihood of teenagers engaging in decision-making processes about sexual activity. Professional and lay literature contains many articles about sex education in the public schools. Fortunately, the focus seems to be on the process of shifting from whether it should be taught to how and what should be taught. A recent issue of the *Journal of School Health* was devoted to the topic of sex education in schools.[15]

A similar shift is occurring in schools of nursing and medicine. Clarifying values, increasing self-acceptance, and increasing communication skills are included with more traditional cognitive objectives. A set of goals proposed for medical students at the Indiana University Medical Center focuses on the need to help students be more tolerant not only of their own sexuality but also that of others. Encouraging students to think about various opinions on controversial sexual issues is an important outcome of sex education. The Indiana program proposed that students be desensitized to sexual stimuli and resensitized in a more humane way to understand the sexuality of others.[38]

Another important outcome of the sex education process is skill in communicating about sexual topics. Cultural taboos have, until recently, relegated conversation about sex and related topics to secret discussions among same-sex individuals. The implications of a climate of secrecy for an intimate relationship are ominous: partners are expected to share the most intimate form of communication, intercourse, but frequently cannot verbalize their feelings about sex to one another.[38] A major outcome of sex education, then, is the prevention of sexual dysfunction.

Approaches. If health professionals are to assume responsibility for sex education, they need an adequate knowledge base in the physiologic, psychologic, and sociologic aspects of sexuality. Of equal importance to sex educators is an awareness of their own sexual attitudes, comfort with and acceptance of their sexuality, and an ability to communicate openly and comfortably about sexual topics. In addition, educators need to have the knowledge and skills to plan, implement, and evaluate teaching activities. After finding that little information on sexuality was being taught in schools of medicine and nursing throughout the world, the World Health Organization (WHO) published "The Teaching of Human Sexuality in Schools for Health Professionals" in 1974. The concept of sexual health advocated by WHO points out areas for health professional education and intervention[22]:

1. A capacity to enjoy and control sexual and reproductive behavior in accordance with a social and personal ethic
2. Freedom from fear, shame, guilt, false beliefs, and other psychologic factors inhibiting sexual response and impairing sexual relationships
3. Freedom from organic disorders, diseases, and deficiencies that interfere with sexual and reproductive functions

Preparation of the health professional

WHO reported that "a growing body of knowledge indicated that problems in human sexuality are more pervasive and more important to the health and well-being of individuals than has been previously recognized" and stressed that "education in human sexuality should be introduced at the earliest possible stage of training programs for health science professionals and should be continued at all subsequent stages."[44] In 1980 the Sex Information and Education Council of the United States (SIECUS) published a list of 19 principles basic to education for sexuality. Among the principles were the following, which are of particular relevance to health professionals. The principles stated that sensitive sex education can be a positive force in promoting physical, mental, and social health; that the three levels of learning—affective, cognitive, and operative—should be covered; and that "all health, social science, religious, teaching and counseling professionals should receive education in human sexuality."[35] Calderone, founder and president of SIECUS, has stated what the sexual rights of health care recipients are. Her statement is a challenge for health professionals to meet[6]:

> Health care consumers have the right to receive health care by informed and humane professionals whose diagnostic, treatment and human relations skills have been developed by systematic and thoughtful preparation in sexual health care. Such preparation confronts the very nature of a person's sexual beliefs and practices, and should facilitate better understanding of self as well as an appreciation of a more holistic approach to the consumer in need of sexual health care.

Are health professionals prepared to meet this challenge and promote sexual health? Although improvements are being made, the literature continues to make references to the inadequate preparation of health professionals in the area of sexuality. In 1961 Greenbank[10] found that 50% of graduates of a Philadelphia medical school believed that mental illness was frequently caused by masturbation; furthermore, one out of five faculty members concurred. More than 10 years later Ebert and Lief[7] found that there had been an increase in knowledge since Greenbank's findings but that 15% of male medical students and 15% of female medical students continued to believe the myth that masturbation causes certain kinds of mental and emotional instability. Lief[19] found that entering medical students have misconceptions, misinformation, and anxieties about sex similar to those of any group of comparably educated people. He concluded that conventional medical training in anatomy and physiology does not equip physicians to counsel the laity in sexual matters. The Center for the Study of Sex Education in Medicine at the University of Pennsylvania School of Medicine conducted a survey that shows faculty are aware of the need for more than anatomy and physiology information. Of the medical sex educators, 68% reported that attitude modification was the most important need of their students; 18% stated that the acquisition of knowledge was most important; and almost 15% reported that the development of treatment skills was the primary need. In addition to the knowledge component, attitude modification, value clarification, and communication and treatment skills are important in the education of other health professionals, as well as medical students.[20]

Sheppe and Hain[36] administered the Sex Knowledge Inventory* to evaluate entering medical and law students' knowledge of human sexuality. Comparing these findings with those from students about to complete both professional programs, they found no significant difference between the knowledge of first-year medical students and first-year law students. There was a significant increase in sexual knowledge among the sample of fourth-year medical students but not in knowledge scores of third-year law students. Results of the study also showed that senior-year medical students still missed 10 of 80 questions on an instrument designed for "average lay persons."

McCreary-Juhasz[27] constructed a 30-item multiple-choice questionnaire to evaluate college students' knowledge of sexual physiology, including knowledge about sexually transmitted disease, conception, contraception, menstruation, and nocturnal emissions.

---

*McHugh, G.: Sex knowledge inventory, form X, Durham, N.C., 1950, Family Life Publications, Inc.

Of the undergraduate students tested, 80% did not demonstrate sufficient knowledge of sexual physiology to enable them to teach sex education classes. Furthermore, graduate nurses who were candidates for bachelor's degrees were able to answer only five out of six questions correctly. McCreary-Juhasz concluded that members of the nursing profession do not have sufficient knowledge to equip them to teach about the physiology of sex.

In a later study of students' perceptions of the extent of their knowledge about sexuality McCreary-Juhasz[26] found that self-ratings of 893 university students did not correlate with their performance on a sex knowledge test. There was no topic on which all students were "well informed." McCreary-Juhasz concluded that a basic course in sexuality should be provided for teachers in training.

Knowledge base. A study of 109 senior and graduate nursing students conducted by Mims and Swenson[28] confirmed "that there is considerable misinformation or lack of information regarding sexual matters among nursing students, both graduate and undergraduate." One of the findings of Woods and Mandetta's 1974 survey[43] of baccalaureate programs in nursing was that human sexuality concepts included in the nursing curriculum are primarily related to reproduction and are presented in the maternal and child health component of the curriculum. This could account for a lack of information about sexuality as it relates to other areas of practice. Solomon[37] surveyed baccalaureate nursing programs of the Western Interstate Council for Higher Education in Nursing in 11 western states and Hawaii to determine whether, where, and how human sexuality was taught in these programs. Responses were received from 34 of the 43 schools polled, a 79% return. The findings indicated that 83% of respondents advocated human sexuality education as a necessary part of nursing education. All of the responding schools dealt with human sexuality to some extent in their curriculum. Over half (56%) reported that sexuality was integrated into another course.

More recently emphasis has been placed on disseminating knowledge about sexuality. Carrera[5] studied the specific skills, competencies, and experiences that highly qualified specialists identified as priorities in the preparation of a senior high school sex educator. Specific areas of knowledge about sexuality were rated according to their priority by a panel of experts. Carrera listed guidelines for the preparation of those responsible for teaching sex education, including knowledge of human reproduction; pregnancy; childbirth; psychosexual and psychosocial aspects of behavior; cultural influences on sexuality, attitudes, and values; and sexual vocabulary. Although these guidelines were not designated specifically for the health practitioner, they represent principal areas of concern in teaching human sexuality to the general public. An educational program for health professions should include additional topics, such as human sexual response, sexual dysfunctions, effects of illness and drugs on sexual functioning, and communication and counseling skills. In a study involving family planning nurses and senior nursing students Payne[32] found that with increased knowledge of sexuality, increased comfort in professional situations with sexual overtones resulted.

Values and behavior. Perhaps the most difficult aspect of preparation for sex educators is development of a healthy attitude toward themselves and their own sexuality. Unless educators can accept their own sexuality and be comfortable with their own behavior, it is difficult to convey comfort to students or clients. Development of a nonjudgmental and accepting approach follows self-acceptance.[1] However, frequently insufficient time is spent constructively exploring the feelings of health professional students with regard to their sexual attitudes and values.[18]

For some health professionals, discussion of aspects of the human sexual anatomy may cause acute discomfort. For others, some aspects of sexual development may lead to anxiety or guilt, resulting in an inability to freely discuss topics such as masturbation, menstruation, menopause, and alternative sexual practices.

Among the topics likely to cause consternation for health professionals are sexual variations, such as homosexuality. Another area that may require health professionals to acknowledge personal biases is alternative life-styles, such as mate swapping or group sex. The issue of abortion may arouse feelings in professionals that need to be identified before they become involved in the educative process. These are only a few examples of a variety of sexual topics that it is useful for health professionals to explore in terms of their own attitudes and values.

It is useful for individuals who are going to teach sex education programs to participate as learners in courses or workshops that include affective objectives. These will provide an opportunity for participants to develop an awareness and appreciation of their sexuality by helping them (1) gain an increased awareness and comfort with personal sexual feelings, attitudes, and behaviors; (2) begin to clarify personal values related to sexuality; (3) become more aware of sexual ideas, opinions, concerns, attitudes, feelings, and values of others; and (4) increase acceptance of the variety of sexual opinions, attitudes, values, and behaviors of others.

Hogan[12] states that nurses who are able to promote sexual health need "knowledge of subject matter, skill in assessing and interviewing, awareness of beliefs, attitudes and values, and finally, awareness of how these beliefs, attitudes and values affect practice." The latter two are essential for health practitioners.

Most health practitioners have biases and believe that certain forms of sexual expression are not acceptable for them. It is useful to recognize and accept these biases and beliefs to avoid imposing them on students or clients. In this way it is possible for health professionals to maintain a supportive climate that encourages clients to share their feelings without fear of censure, while acknowledging the validity of their own beliefs, even though they are at variance with those of the clients. Through self-examination and training experience, negative attitudes can be overcome.[30] If these negative attitudes or a feeling of discomfort about a particular sexual issue or situation persists, it is usually best to let another practitioner interact with an individual or teach about that topic. If this is not done, the negative attitudes or discomfort is often communicated.

Educational skills. If health professionals are to function as effective teachers, then skill in the educative process is essential. Skills most valuable in sex education have been outlined in depth by AASECT and include public education and classroom work. Involving students or clients in the learning process implies the need for skill in establishing rapport and a trusting atmosphere. Selecting appropriate teaching materials is essential in view of the voluminous array available. Specific teaching methods can be designated on the basis of age level of clients and the type of information they need. Educational skills needed will also vary according to the type of objectives. The skills required to meet cognitive objectives are often different from the skills needed to achieve affective objectives. Skill in evaluating the impact of the educational programs is essential to prevent repeating previously ineffective programs and to make changes that continue to improve current ones.

In view of the need to disseminate information about sex to large segments of the population, a group approach is probably the most efficient. Furthermore, grouping of people with homogeneous problems or needs is likely to help the group and its individual members focus on issues with which they may initially be uncomfortable. The resulting climate of acceptance may facilitate discussion of fears or concerns that clients could not deal with on an individual basis. Descriptions of group approaches and programs about sexuality for a wide variety of groups, including the elderly (Guarino and Knowlton[11]), paraplegics (Banek and Mendelson[3]), and the mentally retarded (Kempton[17]), have appeared in professional journals.

Sex educators who operate in the context of a group in which discussion is encouraged cope with both content and process. Initially, educators assume a great responsibility for leading the group, but as an atmosphere of trust develops, their role more clearly resembles that of a resource person or facilitator.

Some knowledge of group process and group facilitation skills are very useful for educators working with a group. This is especially true when the focus of the session is on affective and communication skills objectives. While teaching a one-semester human sexuality course for college students, we[24] followed some simple guidelines that facilitated meaningful group interaction. The methods used in our course can be adapted to the needs of many different groups. Initially we share clear behavioral objectives with the group and describe the types of activities that will be included in the course. When appropriate, it is useful for students to help generate the course objectives or decide which objectives will be emphasized. Next, we ask students to reflect on what they already know and what they want to gain from taking the course. They are asked to consider affective and cognitive objectives. We often ask all students to share their answers to the following questions with the entire group:

1. What do you want to gain or learn from this class?
2. What topics or issues do you want to be discussed?
3. What concerns do you have about the group discussion sessions?
4. What can you and other group members do to hinder open honest discussion during group sessions?
5. What can you and other group members do to help open honest discussions during group sessions?

After sharing and discussing the responses to these questions we draw guidelines for group discussions from what students have said. We add other guidelines that we believe are useful. Sample guidelines include the following:

1. Understanding, not agreement, is our goal. Everyone's opinion is respected, and no one is belittled for expressing differing views.
2. It is the individual's responsibility to determine what is private for him or her. Members may always pass when they do not wish to share.

To help the group members get to know each other initially, ice-breaker games are used. These and other group activities that focus and facilitate discussion have been described by Wilson,[42] Kempton,[16] and Morrison and Price.[30] We have found planned group activities valuable in helping students gain an increased awareness of and comfort with their sexual ideas, concerns, attitudes, feelings, and behaviors and those of others; in clarifying their sexual values; in becoming more accepting of a variety of sexual opinions, attitudes, and behaviors; and in improving their ability to communicate about sexual topics with others comfortably. These group activities use techniques such as role playing, response to the values in popular music, and construction of group value continuums. Polling attitudes and sharing results may also spark further discussion among members.[16]

There are a number of advantages associated with sex education in a group setting. For example, individuals are exposed to several sides of an issue and may eventually feel that they can trust group members sufficiently to share their own views, questions, and concerns. It may be possible for clients to test out their feelings in the context of the group or ask questions of one another about sexual knowledge and attitudes in a ''safe'' atmosphere.

Although the group approach can provide clients with an exposure to other perspectives, a one-to-one approach is appropriate in instances that do not permit contact with the health professional at regular intervals or in which the client's learning needs can be met in a single session. The group model is possible in a variety of settings and can be modified to meet the needs of specific clients.

Evaluation of programs

To what extent can the health worker determine the success of an educational program? Rarely is an attempt made to formally evaluate the effectiveness of education for sexuality, even in institutions of higher learning. In some instances an attempt is made to obtain narrative comments from students about their subjective response to the course.[5,30]

Although a seemingly monumental venture, a program to evaluate the effectiveness of the health professional's endeavors can be designed. Data can be obtained from clients regarding their knowledge and attitudes both before and after the educative process. The approach might be as simple as asking clients to respond either verbally or in writing to a few well-chosen questions on a single topic such as sexually transmitted disease. Questionnaires reflecting the sophistication of the educational program may be devised to collect data about several variables throughout the learning process.

Behavioral criteria may be defined to indicate the presence or absence of learning. In a sexually transmitted disease education program one might collect data about the incidence of recidivism. In the inpatient care area one might use an interview or a paper-and-pencil test to gather data about a client's understanding of limits on sexual activity after myocardial infarction.

In the educational setting one can obtain immediate feedback from clients about their attitudinal response to teaching. Often this practice can provide the health professional with cues about individual or cultural values and perhaps about the process by which knowledge does or does not result in attitudinal change.

Resources

A number of resources are available to help health professionals build a knowledge base for teaching about sexuality. A brief list follows:

Books—General Background on Sexuality and Sex Education

Delora, J., and Warren, C.: Understanding sexual interaction, Boston, 1977, Houghton Mifflin Co. *A useful college text and reference on psychologic aspects of sexuality.*

Kolodny, R., Masters, W., and Johnson, V.: Textbook of sexual medicine, Boston, 1979, Little, Brown & Co. *A comprehensive book on many aspects of medicine and sexuality.*

Lief, H., editor: Sex education in medicine, New York, 1976, Spectrum. *A book on training physicians in sexual health. Much of content is applicable to other health professionals.*

Lief, H., editor: Medical aspects of human sexuality: 750 questions answered by 500 authorities, Baltimore, 1975, The Williams & Wilkins Co. *This book accurately answers questions that are often asked of health practitioners.*

Masters, W., and Johnson, V.: Human sexual response, Boston, 1966, Little, Brown & Co. *The classic book on this topic.*

McCary, J.: Sexual myths and fallacies, New York, 1975, Shocken Books, Inc. *A book that presents sexual myths and facts.*

McCary, J.: Human sexuality, New York, 1978, D. Van Nostrand Co. *A useful college text and general reference.*

Morrison, E., and Price, M.: Values in sexuality: a new approach to sex education, New York, 1974, Hart Publishing Co., Inc. *A useful teaching aid that contains group learning "exercises" for sexuality.*

Sexuality Journals

Medical Aspects of Human Sexuality
Sexual Medicine Today

Nursing Journals—Special Issues on Sexuality

Clinical Nursing, Jan. 1980
Imprint, Dec. 1980
Nursing Clinics of North America, Sept. 1975
Nursing Outlook, Nov. 1970

Other Journals—Special Issues on Sexuality

The Journal of School Health, April 1981. *Contains a useful bibliography for professionals with a focus on schools.*

Sources For Additional Information

American Association of Sex Educators, Counselors and Therapists (ASSECT)
600 Maryland Ave., S.W.
Washington, D.C. 20024

National Clearinghouse for Family Planning Information
P.O. Box 2225
Rockville, MD 20852

Planned Parenthood Federation of America, Inc.
810 Seventh Ave.
New York, NY 10019

Sex Information and Education Council of the United States (SIECUS)
80 Fifth Ave.
New York, NY 10011

Summary

This chapter has focused on the health professional's role as sex educator as a means of preventing sexual problems. Some key points for the health professional include the following:

1. Media have created a new climate of openness about sex that may result in many more clients confronting health professionals with sexual questions and problems.
2. Individuals' needs for sex education continue throughout the life cycle as they cope with changes in their sexuality and sexual function.
3. One outcome of sex education may be the prevention of sexual dysfunction.
4. Health professionals need special training in the area of sex education to provide these services in a competent fashion.
5. Health professionals need a healthy attitude toward their own sexuality and sexual functioning before being able to deal with that of others.
6. The group approach to sex education has specific advantages: it provides clients with an exposure to the attitudes and feelings of others, and it provides an arena for clients to share their concerns.
7. Evaluation is an essential component of the sex education process.

Questions for review

1. Select a part of the life cycle that is of particular interest to you or especially relevant to your practice. Consider the sexual issues of particular concern to this population. Describe the sex education needs of this group. Outline objectives that encompass gains in knowledge, as well as assessment or reassessment of attitudes and values. Briefly outline topics that might be included in a short course for this population.
2. What aspects of human sexuality were included in your educational preparation as a health professional? In what area was there little preparation for the clinical situation you have encountered? What recommendations would you make for curriculum revision?

References

1. American Association of Sex Educators, Counselors, and Therapists: The professional training and preparation of sex educators, Washington, D.C., 1972, AASECT.
2. Bahr, R.: Sexuality education: a need in health care. In Bernard, M.U., Clancy, B.J., and Krantz, K.E.: Human sexuality for health professionals, Philadelphia, 1978, W.B. Saunders Co.
3. Banek, S.N., and Mendelson, M.A.: Group psychotherapy with a paraplegic group with an emphasis on specific problems of sexuality, International Journal of Group Psychotherapy **28:**123-128, 1978.
4. Bart, P.B.: From those wonderful people who brought you the vaginal orgasm: sex education for medical students, Paper presented at the meeting of the American Sociological Association, New York, 1976.
5. Carrera, M.A.: Training the sex educator: guidelines for teacher training institutions, American Journal of Public Health **62:**233-243, 1972.
6. Carrera, M.A., and Calderone, M.: Training of health professionals in education for sexual health, SIECUS Newsletter **4:**2, 1976.
7. Ebert, R.K., and Lief, H.I.: Why sex education for medical students? In Green, R. editor: Human sexuality: a health practitioner's text, Baltimore, 1975, The Williams & Wilkins Co.
8. Evaluation in sex education: realism or rhetoric?: American Association of Sex Educators, Counselors, and Therapists Newsletter **7:**8-10, 1974.
9. Gordon, S.: What adolescents want to know, American Journal of Nursing **71:**534-535, 1971.
10. Greenbank, R.K.: Are medical students learning psychiatry? Pennsylvania Medical Journal **64:**989-992, 1961.
11. Guarino, S.C., and Knowlton, C.N.: Planning and implementing a group health program on sexuality for the elderly, Journal of Gerontological Nursing **6:**600-603, 1980.
12. Hogan, R.M.: Nursing and human sexuality, Nursing Times **76:**1296-1300, 1980.
13. Jacobson, L.: Illness and human sexuality, Nursing Outlook **22**(1):50-53, 1974.
14. Johnson, W.R.: Sex education and the nurse, Nursing Outlook **18:**26-29, Nov. 1970.
15. Journal of School Health **15**(4):1981.
16. Kempton, W.: Techniques for leading group discussions on human sexuality, Philadelphia, 1972, Planned Parenthood of Southeastern Pennsylvania.
17. Kempton, W.: A teacher's guide to sex education for persons with disabilities that hinder learning, North Scituate, Mass., 1974, Duxbury Press.
18. Krizinofski, M.: Human sexuality and nursing practice, Nursing Clinics of North America **8:**673-681, 1973.
19. Lief, H.I.: Sexual knowledge, attitudes and behavior of medical students: implications for medical practice. In Abse, D.W., Nash, E.M., nad Louden, L.M.R., editors: Marital and sexual counseling in medical practice, ed. 2, New York, 1974, Harper & Row, Publishers, Inc.
20. Lief, H.I., and Ebert, R.K.: A Survey of sex education in United States medical schools, Paper presented at the World Health Organization sym-

posium on Education and Treatment in Human Sexuality: The Training of Health Professionals, Geneva, Feb. 4-12.

21. Lief, H.I., and Reed, D.: Sex knowledge and attitude test, ed. 2, Philadelphia, 1971, Division of Family Study, Department of Psychiatry, University of Pennsylvania School of Medicine.

22. Mace, D.R., Braverman, R.H.O., and Burton, J.: Teaching human sexuality in schools for health professionals, Geneva, 1974, World Health Organization.

23. Malo-Juvera, D.: What pregnant teen-agers know about sex, Nursing Outlook **18:**32-35, Nov. 1970.

24. Mandetta, A.F., and Woods, N.F.: Learning about human sexuality—a course model, Nursing Outlook **22:**525-527, 1974.

25. Marram, G.D.: The group approach in nursing practice, ed. 2, St. Louis, 1978, The C.V. Mosby Co.

26. McCreary-Juhasz, A.: How accurate are student evaluations of the extent of their knowledge of human sexuality? Journal of School Health **37:**409-412, 1967.

27. McCreary-Juhasz, A.: Sex knowledge of prospective teachers and graduate nurses, Canadian Nurse **63:**48-50, July 1967.

28. Mims, F.H., and Swenson, M.: A model to promote sexual health care, Nursing Outlook **26**(2):121-125, 1978.

29. Mims, F.H., et al.: Effectiveness of an interdisciplinary course in human sexuality, Nursing Research **23:**248-253, 1974.

30. Morrison, E.S., and Price, M.V.: Values in sexuality: a new approach to sex education, New York, 1974, Hart Publishing Co., Inc.

31. Nelson, S.E.: All about sex education for students, American Journal of Nursing **77:**611-612, 1979.

32. Osofsky, H.J., and Osofsky, J.D.: Let's be sensible about sex education, American Journal of Nursing **71:**532-535, 1971.

33. Payne, T.: Sexuality of nurses: Correlations of knowledge, attitude and behavior, Nursing Research **25:**286-292, 1976.

34. Roesel, R.: The nurse's role in primary prevention in sexual health, Imprint **27**(5):27-28, 1980.

35. Sex Information and Education Council of the United States: The SIECUS/New York University principles basic to education for sexuality, SIECUS report, New York, Jan. 1980.

36. Sheppe, W., Jr., and Hain, J.D.: Sex and the medical student, Journal of Medical Education **41:**457-464, 1966.

37. Solomon, J.: Human sexuality content: should this be included in baccalaureate nursing programs? Imprint **27**(5):29-31, 1980.

38. Tyler, E.A.: Introducing a sex education course into the medical curriculum, Journal of Medical Education **45:**1025-1031, 1970.

39. Vincent, C.E.: Human sexuality in medical education and practice, Springfield, Ill., 1968, Charles C Thomas, Publisher.

40. Vincent, C.E.: Sexual and marital health: the physician as consultant, New York, 1973, McGraw-Hill, Inc.

41. Walker, E.: Study of sexuality in the nursing curriculum, Nursing Forum **10**(1):18-30, 1971.

42. Wilson, R.R.: Sexual counseling skills workshop: a trainer's handbook, Chapel Hill, N.C., 1977, Carolina Population Center.
43. Woods, N.F., and Mandetta, A.F.: Sexuality in the baccalaureate nursing curriculum, Nursing Forum **15:**294-313, 1976.
44. World Health Organization: Education and treatment in human sexuality: the training of health professionals, WHO Technical Report Series no. 972, Geneva, 1975, WHO.

7

Nursing practice and sexual health care: an overview

The purpose of this chapter is to describe nurses' roles in the delivery of sexual health care, including both the current roles for nurses and those envisioned for the future. Before exploring the nursing profession's involvement in the delivery of sexual health services, a nursing perspective on human sexuality and sexual health will be examined. Next, the types of roles that nurses are currently playing and clinical illustrations will be considered.

A nursing perspective

Nursing is concerned with human responses to actual and potential health problems. Common to both clinical practice and nursing research is emphasis on the health of whole human beings and the recognition that individuals are in constant interaction with their environment. Fostering self-caring behavior that leads to health and well-being is a primary goal of nursing service.[2,6,9]

As one might anticipate, nursing's view of human sexuality is shaped by the view of the discipline, in this case, a holistic view of clients. Human sexuality is viewed as a complex phenomenon; its biologic, psychosocial, and cultural aspects are seen as interrelated. Nursing's concept of sexual health is thus consistent with the integrative and holistic aspects of the definition of sexual health recently accepted by WHO[26]: "Sexual health is the integration of the somatic, emotional, intellectual, and social aspects of sexual being, in ways that are positively enriching and that enhance personality, communication, and love." With this definition in mind, we shall now examine the scope of sexual health services and nursing's involvement in these services.

The report of the 1975 WHO meeting dealing with education and treatment in human sexuality acknowledged that a variety of sexual health services is needed, ranging from education or dissemination of information to the community to intensive therapy for complex sexual dysfunctions. Participants in that conference recommended that first priority be given to the education of persons in the community and to health practitioners, since this approach might be both preventive and therapeutic. Next, the group recommended that health professionals, including nurses and other practitioners, be able to

117

provide counseling for individuals and couples with sexual problems. Finally, provision of sex therapy by those professionals with special preparation was seen as an essential health service for those persons with complex problems. With this scope of sexual health services in mind, we will now examine the roles for the nurse in the delivery of sexual health care.

Nursing roles

Role has been defined as "the interaction unit between two self systems." Roles develop from a set of norms and reflect goals, values, and sentiments. The way in which one enacts a role depends on that individual's conception of the role and the influence of that person's self-system. Roles are not single-person phenomena but are dyadic or complementary. The kinds of role transactions in which nurses are, or can be, involved are influenced by three sets of variables. These variables relate to nurses, clients, and settings. We will consider each of these sets of variables one at a time.

Nurse variables. The first set of variables relates to nurses. These include the level of nurses' preparation and the requisites for intervening on behalf of the person with a sexual concern or problem. With the range of sexual health services in mind, it is easy to see that each level of intervention requires slightly different professional preparation. However, three prerequisites are common to each level of intervention. First, a knowledge base is required, including an understanding of human sexual response; awareness of the variety of sexual behaviors existing in society and their prevalence; an understanding of the types of sexual dysfunctions; and an awareness of the relationship of age, life events, pathologies, behavioral problems, pharmaceutical agents, and sexual function. Without such a knowledge base, the practitioner has no basis for discriminating between healthy and unhealthy responses, or for the interpretation of clients' concerns, and thus has no basis for teaching or counseling.

Although a knowledge base is essential to effective intervention, an awareness of professionals' value systems, including the biases and beliefs about appropriate and inappropriate sexual behavior, is not unimportant. Unless professionals can accept their own sexuality and are comfortable with their own behavior, it will be difficult to convey comfort to clients. Self-acceptance is seen as prerequisite to the development of a tolerant approach in the care of clients. However, nurses have belief systems about sexual phenomena, and so do clients. Does this imply that nurses or other professionals must condone every variety of sexual activity for themselves? It is essential that professionals be aware of their own feelings and values and attempt to keep them in perspective by acknowledging them. This strategy would allow professionals to maintain a supportive climate that encourages sharing of feelings by clients yet simultaneously permits professionals to acknowledge the validity of their own beliefs. In some instances awareness of professionals' own values would lead them to refer patients to more objective practitioners.

Finally, professionals need to be able to communicate genuinely and therapeutically with clients. Often this involves using clients' language, which may be quite different from that of health professionals. Without the ability to accurately and empathetically interact with clients, the most sophisticated knowledge base and objective attitudes are of little benefit. Skills supportive of sex education and counseling include the progression from active listening techniques to sophisticated psychotherapeutic skills. Some of the basic requirements provided in most professional nursing programs include active listening strategies, communication techniques designed to elicit feelings, strategies for showing acceptance, goal setting, and problem solving. These skills provide a strong base for nurses providing sex education or counseling as a part of their practice. Mims and Swenson[22] point out that if nurses attempt to provide sexual health care based on their life experiences, their behaviors may be both destructive and intuitively helpful. Because nurses are exposed to the same confusing messages and misinformation about sexuality as others, they may perpetuate incorrect or destructive ideas about sexuality. Mims and Swenson describe three levels in the provision of sexual health care that are based on an increasingly sophisticated preparation. The first level is characterized by increasing awareness on the part of the nurse. Awareness is a product of the interactions between perceptions, attitudes, and cognitions; in other words, it is a consciousness-raising process. The next level incorporates communication, counseling, and teaching skills to give permission and give information. The most advanced level includes suggestion giving, therapy, educational programs, and research projects. A basic course in human sexuality would permit many nurses to capably provide specific suggestions, whereas postbaccalaureate education is seen as necessary preparation for providing sex therapy, planning and conducting educational programs, and conducting sex research.

Setting variables. The second set of variables deals with the settings in which nurses practice. These settings may be primary, secondary, or tertiary treatment settings, as well as the community at large. To some extent, the setting helps delineate the client population, the third and most important variable. The setting may also determine the extent to which nurses deliver sexual health services. Some settings facilitate delivery of services, and others preclude it.

Client variables. Nursing practice may be directed toward clients as individuals, families, groups, organizations, or communities. The nature of the client's actual or potential problem in turn usually implies specific needs or concerns with regard to sexuality. These needs or concerns may range from prevention to therapy. It is out of these potential or real concerns that nursing roles have emerged.

Types of roles. Following are several roles that nurses enact in the delivery of sexual health services:
1. Facilitator of a milieu conducive to sexual health
2. Provider of anticipatory guidance
3. Validator of normalcy
4. Educator (including the cognitive, attitudinal, and communication components of sexuality)
5. Counselor of clients who must adapt to changes in their usual forms of sexual expression
6. Provider of intensive therapy for clients with complex problems
7. Consultant to other helpers

We shall consider each of these roles and some examples of each from nursing practice.

Facilitating a milieu conducive to sexual health may occur at the individual, family, group, organization, and community level. One approach useful in developing such a milieu includes minimizing guilt and anxiety that clients experience in conjunction with their sexual thoughts, attitudes, feelings, and behavior. Nurses can assist clients to solve problems, objectively examining their behavior and its consequences within a reality-oriented framework. Fostering open communication about sexuality within the family and other social systems can enable individuals to participate in open interchange about their concerns.

In the nursing setting nurses can assist families to establish a milieu that encourages openness with their children. Use of role modeling for the parents, or even role plays to "try out" various responses to children's questions, may be helpful.

Another important aspect of fostering a milieu conducive to sexual health is supporting parents as they attempt to set limits with their children. One mother shared that her 4-year-old son was making her feel very anxious because he often touched his penis and acted as if he were about to masturbate in public. When asked about the family rules for masturbation, she replied that the children could masturbate in their bedrooms and knew that their privacy would not be invaded. This woman was perplexed because she did not want to make her child feel uncomfortable about his sexuality yet did not want to expose him to the negative responses he might well hear from the neighbors. After a discussion of family rules and social boundaries for sexual expression this woman asserted that she did not think it was appropriate for her son to masturbate in public and that it would be perfectly appropriate for her to establish the limit that masturbation was not appropriate outside of the child's bedroom. In this instance the child's mother was fearful of creating a negative environment for the child but initially had not considered that society might provide some even more negative messages to him about his sexuality if he did not abide by these limits.

Another strategy that can be implemented in nursing practice settings is including material regarding sexual health in the history and physical examination. During an initial workup the clinician has the opportunity to establish that the client's sexuality is a valid component of health. By including this material in the earliest contacts with clients, practitioners convey their willingness to pursue discussion about sexual topics. This openness also fosters a milieu conducive to sexual health.

Providing anticipatory guidance is frequently a component of nursing practice. This involves providing the client with information about what to expect or what phases of experience are likely to occur. Adolescence and middlescence are two life periods during which anxiety about sexuality is likely to surface. By discussing the usual changes experienced at these points with clients, nurses can assist them to cope realistically with major changes in their bodies and their feelings.

Young adolescents, when given the opportunity, frequently voice concerns about masturbation, nocturnal emissions, menstruation, and their changing body configurations. When possible, sharing with them the phasing or timing of these bodily and affective changes will give them a notion of what to expect.

Middlescent women frequently benefit from anticipatory guidance with regard to menopause. Generally, the more informed these women are with regard to their changed physiology, the more likely it is that they will be able to cope with what could be a maturational crisis. For example, some women assume that since their reproductive days are over, they will no longer be capable of having sexual feelings, that they will no longer be able to have intercourse, or that their spouses will no longer find them attractive. If the woman recognizes that she may have diminished vaginal lubrication, but that this can be overcome with the use of a water-soluble lubricant and by a sensitive partner, she can anticipate coping with her changing body.

Validating normalcy is a function that nearly all health professionals perform but sometimes undervalue. Often the focus is on finding out what is wrong, what the patho-physiologic process is, and what therapy to prescribe to correct the malfunction. As mentioned earlier, the primary goal of the nursing profession is health maintenance rather than treatment of pathology. Often family members approach health professionals to find out whether they are normal, acceptable, and not perverted. They seek out the health professional for validation of their sexual normalcy. People may be concerned about their thoughts, fantasies, dreams, and feelings, as well as overt sexual behaviors. In the process of validating normalcy nurses often help clients exchange labels. Often labels bearing negative connotations such as "dirty," "perverted," or "abnormal" are exchanged for labels such as "healthy" and "okay."[1] Although most sexual acts could be considered normal in some sense—that is, statistically or phylogenetically—clients do need to be made aware of the consequences of their behavior. The health professional cannot ignore clients' ethical codes or the legal code.

One situation sometimes encountered in nursing practice is the adolescent questioning whether it is "normal" not to be sexually active. Recently a nursing colleague saw a young woman in the clinic who was requesting a prescription for an oral contraceptive. The physician who saw her did a pelvic examination and gave her a prescription. The nurse, who had been with her during the examination, noted that she was quite anxious about the procedure and was very hesitant to leave the examining room after the examination was completed. After pursuing the reason for her obvious discomfort with the situation the nurse found that the woman was seeking a prescription at her boyfriend's insistence; furthermore, she was *not* convinced about her desire to become sexually active, but she feared that the relationship would end if she did not meet the young man's demands. She wanted some reassurance that she was "normal" for having these reservations and that *not* being sexually active was okay.

Another occasion for validating normal sexual attitudes is during the physical examination. Many nurses who perform pelvic examinations are beginning to make these an educational experience for their patients. At the beginning of the examination the examiner asks the woman whether she would like a mirror so that she can watch the examination as it is being performed. As the examiner inspects the external genitals, it is possible to identify the anatomic parts, pointing out how healthy the genitals appear. As the speculum is inserted, the examiner, who may use a lighted speculum, can identity the woman's internal pelvic structures. For many women, this is the first time they have been able to see their external genitals, to say nothing of their cervices and other internal structures.

Families often encounter disabling diseases or injuries that interfere with usual forms of sexual expression. Couples may be asking nurses to validate the normalcy or health of the adaptations they make, such as the exploration of new types of sexual expression.

Educating clients about their sexuality implies more than merely disseminating data. "Teaching is the process of assisting clients to acquire the health-related knowledge, skills and values which foster and maintain cognitive, interpersonal and psychomotor functioning.''[3] It implies helping clients explore their attitudes and values, inasmuch that they shape their sexual behavior, and helping clients communicate comfortably about sexual phenomena.

In the context of nursing practice there are many areas of client concern in conjunction with childhood and adult sexuality, sexual behavior during pregnancy, and sexual adaptation to illnesses. One of the most frequently encountered problems is pregnancy. To cope with the multitude of strains that appear during pregnancy, labor, and delivery, many health care agencies have designed childbirth or parenthood preparation courses. Often the individual providing this course is a nurse. A knowledge base regarding sexual expression during pregnancy is now commonly included as part of childbirth preparation courses. This material indicates to couples that unless there are complications of pregnancy, such as bleeding, infection, ruptured membranes, or a history of habitual abortion, there is no need to discontinue the couple's usual sexual activities, unless, of course, that is the preference of the couple. In addition, couples are helped to communicate authentically with one another with regard to their sexual feelings and to the pregnancy in general. Attitudes and values are explored: often women in these groups will express feelings relative to the changes in their bodies and how they perceive themselves as sexual beings as a result of the pregnancy. Male partners will often express fear or hesitancy about sexual encounters out of deference to the pregnancy (see Chapter 9).

This same strategy may also be applied to couples who are adapting to illnesses. Often working with the couple before a surgical procedure can be preventive as well as therapeutic. Women who are about to have hysterectomies are often concerned that they will no longer be able to have intercourse or that they will have no more sexual feelings. Informing these women and their partners before the surgery may remove unnecessary barriers from the resumption of their sexual relationships. Similar information would be helpful to men having a transurethral resection. Following this procedure, men usually experience retrograde ejaculation, or a "dry ejaculate." If the couple is aware of this before surgery, they are less apt to be concerned about this phenomenon when they resume their sexual relationship.

Often providing limited information can free clients from anxieties connected with sexual performance or assumptions about the negative effects of health or illness conditions. However, education is not synonymous with information giving. Nurses must be aware of the meaning of this information in the context of clients' value systems and be willing to assist clients to communicate more comfortably about their sexual concerns.

In *counseling clients regarding their sexuality* nurses attempt to help clients change their behavior to reach a designated goal. The process involves helping clients achieve a more satisfying level of functioning.

As a basis for counseling, a sexual problem history would usually be obtained. This would include data such as that discussed in Chapter 5.

1. A description of the current problem or concern in the client's own words: "I can't get an erection." "I hate it when it takes me so long to have a climax."
2. The onset and course of the problem, including the following:
   a. Age at onset—"Right after I had my tubes tied . . . " "When I was 13 . . ."

      b. Nature of the onset—"I felt this coming on for a long time." "All of a sudden . . ."

      c. Precipitating events—"After a few drinks . . ."

      d. Other life events associated with the problem—"About the time I lost my job . . ."

  3. The client's concept of the cause and persistence of the problem: "Guess I'm getting older." "Seem to be too tired." "Not as exciting as it once was."

  4. Past attempts at treatment and their results, including the attempts at treating initiated by the client as well as those of other professionals: "I tried having a few drinks."

  5. Examination of the client's current expectations and the goals for treatment. (These may be impossible or incongruous with the way nurses practice.)

These data would be supplemented by the results of the usual history and review of systems.

Some of the suggestions made by the nurse in the role of counselor may relate to the conditions conducive to optimal sexual functioning, specific approaches to use given certain illnesses or surgeries, and directives for coping with some sexual dysfunctions.

Several areas in which counseling may be needed have been defined by the American Association of Sex Educators, Counselors, and Therapists (AASECT). The first area, that of assisting youth to deal with problems associated with sexual development, is one in which clinicians practicing in a school system or in a pediatric or family care setting are often involved. Anxiety about normal physical development may manifest itself to practitioners, who then assist youth to work through feelings about menstruation, masturbation, nocturnal emissions, sexual fantasies, and changes in body image and function. Adolescents who must deal with pregnancies also need counseling about their own sexuality, as well as about the experience of pregnancy, delivery, and subsequent decisions regarding the child's future or, alternatively, about abortion.

Since many problems seen in youth are also problems to parents, clinicians have an opportunity to work with and through a family unit. Frequently, parents have questions about the sexual development of their children. In a clinic setting one may encounter parents who are anxious about the child's sexual play, their communication with the child on sexual topics, and dealing with the child's questions. Often parents seek validation of their child's normal state. Sometimes parental anxieties may create problems for the child. Parents who are uncomfortable with their own sexuality and sexual development may need to be reassured that masturbation and nocturnal emissions are normal components of sexual development. The family who must deal with teenage pregnancy, abortion, or a child who has been sexually assaulted may require both crisis intervention and long-term follow-up care to assist in restoration of family health.

Practitioners working in a family planning setting are often confronted with questions related to sexual aspects of relationships. Many adults require counseling about pregnancy problems, including promotion and prevention. Practitioners may find that anxieties about infertility problems may seriously affect self-esteem. Lack of knowledge of the reproductive processes and sexual behavior may be intensifying the problems of couples who are unable to conceive. Contraception and voluntary sterilization are two additional issues often requiring counseling.

Couples may seek help concerning their relationships. Frequently, nursing practitioners are in a first-line position to initiate counseling, since they are usually more accessible than other health team members. Publicity related to sexual dysfunction has made it easier for some adults to request counseling for orgasmic dysfunction, dyspareunia, vaginismus, premature ejaculation, and impotence. In addition, some adults may need the help of professionals to resolve differences related to explicit aspects of sexual behavior, such as frequency, positions and techniques, and inhibitions and anxieties about sexual functioning.

Concerns are frequently voiced regarding sexual behavior that is at variance with cultural and societal norms. Some people may be anxious about behavior that they enjoy but think is perverse.

Another area in which the practitioner may provide counseling is with the aging population. Menopause and age-related changes in sexual functioning may present problems for the older segment of the population. These problems may be compounded by the popular myth that sexual desire and functioning are nonexistent among the aging. Many older people may be unaware of the effects chronic illness may have on their sexual functioning.

Practitioners may provide anticipatory counseling to those people who have had illnesses or medical-surgical interventions that may cause sexual dysfunction. Frequently, people are not aware of the effects that surgery, degenerative diseases, and drug therapy may have on sexual desire and expression.

Finally, AASECT has designated gender identity as another area in which counseling is important. Nurses may be a part of a team to support persons desiring transsexual surgery and gender reorientation.

Some rather simple directives for coping with sexual dysfunction can be provided in the context of a counseling relationship. The man who ejaculates prematurely can be taught to use the "squeeze technique," or the partner may learn to apply the technique. Women who have difficulty with lubrication and who experience painful intercourse as a consequence of steroid alteration during the postpartum or menopausal period may benefit from the use of a water-soluble lubricant in conjunction with the suggestion to explore alternative kinds of sexual pleasuring.

One suggestion often incorporated in sexual counseling for a couple having difficulties with intercourse is that the couple abstain for a specified period of time. This admonition is designed to reduce the "pressure to perform" perceived by the dysfunctional couple. This suggestion often has paradoxic results. The couple might violate the admonition and have a positive experience. In some instances the anxiety directed at the sexual difficulty dissipates, permitting the couple to function comfortably.

As implied in the discussion about the educational role of the nurse, it is equally as important to examine attitudes, values, and feelings and foster open communication as it is to provide information. The counseling strategy implies, then, that couples or individuals be helped to identify methods of coping that are consistent with their value systems and that can be communicated about with comfort.

AASECT has proposed an explicit set of criteria for preparation of those who provide comprehensive sexual counseling. Knowledge of the process of reproduction, sexual development, sexual functioning and behavior, and sex and gender issues is recognized as essential for those engaged in sexual counseling. In addition, marriage, family, and interpersonal relationships; sex and health; and sexology are relevant areas of knowledge for the counselor. AASECT also emphasizes the importance of counseling theory and methodology and knowledge of various patterns of counseling, such as one-to-one and co-counseling approaches.

Interviewing skills, as well as collaboration and consultation skills, are also important for counselors' practices. It is recommended that counselors be skilled in more than one method, since no single method may be appropriate for the variety of client needs that may be encountered.

Attitudes and professional behavior are also significant considerations in the preparation of sex counselors. It is suggested that counselors have mature, healthy attitudes toward themselves, their own sexuality, and their roles as counselors. An accepting, nonjudgmental attitude toward clients is essential, as is the willingness to provide direction to clients when necessary and to avoid doing so when it would limit the growth of clients.

To assist with sexual problems, counselors need adequate knowledge of sexual phenomena from psychosocial and biologic perspectives. In addition, it is necessary that counselors be aware of their own feelings, attitudes, and values. Comfort with one's own sexuality is as integral a part of sexual counseling as are the basic therapeutic skills of the counseling process.

Some nurses function as *providers of intensive therapy.* Some persons with complex sexual dysfunctions may require referral to individuals who have added preparation psychotherapy and special approaches to intervention with sexual dysfunctions. This may be a component of practice that most nurses do not offer to clients. An awareness of such sexual dysfunctions may prompt nurses in many settings to make referrals to specialists in sexual health. There are, however, some nurses in psychiatric, obstetric, and gynecologic settings who currently provide this intensive therapy (see Chapter 8).

A final role that some nurses enact is that of a *consultant.* The focus for consultation might be the community, an organization, such as a school, and other professionals. "Consulting is an interactional process between professionals in which the consultant shares specialized expertise to assist the consultee to solve work problems in the framework of the consultee's professional functioning."[9]

Nurses may extend their expertise to other professionals and to the lay public through their participation in the community planning for educational experience in schools, churches, and other social systems. The nurse may consult with other practitioners who are having difficulty managing the sexual concerns of their patients.

There is one final note about nurses' roles in the delivery of sexual health services: they are often of a collaborative nature. For example, the client with a sexual dysfunction may require the care of a medical practitioner, as well as a physical therapist and social worker. Rather than fragmenting care by treating the person's sexual concerns as an entity unrelated to the medical regimen, problems with the social system, or physical disability, nurses seek to coordinate these efforts.

Sexual concerns and problems and sexual health care

People have a variety of sexual problems ranging from concerns about sexual phenomena to sexual dysfunctions. Each type of problem is the consequence of different antecedents, and each requires somewhat different therapeutic approaches. *Sex-*

ual concerns constitute a source of worry, dissatisfaction, or discomfort for clients but do not produce difficulty in sexual function, profound problems in the sexual relationship, or a greatly altered sexual self-concept. Sexual concerns often arise because of misinformation or lack of information, conflicting values, difficulty in communicating about sexual issues, and anxiety or guilt about sexual phenomena. These concerns are usually amenable to sex education strategies such as permission giving, provision of limited information, values clarification exercises, rehearsal of communication, validation of normalcy, and provision of anticipatory guidance.

Sexual difficulties create discomfort in the sexual relationship, may occasionally interfere with sexual function, and may sometimes challenge the person's sexual self-image. Sexual difficulties include the inability to relax, disinterest in sexual activity, sexual dissatisfaction, inability to please or be pleased by a partner, and problems in the timing of sexual activities. These difficulties are amenable to counseling approaches, including relaxation training, exploration of alternatives in the sexual repertoire, provision of specific suggestions, and training in communication skills.

Sexual dysfunctions usually result not only in disruption of sexual function but also in severe strains on the sexual relationship and a threatened sexual self-image. There are three categories of sexual dysfunctions[14]:

- Disorders of sexual desire
- Disorders of arousal
- Disorders of orgasm

Sexual dysfunction is usually treated by a sexual counselor or therapist. In addition, there are two other categories of sexual dysfunction. The first includes disorders that result from involuntary painful spasms of genital and reproductive organ muscles, resulting in vaginismus in women and ejaculatory pain in men. Sexual phobias constitute the second.

Disorders of the desire phase include hypoactive sexual desire and inhibited sexual desire. Persons with hypoactive sexual desire lose interest in sexual matters, do not pursue sexual gratification, and are not likely to avail themselves of sexual opportunities. Individuals with inhibited sexual desire may be able to experience lubrication or erection but do not experience much pleasure.

Disorders of the excitement phase include inability to have an erection in men and difficulty with lubrication and swelling in women (general sexual dysfunction). Erectile dysfunction probably affects most men at least once in their lifetimes, and transient episodes are estimated to occur in 50% of all men. These fleeting episodes are considered within the range of normal. Erectile dysfunction (sometimes referred to as impotence) occurs in varying degrees. Some men experience total inability to attain an erection of sufficient hardness. This frustrating, humiliating condition may lead to decreased self-esteem and consequent depression. Erectile dysfunction is described as primary if the man has never been able to achieve or maintain an erection that would permit intercourse. Secondary erectile dysfunction, a more common phenomenon, occurs situationally and is likely to be of the variety seen in conjunction with pathophysiologically and pharmacologically induced states. The penile prosthetic implant has recently been devised as a method of treatment for organic impotence in men. There are two types of penile prostheses. The older type consists of the implantation of two sponge-filled silicone rods in the corpora cavernosa. This maintains the penis in a constant semierect position. The newer and more acceptable method for many men is the inflatable penile prosthesis. Both types of prostheses are implanted surgically and do not interfere with normal urinary elimination. The silicone implants are inserted through perineal or penile incisions and the inflatable prostheses through perineal and abdominal incisions. Penile edema is minimal, but scrotal edema may occur with the inflatable type. Pain may be severe during the first week, and mild pain may continue for several weeks after surgery. As with any prosthetic device, there is a need to integrate it with one's self-image *and* the relationship.

Disorders of the orgasm phase include inadequate ejaculatory control or premature ejaculation, retarded ejaculation, and orgasmic dysfunction in women. Premature ejaculation is the inability of a man to control the ejaculatory reflex. This is thought to be a conditioned response to hurried circumstances and is treated quite successfully by means of the "squeeze technique." This technique requires the man or his partner to place the thumb and second and third fingers at the coronal ridge of the glans, exerting enough pressure over this area for 3 or 4 seconds to relieve the feeling of ejaculatory inevitability. Retarded ejaculation, also known as ejaculatory incompetence, implies that despite the amount and quality of stimulation of the penis, intravaginal ejaculation either does not occur or is so delayed that the couple experiences pelvic irritation and fatigue as a result.

Primary orgasmic dysfunction occurs in the woman who has not had orgasm with sexual activity, including intercourse or masturbation. Secondary orgasmic dysfunction is characterized by inability to experience orgasm under certain conditions. The woman with secondary orgasmic dysfunction has experienced orgasmic sensations with one form of stimulation at some point in her life. This problem does not preclude the woman from experiencing sexual arousal and its physiologic accompaniments; rather, only the orgasmic portion of the sexual response cycle seems impaired. Vaginismus is a relatively rare sexual problem characterized by an involuntary, conditioned spasm of the vaginal outlet, thus causing it to shut tightly. This problem precludes sexual intercourse, but vaginismic women may be orgasmic with alternative methods of sexual stimulation. Dyspareunia, painful intercourse, may be attributable to a number of factors ranging from a full lower bowel to feelings of aversion toward sexual intercourse. It is sometimes experienced by women with steroid alterations, for example, the postpartum mother and the postmenopausal woman.

Masters and Johnson[19] have also conducted clinical studies with homosexual men and women who had a sexual dysfunction or were sexually dissatisfied. There appeared to be more similarity than difference in the kinds of sexual dysfunctions homosexuals and heterosexuals experienced. For a highly motivated segment of the homosexual population that desires conversion or reversion to heterosexuality, a therapy approach was described that may be effective.

Summary

The nurse's role in sexual health care are influenced by the following:
1. The nurse's level of preparation
2. The setting of the practice
3. The clients and/or the concerns and problems they experience

There are a number of ways in which nurses can foster sexual health and prevent sexual problems.

Key considerations for professional nurses in the delivery of sexual health care include the following:

1. A variety of roles exist for provision of sexual health services.
2. Clients may be individuals, families, groups, organizations, or communities.
3. Collaboration with other helpers can prevent fragmentation of health care.

Questions for review

1. During this next week, pay particular attention to your relationships with other health professionals. Include those encounters you have with members of the same sex, as well as those of the opposite sex. Describe one relationship you have with another professional in your practice area. What sexual overtones enter into your relationship? To what extent is touching permitted or discouraged? What boundaries exist between you because of sex? What sex-linked limits exist in your *roles?* Repeat the above exercise in relation to a patient or client versus a colleague. Decide which aspects of this exercise you would like to share with your colleagues.
2. Please think about each of these situations, and record your immediate responses and subsequent thoughts in your journal.

Situation	My immediate response (how I felt)	Subsequent thoughts (how I might respond)
Mrs. N., who is in her third trimester of pregnancy, tells you, "I hate my body! My husband refuses to sleep with me anymore and has been staying out all night for the last 2 weeks. I want this baby, but it's played havoc with my marriage."		
Mr. T., who is recovering from a myocardial infarction, caresses your breast while you are taking his blood pressure and then pinches you on the buttocks as you turn around to leave his bedside.		
Ms. W., a model, says she will not consent to any treatment at all for		

Situation	My immediate response (how I felt)	Subsequent thoughts (how I might respond)
breast cancer. She has a small lump but says, "I could not tolerate the change in my body."		
Mrs. F. asks, "What should I do for my daughter? She is asking about sex, and I think she has had intercourse at least once. Should she be on the pill?" Mrs. F.'s daughter is 19 and mentally retarded but lives at home.		
Mr. P. tells you, "I threw away those high blood pressure pills. They took away my manhood." His blood pressure is 220/170 today.		
Mrs. H. tells you, "Since my hysterectomy, orgasm feels different. I really have a completely different sensation."		
Mrs. J. tells you, "I like to have intercourse while I'm having my period. I don't flow very much and feel really sexy then. Is that normal?"		
A nursing student asks you, "Why does Mrs. J. have gonorrheal pharyngitis? Is that a mistake on the lab report? How would that happen?"		
Mr. B., a patient on the psychiatric ward, says, "I'd really like to marry you."		
Mr. C,. a quadriplegic, has an erection while you are caring for his catheter.		

References

1. American Association of Sex Educators, Counselors, and Therapists: The professional training and preparation of sex counselors, Washington, D.C., 1973, AASECT.
2. American Nurses Association: Nursing: a social policy statement, Kansas City, Mo., 1980, ANA.
3. Annon, J.: The behavioral treatment of sexual problems, Honolulu, 1974, Enabling Systems, Inc.
4. Baldwin, B.A., and Wilson, R.A.: A campus peer counseling program in human sexuality, Journal of the American College Health Association 22:399-494, 1974.
5. Barnard, M., Clancy, B., and Krantz, K., editors: Human sexuality for health professionals, Philadelphia, 1978, W.B. Saunders Co.
6. Donaldson, S., and Crowley, D.: The discipline of nursing, Nursing Outlook 26(2):113-120, 1979.
7. Elder, M.S.: Nurse counseling on sexuality—the unmet challenge, Nursing Outlook 18:38-40, Nov. 1970.
8. Goodwin, T.: Sexual concerns and questions which patients present to registered nurses in selected area of nursing practice, unpublished master's thesis, Cincinnati, 1975, University of Cincinnati.
9. Hall, J.: Nursing as process. In Hall, J., and Weaver, editors; Distributive nursing practice: a systems approach to community health, Philadelphia, 1977, J.B. Lippincott Co.
10. Heit, P.: A high school peer sexuality information and referral program, Journal of School Health 44:572-574, 1974.
11. Hogan, R.: Human sexuality: a nursing perspective, New York, 1980, Appleton-Century-Crofts.
12. Jacobson, L.: Illness and human sexuality, Nursing Outlook 22:50-53, Jan. 1974.
13. Kaplan, H.S.: The new sex therapy, New York, 1974, Brunner/Mazel, Inc.
14. Kaplan, H.S.: Disorders of sexual desire, New York, 1979, Simon & Schuster, Inc.
15. Krizinofski, M.T.: Human sexuality and nursing practice, Nursing Clinics of North America 8:673-681, 1973.
16. Lion, Ed., editor: Human sexuality in nursing process, New York, 1982, John Wiley & Sons, Inc.
17. Mandetta, A., and Gustaveson, P.: Abortion to zoophilia, Chapel Hill, N.C., 1976, Carolina Population Center.
18. Masters, W., and Johnson, V.: Human sexual inadequacy, Boston, 1970, Little, Brown & Co.
19. Masters, W., and Johnson, V.: Homosexuality in perspective, Boston, 1979, Little, Brown & Co.
20. Masters, W., Johnson, V., and Kolodny, R.: Ethical issues in sex therapy and research, Boston, 1977, Little, Brown & Co.
21. Mims, F.: Sexual health education and counseling, Nursing Clinics of North America 10(3):519-528, 1975.
22. Mims, F., and Swenson, M.: Sexuality: a nursing perspective, New York, 1980, McGraw-Hill, Inc.

23. Schiller, P.: Creative approach to sex education and counseling, New York, 1977, Association Press.
24. Vincent, C.E.: Sexual and marital health: the physician as consultant, New York, 1973, McGraw-Hill, Inc.
25. Wilson, R.: Introduction to sexual counseling, Chapel Hill, N.C., 1974, Carolina Population Center.
26. World Health Organization: Education and treatment in human sexuality: the training of health professionals, Report of a WHO Meeting, Technical Report Series no. 572, Geneva, 1975, WHO.

8

Sexual dysfunction: etiology and treatment

**CAROLYN A. LIVINGSTON, MARILYN C. McINTYRE, and
CATHERINE INGRAM FOGEL**

Masters and Johnson[6] have stated that "a conservative estimate would indicate half the marriages [in the United States] are either presently sexually dysfunctional or imminently so in the future." To further make the point, Maddox[22] has stated that "nearly everyone needs short-term sexual counseling at some point in his or her life." Clearly there is a need for the health care professional to consider sexual dysfunction as a legitimate area for professional intervention.

In view of the need for qualified practitioners to help clients who have problems with sexual function, this chapter has the following purposes:

1. To examine the etiology of sexual dysfunction
2. To identify and review general treatment modalities for sexual dysfunction
3. To discuss the common male sexual dysfunctions and their specific treatment
4. To discuss the common female sexual dysfunctions and their specific treatment

The focus of this chapter will be primarily on heterosexual dysfunction, for very little is known about homosexual or bisexual dysfunction, although it is thought that similar principles may apply.

Etiology

Physiologic influences. Physical illness may influence sexual function by systemic and nonspecific effects on the patient and/or by interference with neural, vascular, and hormonal components of the sexual response (see Chapter 15).

Any illness that brings about fatigue, fever, or pain can be expected to limit sexual desire and activity.[7] General or localized infections and hepatic, pulmonary, and renal disease are usually associated with a decrease in sexual desire and difficulty in sexual performance. It is not unusual that following the acute phase of the illness the sexual symptoms subside; however, patients with chronic hepatic insufficiency are frequently aware of a progressive decrease in sexual desire and a decrease in erectile and orgasmic response. These sexual problems may also occur in patients receiving hemodialysis or may follow renal transplantation. Patients with coronary disease frequently avoid sex because of the fear that sexual activity may cause inordinate stress on cardiac functioning.

For patients with diabetes mellitus there are transitory periods of loss of sexual desire, and as the disease progresses, there may be irreversible sexual impairment.[30]

Neural factors. Sexual dysfunction may result from various diseases that affect the brain, spinal cord, or peripheral nervous system. Psychomotor epilepsy that disturbs the limbic sexual circuits, sometimes decreases libido and sexual activity.[15,30] Multiple sclerosis and other degenerative diseases of the spinal cord may cause orgasmic and erectile problems. Diseases such as diabetes or certain types of prostatic or abdominal surgery may impair the autonomic and somatic innervation to the sexual organs, resulting in problems in sexual performance.[30]

Vascular factors. Vascular disorders that affect the blood supply to the genital tissues may disrupt erection in men. Women seem far less disabled by disorders of the genital blood vessels.[15] Vascular problems that may cause sexual dysfunction include occlusive vascular diseases of the lower aorta and internal iliac branches, thrombosis of the vessels to the penis, and systemic vascular disorders such as leukemia or sickle cell anemia.[30]

Hormonal factors. Hypogonadal disorders are frequently accompanied by disturbances in sexual desire and activity. Primary disorders such as mumps, orchitis, and cryptorchidism or secondary disorders such as postpubertal panhypopituitarism bring about a decrease in gonadal hormone production that results in sexual dysfunction. Other endocrine disorders, such as hypothyroidism, acromegaly, and Addison's disease, cause depressed sexual desire and erectile and orgasmic problems.[30] Long-term alcohol abuse affects the hypothalamic pituitary axis and gonads and most likely will cause a decrease in sexual desire, genital sensation, and ability to respond sexually (see Chapter 22).

Psychologic influences. In many instances the cause of sexual dysfunction can be traced to a lack of knowledge about sexuality, ignorance of sexual techniques, or general misinformation about sexuality. For example, unsatisfactory lovemaking can be the result of a lack of information about sexual anatomy. This is hardly surprising in a society that generally places strong prohibitions on sexual behavior. Traditionally, open discussions about sex between partners or individuals are not encouraged and, unfortunately, are actively discouraged.

Another factor operating is the destructive belief that the ability to perform sexually is inherently learned by adulthood—that somehow sexual performance is instinctual and mysteriously understood when people "come of age." If there is a lack of knowledge with respect to sexual function, it is seldom assumed that one needs to be taught, and ignorance and silence prevail. Myths about sexuality, as well as outright misinformation, exacerbate an already existing paucity of knowledge available to the individual.

It is important to understand how the phenomena of ignorance and avoidance of sexual issues have developed in society. Human sexuality is a basic drive that is frequently accompanied by intense and conflicting emotions. Society has therefore developed standards that serve to provide individuals with guidelines for sexual behavior. These guidelines prescribe roles that can often minimize fears and confusion. Unfortunately, they can also create unrealistic expectations, demands, and restrictions that are internalized by individuals and become a part of their value systems.

Forces that prevent violation of sexual rules in many cultures are guilt and anxiety.[34] When guilt and anxiety become associated with early sexual learning, a prototype for inhibited sexual response develops and carries through to adulthood. For instance, a woman may have been actively discouraged from sexual stimulation in early childhood and as an adult finds that she not only has to learn how to enjoy sexual stimulation but also is required to work through negative feelings associated with her sexual self-concept.

There are other sources of sexual anxiety that can be destructive to satisfactory sexual functioning. Fear of failure, demand for performance, and fear of rejection are most commonly identified. Anticipation of the inability to perform is one of the causes of erectile dysfunction and perhaps, to some extent, orgasmic dysfunction. Once an episode of failure has been experienced, the fear of recurrence increases. Anticipatory anxiety related to sexual performance can start a self-defeating cycle of fear that escalates a single transient failure into a state of serious chronic dysfunction.[12] The phenomenon that maintains this cycle is called *spectatoring:* the individual remains outside himself or herself and observes his or her sexual responses. This results in poor performance, which reconfirms anxieties and fear of failure.[13,24]

Fear of rejection by the partner or an excessive need to please may also generate anxiety. To wish to give enjoyment and share pleasure with a partner is desirable and healthy. It is when this becomes a compulsive need "to please, to perform, to serve, to not disappoint"[12] that the emotion becomes dysfunctional.

Poor communication is a factor frequently associated with sexual dysfunction. Communication problems contribute to an inability to talk about sex, which in turn leads to limited knowledge and subsequent restrictive standards of acceptable sexual behavior. This becomes a self-defeating cycle in which partners perpetuate ignorance, lack of understanding, and misinformation about their sexual and emotional needs. To communicate effectively about sex, partners must openly share information about their interests, desires, and wishes. Negotiation and compromise are frequently the outgrowth of effective communication patterns.

Other relationship issues often play a large part in sexual dysfunction. Anger, power struggles, and unresolved conflict within the relationship are important causes of sexual dissatisfaction. Fear of pregnancy may be another factor, since many women find it difficult to relax if fear of pregnancy is a dominant concern.

A history of sexual abuse may have an impact on a woman's sexual functioning. Anger, guilt, and a need for control are emotional sequelae to abuse and often underlie the development of sexual problems, including inhibited desire and avoidance of sexual contact.[28] Research has begun to examine the variables associated with molestation that contribute to adult sexual adjustment.[32] These variables include age of molestation, frequency and duration, and negative feelings associated with molestation. These findings help explain the variations in sexual functioning that exist among women with abuse histories. Further investigation is needed to help clinicians understand and effectively treat the population of abused women with sexual difficulties.

General treatment modalities

A variety of therapeutic approaches are being used today to treat sexual dysfunction. This section will discuss the more commonly used and/or more effective therapy modalities: those of Annon, Masters and Johnson, Kaplan, and group therapy.

Annon. The behavioral method of treatment of sexual dysfunction is based on the assumption that human sexual behaviors are primarily the result of learning or conditioning. In the absence of any physical pathology sexual dysfunction is viewed as a learned phenomenon, maintained by performance anxiety and environmental factors. Learning theorists have identified precise conditions under which sexual symptoms may be acquired or developed. Behavioral therapists apply this knowledge to modify the dysfunctional behavior and replace it with more desirable responses. To do this, techniques based on learning principles are used. The concept of sexual tasks is an important behavioral therapy technique. In this case specific therapeutic sexual exercises are designed, structured, and assigned to teach new and satisfying responses.

Annon's PLISSIT model[1] is based on a behavioral approach. He delineates four levels of intervention: P—permission giving; LI—limited information; SS—specific suggestions; and IT—intensive therapy. The counselor can use this approach for varying levels of client need. The model assumes that many sexual problems can be managed by using methods that do not require intensive therapy. Therefore some clients may simply need information and permission to reverse dysfunctional patterns. Other clients need further direction and suggestions to alleviate problem areas, but still others do require more intense, long-term therapy. It is important for counselors to be cognizant of their own comfort and skill levels to determine how to intervene and when to refer.

All of the following therapy approaches incorporate elements of Annon's PLISSIT model with modifications that focus on the development of effective techniques at the level of intensive therapy.

Masters and Johnson. Perhaps the greatest contribution to the treatment of human sexuality was made by Masters and Johnson. Their pioneer research regarding the physiology of human sexual response cannot be overestimated. Their studies finally gave an accurate picture of the basic pathophysiology of human sexual functioning. This information opened the door to the development of effective treatment of sexual disorders.

Basic to their approach is the underlying premise that any organic factor causing sexual problems must be ruled out by a thorough physical examination before treatment. Once it is established that there is no organic cause for the dysfunction, the therapy begins.

The second basic treatment tenet is the emphasis on the couple: the belief that the couple is the client and that there is no such thing as an uninvolved partner in a relationship in which there is sexual dysfunction. Although it is recognized that a sexual dysfunction can be an isolated facet of a healthy relationship, their major contribution is that sexual distress usually arises from hostility, poor communication, double standards, unrealistic expectations, and other factors. Therefore therapy must focus on the relationship as a whole, or important treatment dynamics may be overlooked.

The third basic tenet is that of a male and female therapy team. The dual-sex therapy team serves as a role model for effective communication between partners. Masters and Johnson assume that factual sexual knowledge relieves a significant amount of sexual dysfunction. In addition, the couple study the dynamics of their relationship—a mutual educational model that allows the co-therapists to educate by modeling healthy interaction, interpreting material from both male and female perspectives, and reinforcing therapeutic content in different teaching styles.

Education is only one component of the therapy and is considered more valuable when combined with some degree of insight. Techniques of directly confronting fears of sexual performance and giving specific suggestions to overcome these fears are an integral part of this approach. Structured exercises that provide opportunities for sexual feelings to be experienced without any demands help to decrease performance anxiety and spectatoring.

The exercises are aimed at reestablishing positive, pleasurable sensations and attitudes toward sexuality and improving communication within the relationship. Masters and Johnson believe that satisfactory sexual activity is a means of enhancing communication, since it is a medium for exchanging trust and vulnerability. With this belief in sex as a form of communication, they developed techniques to improve communication skills. The focus first was on nonverbal aspects of communication and particularly the sense of touch. From this came their concept of sensate focus, which is defined as a "therapeutic technique which emphasizes the sense of touch in which body surfaces are gently, manually explored by one's self or partner."[26,27] Sensate focus is usually carried out in a three-step program. In phase I purposeful erotic arousal (genital and breast stimulation) is avoided. Tender, gentle stroking is used to reestablish sensory reaction, remove fear of failure, and increase intimacy and mutual involvement. Intercourse is forbidden at this point. In phase II the couple is instructed in genital pleasuring, which involves gentle, teasing stimulation. The intent is to produce sexual arousal but not orgasm. In phase III the aim is to produce orgasm by noncoital or coital means.

The Masters and Johnson sexual therapy modality is very successful; their success rates for specific dysfunctions are high (see results discussed under each dysfunction). Their selection process is stringent and may be one reason for their high success rates. Their type of therapy is expensive. The increased cost resulting from large amounts of therapist time when a co-therapy approach is used is one factor. The removal of the couple from the home into a motel is another. One additional disadvantage is the fact that this approach is not applicable to a large part of the population—individuals and the poor, to cite only a few. Because it is produced by Masters and Johnson, it is a highly selective therapy modality and very successful for those who qualify and can afford it.

Kaplan. Kaplan's approach to sex therapy combines a dynamic interaction of specific sexual techniques and psychotherapy to relieve sexual dysfunction. There are some commonalities with Masters and Johnson's approach, but there are essential differences as well.

On the basis of the initial evaluation, which includes a psychiatric examination, medical history, and physical examination if indicated, a provisional diagnosis of the sexual problem is made, as well as the possible underlying causes. The initial interventions of therapy are aimed at modifying the immediate causes and defenses against sexuality. The remote issues are dealt with only to the extent necessary to relieve the sexual symptom and to ensure that the disability will not recur.

Kaplan's therapy modality was modeled after Masters and Johnson; however, individual therapists of either gender are used. She employs a framework that appears to be more strongly rooted in a psychodynamic model and more committed to the resolution of underlying conflicts. Furthermore, Kaplan employs a multicausal approach to sexual dysfunctions. For her the immediate causes seem more specific and similar for each of the sexual dysfunctions. It is when the deeper causes are considered that more individual variation is taken into account.

Kaplan states that 80% of sexually dysfunctional clients can become symptom free using this approach to sex therapy. The prescribed sexual experiences appear to be effective for the following reasons:

1. They alter the previously destructive sexual system and create a secure sexual environment in which the couple learns to make love in a freer, more enjoyable way.
2. The resolution of conflict is facilitated when previously avoided sexual activity is carried out.
3. The tasks bring to the surface psychologic and interpersonal conflicts, which are then available for psychotherapeutic intervention and resolution.

Group therapy. Recently group approaches to sex therapy have been used with good results. Barbach,[2] Labowitz and LoPiccolo,[19] and Zilbergeld[35] have all developed group approaches to treating sexual dysfunction. The group therapy modalities have used time-limited, predominately behavioral approaches. The groups have been all women, all men, and heterosexual couples and have dealt with such problems as preorgasmic difficulties, dissatisfaction with sexual functioning, and partnerless men experiencing sexual dysfunctions. Group therapy has high success rates, the cost is relatively low, and it offers therapy to an otherwise neglected population group—the individual with a sexual dysfunction who either does not have or cannot involve a partner.

Male sexual dysfunction

The four most common sexual dysfunctions for men are inhibited sexual desire, erectile dysfunction (impotence), premature ejaculation, and retarded ejaculation.

Inhibited sexual desire

Description. Masters and Johnson[23] established four stages of the human sexual response cycle: excitement, plateau, orgasm, and resolution (see Chapter 1). Kaplan[15] later modified the stages of response into a triphasic model consisting of desire, vasocongestive reaction, and orgasm. Analyzing the cycle from this point of view, sexual dysfunction occurs in one (or more) of the three phases. In assessing a desire phase disorder one asks the questions, Is the person interested in having sex, and if so, how often? Inhibited desire involves some degree of loss of interest in pursuing sexual contact or gratification and in itself may not be perceived as a problem by the individual. Often, however, if the partner of a man with inhibited sexual desire is interested in sexual contact, a problem emerges, and the relationship is subject to stress.

Causes of inhibited sexual desire include any or all of the factors mentioned in the previous section on etiology. Particular attention should be paid to kinds and doses of medication the man may be taking, especially antihypertensive medication (see Chapter 23 for a more detailed list of medications that affect sexual functioning). Alcohol and drug use must be assessed thoroughly, since their prolonged abuse can have a detrimental effect on sexual desire (see Chapters 22 and 23). Since libido is an appetite regulated by the autonomic nervous system, depression or stress may be the primary cause of a person's lack of desire. A myriad of other psychologic, relationship, and life-style issues may influence a man's sexual desire as well. Chronic anger and unresolved conflict within the couple's relationship frequently contribute to inhibited desire. Many men who question their sexual performance and adequacy learn to associate anxiety with sexual contact and then predictably lose desire for sex altogether. Since each situation is unique and often complex, a thorough assessment is essential before treatment is advised.

Treatment. Treatment for inhibited sexual desire is still in its exploratory stages. After physiologic influences are ruled out, some form of relationship and/or psychodynamic counseling invariably needs to be incorporated into the sex therapy format to promote effective treatment. Through the structured process of sex therapy, the immediate distress in the relationship is alleviated, and the dynamics that are contributing to the problem can then be understood and modified by both partners.

Since the many issues and therapeutic approaches involved with inhibited sexual desire do not fit within the scope of this chapter, the reader is referred to Kaplan's book *Disorders of Sexual Desire.*

Erectile dysfunction (impotence)

Description. The incidence of reported erectile dysfunction varies depending on severity. The less severe forms occur more frequently than the severe. It has been estimated that approximately half the male population has experienced occasional transient episodes of the inability to achieve erection. These are considered to be within the limits of normal sexual behavior. Erectile difficulties can occur in men of all ages from adolescence to old age; furthermore, neither race nor socioeconomic class appears to affect incidence rates.[13]

The term *impotence* has a pejorative flavor to it. *Erectile dysfunction* is less objectionable and technically more accurate and therefore will be used, although the term impotence is well accepted in the literature. Erectile dysfunction is defined as the male's inability to attain or maintain an erection of sufficient strength to enable him to attain vaginal penetration.

A major difficulty in defining erectile dysfunction lies in determining when the failure of erection, at any point during sexual activity, is sufficient to constitute a problem. If dysfunction means an inability to obtain and maintain an erection firm enough to complete intercourse to male and female satisfaction, then therapists are faced with the dilemma of considering self-report data that are highly subjective. In addition, there are no absolutes that act as reference points in judging male erotic drive and capacity.

Erectile dysfunction has been classified as either primary or secondary. Primary erectile dysfunction means that the man has never been able to achieve or maintain an erection long enough to have intercourse. Secondary erectile dysfunction occurs when the man has had at least one successful coital experience but is currently unable to achieve an erection. Primary erectile dysfunction is the rarest and most severe form of the disorder; men who experience it may be able to attain good erections during masturbation but never with a partner. Secondary erectile dysfunction is less severe but still debilitating. Prognosis for treatment depends on the length of time the man has suffered from it and the severity.[26]

There is probably no other sexual problem for men that is as potentially frustrating, humiliating, and devastating as erectile dysfunction. In almost all cultures and socioeconomic groups male self-esteem is tied to the capacity to achieve erection. Consequently, depression is commonly seen with erectile dysfunction. Depression in itself can also be a cause of erectile dysfunction, resulting in a ''chicken-versus-egg'' dilemma in which it is unclear which factors originally contributed to the problem. Another reciprocal relationship exists between erectile dysfunction and relationship difficulties. Obviously, erectile difficulties can have a deleterious effect on a relationship, but the reverse can also be true; destructive relationships can be a cause of dysfunction. The effects of erectile dysfunction can have a far-reaching impact on a man's self-concept and his relationship with intimates.[13]

It is important for treatment purposes to understand the causative factors associated with erectile dysfunction. Levine[20] suggests the use of four basic questions to determine the differential diagnosis. He believes the description by the client in response to these questions will allow the therapist to distinguish between cases of primary organic determinants and those of purely psychologic origin:

1. What is the physiologic impairment? Is it the inability to obtain an erection, the inability to maintain an erection during intercourse, or some combination?
2. How firm does the penis become: not firm at all, slightly firm but erection not self-supporting, decreased firmness with coitus still possible, or fully turgid?
3. Is the impairment constant or episodic? Under what circumstances is the pattern not present: with other partners of either sex, with masturbation, with sleep, on awakening, during the day, or when engaging in other erotic activity?
4. What life events were occurring when the dysfunction initially appeared?

A brief discussion of organic erectile dysfunction is included here, since organic causation must always be considered before a diagnosis of psychogenic dysfunction can be made. Organic dysfunction is not always easy to determine, since psychologic problems can mimic organic patterns, or, in some cases, the dysfunction may be a combination of the two. However, in organic dysfunction the following points are usually present:

1. There is a similar degree of erectile dysfunction in all sexual circumstances.
2. Sleep-related erections may be absent or not fully turgid.
3. Onset of the dysfunction is not associated with any significant life events.
4. There is a previous uninterrupted period of normal erectile function.
5. Sexual desire, interest, or libido is intact.

If these points are present, the explanation for the dysfunction is usually thought to be organic. The chart on p. 140 illustrates many of the organic factors that may cause erectile dysfunction.[20]

When the history does not in any way suggest physical causes, as discussed previously, coupled with any indication that the dysfunction is situational or erection has occurred in any form at any time after the dysfunction originally occurred, then the dysfunction is considered to be psychologic in nature. Causation is not always clear-cut but may remain ambiguous.

Treatment. The treatment of erectile dysfunction depends on careful diagnosis, which in turn depends on obtaining a thorough history. Therapy for organic dysfunction is aimed at reversing the cause. Sometimes injury or illness results in the

Organic contributors to erectile dysfunction*

Frequently relevant factors

Aging or idiopathic
Alcoholism: associated with cirrhosis but pathogenesis unclear
Diabetic peripheral autonomic neuropathy
Diabetes: uncontrolled metabolic state
Drugs used for therapy:
    Guanethidine, reserpine, alpha methyldopa
    Spironolactone
    Anticholinergic agents
    Estrogen
    Methadone
    Propranolol
Drugs commonly abused:
    Alcohol
    Heroin, methadone, morphine
    Cocaine, amphetamines, barbiturates
Organ system failure: cardiac, respiratory, renal
Surgical complications: perineal prostatectomy, aortofemoral bypass, sympathectomy
Trauma: spinal cord transection
Vascular disease: of terminal aorta and iliac arteries

Less common factors

Congenital: diphallus, absent phallus, hypospadias, spina bifida, Klinefelter's syndrome
Endocrinologic: acromegaly, Addison's disease, adrenal neoplasias, chromophobe adenoma, hypogonadism, primary and secondary types, infantilism, myxedema, hyperthyroidism
Infectious: prostatitis
Neurologic: multiple sclerosis, spinal cord tumors, amyotrophic lateral sclerosis, peripheral neuropathies, general paresis, tabes dorsalis, temporal lobe lesions, pernicious anemia, nutritional deficiencies
Pharmacologic: phenothiazines, butyrophenones, thiothixenes
    Antidepressants: tricyclics and monoamine oxidase inhibitors
Toxicologic: lead and herbicide
Traumatic: castration
    Pelvic fracture, penile trauma
    Ruptured intervertebral disc
Urologic: Peyronie's disease, hydrocele, varicocele, phimosis
    Priapism: idiopathies or associated with sickle cell anemia or leukemia
    Elephantiasis

From Levine, S.B.: Marital sexual dysfunction: erectile dysfunction, Annals of Internal Medicine **85:**343, 1976.
*An in-depth table illustrating effects of medical illness on male sexuality may be found in Kaplan, H.S.: The new sex therapy, New York, 1974, Brunner/Mazel Inc., pp. 80-81, 98-103.

man's total inability to have erections. Because of recent technologic progress, several types of penile implants are available to help restore sexual functioning. These implants can provide an erection that is firm enough for intercourse, but they cannot restore penile sensations or normal ejaculation if these have been lost because of organic causes.

There are two types of penile devices that can be surgically implanted. The simplest is a pair of semirigid rods that are implanted in the corpora cavernosa of the penis. These rods produce a permanent state of semierection. The more complicated and expensive, yet more realistic in function and appearance, is an inflatable device. Two tapered inflatable cylinders are inserted bilaterally into the corpora cavernosa and are connected by a tubing system to a fluid storage reservoir implanted beneath the right or left rectus muscle superficially. When a simple pump and valve in the scrotum is pinched, fluid moves into the cylinders, causing a natural looking erection. Releasing the valve moves the fluid out of the cylinders back to the reservoir (returning the penis to the flaccid state).

Either device may seem somewhat "artificial" to the man or his partner. However, for many men facing a "hopeless" situation, penile implants can improve self-esteem considerably.[25]

When treating psychogenic dysfunction, it is important for the therapist to obtain a thorough history. The therapist relies heavily on the individual's and couple's assessments of sexual experiences: what they perceive as the signs, symptoms, and causes of the dysfunction. During the intake evaluation process the individual therapy plan is developed.

Of primary importance in treating erectile dysfunction is avoidance of a direct attack on the problem of poor or absent erection. Reassurance is a useful tool: the man does not have to be taught to have an erection, the loss of function is understandable, and there are things that can be done. The main therapeutic goal of sex therapy in treating erectile dysfunction is to decrease performance anxiety by (1) removing the man's fear of failure and (2) stopping spectatoring by reorienting emotions and sensations toward active participation and involvement.

The sex therapy treatment program for erectile dysfunction usually follows, in general, the sensate focus technique and consists of the following five steps:
1. Pleasuring without direct attempts to produce erection
2. Penile erection through genital pleasuring
3. Extravaginal orgasm
4. Penetration without orgasm
5. Full coitus with orgasm

Using sensate focus techniques, the couple learn to relax and give and receive pleasure. Erection is not a specific goal at first; it will occur in time because neither partner feels compelled to produce it. Throughout the five steps, the emphasis is on keeping anxiety at a minimum, increasing confidence in the man's erectile ability, and having no specific time frame. This technique has been used very successfully by Masters and Johnson and by Kaplan. Masters and Johnson report success rates of 59.4% in primary erectile dysfunction and 73.8% in secondary dysfunction. Therapy is not considered a success until at least 5 years have elapsed since treatment without relapse.[27]

Premature ejaculation

Description. Premature ejaculation is one of the most common and easily treatable male dysfunctions. It occurs at all socioeconomic levels, and there does not seem to be any specific sexual conflict or particular form of psychopathology directly correlated with it. Premature ejaculation rarely results from organic causes. Masters and Johnson[25] believe that 15% to 20% of American men have at least a moderate degree of difficulty controlling rapid ejaculation.

Defining premature ejaculation is somewhat difficult; no precise definition exists because no specific criteria can be easily applied. Each individual's experiences are varied. Many attempt to use various time measurements or partner satisfactions as criteria, but these are highly subjective. Kaplan's definition[14] seems the most helpful: "Premature ejaculation is the absence of voluntary control over the ejaculatory reflex, regardless of whether this occurs after two thrusts or five, whether it occurs before the female reaches orgasm or not." The essential problem is not how quickly the man ejaculates but his inability to control the reflex. It is difficult for a man to be responsive and sensitive to his partner if he is fearful that on arousal ejaculation will occur. It is important to understand that at one time or another almost every man has ejaculated more quickly than he wished; the essential thing is that he not become overly anxious about it or about possible future failure. Otherwise, what was normal may become chronic.

Ejaculatory control is assumed to be a learned process and under control of the brain. It is apt to be minimal in adolescence, increase with experience, and decrease as the physiologic drive decreases with age. Causative factors are numerous. Repeated situations in which the individual is in a setting that encourages a "hurry-up-and-get-it-over-with approach"—teenagers in parked cars, for example—can set up a conditioned response of quick ejaculation. When an element of anxiety is added, as it often is in such situations, the individual experiences a blocking of perception in the sensations that signal ejaculatory inevitability.

Kaplan believes that the man does not allow himself to focus on internal pelvic sensations before orgasm, probably because of performance anxiety. Another explanation for the lack of attention may be distraction caused by guilt or fear even more basic than anxiety. Apparently, control is lacking because the man has not received or not allowed himself to receive the sensory feedback necessary to bring the reflex under control.

Treatment. Premature ejaculation is a reversible phenomenon. Treatment consists of learning to control or delay ejaculation by recognizing the signs of imminent ejaculation and then delaying it. Therapeutic principles include promoting the partner's cooperation, allowing the man to concentrate on his genital sensations and receive pleasure, and mastering a series of tasks that progressively provide for more intense genital stimulation.

Some of the most successful methods used to delay ejaculation include using the stop-start technique, changing the sexual position, and changing the tempo of thrusting during intercourse.[21] Each method requires the man to let his partner know when ejaculatory inevitability is reached. Semans' method,[31] or stop-start, requires the sexual partner to cease extravaginal stimulation of the penis until the ejaculation urge has subsided. The partner then renews stimulation. This is repeated at least four times, and then the man proceeds to ejaculate. Coital position is very important, since when the male is in an astride position, he has very little control over his ejaculation. When the man uses the bottom or side-to-side position, his ejaculatory control is definitely increased.[33] It is therefore suggested to the couple that the first coital sessions be done with the woman in the astride position with motionless vaginal containment. When the man can control his ejaculation in this position, female thrusting is included. Finally, male thrusting is included. Once ejaculatory control with the male thrusting is attained, then sexual intercourse in the lateral and man astride position is encouraged. By varying the tempo of thrusting from fast to slow, the man allows himself the time to focus on his internal pelvic sensations. It also gives him a chance to pay attention to what movements he finds overstimulating. Then by changing the activity, varying the position, or slowing down the thrusting tempo, he is more likely to slow down his ejaculatory reflex. Masters and Johnson report a 97.8% success rate in the treatment of premature ejaculation.[27] Kaplan reports almost 100% with Semans' technique.[14]

Retarded ejaculation (inhibited ejaculation)

Description. Retarded ejaculation is less common than premature ejaculation, but the exact incidence is unknown. It is interesting to note that the same fears, performance anxiety, and minimal commitment to the sexual partner will cause erectile difficulties in one man and retarded ejaculation in another.

Retarded or inhibited ejaculation is either primary or secondary. Primary retarded ejaculation is defined as the inability to ejaculate while being sexual with a partner. The cause for this is usually psychologic, such as fear of impregnating the partner or fear of loss of control. Secondary retarded ejaculation is defined as the inability to achieve normal ejaculations with a partner by a man previously able to do so. Secondary retarded ejaculation is usually a symptom of a problem within the relationship, but organic factors must be ruled out.

Organic factors that may cause inhibited ejaculation follow:
1. Neurologic disorders that interfere with the sympathetic innervation of the genitals
2. Diseases, such as Parkinson's, that cause central thalamic dysfunction
3. Antiadrenergic drugs, such as guanethidine and methyldopa, that block the autonomic sympathetic response and impair ejaculation

Treatment. Treatment is aimed at overcoming the mechanisms that inhibit ejaculation and resolving the underlying problems. A series of progressive sexual exercises are used by Kaplan to relieve fear and anxiety. The couple begin by using sexual techniques that are likely to evoke ejaculation. As the man is successful in the easiest and safest situation, he moves to progressively more difficult situations. Concurrently, therapy sessions are directed at developing client insight into fears and assisting with the interaction between the partners.[14] Success rates for Kaplan and for Masters and Johnson are approximately the same: 75% and 82%, respectively.

•   •   •

Zilbergeld's *Male Sexuality* is a very useful self-help guidebook for men experiencing sexual dysfunction. Most men have reported this book to be beneficial in helping them understand that they are not alone. This book provides specific information about and specific suggestions for dealing with male sexual dysfunction.

Female sexual dysfunction

The four most common sexual dysfunctions for women are inhibited sexual desire, orgasmic dysfunction, vaginismus, and dyspareunia.

Inhibited sexual desire

Description. As described in the section on male dysfunction, inhibited sexual desire involves loss of interest in being sexual. A woman's drive to have sex may be inhibited by physiologic, psychologic, interactional, and/or environmental factors. Again, a low sex drive is not necessarily a problem unless one's partner is dissatisfied with the lack of or limitations on sexual contact. When there is a discrepancy in sexual desire, the woman will invariably take responsibility for not meeting her partner's needs and feel guilty for her persistent refusals. In such a case therapy with both partners is advised, and both learn how they are contributing to the sexual distress.

Some assessment variables to consider with women presenting with inhibited sexual desire are use of birth control pills or replacement therapy, use of alcohol and drugs, a history of sexual abuse or incest, pain associated with intercourse, orgasmic dissatisfaction, vaginismus, and depression. All of these factors and many others mentioned under the section on etiology may contribute to a woman's lack of desire.

Treatment. Generally, treatment for women with inhibited sexual desire is the same as it is for men, although, as emphasized earlier, each case is different, and specific variables need to be approached individually. Initially the treatment follows the sensate focus exercises, with emphasis placed on understanding the mechanisms used to decrease and increase sexual desire. Both partners learn how they create and respond to sexual feelings, and communication is enhanced. Initiation and refusal of sexual contact are focused on, and the woman especially is taught how to say "no," as well as to ask for what she wants. The couple may need to develop means of creating the positive sexual tension that is necessary for desire to emerge and in the process may find that their schedules and life-style have not been conducive to creating an effective mental and physical environment. More frequently the couple learn the role that anger and unresolved conflict play in undermining their capacity for generating and maintaining sexual interest.

Behavioral and psychodynamic approaches blend to facilitate the therapeutic process for each couple; however, more research and experience is needed to refine the existing treatment models for this common yet complex presenting problem.

Orgasmic dysfunction

Description. It is estimated that between 30% and 50% of women report they have problems with orgasm.[10,11] Kaplan[13,16] states that in her experience 8% to 10% of women have never experienced an orgasm of any kind (primary orgasmic dysfunction), whereas 90% of women appear to achieve orgasm by some means. She breaks this estimate down as follows: no orgasm at all—10%; no orgasm with partner—10%; orgasm with intercourse plus clitoral "assistance"—50%; and orgasm during intercourse without clitoral "assistance"—30%. What is considered an orgasmic problem varies greatly among women (and their partners). There continues to be confusion about what type of orgasm is "normal" and what type is dysfunctional. Much of this is a residual of the vaginal-clitoral orgasm dichotomy developed by Freud. According to Masters and Johnson, there is considerable evidence to discount the psychoanalytic position of two types of female orgasm. They found all orgasms, whether facilitated by intercourse or direct clitoral stimulation, to be physiologically similar. Furthermore, female orgasms were not "either/or" but rather had both vaginal and clitoral components. There is new evidence (and debate) regarding the Gräfenberg spot, a sensitive area of the anterior wall of the vagina midway between the cervix and the vaginal opening. Recent studies claim that some women reach orgasm and ejaculate fluid through the urethra as a result of stimulation of this vaginal tissue.[29] Further investigation is needed for a definitive understanding of female genital anatomy and sexual response.

Orgasms may be inhibited because of lack of information, inadequate stimulation, or poor communication. Also, orgasm may have acquired some negative connotations for the woman because she fears loss of control, dependence on her partner, or the intensity of the experience. Other factors involved may be ambivalence about the relationship, fears of rejection, or guilt. On questioning a woman about her orgasmic response, it is not uncommon to discover that her expectations about how she "should" be responding are inordinately high. She and/or her partner may be gauging their sexual self-esteem by her "performance." This places pressure on both partners, and if orgasm is not achieved, she feels guilty, and he feels inadequate. Over time these emotions become entrenched, and sexual contact becomes more and more stressful.

Treatment. The easiest way for most women to learn to have orgasms is through self-stimulation while alone. The experience may then be transferred to being sexual with a partner. For most women who want to learn to have orgasms through masturbation, the preorgasmic women's group is the treatment of choice. (If a group is not available, individual counseling is appropriate.) The group provides support, education, and permission to be sexual. Graduated touching exercises are assigned, and the woman learns to focus on actual sensations rather than expected responses. As the woman progresses in her ability to give and receive self-pleasure, sexual fantasy and the use of a vibrator are often incorporated to enhance arousal. Through the combination of obtaining accurate information about their bodies,[8] gaining support and permission from other women, and learning their specific conditions for arousal, 93% of the women in Barbach's groups had an orgasm by the end of 10 sessions.[2] For more detailed information on group treatment for preorgasmic women, the reader is referred to Barbach's books *For Yourself* and *Women Discover Orgasm*.

After a woman is consistently reaching orgasm through masturbation the treatment may then proceed to her learning to have orgasms with a partner. The approach is often gradual—orgasm while he is in the room, to orgasm while he is holding her, to his stimulating her to orgasm. Through this step-by-step process, she learns what the physical, mental, relationship, and environmental components are that keep her from having orgasms with her partner. Areas to assess include the type and duration of stimulation she is receiving, the degree of communication between the partners, her feelings about herself and her partner, and any fears she may have about allowing herself to be sexual in the presence of her partner. Masters and Johnson report a 72.2% success rate in the treatment of secondary orgasmic dysfunction. The reader is referred to Barbach's *For Each Other* for further discussion.

Vaginismus

Description. Vaginismus is a relatively rare sexual dysfunction: approximately 2% to 3% of women experience it.[25] Anatomically, the genitals of a woman with vaginismus are normal, but whenever vaginal penetration is attempted, the muscles surrounding the vaginal orifice go into an involuntary spasm and close so tightly that penetration is impossible. The severity of this dysfunction is highly variable. For some women the vagina is closed so tightly that neither a finger nor a tampon can be inserted. For others, penetration is possible, but the result is severe pain. Apart from the physical pain caused by repeated attempts to penetrate, the woman may feel frightened, frustrated, humiliated, and inadequate. Fears of abandonment may also develop. It is not unusual that with time, the woman attempts to avoid all sexual activity. This helps relieve the anxiety, which then reinforces the avoidance pattern and the maintenance of vaginismus. The partner's reaction may vary depending on his psychologic and sexual vulnerability.

Vaginismus can be associated with other forms of female sexual dysfunction, but this is not always the case. Many women who seek treatment for vaginismus are sexually responsive and orgasmic. It is necessary to treat it as a separate syndrome and to rule out any physical conditions that may be causing it. A careful pelvic examination must always be done by a health care provider who is knowledgeable in detecting physical factors that contribute to sexual problems.

A wide variety of factors may cause vaginismus. The original stimulus can be psychologic or physical. Kaplan[13] believes that any adverse stimuli coupled with penetration can cause the conditioned response that associates pain or fear with sexual activity. Therefore painful penetration or trauma such as rape may lead to vaginismus. Other factors contributing to vaginismus include fear of men and ignorance about sex and childbirth, rigid restrictive attitudes that evoke guilt and anxiety, and hostility toward the partner.[13] For a further detailed discussion of etiology, the reader is referred to Fertel's article.[9]

Treatment. Treatment of vaginismus is aimed at modifying the immediate cause of the conditioned reflex. Psychologic causes are considered as they emerge in the treatment process. The two widely used approaches are those of Masters and Johnson and of Kaplan.

Masters and Johnson[25] believe that the most important step in treatment is to demonstrate the existence of the involuntary vaginal spasm to both partners in a carefully conducted pelvic examination. The woman is then taught exercises that effectively relax the muscles surrounding her vagina. She learns to deliberately tighten and release these muscles. She is then given a set of plastic dilators, ranging from the size of a finger to the size of a penis. She is shown how to insert the dilator herself, and using sufficient lubricating jelly, she keeps the dilator in place for 10 to 15 minutes at a time several times a day. She increases the size of the dilator as she experiences increasing comfort. When she feels ready, she invites her partner to join her in the exercises during which she guides and directs the nonsexual and sexual activity. She is then encouraged to become comfortable with her partner's finger in her vagina, and finally, at her direction, she inserts his penis.[25]

Kaplan believes the unconscious meanings of vaginismus, although interesting, are of limited relevance to treatment. Additionally, the insight-oriented approach is not uniformly effective. Her approach is aimed at modifying the immediate causal agent, and underlying causes are addressed only when they interfere with the therapy progress. The woman is encouraged to do the same vaginal dilation exercises as described by Masters and Johnson. When no muscle spasms occur, the couple is ready for penile penetration. The penis must be well lubricated and slowly inserted with the woman's direction and control. Penile containment lasts for a few minutes, and then the penis is slowly withdrawn. The couple continues to remain close and is directed to discuss what will make subsequent experiences less difficult.

Masters and Johnson[25] report a 98.8% success rate for their 83 cases. Kaplan states that 100% of clients can succeed by combining dilator desensitization with psychotherapeutic interventions.[9]

Dyspareunia

Description. Dyspareunia, or painful penetration, is likely to deter a woman from sexual arousal and orgasm. Pain may occur at any time during sexual activity and is sometimes experienced as a burning, sharp, searing, or cramping sensation. It can be external, within the vagina, or deep in the pelvic region or abdomen. The incidence of dyspareunia is unknown. Masters and Johnson[25] have found that approximately 15% of adult women experience coital discomfort on a few occasions during a year. They estimate that 1% to 2% of adult women have painful intercourse on more than an occasional basis.

Dyspareunia is most likely to have an organic rather than a psychologic origin. One of the major organic causes is a lack of adequate lubrication at the vaginal entrance or intravaginally. Usually this is the result of insufficient arousal, frequently caused by a lack of effective stimulation, cultural inhibitions, or relationship conflicts. Drugs such as antihistamines, certain tranquilizers, marijuana, and alcohol have a drying effect on the vaginal mucosa. Other physiologic causes may be estrogen deficiencies or diseases such as diabetes.

Vaginal discomfort can also be the result of fungal, bacterial, and trichomonal infections that cause the vaginal wall to become inflamed. The possibility of vaginal infections increases when vaginal walls become irritated with penetration and there is inadequate lubrication. The vaginal walls of some women can also become irritated when diaphragms, contraceptive jelly or cream, foam, or condoms are used. Pain at the opening to the vagina may be caused by irritation of Bartholin's glands, scar tissue at the opening, or an intact hymen.

Pain deep in the pelvis during coital thrusting may be caused by a jarring of the ovaries or stretching of the uterine ligaments. A woman may experience this only in certain positions or at certain times.

Other organic causes of dyspareunia may include pelvic disease, such as gonorrhea, neoplasms, endometriosis, cervicitis, clitoral pain, urethritis, or anal and bowel lesions. Organic causes of coital pain should always be investigated before searching for psychologic causes.

The psychologic problems associated with dyspareunia are usually complex and stem from fear or anxiety. The woman may fear becoming pregnant, feeling pain with penetration, and/or losing control. This fear may be experienced as pain, shame, or guilt. Some women may use pain as an "excuse" for not being sexual because they find saying "no" to sex too difficult.

Treatment. Organic causes for dyspareunia must be ruled out first. This is accomplished by obtaining a careful and detailed sex history and conducting a thorough physical and pelvic examination. Usually the organic cause will determine the appropriate treatment.

Psychologic causes are more complex and require exploration of the woman's fears, guilt, or shame about being sexual.

Summary

This chapter has reviewed the etiology and treatment of male and female sexual dysfunction. Key considerations for health care practice include the following:

1. The etiology of sexual dysfunction includes physiologic and psychologic components. In many instances a physical examination needs to be included in assessment.
2. Physiologic factors that may interfere with sexuality include illnesses, surgeries, and drugs that influence neural, vascular, and hormonal functioning.
3. Psychologic factors include fear of failure, guilt, anxiety, anger, fear of rejection, depression, poor communication, relationship conflict, fear of pregnancy, and a history of sexual abuse.
4. The most common therapy modalities used to treat sexual problems are those of Annon, Masters and Johnson, Kaplan, and group therapy.
5. The four most common dysfunctions for males are inhibited sexual desire, erectile dysfunction, premature ejaculation, and retarded ejaculation.
6. The four most common dysfunctions for females are inhibited sexual desire, orgasmic dysfunction, vaginismus, and dyspareunia.

Questions for review

1. Under what circumstances should a medical examination be included in the assessment of sexual dysfunction?
2. List four psychologic influences on sexual functioning.
3. Compare and contrast the general treatment modalities of Masters and Johnson and Kaplan.
4. What are three causative factors associated with erectile dysfunction?
5. Describe the major treatment components for primary orgasmic dysfunction.
6. What are two physiologic causes of dyspareunia?

References

1. Annon, J.S.: The behavioral treatment of sexual problems. I. Brief therapy, Honolulu, 1974, Enabling Systems, Inc.
2. Barbach, L.G.: Group treatment of preorgasmic women, Journal of Sex and Marital Therapy 1(2):139-145, 1974.
3. Barbach, L.G.: For yourself, New York, 1975, Doubleday & Co., Inc.
4. Barbach, L.G.: Women discover orgasm, New York, 1980, The Free Press.
5. Barbach, L.G.: For each other, Garden City, N.Y., 1982, Anchor Press.
6. Belliveau, F., and Richter, L.: Understanding human sexual inadequacy, Boston, 1970, Bantam Books, Inc.
7. Dickman, G., and Livingston, C.: Sex and the female ostomate, Los Angeles, 1982, United Ostomy Association, Inc.
8. Federation of Feminist Women's Health Centers: A new view of a woman's body, New York, 1981, Simon & Schuster, Inc.

9. Fertel, N.S.: Vaginismus: a review, Journal of Sex and Marital Therapy **3**(2):113-121, 1977.

10. Hite, S.: The Hite report, New York, 1976, Macmillan, Inc.

11. Hunt, M.: Sexual behavior in the 1970's, New York, 1974, Dell Publishing Co., Inc.

12. Kaplan, H.S.: The classifications of the female sexual dysfunctions, Journal of Sex and Marital Therapy **1**(2):124-138, 1974.

13. Kaplan, H.S.: The new sex therapy, New York, 1974, Brunner/Mazel, Inc.

14. Kaplan, H.S.: No nonsense therapy for six sexual malfunctions. Annual editions. In Barbour, J.R., editor: Focus: human sexuality 77/78, Guilford, Conn., 1978, The Dushkin Publishing Group, Inc.

15. Kaplan, H.S.: Disorders of sexual desire, New York, 1979, Simon & Schuster, Inc.

16. Kaplan, H.S.: Making sense of sex, New York, 1979, Simon & Schuster, Inc.

17. Kegel, A.H.: Sexual functions of the pubococcygeus muscle, Western Journal of Obstetrics and Gynecology **60**:521-524, 1952.

18. Kinsey, A.C., et al.: Sexual behavior in the human female, Philadelphia, 1953, W.B. Saunders Co.

19. Labowitz, W.C., and LoPiccolo, J.: New methods in the behavioral treatment of sexual dysfunction, Journal of Behavioral Therapy and Experimental Psychiatry **3**:265-271, 1972.

20. Levine, S.B.: Marital sexual dysfunction; erectile dysfunction, Annals of Internal Medicine **85**:342-350, 1976.

21. Livingston, C.: Premature ejaculation in young males, doctoral dissertation, San Francisco, 1981, Institute for Advanced Study of Human Sexuality.

22. Maddox, J.: Sexual health and health care, Postgraduate Medicine **58**(1):54, 1975.

23. Masters, W., and Johnson, V.: Human sexual response, Boston, 1966, Little, Brown & Co.

24. Masters, W., and Johnson, V.: Human sexual inadequacy, Boston, 1970, Little, Brown & Co.

25. Masters, W., Johnson, V., and Kolodny, R.: Human sexuality, Boston, 1982, Little, Brown & Co.

26. McCary, J.L.: Sexual myths and fallacies, New York, 1975, Schocken Books, Inc.

27. McCary, J.L.: McCary's human sexuality, ed. 3, New York, 1978, D. Van Nostrand Co.

28. McGuire, L.S., and Wagner, N.N.: Sexual dysfunction in women who were molested as children; one response pattern and suggestions for treatment, Journal of Sex and Marital Therapy **4**(1):11-15, 1978.

29. Perry, J.D., and Whipple, B.: Pelvic muscle strength of female ejaculators: evidence in support of a new theory of orgasm, Journal of Sex Research **17**(1):22-39, 1981.

30. Schiavi, R.C.: Sexuality and medical illness: specific reference to diabetes mellitus. In Green, R., editor: Human sexuality: a health practitioner's text, Baltimore, 1979, The Williams & Wilkins Co.

31. Semans, J.: Premature ejaculations; a new approach, Southern Medical Journal **49**:353-358, 1956.

32. Tsai, M., Feldman-Summers, S., and Edgar, M.: Childhood molestation variables related to differential impacts on psychosexual functioning in adult women, Journal of Abnormal Psychology 88(4):407-417, 1979.
33. Wabrek, A.J., and Wabrek, C.: Premature ejaculation, Connecticut Medicine 42:214-216, 1977.
34. Wilson, R.: Introduction to sexual counseling, Chapel Hill, N.C., 1974, Carolina Population Center.
35. Zilbergeld, B.: Group treatment of sexual dysfunction in men without partners, Journal of Sex and Marital Therapy 1(3):204-214, 1975.
36. Zilbergeld, B.: Male sexuality, Boston, 1978, Little, Brown & Co.

References for clients

Barbach, L.G.: For yourself, New York, 1975, Doubleday & Co., Inc.
Barbach, L.G.: For each other, Garden City, N.Y., 1982, Anchor Press.
Barbach, L.G., and Levine, L.: Shared intimacies: women's sexual experiences, Garden City, N.Y., 1981, Anchor Press.
Federation of Feminist Women's Health Centers: A new view of a woman's body, New York, 1981, Simon & Schuster, Inc.
Friday, N.: My secret garden: women's sexual fantasies, New York, 1973, Pocket Books.
Kassorla, I.: Nice girls do, Los Angeles, 1980, Stratford Press.
Zilbergeld, B.: Male sexuality, Boston, 1978, Little, Brown & Co.

III

Clinical aspects of human sexuality

9

Sexuality during pregnancy and lactation

NANCY FUGATE WOODS and GRETCHEN KRAMER DERY

Although proscriptions regulating sexual behavior have existed for centuries, perhaps the most commonly accepted, without question, by the medical and nursing professions are those related to the pregnant woman. Maternal sexuality may engender greater anxiety than other areas of sexuality. It has been suggested that in Western cultures there is a split between maternity and sexuality, resulting from the male dominance orientation of these cultures.[70] The taboo against maternal sexuality appears to involve not only the women and their partners but also health care practitioners.[59] The resulting lack of factual knowledge about the topic leads many practitioners to base their counsel on their own value-laden assumptions; others may avoid the topic completely.

Until recently not much was known about a woman's sexuality during pregnancy or the postpartum period. Minimal data were available about the effects of a pregnant woman's sexual practices on the fetus. The sexuality of the woman's husband or partner during the entire childbearing experience was not addressed. In recent years knowledge about the biophysical, intrapersonal, and interpersonal aspects of pregnancy has been advanced. It is the purpose of this chapter to acquaint health professionals with the findings of recent studies and theoretic formulations relevant to an understanding of sexuality during pregnancy and the postpartum period, including lactation, as a basis for rational counseling of the pregnant, postpartal, and lactating woman and her sexual partner.

Sexuality during pregnancy

Despite growing concern over sexuality, the influence of pregnancy on a woman's sexual behavior is not thoroughly understood. As early as the 1940s, investigators began an attempt to identify specific behaviors exhibited during pregnancy, especially those related to sexual functioning. Robertson,[68] in a study of 100 pregnancies, found that unwanted sexual intercourse and an absence of orgasm were frequently associated with the nausea and vomiting of pregnancy. In 100% of the women with severe nausea sexual function was disturbed, as opposed to 9% in the control group. It was not clear whether there was a cause-and-effect relationship.

153

By the 1950s an attempt was made to identify the stage of pregnancy at which the woman and her partner discontinued vaginal intercourse. In a sample of 500 unselected pregnant women in Louisville who delivered between November 1952 and February 1953 the median time for discontinuing coitus was 28 days before delivery and the average time 52 days.[63] A study of 260 women in the Seattle area, conducted nearly 20 years later, indicated that a decrease in coital frequency occurred between the eighth and ninth months of pregnancy: approximately 25% of the women in the sample abstained from coitus during the eighth month, as opposed to nearly 60% during the ninth month.[76]

Although the literature points to the last month of pregnancy as the time during which sexual behavior patterns change drastically, the biologic changes in the woman's body occur gradually throughout her pregnancy. Masters and Johnson[41] documented several changes in the woman's anatomy and physiology directly implicated in her sexual functioning. First, definite enlargement of the breasts is seen with pregnancy as a result of an increase in their vascularity and development of the glandular components of the breasts. It was noted that when nulliparous women responded to sexual stimulation during the first trimester, the venous congestion in their breasts became more obvious than when the women were not pregnant. Women had breast tenderness during advanced sexual tension early in their pregnancies, sometimes reaching severe proportions. This tenderness was usually experienced in turgid nipples and engorged alveoli. During the second and third trimesters breast tenderness tended to decrease.

The pelvic viscera also become markedly vascular during pregnancy, and an awareness of increased sexual tension develops during the first and early second trimester. Six women studied extensively by Masters and Johnson[41] reported extremely high levels of sexual tension during the second and third trimesters. Four women reported abdominal cramping and aching during and after orgasm in the first trimester, and two women complained of low backache. A subjective awareness of increased uterine irritability was reported by these same women. During the second trimester these women revealed an awareness of strong sexual drives marked by an increased interest in coital and manipulative activity. They reported fulminating orgasmic experiences.

Some of the changes reported by Masters and Johnson's sample[41] of pregnant women were phase specific to the human sexual response cycle. During excitement multiparous women experienced impressive engorgement of the labia majora. The labia minora enlarged two to three times their unstimulated size, and during the third trimester the labia minora were chronically engorged with blood. Near the end of the first trimester an increase in vaginal lubrication was noted: this phenomenon was enhanced in both rapidity and amount. All of the subjects complained of a light mucoid vaginal discharge. The tenting phenomenon of the uterus in the transcervical vaginal depth was not demonstrated in these subjects after the first trimester.

During the plateau phase the only change visualized related to the engorgement of the entire vaginal barrel. With more advanced pregnancy, there was more intense venous engorgement.

During the third trimester the orgasmic platform appeared to be so overdistended that any objective evidence of its contractile efficiency was obscured. During orgasm, spasm of the uterus in third-trimester women was observed for as long as a minute. Fetal heart tones were slowed during this period, but there was no further evidence of fetal distress reported.

The resolution phase was altered in the pregnant subjects, since the vasocongested pelvis was frequently not completely relieved. A residual vasocongestion was often translated into a continued feeling of sexual stimulation. The investigators concluded that the residual pelvic vasocongestion, accompanied by pelvic pressure from uteri in second- and third-trimester women, yielded sustained high levels of sexual tension.

Masters and Johnson[41] also interviewed 111 women during their second, sixth, and eighth months of pregnancy. The subjects were young, with an average age of 27 years, and well educated, with an average of 2 years 3 months of college education. The investigators found rather revealing concerns related to pregnancy and sexuality.

During the first trimester a great variation in levels of eroticism and in the effectiveness of the woman's sexual performance was reported. Among forty-three nulliparous women, there was a decrease in sexual functioning and effectiveness that the investigators attributed to nausea, sleepiness, and chronic fatigue. Over half of these women reported fear of injury to the unborn child as a result of intercourse. In unmarried women there was little reported eroticism during the first trimester, probably because they were overwhelmed with the social aspects of the pregnancy. Four of the nulliparous women indicated heightened interest in sex, and six women reported no change. Among the parous women in the sample, sixty-eight reported little change, seven had nausea and vomiting and accompanying decreased sexual interest, and four reported heightened interest.

During the second trimester there was a marked increase in eroticism and effectiveness of sexual performance among this sample. This finding conflicts with those of Solberg, Butler, and Wagner.[76] Eighty-two of the 111 women in Masters and Johnson's sample[41] reported a significant improvement in their sexual performance well beyond that which they had experienced in their nonpregnant state. Even the unmarried women reported feeling heightened sexual awareness during this period.

During the third trimester the nulliparous women experienced a significant decrease in coital frequency, as opposed to the second trimester. For thirty-one of the forty nulliparous women continence had been prescribed by the physician for periods of 4 weeks to 3 months, which may account for the decrease in sexual activity. During this period women reported more somatic complaints, with pelvic tension and backache being of special interest. Thirty-three of the forty nulliparous women reported losing interest in sexual activity gradually throughout the third trimester.

Sexual activity for parous women was restricted by physicians for forty-six of the sixty-one women. Forty-one of these women reported a decrease in sexual interest and frequency of intercourse as their due date approached; sixty-eight of the women were concerned about the medical contraindications for intercourse.

Twenty of the women reported that their husbands withdrew from sex late in the second or early in the third trimester. They attributed the withdrawal to the appearance of their large abdomens, the husband's concern for their personal comfort, and fear of injuring the fetus.

Solberg, Butler, and Wagner's later study[76] of 260 women from the Seattle area who were interviewed in the immediate postpartum period revealed that there was a nearly linear decrease in coital frequency for the women who continued to have intercourse during their pregnancies. The frequency of coitus was significantly age related, with younger women tending to be more active. Length of marriage was also a significant variable, being inversely related to coital frequency. Frequency of intercourse during pregnancy was not related to race, religious preference, education of the woman or her partner, negative feelings about pregnancy, or whether or not the pregnancy was planned. During the last 2 months of pregnancy frequency of intercourse was not related to the length of the marriage. Women who were not frequently orgasmic tended not to have coitus often during the second trimester and the eighth month, but this relationship was not apparent for any other period during their pregnancies. The woman's interest in sex during her pregnancy was the variable most consistently associated with her coital frequency. Those who reported a diminished interest in sexual activity tended to have lower frequencies of coitus than those whose interest level was maintained or increased during pregnancy; in this sample interest level was not associated with age, length of marriage, or parity.

Rates of orgasm with coitus seemed to diminish as the pregnancy progressed. In addition, there appeared to be a decrease in the strength or intensity of orgasm during pregnancy as compared to prepregnancy experience. It was pointed out by the investigators that a percentage of women consistently reported an increase in intensity of orgasm at all stages of their pregnancies. The woman's ability to enjoy orgasm was related to frequency of coitus during the first, second, and early third trimesters. Those women who were orgasmic were more likely to continue coitus during pregnancy. Rate of orgasm throughout the pregnancy was related to sexual interest levels as expressed by the sample.

Other patterns of sexual behavior were studied in addition to intercourse. Of a portion of the sample who masturbated before pregnancy, fewer masturbated during pregnancy. Orgasmic rate subsequent to masturbation did not change during pregnancy. Manual stimulation by the woman's partner was used by some women in the sample, and its frequency of use also decreased during pregnancy. Orgasmic rates from manual manipulation did not change significantly during pregnancy. Oral-genital stimulation was also used by some of the women in the sample, but orgasmic rates from cunnilingus declined with the advanced stages of pregnancy.

Another variable in sexual behavior that changed with pregnancy was coital position. The use of the male-astride position declined as the use of other positions, especially the side-by-side position, increased with the advancement of pregnancy. The variability in coital position also decreased throughout pregnancy, probably because of changes in the woman's contour. There did not appear to be any relationship between coital position and rate of orgasm.

Solberg, Butler, and Wagner[76] queried those women in their sample who reported a change in the degree or intensity of their sexual experience during pregnancy. Of these women, 46% attributed changes in their patterns of sexual behavior to physical discomfort; 27% to fear of injury to the baby; 23% to loss of interest; 17% to awkwardness having intercourse; 6% to reasons unrelated to pregnancy; and 4% to the woman's imagined loss of attractiveness. In only 8% of the sample was a change in sexual activity during pregnancy attributed to the recommendation of a physician. Women who did receive instructions about coital abstention from their doctors were informed to refrain from intercourse anywhere from 2 to 8 weeks before their due dates.

Kenny,[32] in a study of thirty-three women, defined sexual functioning in terms of four parameters: desire, frequency, enjoyment, and orgasm. When comparing the prepregnancy period with the first two trimesters, he found they were similar. During the third trimester he noted a decrease in frequency, desire, and enjoyment, but orgasm remained essentially the same. He also noted that the third trimester might be looked at as two time periods in future studies, since it is essentially the last 6 weeks and not the entire period when there appears to be a decrease in sexual functioning.

Falicov,[16] in a study population of nineteen primigravidas, interviewed the participants at five points during their pregnancies and twice during the postpartum period. The three aspects of sexuality measured in this study were frequency of coitus, degree of sexual desire or interest, and feelings of eroticism and sexual satisfaction. By the end of the first trimester fourteen of the nineteen subjects had experienced a moderate or marked decrease in all three aspects. Certain factors mentioned as affecting this decline were physiologic signs and symptoms, such as nausea, vomiting, and heartburn. Increased severity of symptoms was associated with decreased sexual activity. In addition, somatic complaints directly related to sexual functioning were reported. These included the vagina feeling smaller, making penetration painful, and vaginal numbness, making orgasm more difficult to achieve. Fear of harming the fetus, even though many subjects recognized this as unfounded, persisted and hampered engagement in intercourse for ten of the nineteen subjects.

In the second trimester coital frequency and sexual satisfaction slightly increased relative to the first trimester yet remained below prepregnancy levels. Sexual desire did not change from the decreased levels of the first trimester. Continued factors mentioned by women during this period were tiredness, breast tenderness, and discomfort in the genital area. Beginning need for modification of position and movements was seen as interfering with sexual satisfaction. Fear of harming the fetus remained for nine of the eighteen subjects but appeared to lessen in intensity.

During the seventh and eighth months seven subjects reported fluctuations in sexual desire. Half the women who had previously reported decreased eroticism found intercourse more relaxed and enjoyable than during previous stages. The fear of harming the fetus was diminished at this time. Despite the relative increase in sexual interest, by the eighth month fifteen of eighteen women had stopped sexual intercourse. Two couples subsequently stopped 3 weeks before the due dates, and one couple did not stop.

Husbands' and wives' attitudes related to changes in sexual adjustment throughout the pregnancy were variable and ranged from bland acceptance to intense frustration. However, certain attitudes tended to predominate at certain phases of the pregnancy. The first trimester was characterized by acceptance, the second by a feeling that sexual interaction was an avenue for effective communication, the early third by frustration and resentment at abstinence, and the latter third by acceptance.

Five of the subjects were advised by their physicians to stop coital activity at a time before their due dates, and the general recommendation was 6 to 7 weeks.

Morris[45] reported data from a population sample of 114 pregnant Thai women. The data were originally collected from a cross-sectional field sample of pregnant and non-pregnant Thai women as a part of a fertility survey in 1967 and 1968. The women were interviewed on a weekly basis and asked whether they had had sexual intercourse on the day of interview and on each remaining day of the previous week. Since the focus of the original study was fertility-relevant behavior, the only sexually relevant question related to the occurrence of intercourse. The 114 pregnant women were also compared with 490 nonpregnant women included in the overall sample.

Nonpregnant women reported no intercourse more often than women in the first trimester of pregnancy. There was a consistent downward trend in frequency in the pregnant women as pregnancy advanced. The differences in frequency between the pregnant and nonpregnant women were not statistically significant until the seventh month. The decline was not linear, and a greater decrease was seen in the last trimester than the previous two. In the ninth month 72.7% of the pregnant women reported no intercourse.

Tolor and Di Granzia[80] studied sexual attitudes and behavior patterns that could be associated with pregnancy and childbirth. Included in the subject population were 216 women who were attended by several physicians in an obstetric-gynecologic group practice. Four groups were defined from the population as follows: fifty-four women in their first trimester, fifty-one women in their second trimester, fifty-six women in their third trimester, and fifty-five women in the postpartum period. Each voluntary participant was given a questionnaire seeking information about present and previous sexual behavior. Also administered was an Attitude Toward Sex Scale, measuring sexual conservatism versus liberalism.

At this point only the three groups consisting of pregnant subjects will be considered. A significant between-group difference was obtained when looking at reported desire for intercourse, indicated by a progressive decline in desire for intercourse during pregnancy. There was also a considerably reduced frequency of coitus during the third trimester, wherein almost one of every three women completely abstained. Another significant difference between the three pregnant groups was in the area of preference for sexual relations. Women in the first and second trimester were generally satisfied with the current rate of sexual activity, whereas women in the third trimester were less satisfied and preferred either increased or decreased activity from what prevailed. There was also a significantly greater incidence of occasional multiple orgasms in women in the second trimester and a significantly greater occurrence of complete lack of multiple orgasms in women in the third trimester. There was a significant decline in interest levels in sex as the pregnancy progressed.

The degree of conservatism or liberalism in sexual attitudes was not found to be significantly related to sexual behaviors or attitudes toward sex during pregnancy.

Holtzman[28] conducted a retrospective study of sexual practices during pregnancy. She interviewed twenty-five women during the second to fifth day postpartum. Prepregnancy levels of interest in sexual relations follow: 56% very interested, 40% moderately interested, and 4% not interested. Frequently of intercourse showed a linear decline throughout pregnancy, and frequency of orgasm decreased with advancing pregnancy.

Comparing prepregnancy with pregnancy, there was a decrease in masturbation. Oral-genital sex showed a slight first trimester increase from prepregnancy levels and a decrease in the latter two thirds of the pregnancy. The practice of mutual masturbation never reached prepregnancy levels, but there was a slight rise in this practice during the third trimester when compared with the first or second trimester.

Positions used during pregnancy were varied, but there was a marked decrease in the use of the male-astride position.

Over half the women received counsel from medical personnel. Recommendations included the following: ten women were told to do anything as long as it remained comfortable; three were told not to have sex; one was told not to have intercourse past the twenty-eighth week; and one was told not to have intercourse past the thirty-sixth week.

The reasons the woman's male partner gave for decreasing or stopping intercourse were in order of increasing mention: loss of interest, physical awkwardness, fear of injuring the woman, fear of injuring the baby, and the woman's request.

Twenty-one of the women in this study reported that their partners found them more attractive while pregnant; three women reported no change; and one woman reported that her partner found her less attractive.

Pasini,[59] in a review of his work done in 1974, reports on data from interviews with 100 women during the postpartum period. Sexual desire, sexual satisfaction, and frequency were related. Parity influenced sexuality, as reported by Masters and Johnson (1966), with primiparous women experiencing a decline and multiparous women experiencing an improvement, especially after the first 3 months. Overall, sexual behavior diminished progressively as pregnancy proceeded.

Women attributed the decrease in frequency to physical symptoms such as nausea and vomiting. The psychic state was also influential. Well-adjusted women noted no change. Women who possessed either extremely positive or extremely negative attitudes toward the pregnancy noted that there was a concomitant positive or negative effect on their sexuality.

The women's male partners were influential, with half of them deciding to reduce the frequency of sexual acts. They expressed concern for the safety of the fetus. Changes in behavior toward the pregnant women, such as increased attention and understanding, were generally positive.

Battacchi et al.,[2] in an attempt to replicate Pasini's work, investigated general emotional problems during pregnancy, with special attention directed toward sexual frustration. A questionnaire was administered to 500 women in the first days after delivery. Three aspects of sexuality—satisfaction, frequency of coitus, and libido—were studied. Women noting an improvement in their sex life in the first trimester were a modest part of the sample (satisfaction, 10.4%; frequency, 8.2%; libido, 10.2%). The proportion noting improvement increased slightly in the second trimester (satisfaction, 12.6%; frequency, 10.6%; and libido, 14.2%). The proportion noting improvement then dropped during the third trimester, with 3.0% noting an increase in satisfaction, 2.6% noting an increase in frequency, and 8.2% noting an increase in libido. A larger number of women noted a decrease in these three parameters beginning in the first trimester (satisfaction, 36%; frequency, 44.6%; and libido, 28.2%) and a continuing and increasing drop in the second trimester (satisfaction, 48.8%; frequency, 56.2%; libido, 34.4%) and third trimester (satisfaction, 73%; frequency, 85%; and libido 52.2%).

Of the three dimensions studied, libido underwent the least alteration, and the number of women having a lowered libido was always inferior to the number of women showing lowered satisfaction and frequency.

The influence of previous pregnancy on satisfaction was analyzed for the second trimester. Primiparous women constituted the largest percentage of women noting reduction in satisfaction (49.7%). The highest percentage of women stating no change in satisfaction (45.3%) was among women with one previous pregnancy, and multigravidas constituted the highest percentage (27.8%) of women experiencing an increase in satisfaction.

Fears, including fear of miscarriage and fear of intercourse damaging the fetus or causing abortion, were related to a reduction of satisfaction during the second trimester.

There was a strong and significant relationship between changes in satisfaction and changes in the partner's sexual behavior; 80% of women noting increases in satisfaction also noted behavior changes in their partners, as well as 76.7% of women noting a decrease in satisfaction.

Battacchi et al. also looked at communication and counsel between the pregnant woman and the obstetrician. Only 28% of the pregnant women and 23% of the physicians addressed the topic of sexuality spontaneously. Obstetricians gave advice to 257 women in the study, with only a small percentage of advice begin justified by the woman's physical condition. Often rationale for advice was not included, and the most frequent advice was to refrain from coitus during the entire pregnancy (15%).

Obstetric parameters that influenced frequency negatively were the presence of relevant pathology, previous problem pregnancies, toxemia, and nausea and vomiting.

Lumley[38] reported on a prospective study of twenty-six Australian primigravidas that was conducted as part of a larger study related to attitudes toward the fetus. Interviews were conducted during each trimester, after childbirth, and at 3 months postpartum. At this point only the data related to the pregnancy will be considered. The frequency of sexual intercourse declined progressively from the first to the third trimesters for the majority of the women. There was, however, an increase in libido and frequency noted for 11% during the second trimester.

The two most frequent reasons given for avoidance or dislike of sexual intercourse during the first trimester were fear of harming the fetus and nausea and vomiting. During the second trimester fear of harming the fetus and the general stress of the pregnancy on the marital relationship were the two most frequent reasons offered. During the third trimester physical awkwardness and loss of interest were most frequently cited as reasons for the decline.

Ellis[15] developed a questionnaire to ascertain the sexual needs and concerns of expectant couples. The categories of needs were physical satisfaction and comfort, self-esteem, knowledge and understanding, communication, and love and dependency. Fifteen expectant couples attending prenatal classes completed questionnaires.

Regarding physical satisfaction and comfort, there was a decline in the enjoyment of sexual intercourse over the period of pregnancy for both men and women. Several individuals indicated sexual interest in individuals other than their mates during pregnancy. The majority of the women felt that their bodies were viewed positively by their mates. Couples stated their current source of information about sexual activity, and physicians were a desired source of information but were not being used.

More than a fourth of the respondents indicated a desire for comfortable communication and expression of needs. Twenty-eight respondents indicated that women need more emotional support during pregnancy, and nineteen also felt men needed more emotional support.

Robson, Brant, and Kumar[69] more recently conducted a longitudinal survey of maternal emotional health during pregnancy and the first year postpartum. A total of 119 women were interviewed at approximately 12, 24, and 36 weeks' gestation and at 1, 12, 26, and 52 weeks after delivery.

The women retrospectively reported higher rates of intercourse during the month before pregnancy than at any other time during the survey. Changes in frequency occurred throughout the pregnancy but in a nonlinear manner. Seven women reported an increase in frequency of sexual intercourse during the first trimester. Forty-three women reported an increase between the first and second trimester, but a similar number reported a decrease, making the overall pattern for the first and second trimester very similar. There was a sharp reduction in sexual activity in the third trimester.

Twenty-five of the women in this sample derived little or no pleasure from sexual intercourse before pregnancy. These women were more likely to stop engaging in intercourse in the first trimester or to continue experiencing minimal pleasure. The proportion of women not enjoying sexual intercourse during the second trimester fell from 41% to 24%. The most marked change occurred during the third trimester, when only 40% of the women continued to find intercourse pleasurable.

Overall, the two variables, frequency of sexual intercourse and enjoyment of sexual intercourse, were significantly related throughout pregnancy.

Orgasm before pregnancy occurred on at least half the occasions of intercourse for 74% of the women. During the first and second trimesters this decreased to 60%. During the third trimester 42% of the subjects who were still having intercourse had orgasms at least half of the time.

Libido during early pregnancy was described as reduced in sixty-five women, unchanged in thirty-eight, and increased in sixteen.

Effects of pregnancy on the need for closeness. It has been noted[6] that an increased need for noncoital touching, cuddling, and closeness may be experienced during pregnancy by some women or couples. Hollender and McGehee[27] analyzed the wish to be held during pregnancy. Thirty-five women were asked to recall their feelings about being held during pregnancy. Half of these women remembered a change in desire for body contact, and for two thirds of these the change was toward an increased wish to be held.

Information was also obtained from fifty women in the prenatal period during their first medical examination. These women were asked whether the current pregnancy affected their wish to be held. Twenty-three reported an increase, nineteen reported no change, and eight reported a decrease. These findings were consistent with those obtained during retrospective questioning.

Thirty women in this study had been pregnant before. When asked about their previous pregnancy and their desire to be held, ten women reported an increase, six reported a decrease, and fourteen stated that there was no change.

Thus, when women did report a change, they were two to three times more likely to report an increase. This was consistent in situations in which pregnant women reported on past or current pregnancies or when nonpregnant women reported on a previous pregnancy.

Tolor and Di Granzia's study[80] of 216 pregnant and postpartal women also documented a high need for close physical contact during pregnancy that continued into the early postpartum period. Along with this finding they also noted that when these women did not want to have intercourse, being held was the most frequently selected preferred alternative.

Effects of body image on the expectant woman/couple. Another variable influencing the woman's psychologic outlook during pregnancy, and in turn her sexuality, is the image she has of her changing body. Pigment changes, breast alterations, the growth of her abdomen, and uncertainty about her future sexual function may all cause her to question her body competence or conversely find increasing pleasure in it. It follows that the woman's altered self-image may in turn influence her sexual self-concept and sexual behavior.

In one series 200 patients who requested treatment of nausea and vomiting during pregnancy, eighty patients with excessive weight gain, and fifty patients who had no nausea with their past or present pregnancies were evaluated by means of a psychosociosexual questionnaire. Patients in the group plagued by nausea evaluated their sexuality in a favorable fashion similar to that of the control group. The women who gained weight rated themselves poorly: only 50% considered themselves attractive, as compared to 85% in the other groups. The women in the "weight-gaining" group were also concerned regarding their husbands' fidelity: 16% questioned it.[73]

Most of the women who experienced nausea and vomiting and those who gained excessive weight enjoyed coitus (92% and 93%, respectively). More women (75%) in the groups with nausea and vomiting tended to experience orgasm than those in the weight-gaining group (60%). These findings contrast sharply with earlier theories that the nausea and vomiting of pregnancy were linked to the threat of coitus and the disgust experienced immediately after intercourse. The patients in the weight-gaining group, in contrast, were thought to experience conflict, best exemplified by their poor concepts of their own sexuality.[73] These findings lend credence to the relationship previously proposed between body image and sexuality.

Interpersonal aspects of sexuality and pregnancy. Throughout pregnancy, society and culture shape many of the woman's feelings and behavior. It is significant that values and mores also influence the nature of the relationship between the future mother and father.

Response to pregnancy. Mead and Newton[43] report that cultural patternings significantly shape the couple's reaction to pregnancy. First, there is usually a sense of responsibility for the growth of the unborn child. Beliefs often link parents' behavior to the health and welfare of the fetus, thus providing grounds for parental guilt associated with malformation or illness of the child. That coitus might harm or endanger the fetus is a fear common to many of the women interviewed in studies mentioned earlier in this chapter.

In several societies a solicitous approach to the pregnant woman is evident. Protective tendencies, especially those seen among men, may contribute to intercourse prohibitions at varying points in the pregnancy.

Among some cultural groups, pregnancy may be seen as evidence of sexual adequacy. In fact in some societies marriages are not finalized until the bride proves her fertility by becoming pregnant. In many cultures pregnancy may be welcomed, especially if it is highly prized by polygamous husbands. In Western society pregnancy may be used in an attempt to solidify a marriage or ward off divorce.

In yet other societies pregnancy may be viewed as a time of debilitation, with the woman seen as being particularly vulnerable. Western culture has subtly moved to regarding pregnancy as an illness and has devised an elaborate system of prevention and treatment for the "condition."[26]

Finally, pregnancy may be seen as a time for reticence or shame. This feeling may be related to fear that evil spirits will harm the fetus if the pregnancy is publicized or to the fact that the woman must publicly acknowledge the coitus that produced it.[43] In many instances pregnancy is politely ignored to spare the mother-to-be embarrassment about her "condition."

Marital and maternal roles. The social relationship most affected by pregnancy is usually that between the marital partners. In a review of parental attitude development during pregnancy Jessner, Weigert, and Foy[31] point out that role conflicts exist from the start. Humans are the only mammals capable of enjoying sexual activity and mothering a relatively dependent infant simultaneously; however, the mother/lover conflict arises from this ability.

Weisskopf[84] proposes the existence of an ideology of "asexual motherhood" as a cultural belief system in the United States. This belief system purports that mothers, especially good mothers, are not and should not be sexual persons. A substantial group of women have internalized this ideology, which results in considerable psychologic pain. Weisskopf notes that the psychoanalytic theorists and the biosocial theorists differ dramatically as to what they feel the proper relationship between maternity and sexuality should be. Psychoanalytic theorists argue that a mature woman's sexuality is harnessed for, or separated from, motherhood. Biosocial theorists propose that sexual gratification can and should be an important bonus accompanying motherhood.

LaRossa[35] conducted a study related to the workings of the husband-wife system during the first pregnancy. As part of this study, he addressed husbands' and wives' reasons for changes in prenatal sexuality. Using a symbolic interactionist framework, he described reasons or motives as basically consisting of aligning actions that orient people toward each other and integrate deviant conduct with the existing culture. Sexual changes (especially decreases) occurring during pregnancy had potential for being perceived as a form of deviance and a violation of the rules of the marital game unless a husband and wife could construct an acceptable "why" (an aligning action) to make sense of their behavior. Sixteen couples were conjointly interviewed during the twelfth, twentieth, twenty-eighth, and thirty-sixth weeks of the women's first pregnancies. The researchers categorized the couples' reasons for changing sexuality into *excuses* and *justifications*. Excuses were defined as accounts by which one admits an act is bad but denies full responsibility for it. Justifications were described as accounts by which a person accepts full responsibility for an act, while denying the negative quality associated with it. Excuses were divided into physiologic/anatomic types and biographic/sociocultural types. Justifications were divided into appeals to self-fulfillment and appeals to priorities. Twelve couples experienced a decline in frequency, and two couples reported no sexual change. A qualitative analysis of the interview transcripts resulted in the identification of four types of explanations: biographic/sociocultural excuses (40% of reasons given by husbands and wives), appeals to priorities (28%), physiologic/anatomic excuses (22%), and appeals to self-fulfillment (10%). This distribution conflicts with the previously mentioned Solberg, Butler, and Wagner[76] study, in which women emphasized physiologic/anatomic reasons.

One of the major role changes seen frequently in the couple who await the birth of a child is a tendency toward increased dependency on the part of the wife. This tendency, along with physiologic changes, may elicit protective behavior on the part of the husband.

To add to the complexity of role alterations, the childhood concepts of both husband and wife may lead to changes in sexual behavior patterns. The idea of intercourse may be irreconcilable with a puritanic concept of "motherhood."[31] Breast-feeding, with breasts as an either/or phenomenon—either as sexual objects *or* as mechanisms for feeding or nurturing—further adds to the confusion.

Selby and Calhoun[72] considered sexual desire and behavior of couples as a function of marital satisfaction. Twenty-five couples were divided into high, moderate, and low satisfaction groups. In this study women reported a decrease in sexual desire over the pregnancy, whereas men reported an increase. Both men and women reported decreased frequency in sexual behavior. In general, for women, the highest marital satisfaction was associated with highest sexual desire and highest frequency of sexual behavior. Men with high sexual desire and high satisfaction appeared to have moderate levels of marital satisfaction. This pattern appeared to be stable across pregnancy. Selby and Calhoun indicate that this pattern may suggest that in many cases the sexual desire of the woman is the controlling influence on the occurrence of sexual behavior in expectant couples.

Overall, there is little information and considerable confusion about motherhood, including breast-feeding, and sexuality. Reinforcing a split between sexuality and motherhood fragments a woman's experience. To be both a mother and a sexual being is a woman's right. There are few studies of what constitutes harmful erotic interaction between mothers and children. Research questions are numerous, since the topic has not been investigated thoroughly.

Since the extended family is no longer geographically near, some of the cultural supports associated with pregnancy are no longer available. This situation may provide part of the impetus for involving the father in more of a "participant" role in the birth process.

Historically men have experienced couvade in many cultures. This mimicry of labor pains and postpartum weakness on the part of the father supposedly provided for a closeness between father and child. An interesting parallel might be the new trend of encouraging the father to be actively involved in the delivery of his child. Formal preparation and attendance at delivery can positively influence the father's perception of his role and his relationship with his wife.[14]

Taylor and Langer[79] suggest that reactions in pregnancy very closely simulate reactions to physically stigmatized persons. They designed two experiments to support their hypotheses. The first dealt with avoidance, and they hypothesized that when strangers interact with a pregnant woman, they increase their interpersonal distance by standing farther from her than they would a nonpregnant woman. In a forced choice situation there was a strong preference demonstrated for standing next to a nonpregnant experimenter, and men avoided the pregnant experimenter significantly more than women did.

A laboratory experiment was also performed to assess the effect of the pregnant woman's behavior as well. Making the assumption that the traditional role of women is passive versus assertive, they hypothesized that for pregnant women, role proscriptions would be more rigid. They predicted that a passive pregnant woman would be more accepted than an assertive one and that passiveness and assertiveness would not predict as strongly the acceptance of the nonpregnant woman. Results demonstrated that the pregnant women was liked more by women if she was passive, whereas the nonpregnant woman was liked more by women if she was assertive. The assertive woman, regardless of her state, was preferred by men.

These authors propose that the pregnant woman is traditionally expected to withdraw from many activities where she would ordinarily interact with others. Consequently, pregnant women are infrequently seen. When they do appear in public, a common response might be male staring and female disapproval. These responses could cause a pregnant woman discomfort and embarrassment and lead to further withdrawal on her part, promoting a cyclical phenomenon.

Summary. There remains controversy in the literature about a woman's sexual behavior during pregnancy. Some theorists suggest that pregnancy enhances the woman's sexual pleasure, whereas others believe that pregnancy has an overall deleterious effect on a woman's sexual activity. Multiple factors appear to be implicated in influencing a woman's sexual behavior during the pregnancy experience. The fact remains that in most studies, despite trends in sexual appetite and practices during pregnancy, there consistently remains a wide variability in individual differences in all areas studied.

Intrapartum sexuality

In a comparison of coitus and undisturbed, undrugged childbirth, Newton[55] notes several similarities. First, breathing becomes deeper during sexual excitement and early labor; it may be interrupted, however, in coitus as orgasm approaches, and the breath may be held during the second stage of labor. Next, the woman tends to make gasping noises as orgasm approaches, much as she does during the second stage of labor. As orgasm approaches, the woman tends to have what might appear to be a "tortured expression"; a strained look may appear on the face of the mother as birth approaches. It is interesting to note that twelve of Masters and Johnson's subjects[41] described sensations during late labor that progressed through orgasm.

Baxter,[3] in the previously mentioned study, reported a positive correlation between an increase in coital orgasm rate and the length of the second stage of labor. This relationship persisted when controlling for forceps-assisted delivery, which was also positively correlated with increased length of the second stage and an increased coital orgasm rate. Baxter suggests that perhaps orgasm and delivery may share a common mechanism.

In both childbirth and orgasm the uterus contracts rhythmically, and the mucous plug from the cervix loosens. Contraction of abdominal muscles during orgasm is not unlike the bearing down as delivery approaches. Positions for childbirth and coitus are not dissimilar for women in the United States, and in both cases women become less inhibited. Muscle strength and flexibility are both enhanced during coitus and childbirth. Finally, sensory perception may be dulled as delivery and orgasm approach, but both are usually followed by feelings of well-being or joy.

Newton[55] maintains that women are trebly sensuous: they enjoy aspects of parturition and lactation, as well as coitus. Newton bases her thesis on the premise that these three activities are interrelated both physiologically and psychologically. First, all three are based on closely related neurohormonal reflexes; oxytocin is believed to be involved in all three processes. Next, in all three activities the woman is sensitive to her environment, and certain stimuli may inhibit labor, coitus, or breast-feeding. Finally, all three seem to trigger caretaking.

Sexuality of postpartal and lactating women

Masters and Johnson's sample[41] was also studied during the postpartum period. In general there was decreased sexual tension during this period, attributable to fatigue, weakness, pain, vaginal discharge, and personal fear of permanent physical injury.

During the fourth to fifth week postpartum, sexual tensions were described as similar to nonpregnant levels. During coitus the physical reaction of the target organs appeared to decrease in rapidity and intensity of response; lubrication occurred more slowly and was not so profuse as during pregnancy. Vaginal distention also occurred more slowly and was less marked; the vaginal walls themselves appeared thinner than before pregnancy, possibly as a result of steroid starvation during this period. The sex skin appeared much less colorful, and the orgasmic platform was not nearly so vasocongested.

By the third month postpartum, vaginal rugae had returned, the uterus had descended into the pelvis, the labia majora and minora began to respond more readily, and vaginal lubrication had returned to nonpregnant levels. Expansion of the vaginal barrel had returned to prepregnancy dimensions.

Masters and Johnson reported that in their sample, nursing mothers resumed intercourse 2 to 3 weeks after delivery, probably as a result of experiencing higher sexual tension than in the nonpregnant state. The only deterrents to intercourse for these women were perineal pain or irritation of the vaginal barrel after intercourse. Interestingly enough, eleven women described increased sexual pleasure from tenderness of the episiotomy site or tightness of the postpartum vaginal barrel.

Some of the nursing mothers reported receiving sexual stimulation to plateau or orgasmic levels as a result of breast-feeding their infants. Some also indicated they felt abnormal or perverted about this response.

From 2 to 3 months postpartum, many women who were nursing reported losing milk in uncontrollable spurts when they were stimulated sexually; this phenomenon was more common during and after orgasm.

Fifty-eight of the 111 women in the total sample were concerned about their husband's sexual outlet, especially when intercourse had been contraindicated for a long period before and after delivery. Many of the husbands wished that physicians had better interpreted the reasons for abstinence to them before their wives' deliveries. They also would have preferred to have been informed about the time after pregnancy when intercourse could be safely resumed.*

Kenny[32] studied the reports of women's sexuality during the breast-feeding and weaning phases. Thirty-two women out of the original sample of thirty-three had breast-fed or were currently breast-feeding. Thirty percent of the women reported that the childbirth experience made them more interested in sex, 52% reported no difference, and 18% felt less interested than before pregnancy. Sexual functioning during the breast-feeding period was reported to be similar to prepregnancy levels by 75% of the women. Fifty-two percent of all subjects believed that intercourse could be safely resumed when vaginal discharge stopped, even when this occurred before the first postpartum visit with the physician. Forty-two percent of the women desired to resume intercourse at a time when only 12% felt it safe to do so. None of the subjects felt it unsafe to resume sexual intercourse after 6 weeks; however, 18% were still disinterested at this time. Women who had been married longer, had more children, and had longer breast-feeding time reported a faster return of sexual interest and felt safe resuming intercourse earlier. All breast-feeding women in this study reported the experience as enjoyable, and 72% found it "exceptionally meaningful." After weaning their infants most women reported essentially unchanged sexual interest, and no one reported a decrease in interest after weaning.

Falicov[16] examined sexuality at 2 and 7 months postpartum. Twelve of the eighteen couples had resumed sexual intercourse within 2 months of delivery. Six of these twelve did not return to their previous level of sexual interaction because of physical discomforts such as breast soreness or engorgement and soreness of the episiotomy site. Five of the eighteen women reported increased eroticism, primarily as a result of increased sensitivity of the breasts. The nursing experience appeared to heighten breast eroticism for six of the thirteen women who were breast-feeding, but two women who were not breast-feeding also experienced it. Most women who had resumed intercourse reported increased difficulty in experiencing orgasm compared to prepregnancy experiences. Responsible factors noted by these women included tension, fatigue, and some anxiety about perceived changes in their sexual organs. The six couples who had not resumed intercourse by the 6- to 8-week postpartum period included four of the five women in the sample who were bottle-feeding. Reasons advanced for nonresumption were fatigue, lack of interest, tenderness of episiotomy site, and lack of time.

Tolor and Di Granzia[80] reported data related to fifty-five women seen for the 6 weeks' postpartum physician examination. Comparisons were made between the postpartum women and 125 women in varying stages of pregnancy. Several significant differences in behavior and attitudes were noted. The decline in desire for intercourse seen in the pregnant women was reversed in the postpartum phase. There was a relatively high incidence of intercourse following childbirth, with one out of every three women reporting having intercourse four or more times each week. Postpartal women were more satisfied than third-trimester women with the prevailing level of sexual activity, but 31% of these women preferred still higher levels of activity. The postpartum group reported occasional

*It is interesting to note that the first pregnancy was often noted to coincide with men's first extramarital affairs.

multiple orgasms but less frequently than the pregnant group. There was increased preference for oral sexuality and decreased preference for clitoral stimulation in the postpartal women. Interest in sex demonstrated a decline in the pregnant group until the postpartum period, when interest peaked.

Seven months postpartum found sexual intercourse still considerably less frequent than prepregnancy levels for ten of sixteen couples. However, sexual desire and eroticism had returned to normal or heightened levels. Nine women reported an increased capacity for arousal and orgasm relative to prepregnancy levels. Four of the six women who continued to nurse their children at this time reported increased sexual desire and expressed frustration at the infrequency of sexual intercourse.

Richardson et al.[67] reviewed over 800 consecutive records of women who had vaginal deliveries with episiotomies, primarily median, from 1972 through 1974. All repairs were done with PGA 4-0 or 5-0 suture and a small needle. The majority of women in this group were resuming coitus with reasonable comfort between the fourteenth and the twenty-first day postpartum. The earliest resumption was on the fifth day postpartum, with a few women waiting until after a fourth week postpartum examination.

There was no evidence that resumption of sexual activity adversely affected healing of the perineum in any way. Healing occurred by primary intention, and there were no breakdowns or fistulas. Anatomic results after healing were uniformly satisfactory.

Baxter[3] interviewed fifty-four British primiparous women during the eleventh and fifteenth weeks postpartum and examined delivery data about their births from their hospital records. All the women were in stable sexual relationships. Four of the fifty-four women had not resumed intercourse at the time of interview.

Changes in interest in intercourse (in fifty-one women) were as follows: nineteen (37.2%) reported an increase; eighteen (35.3%) reported a decrease; and fourteen (27.5%) remained unchanged.

Changes in coital orgasmic rate (in forty-eight women) were as follows: sixteen (33.3%) reported an increase; fourteen (29.2%) reported a decrease, and eighteen (37.5%) remained unchanged.

Changes in frequency of intercourse (in forty-eight women) were as follows: eight reported an increase; twenty-four reported a decrease; and sixteen reported no change. Changes in coital orgasmic rate were significantly related to changes in interest in intercourse, but there was no relationship between either of these measures and changes in intercourse frequency.

Changes in coital orgasmic rate were not related to the woman's age, educational level, or length of marriage. There was no relationship between coital orgasmic rate in women who experienced nausea or vomiting (46.3%), heartburn (48.5%), preeclamptic toxemia (46.0%), or unplanned pregnancy (36.2%). Neither the sex of the child (30.8 were male) nor the major direction or change of interest in intercourse during pregnancy was related to coital orgasmic rate.

Women who had at any time attempted breast-feeding were significantly more likely to experience a decreased coital orgasmic rate than were women who had never attempted breast-feeding. This relationship did not appear at the time of interview with women who were currently lactating.

Dyspareunia at the resumption of intercourse and at the time of interview was significantly associated with decreases in coital orgasmic rate. Decreased coital orgasmic rates were related to the women's perception of their vaginas being slacker during intercourse than previously, and increased rates were related to a feeling that the vagina was tighter.

Changes in interest in intercourse were related to the previously mentioned variables in a manner similar to the coital orgasmic rate.

In Lumley's sample[38] twenty-six women were also interviewed after childbirth and at 3 months postpartum. She noted a partial return to prepregnancy levels of intercourse by 3 months. The third month postpartum showed increasing ratings of libido when compared to prepregnancy levels in 23% of the women. Libido remained the same in 61% of the women and decreased in 15% of the women. Frequency of coitus increased, however, in only 11% of the women, remained the same for 43% of the women, and decreased for 46% of the women.

Thus there was an apparent discrepancy between postpartum sexual feelings and enjoyment of intercourse, which were as great (61%) or greater (23%) than before pregnancy, and the frequency of intercourse, which was reduced among almost half the couples. Pain and tenderness at the episiotomy scar site and fatigue were the two most common reasons given for the decreased frequency of intercourse.

Hames,[24] in a study of forty-two couples following the birth of their first child, examined sexual needs and interest during the postpartum period. Breast changes following delivery had no effect on normal sexual activity for twenty-seven women. Ten women found that breast changes inhibited their sexuality, with tenderness and milk leakage listed as the main problems. Breast changes enhanced sexuality for five women, and these women believed their husbands enjoyed their larger breast size and were sexually stimulated by the increase. Eight men agreed that their partners' increased breast size enhanced their sexuality. Nine men found breast leakage a sexually inhibiting factor, and twenty-five respondents indicated breast changes had no impact on their sexuality. Data indicating how many of the women were breast-feeding were not included in this report.

The presence of vaginal bleeding had no effect on sexual activities for 62% of both male and female subjects. The 38% for whom vaginal bleeding was inhibiting gave reasons such as fear of infection, messiness, the woman's discomfort, and concern about the healing process.

Twenty-six (62%) of these couples resumed sexual intercourse before the sixth week postpartum, with the mean time interval for resumption being 4.4 weeks.

Twenty-three women (54.8%) stated that pain in the sutured area was the greatest factor preventing resumption of intercourse, followed by fear of harming the incision (17), physician's orders (15), tiredness (11), vaginal bleeding (11), fear of pregnancy (8), and fear of infection (1). Twenty-seven men stated that fear of hurting their wives prevented the resumption of intercourse, followed by fear of harming the incision (21), physician's orders (12), vaginal bleeding (10), fear of pregnancy (6), disinterest in intercourse (3), and fear of infection (1).

Most women described their husbands' behavior after the delivery of the baby as understanding, close, sympathetic, and gentle.

Robson,[69] as a part of the previously mentioned study, again interviewed 118 primiparous women during the first postpartum week. She repeated interviews at 12 weeks (113 women), 26 weeks (110 women), and 52 weeks (98 women) postpartum.

About one third of the women had resumed intercourse by the sixth week, with nearly all of the women resuming by the twelfth week. There was, however, a persisting fall in frequency of intercourse over the entire year when compared to prepregnancy levels.

Intercourse was found enjoyable at 12 weeks by over two thirds of the women. At 12 weeks 40% of the women complained of soreness or painful intercourse at times, and one fourth of the subjects found tiredness interfering with their enjoyment of sex or reducing their libido.

One year after delivery, 80% of these women were experiencing sex as predominately pleasurable, which was close to prepregnancy figures. In fact one fourth of the women said that they were enjoying sex more than they did before conception. Achievement of orgasm gradually returned to prepregnancy levels by the end of the first year. Libido was described as reduced compared to prepregnancy levels by 57% of the women, whereas 10% described an increased libido, and 33% stated there was no change.

Body-mind interaction. Bardwick,[1] in her study of the psychology of women, calls to mind a possible relationship between hormonal levels and the feelings of patience and nurturance. Perhaps there is also a relationship between hormonal levels and sexual appetite, but this theory was not borne out in the findings of Masters and Johnson.[41] Women in their sample with the highest postpartum eroticism were nursing mothers, who probably had the lowest levels of sex steroids.

In a discussion of female sexuality Sherfey[74] explores the "pregnancy effect." She relates the vascularization of the labia majora and other pelvic tissues to the hormonal influence of pregnancy; this increased vascularization results in marked engorgement that requires several hours of resolution after intense sexual arousal. Pointing out that many women have their first orgasmic experience after their first pregnancy, Sherfey attributes this phenomenon to the greatly increased vascularity of the entire pelvic region. Although the effects of a decrease in anxiety after the first pregnancy and the benefits of the maturing experiences of labor, birth, and care for a newborn infant cannot be discounted, the hormonal influences and resultant growth of new blood vessels and varicosities in the female pelvis are thought to be of primary importance in creating heightened sexual arousal. In addition, Sherfey postulates that androgen and androgen-related activities of the end products of progesterone metabolism, both of which are secreted during pregnancy, probably influence the responsivity of the coital system and the strength of the muscles of the orgasmic platform. She concludes that as long as there is no obstetric damage, pregnancies will only increase the volume capacity of the venous bed of the pelvis, thus enhancing the woman's capacity for sexual tension and probably improving her orgasmic frequency, intensity, and pleasure. It is theorized that this mechanism may be designed to enhance sexual pleasure to ensure that motherhood will continue, and with it the propagation of the human species.

Unfortunately, obstetric damage does occur, and with it there may be accompanying sexual dysfunctions. It is debatable whether the varicosities found after delivery are adaptive or maladaptive, since in some women they may cause discomfort sufficient to interfere with intercourse and in others only serve to enhance vasocongestion. Most moderate-to-mild trauma rarely interferes completely with the woman's ability to enjoy orgasm, but it may lessen her capacity.

Sherfey[74] maintains that there are three essential ingredients in the production of orgasmic levels of vasotension: the gripping of the shaft of the penis, the production of friction on the tightened lower third of the vaginal barrel and the upper labia, and the labial-preputial glandular action. With tears to the bulbar system, the woman may experience a decreased orgasmic reaction, even with only one malfunctioning bulb. With a torn or stretched perineal body, there may be a gaping vaginal orifice. It is easy to see how these two obstetric traumas may interfere with the three components of orgasmic production. With moderate degrees of trauma, orgasm may occur, but conditions must be optimal.

Bentovim[5] uses a systems approach to describe the breast-feeding or bottle-feeding experience. Sexually related variables in the decision to breast-feed include maternal attitudes toward nudity and tolerance of masturbation and sex play. Sexually related family variables include marital status, length of marriage, and openness rather than modesty concerning sexuality. Societal and cultural variables include views toward the role of the breast as a sexual rather than feeding object and sexual modesty in the community. Sexually related precipitating factors in the decision to breast-feed include the response to breast changes in pregnancy with pleasure versus shame and neurohormonal changes.

Possible sexually related outcomes for the mother are identified as (1) sexual responses such as pleasure or shame, embarrassment and modesty, uterine contractions, and skin temperature changes, (2) breast-feeding as natural contraception, and (3) wish for return to a sexual relationship. Sexually related consequences for the infant include a total body pleasurable response. Consequences for the family and society could vary from marital satisfaction to dissatisfaction and from acceptance to rejection of the breast as a sexual and feeding object.

This approach allows for great flexibility in looking at lactation and sexuality, their interrelations, and their possible influences and consequences. It also provides the possibility of keeping sexually related aspects of lactation in perspective with the other multiple complexities involved in this process. Many of the sexually related factors Bentovim has described will be discussed further in the following paragraphs.

There is a tendency in society to define healthy female sexuality in terms of adaptability to male sexuality[71] and to place special emphasis on the types of female sexual behavior that hold particular pertinence for men.[56] This has resulted in singling out women's responses in coitus for much discussion and research, leaving other aspects of female sexuality minimally attended.

Newton[56] hypothesizes that during early times the survival of the human race depended on two voluntary behaviors, coitus and breast-feeding. These behaviors would need to be sufficiently pleasurable to facilitate their recurrence. Partial explanation for these behaviors has been thought to be biologically based, and oxytocin appears to have a significant role in interpersonal reproductive acts. There has been a general reluctance to study hormones involved in strongly emotional acts of love because of the belief present in society that these acts belong in the private sphere. Researchers have found it easier to gear their orientation toward acts of aggression and stress and the hormonal importance of adrenaline and related substances.[50]

Comparing coitus with breast-feeding, Newton describes several similarities.[56] Uterine contractions and nipple erection are noted to occur during both acts. Nipple stimulation and breast stroking are generally included in breast-feeding and sexual foreplay. Older infants show total body response to nursing: rhythmic movements of hands, fingers, feet, and toes. Erection of the penis is common in male babies. Sexual contact and breast-feeding contact both involve skin changes, and both can trigger the milk letdown reflex. There appears to be a similar emotional component experienced during sexual arousal and unrestricted, unlimited breast-feeding; orgasm has been experienced during breast-feeding. There may be a relationship between an accepting attitude toward sexuality and an accepting attitude toward breast-feeding. There also may be some similarities between "nursing songs"—soft, contented vocalizations made by nursing babies—and the spontaneous noises sometimes made during coitus.[54]

Pryor[62] denies that sustained sexual pleasure in nursing is the usual experience. The nipple, although generally an erogenous area, becomes relatively desensitized during lactation. The areola, generally insensitive to the touch, receives most of the sensations during feeding. Mildly erotic feelings may be felt at the initiation or termination of feedings.

Technologic interference and rigid inhibiting social patterns surrounding childbirth and lactation may be the reason that the sensuous nature of components of parturition and lactation are so seldom recognized or studied.

Potential medical complications from sexual behavior throughout pregnancy and during the postpartum period

Hypothesized links between sexual behavior throughout pregnancy and the postpartum period and medical complications have a long history.[72] Sexual behavior of the pregnant and postpartal woman has been hypothesized to cause miscarriage, premature labor, premature rupture of the fetal membranes, vaginal bleeding, abruptio placentae, amniotic fluid infections, fatal air embolism, and disruption of the episiotomy site. Based on the potential possibility of such complications, women have received recommendations for prophylactic abstinence for varying periods of time.[11] A major area of concern to investigators who have studied sexuality during pregnancy has been the effect of sexual intercourse on the fetus.

In 1953 Pugh and Fernandez[63] found no significant relationship between the time of last coitus before delivery and puerperal infection or premature rupture of fetal membranes in a sample of 500 women admitted to a general hospital in Louisville. There was a statistically significant difference between those women whose last coitus was shortly before delivery who experienced premature labor and all other women. However, the investigators question a cause-and-effect relationship, since the median time of last coitus before delivery was 21 days. There did not appear to be a concrete relationship between late antepartum bleeding and coitus in this sample.

Goodlin, Keller, and Raffin,[20] in a study of 200 women experiencing orgasm during the second and third trimesters of pregnancy, found that the risk of premature labor or ruptured membranes was 15% in those women who experienced orgasm after the thirty-second week of pregnancy. In those women who had previous premature births there was a 21% risk of premature delivery. However, 85% of these women were not orgasmic after the thirty-second week of pregnancy, so their poor reproductive history also appears to be a variable.

Goodlin, Keller, and Raffin also conducted a second study of the effect of maternal orgasm on uterine tension levels and fetal heart rate. One woman, during her thirty-ninth week of an uncomplicated pregnancy, was externally monitored during five orgasmic episodes. Orgasm was achieved by vulvar and vaginal manipulation by the woman and her husband. Increasing uterine tension and associated decelerations of fetal heart rates with uterine contractions were noted. Uterine contractions appeared to increase with intensity with succeeding orgasms, but fetal heart rate decelerations were not constant. Six days after this study the woman delivered her infant, and both did well.

Wagner, Butler, and Sanders[82] studied nineteen women who delivered premature infants at gestational age of less than 37 weeks and/or birth weight of 2500 g or less and a matched control group of nineteen full-term women. There was no significant relationship found between the premature and control group in the percentage of women experiencing orgasm at some time during pregnancy.

Grudzinskas, Watson, and Chard[22] reported data from their interviews with seventy married primiparous women, thirty of whom remained sexually active during the last 4 weeks before their deliveries. There was no association in the thirty sexually active women between gestational age at delivery and the incidence of coitus during the last month of pregnancy. When the women who had coitus during the last 4 weeks of pregnancy were compared with those who did not, the sexually active women had a higher incidence of meconium staining, and their infants had a higher incidence of low Apgar scores at 1 minute. No other associations were noted between maternal sexual behavior and any other indicator of maternal or neonatal conditions.

Perkins[61] reported sexual and obstetric data obtained from 155 postpartal women through written questionnaires. There was no connection between sexual behavior with or without orgasm and complications such as premature labor, premature rupture of membranes, or low birth weight infants. There was a significant association between a last sexual experience less than 24 hours before labor onset and delivering an infant less than 38 weeks' gestational age but no association with orgasmic response and rupture of membranes.

Rayburn and Wilson[65] studied coital activity during pregnancy and its relationship to premature labor and delivery. One hundred eleven women who had spontaneous premature labor were compared with a matched group of women who subsequently delivered at term. Frequencies of coitus with or without orgasm did not vary significantly between the two groups of women. No association was found between the interval from the last coital experience, with or without orgasm, and the risk of subsequent premature delivery. There were no known predisposing factors in eleven of the eighteen women delivering prematurely. This special group of eighteen women did demonstrate an incidence of coital frequency that was significantly higher than that among the control group.

Mills, Harlap, and Harley[44] interviewed 10,477 women the day after delivery on three obstetric units in Jerusalem. Medical records for these women were also examined. Sexual intercourse during the last 3 months of pregnancy did not increase the risk of premature rupture of membranes, low birth weight, perinatal death, or preterm delivery for these women.

Naeye[50] explored the relationship of coitus to antepartum hemorrhage in a longitudinal study of 56,568 pregnancies. Data from this study were collected as part of the Collaborative Perinatal Project of the National Institute of Neurological and Communicative Disorders and Stroke. Recorded information on gestation, labor, delivery, and the neonatal period was gathered on patients at 12 hospitals affiliated with medical schools in different regions of the United States between 1959 and 1966. Coitus was noted to be associated with hemorrhages, and this association was independent of other factors that predispose to bleeding. The frequency of antepartum hemorrhage was 30/1000 births in women reporting coitus since their last clinic visit versus 19/1000 when no recent coitus was reported. Bleeding frequency did increase with the frequency of coitus. This study did not demonstrate a causal relationship between coitus and antepartum hemorrhage.

The question of the relationship between coitus during the last weeks of pregnancy and amniotic fluid infections has received attention. Naeye[46] analyzed data from 27,232 single births that took place between 1959 and 1966 to determine whether coitus was involved in the genesis of amniotic fluid infections. The data were also originally collected as part of the Collaborative Perinatal Project previously mentioned. Data were collected at each antenatal clinic visit and on admission for delivery. Data collected at the last clinic visit or an admission for delivery were used to determine coital activity for the month before delivery. Amniotic fluid infections were diagnosed when there was acute inflammation in the subchorionic plate of the placenta. Infection was rated as mild when 4 to 15 neutrophils were present in the placental plate as observed through high-powered microscopic field. The infection was rated as moderate to severe when more than 15 neutrophils were present.

Fetal and neonatal deaths at any gestational age that occurred after infection were greater when coitus had occurred than when it had not, since infections were more severe when coitus had taken place. However, differences in perinatal mortality between the group having coitus and the group not having coitus were not statistically significant when delivery occurred during the thirty-third to thirty-eighth weeks. Coitus-associated effects were greater in preterm than full-term infants, and the frequent coitus group was skewed in the direction of shorter gestation. Infections occurred in 156/1000 births when women reported coitus at least weekly during the month before delivery. The rate was 117/1000 births when no coitus was reported.

In another paper Naeye[47] analyzed data from the study just mentioned related to 6613 women whose pregnancies ended before term, to determine whether amniotic fluid infections could be a cause as well as a consequence of premature rupture of fetal membranes. He found no relation to the frequency of premature rupture and the number of coital acts in the month before delivery.

Rehu[66] reported the results of a 1-year study of puerperal endometritis rates among 5058 women giving birth at a state maternity hospital in Helsinki, Finland. Of the women in this group, 774 had cesarean sections. There was no significant difference in the puerperal endometritis rate in those who had coitus during the last week before delivery and those who did not. Among the women who had cesarean sections, endometritis was found in 20% of the women having coitus during the final week of pregnancy and in 8.3% of the women who abstained. The highest infection rate occurred in primiparous women and in women under 25 having sexual intercourse during the last week before cesarean section. There was no difference between infection rates in parous women having coitus during the final week before surgery and parous women who did not have coitus.

Also noted under the potential medical complications of sexual behavior during pregnancy is the rare occurrence of fatal air embolism as a result of inflation of air into the vagina during oral-genital sex. Fatteh, Leach, and Wilkinson[17] published a case report of such an incident. These authors reviewed the world literature and found only eight reports of such deaths to date. Maternal deaths have occurred in varying stages of pregnancy and seemingly occur almost immediately after the air inflation.

In view of the fact that prostaglandins administered intravaginally can stimulate uterine contractions,[77] Goodlin, Keller, and Raffin[20] postulate that semen may have the property of inducing labor. The fact that an increase in peripheral oxytocin levels is seen in women experiencing orgasm may also lend credence to the theory that orgasm can precipitate uterine contractions forceful enough to initiate labor.[18] In some women postorgasmic uterine contractions were sufficiently painful to discourage intercourse.[20]

Lavery and Miller[36] studied 220 human chorioamniotic membranes and evaluated their tensile strength after exposure to human seminal fluid and prostaglandins. They concluded that the biochemical constituents of seminal fluid do not have an adverse effect on the strength of human chorionic membranes. The research did not address the potential uterotonic effect of prostaglandins.

In Solberg, Butler, and Wagner's 1973 series[76] of 260 women studied in Seattle only nineteen babies were born prematurely according to birth weight or dates, and only nine infants were premature by both standards. Not one of the mothers noted an immediate onset of labor after intercourse or orgasm. Frequency of coitus or orgasm during the seventh, eighth, and ninth months of pregnancy seemed unrelated to the infant's birth weight, Apgar score at 1 minute, or gestational age at birth.

Health care process

Assessment. Before counseling the pregnant woman and her partner about sexual aspects of pregnancy, the postpartum period, and, if applicable, the period of lactation, it is essential to collect data about personal and social aspects of the pregnancy. Since bodily changes may greatly alter the woman's sexual function, it is important to assess the stage of her pregnancy, body contour, and general feeling tone. If the woman reports discomfort during or after intercourse or other sexual activity, further data can be obtained to determine whether the source of discomfort is anatomic, as in the increase in abdominal size, or physiologic, as in chronic vascular congestion of the pelvis. Feelings of tiredness and nausea may transiently depress sexual interest, but consistent discomfort warrants medical attention.

The woman's responses to the changes in her body provide valuable cues to potential sexual concerns. Assessment of feeling tone is probably most accurate when recorded in terms of the woman's own words.

Interpersonal factors resulting in heightened sexual interest and frequency also need to be considered, since they may imply a need for reassurance of normalcy. Feelings related to the pregnancy, the postpartum period, and the period of lactation, particularly those reflecting ambivalence or a negative response, may be especially significant for the health practitioner, and anticipatory guidance can prevent normal variation from being problematic.

Finally, data related to social aspects of pregnancy, the postpartum period, and lactation may be very revealing. For example, many cues to potential sexual concerns and to the possibilities for intervention may be provided by the woman's feelings about her femininity, her relationship with her partner, her sexual desire and function, and others' responses to her pregnancy. The role of the partner and his or her relationship with the pregnant woman is crucially important and therefore demands consideration. If the prospective father no longer plays a role with the woman, special attention needs to be given to the support systems in which she is involved.

Intervention. Counseling the pregnant woman and her partner about sexuality during pregnancy-related periods is probably most effective when it is done conjointly. This is especially important when, for a specific reason, sexual intercourse must be prohibited.[41]

According to the literature, there is little rationale for prohibiting vaginal intercourse at any time during a normal pregnancy provided the cervix is not ripe and there is not a poor reproductive history.[14,41] If the woman is spotting or bleeding vaginally, if the fetal membranes are prematurely ruptured, or if she has a repeated history of miscarriages, prohibition of intercourse may be necessary.[23] In these instances it is crucial that she be informed that the prohibition is concerned with the orgasmic experience, not merely intercourse. It should be emphasized that masturbating to orgasm may have more deleterious effects on the fetus than intercourse, since the orgasmic experience, when produced by self-manipulation, tends to be more intense than that during intercourse.[41] Presence of an infection in either partner may neccessitate abstinence. There is also limited evidence that in extremely rare instances oral-genital sex may be associated with fatal air embolism *if* air is introduced into the vagina.[17]

Another important aspect of sexual counseling during pregnancy involves the issue of coital frequency. There are no data to suggest that a limitation in frequency is necessary during pregnancy. However, it should be emphasized by the practitioner that either an increase or a decrease in desire is quite normal[41,54] and that frequency may be somewhat altered in either direction. Certain coital positions may become uncomfortable during the later stages of pregnancy. Frequently the female-astride or side-by-side positions offer the woman more satisfaction. However, a number of variations are possible, and the couple may be encouraged to discover what is most comfortable for them.

Vaginal discomfort may sometimes present problems during pregnancy and the postpartum period. Guttmacher[23] suggests use of a lubricant. However, its use should be based on the woman's determination of whether she feels adequately lubricated before intromission.

Postpartally, intercourse can be resumed when it is comfortable for the woman. If there has been an episiotomy, the healing process generally takes 2 to 3 weeks.[41]

Evaluation. When a consistent relationship with the client and her partner exists throughout pregnancy and the postpartum period, it can afford the practitioner special opportunities to evaluate the effectiveness of teaching and counseling. The ability of the health provider can be mirrored to some extent in the quality of the relationship between the woman and her partner if both have been considered in the prenatal period.

One final means of evaluating the effectiveness of the health care process would be a comparison of the woman's perceptions of her relationship with her partner to her personal goals. If counseling is based on a thorough assessment of the individual woman and her significant others and on the findings of the current studies, pregnancy may be a time during which the woman and the expectant couple are offered and experience real growth.

Summary

This chapter has focused on sexuality during pregnancy, the post-partum period, and lactation. Some key considerations for health care professionals include the following:

1. There are fluctuations in the woman's interest in sex and fre-quency of intercourse throughout pregnancy and the postpartum period.
2. In some respects pregnancy may enhance the woman's capacity to be orgasmic both during and after the experience.
3. There are few reasons to contraindicate sexual activity during pregnancy. When it is necessary to do so, clear explanations of the necessary changes in behavior and their rationale should be presented.
4. Changes in the woman's anatomy and physiology during preg-nancy may make some aspects of intercourse uncomfortable.
5. Masturbation and sexual intercourse should be prohibited if there is fear that orgasm will initiate fetal or maternal damage.
6. Mild-to-moderate obstetric trauma should not interfere with sex-ual function after delivery.
7. Changes in body contour may alter the woman's concept of herself as a sexual being.
8. Lactation can enhance a woman's sexuality.
9. Aspects of lactation may appear similar to sexual arousal in some women.
10. Responses to pregnancy and lactation are socially and culturally determined.
11. The marital role and other role relationships are usually altered in some way by pregnancy and childbirth.

Questions for review

1. In what ways may the bodily changes of pregnancy influence the woman's sexual function? At what periods in her pregnancy may her sexual expe-rience be enhanced?
2. How might the woman's changed body structure alter her self-concept?
3. What influence can the woman's changing body have on her sexual rela-tionship?
4. What relationship can pregnancy have to subsequent sexual function?

5. How does coitus affect the fetus? When should a woman be advised to discontinue intercourse during her pregnancy?
6. How might pregnancy affect the woman's sexual partner? What changes might be seen in marital roles?
7. In what ways does culture influence the woman's response to her pregnancy?
8. As a clinician, you may be approached for advice about sexual behavior during pregnancy. Analyze the following excerpts from clinical cases and determine your response to the client:

   - I am very uncomfortable having Joe on top of me now, so we don't have intercourse often.
   - I'm afraid that it (intercourse) might hurt the baby. . . .
   - After we have intercourse I find that I spot for the next few days.
   - Sometimes I get terrible cramps in my stomach after I come to climax.
   - My partner has a urinary infection.

9. How does the undrugged labor experience compare with orgasm?
10. Describe the postpartum sexual experience, comparing nursing and non-nursing mothers.
11. How does the nursing experience compare with sexual arousal and orgasm?

References

1. Bardwick, J.M.: The psychology of women, New York, 1971, Harper & Row, Publishers, Inc.
2. Battacchi, M., et al.: Personality and stress factors in women's sexuality in pregnancy. In Carenza, L., Pancheri, P., and Zichella, L., editors: Clinical psychoneuroendocrinology in reproduction, New York, 1978, Academic Press, Inc.
3. Baxter, S.: Labor and orgasm in primiparae, Journal of Psychosomatic Research 18:209-216, 1974.
4. Benedek, T.: The psychobiology of pregnancy. In Anthony, E.J., and Benedek, T.: Parenting: its psychology and psychopathology, Boston, 1970, Little, Brown & Co.
5. Bentovim, A.: Shame and other anxieties associated with breast-feeding: a systems theory and psychodynamic approach. In Ciba Foundation Symposium: Breast-feeding and the mother, vol. 45, New York, 1976, Ciba Foundation.
6. Bing, E., and Colman, L.: Making love during pregnancy, New York, 1977, Bantam Books, Inc.
7. Blachman, L.: Dancing in the dark. I. Romanticized motherhood and the breast feeding venture, Birth and the Family Journal 8:271-279, 1981.
8. Blachman, L.: Dancing in the dark. II. Helping and not so helping hands, Birth and the Family Journal 8:280-286, 1981.
9. Bloom, M.: The romance and the power of breast feeding, Birth and the Family Journal 8:259-269, 1981.
10. Calhoun, L., Selby, J., and King, E.: The influence of pregnancy on sexuality: a review of current evidence, Journal of Sex Research 17:139-151, 1981.
11. Clark, A., and Hale, R.: Sex during and after pregnancy, American Journal of Nursing 74:1430-1431, 1974.

12. Cohn, S.: Sexuality in pregnancy, Nursing Clinics of North America **17**(1):91-98, 1982.
13. Colman, D., and Colman, L.L.: Pregnancy as an altered state of consciousness, Birth and the Family Journal **1**(1):7-11, 1973-1974.
14. Cronenwett, L., and Newmark, L.: Fathers' responses to childbirth, Nursing Research **23**:210-217, 1974.
15. Ellis, D.: Sexual needs and concerns of expectant parents, J.O.G.N. Nursing **9**:306-308, 1980.
16. Falicov, C.J.: Sexual adjustment during first pregnancy and postpartum, American Journal of Obstetrics and Gynecology **117**:991-1000, 1973.
17. Fatteh, A., Leach, W., and Wilkinson, C.: Fatal air embolism in pregnancy resulting from orogenital sex play, Forensic Science **2**:247-250, 1973.
18. Fox, C.A., and Knaggs, G.S.: Milk-ejection activity (oxytocin) in peripheral venous blood in man during lactation and in association with coitus, Journal of Endocrinology **45**:145-146, 1969.
19. Goodlin, R.C.: Orgasm and premature labor, American Journal of Obstetrics and Gynecology **135**:1122-1123, 1979.
20. Goodlin, R.C., Keller, D.W.F., and Raffin, M.: Orgasm during late pregnancy: possible deleterious effects, Obstetrics and Gynecology **38**:916-920, 1971.
21. Goodlin, R.C., Schmidt, W., and Creevy, D.: Uterine tension and fetal heart rate during maternal orgasm, Obstetrics and Gynecology **39**:125-127, 1972.
22. Grudzinskas, J.G., Watson, C., and Chard, T.: Does sexual intercourse cause fetal distress?, Lancet **2**(8144):692-693, 1979.
23. Guttmacher, A.F.: Pregnancy, birth, and family planning: a guide for expectant parents in the 1970's, New York, 1973, The Viking Press.
24. Hames, C.: Sexual needs and interests of postpartum couples, J.O.G.N. Nursing **9**:313-315, 1980.
25. Herbst, A.: Coitus and the fetus, New England Journal of Medicine **301**:1235-1236, 1979.
26. Hern, W.: The illness parameters of pregnancy, Social Science and Medicine **9**:365-372, 1975.
27. Hollender, M.H., and McGehee, J.B.: The wish to be held during pregnancy, Journal of Psychosomatic Research **18**:193-197, 1974.
28. Holtzman, L.: Sexual practices during pregnancy, Journal of Nurse-Midwifery **21**(1):29-38, 1976.
29. Iffrig, Sr. M.C.: Body image in pregnancy: its relation to nursing functions, Nursing Clinics of North America **7**:631-639, 1972.
30. Inglis, T.: Postpartum sexuality, J.O.G.N. Nursing **9**:298-300, 1980.
31. Jessner, L., Weigert, E., and Foy, J.L.: The development of parental attitudes during pregnancy. In Anthony, E.J., and Benedek, T., editors: Parenthood: its psychology and psychopathology, Boston, 1970, Little, Brown & Co.
32. Kenny, J.A.: Sexuality of pregnant and breastfeeding women, Archives of Sexual Behavior **2**:215-229, 1973.
33. Kyndely, K.: The sexuality of women in pregnancy and postpartum: a review, J.O.G.N. Nursing **7**:28-32, Jan.-Feb., 1978.
34. Lanahan, C.: Eroticism and orgasm in pregnancy. In McNall, L., and

Galeener, J., editors: Current practice in obstetric and gynecologic nursing, vol. 1, St. Louis, 1976, The C.V. Mosby Co.

35. LaRossa, R.: Sex during pregnancy: a symbolic interactionist analysis, Journal of Sex Research **15:**119-128, 1979.

36. Lavery, J., and Miller, C.E.: Effect of prostaglandin and seminal fluid on human chorioamniotic membranes, J.A.M.A. **245:**2425-2427, 1981.

37. Leif, H.: Sexual desire and responsivity during pregnancy, Medical Aspects of Human Sexuality **11:**51-57, 1977.

38. Lumley, J.: Sexual feelings in pregnancy and after childbirth, Australian and New Zealand Journal of Obstetrics and Gynecology **18:**114-117, 1978.

39. Malinowski, J.: Sex during pregnancy: what can you say? R.N. **41**(1):48-51, 1978.

40. Mann, E., and Cunningham, G.: Coital cautions in pregnancy, Medical Aspects of Human Sexuality **6:**14-27, Oct. 1972.

41. Masters, W., and Johnson, V.: Human sexual response, Boston, 1966, Little, Brown & Co.

42. McGee, K.: Sexuality in pregnancy, J.O.G.N. Nursing **7**(3):49, 1978.

43. Mead, M., and Newton, N.: Cultural patterning of perinatal behavior. In Richardson, S.A., and Guttmacher, A.F., editors: Childbearing: its social and psychological aspects, Baltimore, 1967, The Williams & Wilkins Co.

44. Mills, J., Harlap, S., and Harley, E.: Should coitus late in pregnancy be discouraged? Lancet **2:**136-138, 1981.

45. Morris, N.M.: The frequency of sexual intercourse during pregnancy, Archives of Sexual Behavior **4:**501-507, 1975.

46. Naeye, R.: Coitus and associated amniotic fluid infections, New England Journal of Medicine **301:**1198-1200, 1979.

47. Naeye, R.: Seasonal variations in coitus and other risk factors, and the outcome of pregnancy, Early Human Development **4**(1):61-68, 1980.

48. Naeye, R.: To the editor, New England Journal of Medicine **302:**633, 1980.

49. Naeye, R.: Coitus and antepartum hemorrhage, British Journal of Obstetrics and Gynecology **88:**765-770, 1981.

50. Naeye, R.: Safety of coitus in pregnancy, Lancet **2**(8248):686, 1981.

51. Naeye, R., and Peters, E.: Causes and consequences of premature rupture of fetal membranes, Lancet **1:**192-194, 1980.

52. Neubardt, S.: Coitus during pregnancy, Medical Aspects of Human Sexuality **7:**197-198, 1973.

53. Newton, N.: Maternal emotions: a study of women's feelings toward menstruation, pregnancy, childbirth, breast feeding, infant care, and other aspects of their femininity, New York, 1955, Harper & Row, Publishers.

54. Newton, N.: Psychologic differences between breast and bottle feeding, American Journal of Clinical Nutrition **24:**933-1004, 1971.

55. Newton, N.: The trebly senuous woman, Psychology Today **5:**68-71, July 1971.

56. Newton, N.: Interrelationships between sexual responsiveness, birth, and breast feeding. In Zubin, J., and Money, J., editors: Contemporary sexual behavior: critical issues in the 1970's, Baltimore, 1973, The John Hopkins University Press.

57. Newton, N.: The role of the oxytocin reflexes in three interpersonal reproductive acts: coitus, birth, and breast feeding. In Carenza, L., Pancheri,

P., and Zichella, L., editors: Clinical psychoneuroendocrinology in reproduction, New York, 1978, Academic Press, Inc.

58. Parker, L.: Coitus during pregnancy, Journal of Nurse-Midwifery **19:**4-7, 1974.

59. Pasini, W.: Sexuality during pregnancy and postpartum frigidity. In Money, J., and Musaph, H., editors: Handbook of sexology, New York, 1977, Elsevier North-Holland Biomedical Press.

60. Perkins, R.: Reply to Dr. Goodlin, American Journal of Obstetrics and Gynecology **135:**1122-1123, 1979.

61. Perkins, R.: Sexual behavior and response in relation to complications of pregnancy, American Journal of Obstetrics and Gynecology **134:**498-505, 1979.

62. Pryor, K.: Nursing your baby, New York, 1973, Pocket Books.

63. Pugh, W.E., and Fernandez, F.L.: Coitus in late pregnancy: a follow-up study of the effects of coitus on late pregnancy, delivery and puerperium, Obstetrics and Gynecology **2:**636-642, 1953.

64. Quirk, B., and Hassanein, R.: The nurse's role in advising patients on coitus during pregnancy, Nursing Clinics of North America **8:**501-507, 1973.

65. Rayburn, W., and Wilson, E.: Coital activity and premature delivery, American Journal of Obstetrics and Gynecology **137:**972-974, 1980.

66. Rehu, M.: The effect of education, marital status, and sexual behavior on the incidence of puerperal endometritis and bacteriuria, Annals of Clinical Research **12:**315-319, 1980.

67. Richardson, C., et. al.: Decreasing postpartum sexual abstinence time, American Journal of Obstetrics and Gynecology **126:**416-417, 1976.

68. Robertson, G.G.: Nausea and vomiting in pregnancy, Lancet **2:**336-341, 1946.

69. Robson, K., Brant, H., and Kumar, R.: Maternal sexuality during first pregnancy and after childbirth, British Journal of Obstetrics and Gynaecology **88:**882-889, 1981.

70. Rossi, A.: Maternalism, sexuality, and the new feminism. In Zubin, J., and Money, J., editors: Contemporary sexual behavior—critical issues in the 1970's, Baltimore, 1973, The Johns Hopkins University Press.

71. Seiden, A.M.: Overview: research on the psychology of women. I. Gender differences and sexual and reproductive life, American Journal of Psychiatry **133:**955-1007, 1976.

72. Selby, J., and Calhoun, L.: Sexuality during pregnancy. In Ahmed, P., editor: Pregnancy, childbirth, and parenthood, New York, 1981, Elsevier North-Holland, Inc.

73. Semmens, J.P.: Female sexuality and life situations: an etiologic psychosocial-sexual profile of weight gain and nausea and vomiting in pregnancy, Obstetrics and Gynecology **38:**555-563, 1971.

74. Sherfey, M.J.: The nature and evolution of female sexuality, New York, 1966, Random House, Inc.

75. Slate, W.: Coitus as a cause of abortion, Medical Aspects of Human Sexuality, **1**(1):25-32, 1970.

76. Solberg, D.A., Butler, J., and Wagner, N.N.: Sexual behavior in pregnancy, New England Journal of Medicine **288:**1098-1103, 1970.

77. Speroff, L., and Ramwell, P.W.: Prostaglandins in reproductive physiology, American Journal of Obstetrics and Gynecology **107:**1111-1130, 1970.
78. Swanson, J.: The marital sexual relationship during pregnancy, J.O.G.N. Nursing, **9:**267-270, 1980.
79. Taylor, S.E., and Langer, E.J.: Pregnancy: a social stigma? Sex Roles **3:**27-35, 1977.
80. Tolor, A., and Di Granzia, P.: Sexual attitudes and behavior patterns during and following pregnancy, Archives of Sexual Behavior **5:**539-551, 1976.
81. van den Berg, B.: Coitus and amniotic fluid infections, New England Journal of Medicine **302:**632-633, 1980.
82. Wagner, N., Butler, J., and Sanders, J.: Prematurity and orgasmic coitus during pregnancy: data on a small sample, Fertility and Sterility **27:**911-915, 1976.
83. Wagner, N., and Solberg, D.: Pregnancy and sexuality, Medical Aspects of Human Sexuality **8:**44-79, March 1974.
84. Weisskopf, S.: Maternal sexuality and asexual motherhood, Signs: Journal of Women in Culture and Society **4:**766-782, 1980.

10 Sexuality and abortion

MARCIA KILLIEN

Induced abortion is one of the most provocative sex-related issues of this era, for it forces individuals to examine their beliefs not only about sexuality but also about the definition and meaning of human life. The practice of abortion encompasses biomedical, social, ethical, political, and legal considerations about which most individuals feel strongly. Because values and attitudes toward abortion influence health care delivery, the topic needs to be carefully examined by all health care professionals.

An induced abortion is defined as the termination of a pregnancy, by deliberate action, before viability of the fetus.[14] Viability, the capability to sustain extrauterine life, has been individually interpreted by the laws of various countries. Definitions have been based on length of gestation (e.g., 20 to 28 weeks), fetal weight, and fetal length. In the United States length of gestation is the accepted criterion for viability.

It is estimated that over 55 million legal abortions occur annually worldwide.[62] In the United States 1.55 million legal abortions were performed in 1980; one fourth of all pregnancies were electively terminated.[35] Thus abortion-related services represent a significant portion of health care to women and their families.

In view of the need for prepared practitioners to provide such care this chapter has the following purposes:
1. To consider the sexual antecedents of abortion, including biologic, psychologic, and sociologic factors
2. To review the sexual sequelae of abortion in terms of biologic, psychologic, and sociologic phenomena
3. To examine the feelings with which the woman and practitioner deal at the time of her decision to abort and after the abortion
4. To explore the health practitioner's role in helping a woman who has had an abortion and her partner to make a positive sexual adjustment

Antecedents of abortion

Sexual decisions. By the time a woman seeks an abortion she has made a number of decisions related to her sexuality and has been influenced by a variety of biologic, psychologic, and sociocultural factors.

The woman's first decision concerns sexual activity: will she have intercourse or not? Increasing proportions of women are becoming sexually active as teenagers. For example, Kinsey[41] found that although 84% of the women in his study were petting by age 18, only about 10% were having intercourse. Recent survey data of unmarried women residing in metropolitan areas of the United States indicated that 23% of 15-year-olds and 69% of 19-year-olds had had intercourse.[71] It has been estimated that among U.S. women of reproductive age (13 to 44 years), 78% are sexually active: about one third of teenagers and nine in ten women aged 20 and older.[20]

Approximately 10% of women of childbearing age are not fecund, resulting either from surgical sterilization or functional infertility. The remainder are at risk for pregnancy unless the decision to use contraception is made. Data from 1978[20] indicated that about three fourths of sexually active, fecund women used some method of contraception at the time of their last intercourse. The remaining 25% were pregnant, attempting a pregnancy, or at high risk of an unintended pregnancy. There are multiple reasons for nonuse of contraception, which will be discussed later in this chapter in relation to women seeking abortion.

In 1978 (the latest year for which data are available) there were 3.1 million unintended pregnancies; this number represents 55% of the 5.6 million pregnancies that occurred that year. Of these unintended conceptions, 58% occurred in women using some method of contraception. Contraceptive failure rates ranged from 2.3% among oral contraceptive users to 21.3% among users of rhythm, withdrawal, and douche methods.[20,35]

Faced with an unintended pregnancy, a woman may choose to continue the pregnancy or have an abortion; in 1980 slightly less than half of women with unintended pregnancies elected abortion.[35]

Biologic considerations: age and health. Over 1.6 million women under age 20 are estimated to have become pregnant in 1978 in the United States. Of these pregnancies, 71% were unintended, compared to 47% of the pregnancies experienced by older women. Approximately 38% of the teenage pregnancies were terminated by elective abortion, in contrast to 22% of the pregnancies of older women.[20] Contrary to popular belief, however, the majority of abortion clients are not teenagers. In 1978, 30.8% of reported induced abortions were performed on women under 20 years of age. The highest proportion of abortions (34.7%) in that year was for women aged 20 to 24 years. In fact the proportion of teenage abortions declined from the 32.8% rate in 1973.[35,62]

Several biologic factors do, however, place today's teenagers at higher risk for unintended pregnancy than either their parents or their older contemporaries. In the analysis of several previous studies Cutright[16] suggested that changes in fecundity, the ability to conceive, and the capacity to avoid spontaneous abortion may be biologic variables contributing to a higher pregnancy rate among today's adolescents than among previous generations. The fecundity of teenage girls seems to have been modified by improved nutrition and general health in preadolescent years. Notable is the decline in the age of menarche: the (average) age in 1940 is estimated to have been 13.5 years, whereas in recent years it is 12.5 years.[13,69] Cutright's analysis indicated that adolescent girls become fully fecund nearly a year earlier than their mothers did: in 1968 nearly 93% were fecund at the age of 17 years; in 1940 only 80% were fertile at that age. He suggested that the pregnancy rate among 15- to 19-year-olds in 1940 was probably lower by 1.6/1000 births because of adolescents' lower fecundity. Biologic maturity may also influence sexual behavior. In an analysis of the fecundity of adolescents Zabin, Kantner, and Zelnik[68] found that girls who begin intercourse at early ages have also had early menarche.

A decline in spontaneous fetal loss has also been observed during the past 30 to 40 years. Cutright[16] suggested that the birth rate among teenagers in 1940 may have been lower by 3.4/1000 births simply because of higher rates of spontaneous abortion. Today's teenager is not only at lower risk of early spontaneous fetal loss than her mother but is also at lower risk than older women. The frequency of spontaneous abortion increases steadily from its lowest rate at ages 20 to 24 to a rate of one in three at age 35, independent of the woman's obstetric history.[43,50] The high rate of spontaneous abortion among older women is most likely related to a propensity for genetic abnormalities. In addition, 75% of spontaneous abortions occur early in pregnancy, and 40% to 60% of these show chromosomal abnormalities.[30] A higher rate of spontaneous fetal loss, increasing proportions of abnormal menstrual cycles, and a tendency toward decreasing frequency of coitus with age contribute to a lower rate of unintended pregnancy and thus abortion in older women.[4,22,30] However, the increasing risk of chromosomal abnormalities of the fetus associated with increased maternal age places older women at risk for an induced abortion for therapeutic reasons.[37]

These findings cause one to wonder if the better biologic status of young women helps to explain the high pregnancy rates and challenges the belief that changes in sexual behavior patterns among teenagers are solely responsible for a great incidence of pregnancies, abortions, and births. In essence the age of the client seeking an abortion may reflect her increased biologic health rather than a propensity for being sexually promiscuous.

Contraceptive use. One wonders, with the increasing availability and acceptability of effective contraceptives, why unintended pregnancies and resulting abortions continue to occur. In fact the abortion rate has continued to increase*:

Year	Abortion rate	Increase over previous year (%)
1973	16.6	unavailable
1974	19.6	18
1975	22.1	13
1976	24.5	11
1977	26.9	10
1978	28.2	5
1979	29.3	4
1980	30.0	2

Henshaw et al.[35] speculate that the rise in the abortion rate in the first years after abortion was legalized can be attributed to the rapid diffusion of abortion services. They attribute the increased abortion rate since 1975 to increases in unintended pregnancy caused by a shift away from the use of the most effective methods of contraception. For example, the proportion of U.S. women aged 15 to 44 years using oral contraceptives was estimated

*From Henshaw, S., et al.: Family Planning Perspectives **14**(1):5-15, 1982.

to have declined by 25% between 1975 and 1978. Use of the intrauterine device similarly declined.[35,71] Reports of negative health consequences associated with the use of these contraceptive methods have undoubtedly contributed to this shift. As stated previously, 58% of unintended pregnancies in 1978 were attributed to contraceptive method failure.[20,35] Contraceptive failure appears to be a significant factor in repeat abortions (i.e., not the first abortion). In a study of 1505 women obtaining abortions in a freestanding New York clinic 23.7% of repeat aborters reported method failure, compared to 15% of first-time aborters.[38] These figures suggest that abortion is not viewed as a substitute for contraception. At particular risk for pregnancy resulting from method failure are teenagers and low-income women. These groups not only tend to use less reliable contraceptive methods but also have higher failure rates for all methods.[13,20] The contraceptive method used may also be an indicator of the woman's desire to avoid a birth. Dryfoos[20] found that 58% of the women who became pregnant while using the most effective birth control methods obtained abortions, compared to 29% of the women using less effective methods. Similar findings were reported in a survey of abortion facilities in Illinois.[65]

Approximately 60% of the abortions that occurred in 1978 were obtained by women who were not using any method of contraception when they became pregnant.[20] Reasons for nonuse of contraceptives are multiple, including lack of knowledge of pregnancy risk, belief that contraceptive use is wrong or dangerous to health, unexpected intercourse, and belief that contraception interferes with sexual enjoyment.[13,45,70] A study of women having a repeat abortion indicated that medical complications associated with contraception led 32% of repeaters to use no method; these women reported trying one or more methods since their first abortion.[38]

The psychodynamics underlying unprotected intercourse are variable: intercourse may be motivated by fear of physical violence, such as rape, or fear of social consequences, such as loneliness. One may use intercourse without contraception as a way of validating fertility, conveying love for another, or conveying hostility toward a parent, spouse, or the "system." There are individuals whose sexual liaisons may be motivated by masochism, those who feel they are "nobody without somebody," and those who simply take advantage of the opportunity to get close to another human being.[45]

In addition, there are several psychic mechanisms that help to explain why women who are enjoying intercourse outside of marriage do not effectively use contraception. First, there may be guilt in conjunction with sex if one believes that sex is only for procreation. Not using contraceptives may alleviate some of the guilt, since one in essence accepts the risk of pregnancy, or "punishment." There may be intense shame involved in obtaining adequate contraceptives; some of the embarrassment may be iatrogenically transmitted by health professionals who are uncomfortable with aspects of sexuality and contraception. Finally, one may deny that a sexual union will occur, since society discourages intercourse among the unmarried. Being convinced that use of contraceptives can be equated with premeditation of the sex act, some women deny themselves adequate protection.[64]

Among women who have abortions, teenagers are much less likely to have used birth control before conception.[20] Teenagers are particularly vulnerable to the psychodynamics just discussed and are more likely to believe themselves immune from pregnancy. Young teenagers may not have achieved the cognitive development that allows them to plan ahead and consider the consequences of their actions.[13] A recent survey of U.S. urban family planning clinics indicated that 36% of teenagers came to clinics because they suspected a pregnancy; only 14% sought contraceptive services in anticipation of first intercourse. Delay in seeking contraceptive services was related to procrastination and fear of parental notification.[67] Black teenagers have been found to seek clinic services more promptly than whites and are more likely to have used a prescription method at first coitus. Effective use of contraception by teenagers is positively associated with formal sex education,[67,72] perception of parental support of contraceptive use,[65] peer use of contraceptives, and satisfying communication with one's sexual partner.[40]

Psychologic antecedents. Historically, the movement for legalized abortion began after World War I. Feminists proclaimed that women should have control over their bodies, psychiatrists warned of suicidal depressions in young pregnant women, and those who favored social reform saw abortion as an end to the cycle of poverty.[20] Danger to life or health were the only grounds for abortion until the more liberal legislation was passed in the early 1970s. Until this legislation was passed, women who were medically ill or were in danger of having an acute and incapacitating emotional problem were the only ones who had access to abortion. As one author[2] put it, women had to be crazy, or in danger of becoming crazy, to have an abortion.

Before more liberal legislation, the most frequently identified antecedents of abortion were usually those related to existing psychopathology, such as depression, personality disorder, and drug abuse. In a more recent sample of 268 women having induced abortions no significant differences between women who had abortions and women having term deliveries appeared on the Minnesota Multiphasic Personality Inventory (MMPI). Furthermore, on tests for anomie (Srole Anomie Scale), self-esteem (Rosenberg's Self-Esteem Scale), and somatic complaints, no differences between the two groups were found in the scores obtained either before or after the abortion or delivery.[2] Gispert and Falk[26] found no differences on the MMPI between 125 teenage abortion candidates and nonpregnant controls. In view of the 1973 legislation making abortion available on demand the psychologic antecedents reported in earlier studies may be invalid.

A study comparing 100 women who applied for hospital abortion and chose not to follow through with 100 women who proceeded with abortion cites characteristics of those who dropped out. The women who chose not to have the abortion tended to be more indecisive; they expressed greater concern about the procedure and its moral implications; they and their partners were less educated; and when telling their partners of the anticipated abortion, the women received more negative responses.[61] A number of investigators who have compared the mental health status of aborters and nonaborters have concluded that the former group tends to be psychologically healthier.[24,54]

Social variables. To fully comprehend sociologic antecedents to abortion, one can consider the strange and often conflicting sociodynamics in the world today. People debate the value of a single human life lost in a war and yet have worldwide population control programs underway. In developed countries the value of a child as a contributor to the family's welfare has come to exist only in rare circumstances; children are now thought to limit a family's economic and social achievement. It is no wonder that there exists neither clear-cut universally acceptable social guidelines regarding abortion nor a list of social variables that reliably predicts who is likely to seek an abortion.

The likelihood of obtaining an abortion is influenced by legal availability of services, economic factors, and sociocultural attitudes. Among the countries of the world, the legal status of induced abortion ranges from complete prohibition to abortion at the request of the pregnant woman. As of late 1980, the world situation can be summarized as follows: of the 4.4 billion people living in the world, 9% live in countries totally prohibiting abortion for any reason; 19% live where abortion may be performed only to save the mother's life; for 10% abortion is permitted for broader medical reasons; for 24% abortion is permitted for social factors as additional threats to health; 38% live where abortion is available on demand. The most restrictive countries include the Muslim countries of Asia, two thirds of Latin America, most of Africa, and five European countries (Belgium, Ireland, Malta, Portugal, and Spain). Opposition to liberalization of abortion laws has come from conservative groups on moral and religious grounds (e.g., Roman Catholic church) and from groups concerned about low birth rates.[62] The enforcement of abortion statutes varies.

The United States is currently among the countries with liberal abortion statutes. Before 1967 most states restricted abortion to those pregnancies that presented a threat to the mother's life. In that year Colorado (followed by other states) adopted legislation permitting abortion if the pregnancy (1) posed a threat to the physical or mental health of the mother, (2) would result in a physically or mentally defective child, or (3) resulted from rape or incest.[62] In 1970 laws were enacted in Alaska, Hawaii, Washington, and New York that did not specify indications for abortion, thus authorizing pregnancy termination on request. These laws initiated considerable debate in states with more restrictive legislation and led to two landmark decisions by the Supreme Court in January 1973. In one case, *Roe v. Wade,* the court ruled that during the first trimester, "the abortion decision and its effectuation must be left to the medical judgment of the pregnant woman's attending physician" in consultation with the woman. After the first trimester "the state . . . may . . . regulate the abortion procedure in ways that are reasonably related to maternal health." After the fetus has reached viability "the state . . . may . . . proscribe abortion except where necessary . . . for the preservation of the life or health of the mother." The second case, *Doe v. Bolton,* involved the elimination of procedural restrictions, such as authorization for abortion by a special committee and residency requirements.[62]

Since the 1973 Supreme Court decisions, ethical and moral issues concerning abortion have been debated. The ethical issues focus on the respect for human life and a determination of when life begins. Supporters of the antiabortion movement assert that since abortion is a moral issue, it should not be legislatively sanctioned. In a pluralistic society such as this one can such moral positions be legislated? The Right to Life movement appears to be a highly organized, well-financed group of people whose primary purpose is to stop abortions. Their strategies to accomplish this goal have varied from supporting restrictive state legislation interfering with delivery of abortion services, to proposing an antiabortion amendment, to calling for a constitutional convention. They exert pressure on candidates at local, state, and national levels of government to take a stand on the abortion issue.

Legislative attempts to prevent or delay implementation of liberal abortion laws have been challenged in the courts. In 1976 the U.S. Supreme Court struck down state laws requiring spousal and parental consent for abortion.[53,62] However, in March 1981 the authority of a state to require parental notification for abortion for a dependent minor living at home was upheld. In that year eight states passed laws requiring a minor seeking abortion to have consent of her parents or a judge or to notify her parents of her intentions.[19]

In June 1977 the Hyde Amendment was attached to the Department of Health, Education, and Welfare's labor appropriations bill. It prohibited the use of federal funds to pay for or to promote or encourage abortions after October 1977. Federal funding remained available only when the life of the mother was endangered by carrying the fetus to term and in some cases of rape or incest. Many states followed the lead of the federal government by restricting funding for abortion. As a result, the numbers of abortions funded by either state or federal governments fell by one third between 1977 and 1978 from 294,000 to 193,800.[27] There have been several attempts to determine the impact of this legislation on pregnancy outcomes. A study of two states, Georgia and Ohio, indicated that when medicaid abortion funding was restricted, between 18% and 23% of the women who would have terminated their pregnancies instead had unwanted births.[63] In a comparison of states with and without public funding of abortion Selik, Cates, and Tyler[57] found that medical complications from illegal abortions have not significantly increased as a result of funding restrictions but that legal abortions performed on poor women have declined. However, a report from the Centers for Disease Control (CDC) indicated that the absence of public funding and lack of abortion services played a primary role in six of the seventeen illegal abortion deaths occurring between 1974 and 1979.[5] These findings support the view that the primary result of the Hyde Ammendment has been an increase in unintended births among certain groups of women.[33,56,57]

The results of 1978 and 1979 national surveys of abortion services in the United States by the Alan Guttmacher Institute indicated that 34% of women needing abortion services in 1978 and 29% in 1979 were unable to obtain them. This deficit in health care was attributed to inaccessibility of abortion facilities and withdrawal of public funding. In 1978, 77% of U.S. counties had no abortion services; 27% of women in need of abortions resided in these counties. Only 18% of all public hospitals (on which many poor people depend for medical care) offered abortion services.[33,56]

Women who obtain abortions are primarily young, white, unmarried, and childless. In 1978 two thirds of abortion clients were under age 25, 69% were white, 75% were unmarried, and 57% were childless. Between 1977 and 1978 the abortion rate declined slightly for nonwhite and unmarried women, probably reflecting the decreased financial accessibility of these women to abortion.[33] It is important to keep in mind, however, that women of all ages, ethnic backgrounds, socioeconomic levels, and marital statuses do seek and obtain abortions.

Public attitudes toward abortion have become increasingly liberal since the mid-1970s. In a 1980 survey sponsored by the National Opinion Research Center of the University of Chicago, 41% of respondents indicated approval for legal abortion for "any reason," compared to 33% who gave "blanket approval" in 1978. Approval rates based on six circumstances varied from 83% to 90% approval for reasons such as threat to the woman's life, rape, and serious fetal defects to 47% to 52% approval for reasons of low income, unmarried status, or not wanting additional children. Only 7% of respondents disapproved of abortion for all reasons.[29] What are the factors that influence a person's attitude toward

abortion? Data from several studies[29,34,58] have indicated that attitudes are closely associated with education, religious affiliation and religiosity, and other social values. The
more highly educated, non-Catholics, and those who attend church less frequently tend
to be more supportive of legal abortion than their counterparts. Sex, age, race, occupational prestige, and income do not seem to be strong predictors of attitudes. Conservative
attitudes toward abortion are related to conservativism in other values, such as disapproval
of nonmarital sex and women's rights. At this time antiabortion groups are attempting
to restrict abortion through passage of a Human Life Amendment, which would propose
that human life begins at conception. Such an amendment would nullify the 1973 Supreme
Court decision. Some proposed legislation would prohibit abortion even to save the
mother's life. Such conservatism is inconsistent with national public attitudes. A 1981
national telephone survey indicated that only 32% of women favor a law that says that
human life begins at conception, and 92% favor legal abortion if the mother's health is
at risk.[34] However, survey data have indicated that people who oppose abortion are more
likely to give financial or other support to political action activities related to abortion
than advocates are.[58]

Sequelae of abortion

Biologic sequelae. After abortion there are no known physical consequences that directly preclude the woman's return to functional sexual behavior. However, induced abortion does expose the woman to a risk of physical complications that
can indirectly affect her later sexual functioning.

The severity of potential complications ranges from mild symptoms to the rare fatal
outcome. Risk of these complications depends on the woman's general health status, the
gestational period during which abortion is performed, and the abortion techniques used.
Complications can be divided into two categories: early complications that occur during
or immediately following the abortion and up to 1 month after abortion, and late complications that occur after the first month.

Among the serious complications that can occur during or within several hours after
induced abortion are hemorrhage, cervical injury, uterine perforation, and embolism
(thrombus, air, and amniotic fluid). Additional complications occurring primarily with
procedures used in late abortions are severe disturbances in blood coagulation and hy-
pernatremia associated with saline instillation, water intoxication resulting from high
doses of oxytocin, and anesthesic complications. The most frequent delayed complications
include retention of placental fragments, which results in bleeding, infection ranging from
mild endometritis to severe pelvic inflammatory disease, peritonitis and septicemia, and
thromboembolic disease.[31,62] Minor complaints that are common within the first days after
abortion include mild fever, nausea, and uterine cramping.

The most comprehensive investigation of early complications of legal abortions in
the United States was undertaken by the Joint Program for the Study of Abortion, sponsored by the Population Council during 1970 and 1971 and continued by the CDC from
1971 to 1975. The rate of major complications for 66,763 women without preexisting
conditions or concurrent sterilization was 0.7/100 abortions. The risk of major morbidity
increased with advancing gestational age from 0.3/100 abortions at 7 to 8 menstrual

weeks to 2.26/100 abortions at 21 to 24 weeks. Similarly, the incidence of total complications (major and minor) was higher at 6 weeks' gestation or earlier than 7 to 10
weeks. The risk of complications from abortion is best described as a continuum, increasing by about 20% with each week of gestation from 7 through 20 weeks.[31,62] In
1978, 50% of all abortions were performed before 9 weeks' gestation, and 91% were
performed before 13 weeks' gestation; less than 1% occurred at greater than 20 weeks'
gestation. The timing of the abortion is closely associated with the method used and thus
the risk involved. Of all abortions in 1978, 95% were performed by suction or sharp
curettage, 3.6% by saline instillation, 0.1% by hysterotomy or hysterectomy, and 1.3%
by other methods (e.g., prostaglandins). Since 1973, there has been a steady increase in
the proportion of abortions induced at early gestation and with less hazardous techniques.[33]
The joint effects of delay and method compound abortion morbidity. Grimes and Cates[31]
estimated that delay of suction curettage from 8 to 10 weeks' gestation increases the risk
of major complication by 60%; delay from 8 to 16 weeks' gestation increases the risk
by 300% to 1300%, depending on the abortion method used. Women who delay abortion
may also be at increased health risk because of personal and social characteristics. In a
study of women seeking abortion in Washington, D.C., delay was found to be associated
with lower education, irregular periods, nonacknowledgment of pregnancy symptoms,
and shorter duration of relationships with a sexual partner.[10] The investigators concluded
that biologic factors, knowledge, and psychologic maturity are important influences in
postponement. These factors may also be indicators of the woman's general health status
and ability to promote her own health after abortion.

The probability of dying from abortion is very small. According to Cates,[12] legal
abortion provides a safer option for women faced with an unwanted pregnancy than
carrying the pregnancy to term. The mortality associated with abortion has steadily
declined since 1970; in 1978 the National Center for Health Statistics reported 16 abortion-
related deaths. The risk of dying from term birth is about sevenfold greater than from
abortion.[31] Mortality is increased with advanced gestational age and second-trimester
procedures. In the United States abortions performed at 12 weeks' gestation or earlier
have only 1.6 deaths per 100,000 procedures. Infection is the leading cause of abortion-
related death, followed by embolic events and anesthesia-associated reactions.[31] Despite
availability of legal abortions, illegal abortion deaths continue to occur. The CDC reported
63 such deaths between 1972 and 1974 and 17 deaths between 1975 and 1979. These
latter women were disproportionately black and hispanic; the majority died of infection.[5]

The late-occurring consequences of abortion have been the subject of much concern
and investigation. Long-term morbidity is difficult to document, since many years may
be required before any effect can be noted and because such sequelae are relatively rare
occurrences. As several investigators have noted, studies of long-term sequelae have
suffered from several methodologic limitations that limit their generalizability: (1) inadequate documentation of the abortion history in either the study or comparison group,
(2) inadequate information about the abortion procedure, and (3) failure to control for
confounding variables common to both the risk factor of abortion and the complication
being studied (e.g., age, parity, socioeconomic status).[7,11,31,62] Because many women who
have abortions are young and may desire future childbearing, the effect of abortion on
menstrual patterns, fertility, and subsequent pregnancy outcome has been examined. To

date, the available case control and cohort studies have yielded inconsistent findings. Although increased menstrual disorders, including infertility, dysmenorrhea, and perimenstrual distress, have been noted, subsequent studies fail to support these findings.[31] Reviews of available research conducted in the United States and internationally report some findings of association between previous induced abortion and subsequent spontaneous abortion, ectopic pregnancy, premature and low birth weight infants, Rh sensitization, and birth defects. However, a number of other studies report no such association.* There is some evidence that subsequent pregnancy loss or perinatal complications are related to abortion method and number of previous abortions. Specifically, abortions using dilation and curettage may pose some increased risk of later cervical incompetence leading to spontaneous abortion or premature birth. The risk of these complications appears to be increased by multiple previous abortions.[7,31,44,47] It should be emphasized that the absolute risk of these complications is small and that these findings are preliminary.

Although the preceding biologic sequelae of abortion normally do not directly interfere with the woman's sexual function, it is important to examine the indirect influence they may exert on her sexual self-concept and subsequent sexual behavior. The immediate complications of induced abortion may be life threatening. If these complications are seen as punishment for a sexual relationship, chances are their occurrence will reinforce the woman's guilt feelings. If sterility results from sepsis, hemorrhage, or uterine perforation that may warrant hysterectomy, it is possible that the guilt reaction may be profound, especially if the woman desires a child at a future time. Guilt may also be intense if subsequent perinatal complications occur, such as spontaneous abortion or prematurity. Guilt and fear of such problems may interfere with satisfying sexual relationships. It is possible that the woman's body image or concept of herself may be altered: she may wish to dissociate herself from her sexual behavior and may alter her sexual behavior to avoid heterosexual relations. To compensate for her feelings, she may also seek validation of her sexual identity with a number of partners.

Psychologic sequelae. The woman who finds herself pregnant and decides to terminate the pregnancy faces a number of stressful situations. Five potentially traumatic events will be confronted: the realization of an unwanted pregnancy, the decision to terminate the pregnancy, the negotiations for the abortion, the experience of the abortion, and the acceptance of the decision and its consequences. Depending on their own resources, their coping abilities, and the support available from others, women will experience varying degrees of crisis.

It has often been assumed that women undergoing abortions experience emotional distress and psychiatric disturbance. This assumption has been largely based on impressionistic case reports and on studies of women who had abortions before the 1973 Supreme Court decision. In the latter situation emotional disturbance may have been iatrogenically enhanced, since abortion was conditional on establishing a physical or mental disease. Depression, guilt, or inability to cope may have been exaggerated by the medical screening process or circumstances under which the abortion was performed.

A World Health Organization review of data reported from many countries concluded that there was a low incidence of adverse psychologic sequelae from abortion, and

---

*References 6, 7, 11, 31, 46, 47, and 62.

frequently psychologic benefit resulted.[62] The U.S. literature offers similar conclusions. Immediate emotional responses to abortion commonly include anger, guilt, fear, sadness, and relief.[1,6,25] Because abortion does involve a loss, grief responses are not unexpected. Long-term or severe negative psychologic responses are rare.[6,48,56,62] For example, in a study of 125 St. Louis women who sought abortion 78% had no immediate negative psychologic response, and 90% reported no negative sequelae 1 year later.[60]

A follow-up study of women who had first-trimester abortions at a Boston outpatient clinic found that the majority of women who reported sadness, regret, or guilt immediately after abortion no longer reported these feelings 1 year later.[1]

Several factors have been identified as influencing emotional response to abortion. Negative psychologic sequelae have been associated with a history of emotional problems,[1,48] negative or absent relationships with family or sexual partners,[1,18,25,48,59] strong ambivalence about the abortion decision,[1,59] and negative religious or cultural sanctions for abortion.[1,6] These findings suggest that the negative psychologic sequelae of abortion are usually short-term and tend to reflect the circumstances surrounding the abortion and the attitudes and support conveyed by significant others in the peer group, family, and health care setting.

Few studies have compared the psychologic outcome of women who abort with those who carry an unwanted pregnancy to term. As Fogel[23] suggests, although an abortion may evoke feelings of guilt, sadness, and regret, the alternatives of adoption, single parenthood, forced marriage, or unwanted children also carry psychologic burdens. In one Danish study[18] no differences in psychiatric hospital admission rates were found between women who had abortions and those who had full-term pregnancies. However, the highest rates of psychiatric disturbance were among those women who were separated or divorced, regardless of pregnancy outcome, again emphasizing the important mediating effect of social support.

That some women are more vulnerable to unwanted pregnancy and resultant psychologic difficulties is supported by studies of women who seek repeat abortions. Women who seek a repeat abortion display three characteristics more often than those seeking a first abortion: being more dissatisfied with themselves, perceiving themselves as victims of bad luck, and expressing negative feelings toward the current abortion.[42] The dynamics of their sexual relationships may be associated with unprotected intercourse.[6] Freeman et al.[25] found that after pregnancy termination repeat aborters had significantly higher emotional distress scores related to interpersonal relationships than did women having first abortions.

Abortion may also have positive psychologic outcomes for the woman. The experience of making and carrying out a major life decision can be a maturing experience. Abrams, Di Biase, and Sturgis[1] reported that over one third of women in their study felt they were better able to deal with problems and had learned more about their coping abilities as a result of the abortion experience. In addition, they had become more responsible about contraceptive use; 76% of the women were using effective birth control 1 year after abortion, compared to 21% who used contraception before the abortion. In another study teenagers who had abortions were more likely to be using contraceptives at 6-month follow-up than teenagers who had a negative pregnancy test.[21]

The absence of significant negative emotional distress for most women and the potential for positive reactions are important for health professionals to recognize. A 1980 study[3] of three professional groups (physicians, nurses, and social workers) found that these professionals tended to assume that women who undergo abortions are extremely anxious, guilty, and depressed. Experience with abortion clients did not influence these expectations. If health care professionals expect negative responses from their clients, they may inadvertently introduce stress into the situation.

Sexual sequelae. The woman's sexual partner may exert a profound effect on the woman's decision to abort and on her psychologic response to abortion. Shusterman[59] reported that the degree of intimacy between the woman and her male partner and his participation in the experience were major factors explaining emotional reactions to abortion. The importance of the partner's support has already been discussed. Little is known about the man's response to the abortion or the impact of his feelings on the woman. Gordon[28] found that men accompanying their partners seeking abortion experienced anxiety, which decreased when group counseling was provided to them.

Abortion may affect sexual relationships in a variety of ways. One study found that 44% of the unmarried women in the sample had discontinued contact with the partner at the 1-year follow-up; 33% maintained a form of friendship with the partner; and 13% subsequently married him. Another 9% were steadily dating their sexual partner. Also, 67% of the women had positive regard for the partner, and 8% had negative feelings; there was no subsequent change in the marriage status. Most of the women had discussed the abortion with their partners. Furthermore, 81% of the women had resumed intercourse at follow-up. Women younger than 20 years of age were more likely to observe abstinence because of fear of pregnancy or loss of interest in sex.[60]

In another study two thirds of the women reported no change in their feelings about sexual activity 6 months after abortion. The majority of women who reported a change in feelings cited greater feelings of responsibility about sexual activity or increased awareness of sexual feelings. The most frequent negative change was inhibition caused by fear about pregnancy.[1] A comparative study[2] of women having abortions and those with term pregnancies found no significant differences in the frequency of intercourse after the procedure, the number of sex partners before or after hospitalization, changes in orgasm frequency, or changes in the enjoyment of sex. In addition, there were no differences in happiness in their relationship.

Health practitioner: feelings, attitudes, and practice

The root of the conflict experienced by many health professionals caring for the woman who seeks an abortion probably lies in the individual practitioner's attitudinal framework. Unless one is truly convinced of the morality or legality of induced abortion, it is difficult to convey support to the woman involved. The first step in providing care for the woman having an induced abortion is clarification of the clinician's own values. It is essential to determine whether one can be therapeutic while disapproving of abortion for oneself. If one is truly convinced that abortion under any circumstances is immoral, then these feelings will undoubtedly be conveyed to the woman at a time when she requires reassurance that she has made the best possible decision for her. The wisdom of involving oneself in abortion counseling without the conviction that abortion is morally acceptable might be questioned.

For health practitioners to examine their attitudes toward abortion, they can consider a number of relevant questions:

- What is human life?
- When does it begin?
- To what extent does the embryo/fetus develop before it can be considered a live human being?
- To what extent does the quality of a future life influence one's concept of "life"?
- Does an embryo/fetus have rights? Human dignity?
- At what point do the woman's rights supercede those of the embryo/fetus?
- Should the father have any input into the decision to abort the embryo/fetus?

These questions undoubtedly occur to practitioners who perform or assist with abortions and to the woman who seeks the abortion. The manner in which one responds will be influenced by a number of variables: one's religious or ethical commitments, current personal and societal definitions of morality and crime, a society's sanctions of feticide or infanticide, and current social emphasis on the desirability of birth and the practice of fetal medicine. These reference points may yield some personal guidelines for the practitioner to use in those situations in which values are challenged or questioned in a changing world.

Since health professionals practice within the framework of society and culture, it is important to consider the social climate in which abortion occurs. Even among population researchers, divergent opinions exist. Some researchers cast the blame for current ecologic problems in the direction of the American economy. Some authorities believe that population control is desirable and that conception should be the result of a deliberate choice.[49] Some even advocate a policy in which couples are required to pay part of the externalities that another human being imposes on society.[15] Another authority[31] advocates mutual coercion, mutually agreed on, to limit the population, warning that no technical solution will be sufficient to rescue the world from the problems of overpopulation.

In view of the conflict voiced among professionals the Nurses Association of the American College of Obstetricians and Gynecologists (NAACOG) published a statement on the nurse's role with the abortion client. In this statement they urged genuine concern and compassion for the woman having an abortion. Simultaneously they stated that nurses have the right to refuse to assist with abortions or sterilizations in keeping with their own moral, ethical, or religious beliefs except when the patient's life is clearly in danger. The NAACOG also emphasizes that failure to assist with abortions should not jeopardize one's employment; employers are encouraged to describe their policies regarding abortion to employees, and the nurse is encouraged to reciprocate.[51]

Perhaps the most crucial component of the NAACOG statement is the portion affirming that nurses should not impose their personal views on clients or other personnel. In view of the need to respect and safeguard an individual's rights staff members caring for abortion clients are faced with special challenges if their interactions are to be genuine.

Without congruence of attitudes, knowledge, and behavior, the professional cannot present a consistent approach to the client who is most vulnerable to the positive or negative responses of staff persons.

Health care process

Assessment. The counselor's initial response to the client is a critical variable in the relationship to follow. It is during the assessment process that the health practitioner gathers data about the woman's counseling needs; simultaneously the client gathers data about her counselor's genuine acceptance and understanding.

In the initial interview one who provides abortion counseling may be helping a woman who has firm convictions that abortion is her only choice or who is ambivalent about the outcome of her pregnancy and requests assistance with decision making. Once the client has decided to have an abortion, her feelings about the crisis she faces need attention. Anxiety and ambivalence are not unusual responses.

Data about the woman's attitudes toward the abortion itself often reveal conflicts between intellectual and attitudinal dimensions of her thinking. The woman may intellectually believe that abortion is the correct alternative for her at this time, but her gut-level emotions may say just the opposite. Family, education, religion, and cultural background may be strong influences. The woman may verbalize that abortion is murder but still intellectually desire the procedure.

The support offered by significant others is crucial to resolution of the abortion crisis. Does the partner agree that abortion is the best alternative? What effect will it have on the relationship? How will her family and close friends react? Thinking about these potential reactions may help the woman decide whom to tell and what sort of approach to use.

Conflicts about sexuality may become apparent during counseling. These problems may even contribute to this and subsequent unwanted pregnancies. Women who have had previous unwanted pregnancies may be attempting to meet some need. If a precipitating factor can be identified, perhaps recidivism can be prevented.

If the woman is married, the husband can also provide valuable data. Is he supportive of his wife's decision? What are the familial and socioeconomic reasons that abortion was considered? Of what consequence is the abortion to the woman's sexuality? To her sex partner's?

Intervention. Once one has assessed the presence or absence of crisis, the degree of guilt involved in choosing abortion, the potential for support from significant others, and the effectiveness of the woman's coping mechanisms, it is possible to determine the manner in which the counselor intervenes. In some institutions or agencies the counselor can become involved with the woman at the intake interview, observing her throughout with supportive care until the crisis has resolved.

In many instances the practitioner's role becomes one of crisis intervention. The client is assisted to mobilize her own resources to face the abortion and accept her decision. In states where teenagers must have the consent of their parents to have an abortion the counselor may become involved in providing services to the entire family.

Since some women do present with unwanted pregnancies as a result of psychopathology, they may need to be referred to a psychiatrist for help. Women who become pregnant as an act of self-jeopardy are able to gain insights from psychotherapy. The counselor can review the assessment for indications of practices that require referral for psychiatric help.

Another important aspect of the abortion counselor's role is education. In spite of sex education programs in public schools considerable ignorance exists among sexually active adolescents. The use of contraceptives is not always consistent with current knowledge about their relative effectiveness. The fear regarding obtaining contraceptives may be linked to guilt about sexual activity.

Contraception is one very important aspect of teaching for the abortion client but not the only one. The health practitioner has an opportunity to provide counseling for a healthy sexuality. Many women have unanswered questions about their sexuality—both psychologic and biologic aspects. Some women may have aversive feelings toward men and may require help to deal with their feelings in a healthy way. Some may have poor images of themselves as people and/or sexual beings. For the woman whose guilt is reflected in derogatory comments about herself, further sexual relationships may be motivated by a desire to overcompensate for these feelings, or she may avoid heterosexual relations altogether.

In addition to counseling the woman about her sexual function, the practitioner can help her examine ways of promoting sexually responsible behavior in the future. Burchell[9] enumerates nine ways in which one can examine the meaning and uses of sex. He suggests exploring the presence of a conscious decision for sexual involvement, adequacy of the client's knowledge about sexual psychology and physiology, her understanding of contraception and sexually transmitted disease, and her knowledge of and feelings about abortion. He also suggests exploring to what degree vulnerability or exploitation was involved in this pregnancy, the dynamics of the sexual relationship, the congruence of the behavior with the woman's value system, and her ability to achieve joy through sex. Discussion of these components of sexual decision making can give the counselor cues about the issue of responsibility in a sexual relationship. Does the woman use her authority appropriately? Can she accept the consequences of her behavior?

An important aspect of counseling the client who has had an abortion is imparting some guidelines for resuming sexual intercourse. Because of the risk of infection, women are asked to avoid intercourse for 2 weeks, as well as refrain from douching or using tampons.

For the woman who wanted a child, a therapeutic abortion may be synonymous with loss. In this case the counselor may intervene by helping the woman grieve for the lost child. It is also possible that the same woman will feel guilty about having the abortion: she may blame herself for her own ill health or for the problem that caused the fetus to be abnormal.

The abortion counselor is confronted with a variety of women whose problems are unique. How the counselor intervenes will, of course, depend on thorough assessment of the presence of a sexual crisis, the woman's coping mechanisms, and support of significant others.

Summary

This chapter has explored the biopsychosocial aspects of sexual antecedents and sequelae of abortion, the feelings with which the client and counselor deal during abortion counseling, and the clinician's role in helping the woman who has had an abortion make a positive sexual adjustment. Key considerations based to health care include the following:

1. The woman who chooses the abortion alternative cannot be typified: antecedents to abortion may depend on biologic variables, such as contraceptive failure; psychologic variables, such as low self-concept; and social variables, such as unsatisfying interpersonal relationships that precipitate unwanted pregnancy.
2. Biologic sequelae of abortion do not usually preclude future sexual functioning.
3. Psychologic sequelae of abortion usually include relief, sadness, and depression, are not usually profound, and tend to be self-limiting.
4. Sexual sequelae of abortion may be salutary, in that family stress may be reduced and heterosexual relationships may improve, or unhealthy if the sexual relationship is disrupted.
5. Abortion counselors need to determine whether their knowledge, attitudes, and behavior with regard to abortion are congruous.
6. The woman seeking abortion may require crisis intervention services, assistance with feelings of guilt, and help in grieving for a loss.

Questions for review

1. What populations have abortions in the area in which you practice? On what data do you base your response?
2. Since attitudes are extremely contagious and the client having an abortion is vulnerable to them, it is important to sort out your feelings before caring for her. Rate each of the following statements:

	STRONGLY AGREE	AGREE	DISAGREE	STRONGLY DISAGREE
Life begins at conception	☐	☐	☐	☐
Life begins at birth	☐	☐	☐	☐
Abortion will encourage sexual promiscuity	☐	☐	☐	☐
Abortion should never be performed	☐	☐	☐	☐
Abortion should be available to women on demand	☐	☐	☐	☐
Abortion should be available only to women whose physical condition makes completion of pregnancy life threatening	☐	☐	☐	☐
Public funds should be available for abortions	☐	☐	☐	☐

On the basis of your ratings, is it likely that you can be therapeutic with women who are seeking abortion?

3. Discuss the following statement: Women who seek abortions are usually sexually promiscuous. Use data from the chapter to support or refute it.
4. For what reasons do women have intercourse without adequate contraception?
5. What social variables are associated with favorable attitudes toward abortion?
6. What physical consequences of abortion may influence the woman's future sexual function?
7. Of what consequence is having an abortion to the woman's mental health? How can the health professional limit psychic trauma?
8. Analyze the following case studies to determine which person is at greatest risk. Use the following criteria to evaluate how the woman is coping:

- Realistic understanding of her situation
- Supportive others to help her deal with her problem pregnancy
- Past patterns of coping well with stressful situations

How can you best help these women cope with the abortion?

■ **Case A:** Rose Thompson, a 15-year-old high school student, seeks problem pregnancy counseling when she is 5 months pregnant. She says she postponed getting help because she "just couldn't believe she was pregnant." She links her pregnancy to a beach weekend with a casual acquaintance who has since moved to another city.

■ **Case B:** Martha McClure, 45 years old, seeks an abortion on the referral of her physician, who has determined that her unborn child has a genetic defect. Martha has been a devout Catholic to this point but says she cannot accept a retarded child. Her husband is against the abortion, but Martha says she has had to face many problems without his support in the past, since he is in the armed forces and is frequently away from home.

■ **Case C:** Jane Carlson is a 22-year-old single secretary whose pregnancy resulted from a relationship with her married boss. Although she wanted to keep the child, he insisted that she obtain an abortion or he would terminate their relationship. Jane maintains that "everything will be okay after the abortion."

■ **Case D:** Laura Olson is a 38-year-old, recently divorced attorney. She reports her pregnancy is a result of contraceptive failure. She fears a child at this time will interrupt her career plans yet is concerned she may never have another opportunity for pregnancy because of her advancing age.

References

1. Abrams, M., DiBiase, V., and Sturgis, S.: Post-abortion attitudes and patterns of birth control, Journal of Family Practice **9:**593-599, 1979.
2. Athanasiou, R., et al.: Psychiatric sequelae to term birth and induced early and late abortion: a longitudinal study, Family Planning Perspectives **5:**227-231, 1973.
3. Baluk, W., and O'Neill, P.O.: Health professionals' perceptions of the psychological consequences of abortion, American Journal of Community Psychology **8**(1):67-75, 1980.

4. Barrett, J.C., and Marshall, J.: The risk of conception on different days of the menstrual cycle, Population Studies **23:**455, 1969.

5. Binkin, N., Gold, J., and Cates, W.: Illegal-abortion deaths in the United States: why are they still occurring? Family Planning Perspectives **14:**163-167, 1982.

6. Bracken, M.B.: Psychosomatic aspects of abortion: implications for counseling, Journal of Reproductive Medicine **19:**265-271, 1977.

7. Bracken, M.B.: Induced abortion as a risk factor for perinatal complications: a review, Yale Journal of Biological Medicine **51:**539-548, 1978.

8. Bracken, M.B., and Holford, T.: Induced abortion and congenital malformation in offspring of subsequent pregnancies, American Journal of Epidemiology **109:**425-432, 1979.

9. Burchell, R.C.: Promoting responsible sexual behavior. In Wilson, R., editor: Problem pregnancy and abortion counseling, Saluda, N.C., 1973, Family Life Publications.

10. Burr, W., and Schulz, K.: Delayed abortion in an area of easy accessibility, Journal of American Medical Association **244**(1):44-48, 1980.

11. Cates, W., Jr.: Late effects of induced abortion—hypothesis or knowledge? Journal of Reproductive Medicine **22:**207-212, 1979.

12. Cates, W., Jr.: Abortion myths and realities: who is misleading whom? American Journal of Obstetrics and Gynecology **142:**954-956, 1982.

13. Chilman, C.: Adolescent sexuality in a changing American society: social and psychological perspectives, Department of Health, Education, and Welfare Pub. no. (NIH) 79-1426.

14. Clark, A., and Affonso, D.: Childbearing: a nursing perspective, ed. 2, Philadelphia, 1979, F.A. Davis Co.

15. Coale, J.: Man and his environment, Science **170:**132-136, 1970.

16. Cutright, P.: The teen-age sexual revolution and the myth of an abstinent past, Family Planning Perspectives **4:**24-31, Jan. 1972.

17. Daling, J.R., and Emanuel, I.: Induced abortion and subsequent outcome of pregnancy, Lancet **2:**170-173, 1975.

18. David, H., Rasmussen, N., and Holst, E.: Postpartum and postabortion psychotic reactions, Family Planning Perspectives **13**(2):88-91, 1981.

19. Donovan, P.: Fertility-related state laws enacted in 1981, Family Planning Perspectives **14**(2):63-67, 1982.

20. Dryfoos, G.: Contraceptive use, pregnancy intentions and pregnancy outcomes among U.S. women, Family Planning Perspectives **14**(2):81-94, 1982.

21. Evans, J., Selstad, G., and Welcer, W.: Teenagers: fertility control behavior and attitudes before and after abortion, childbearing or negative pregnancy test, Family Planning Perspectives **8:**192-200, 1976.

22. Federation CECOS, Schwarts, D., and Mayaux, M.: Female fecundity as a function of age, New England Journal of Medicine **306:**404-406, 1982.

23. Fogel, C.I.: Abortion. In Fogel, C.I., and Woods, N., editors: Health care of women: a nursing perspective, St. Louis, 1981, The C.V. Mosby Co.

24. Freeman, E.W.: Abortion: subjective attitudes and feelings, Family Planning Perspectives **10:**130-133, 1978.

25. Freeman, E.W., et al.: Emotional distress patterns among women having first or repeated abortions, Obstetrics and Gynecology **55:**630-636, 1980.

26. Gispert, M., and Falk, R.: Adolescent sexual activity: contraception and abortion, American Journal of Obstetrics and Gynecology **132**:620-628, 1978.

27. Gold, R.: After the Hyde Amendment: public funding for abortions in FY1978, Family Planning Perspectives **12**:131-134, 1980.

28. Gordon, R.H.: Efficacy of a group crisis-counseling program for men who accompany women seeking abortions, American Journal of Community Psychology **6**:239-246, 1978.

29. Granberg, D., and Granberg, B.: Abortion attitudes, 1965-1980: trends and determinants, Family Planning Perspectives **12**:250-261, 1980.

30. Gray, R.H.: Biological and social interactions in the determination of late fertility, Journal of Biosocial Science Suppl. **6**:97-115, 1979.

31. Grimes, D.A., and Cates, W.: Complications from legally-induced abortion: a review, Obstetric and Gynecology Survey **34**(3):177-191, 1979.

32. Hardin, G.: The tragedy of the commons, Science **162**:1243-1248, 1968.

33. Henshaw, S., et al.: Abortion in the United States, 1978-1979, Family Planning Perspectives **13**(1):6-18, 1981.

34. Henshaw, S., and Martire, G.: Abortion and the public opinion polls, Family Planning Perspectives **14**(2):53-62, 1982.

35. Henshaw, S., et al.: Abortion services in the United States, 1979 and 1980, Family Planning Perspectives **14**(1):5-15, 1982.

36. Hoffmeyer, H.: Psychological aspects of legal abortion and contraception, Journal of Sex Research **4**:7-15, 1968.

37. Hook, E.B.: Rates of chromosome abnormalities at different maternal ages, Obstetrics and Gynecology **58**:282-285, 1981.

38. Howe, B., Kaplan, H.R., and English, C.: Repeat abortions: blaming the victims, American Journal of Public Health **69**:1242-1246, 1979.

39. Jorgensen, S.: Contraceptive attitude-behavior consistency in adolescence, Population and Environment **3**:174-194, 1980.

40. Jorgensen, S., King, S., and Torrey, B.: Dyadic and social network influences on adolescent exposure to pregnancy risk, Journal of Marriage and the Family **42**:141-155, Feb. 1980.

41. Kinsey, A., et al.: Sexual behavior in the human female, Philadelphia, 1953, W.B. Saunders Co.

42. Leach, J.: The repeat abortion patient, Family Planning Perspectives **9**(1):37-39, 1977.

43. Leridon, H.: Patterns of fertility at later ages of reproduction, Journal of Biosocial Science Suppl. **6**:59-74, 1979.

44. Levin, A.A., et al.: Association of induced abortion with subsequent pregnancy loss, J.A.M.A. **243**:2495-2499, 1980.

45. Luker, K.: Taking changes: abortion and the decision not to contracept, Berkeley, 1975, University of California Press.

46. Madore, C., et al.: A study on the effects of induced abortion on subsequent pregnancy outcome, American Journal of Obstetrics and Gynecology **139**:516-521, 1981.

47. Maine, D.: Does abortion affect later pregnancies? Family Planning Perspectives **11**(2):98-101, 1979.

48. Moseley, D.T., Follingstad, D., and Harley, H.: Psychological factors that predict reaction to abortion, Journal of Clinical Psychology **37**:276-279, 1981.

49. Muller, C.: Fertility control and the quality of human life, American Journal of Public Health **63:**519-524, 1973.

50. Naylor, A.F.: Sequential aspects of spontaneous abortions: maternal age, parity, and pregnancy compensation artifact, Social Biology **21:**194-204, 1974.

51. The Nurses Association of the American College of Obstetricians and Gynecologists: Standards for obstetrics, gynecologic, and neonatal nursing, ed. 2, Washington, D.C., 1981, NAACOG.

52. Olley, P.C.: Age, marriage, personality, and distress: a study of personality factors in women referred for therapeutic abortion. In Sloane, R.B., editor: Abortion: changing views and practice, New York, 1971, Grune & Stratton, Inc.

53. Paul, E., and Pilpel, H.: Teenager and pregnancy: the law in 1979, Family Planning Perspectives **11:**297-302, 1979.

54. Phipps-Yonas, S.: Teenage pregnancy and motherhood: a review of the literature, American Journal of Orthopsychiatry **50:**403-445, 1980.

55. Ramsey, P.: Reference points in deciding about abortion. In Noonan, J.T.: The morality of abortion, Cambridge, Mass., 1970, Harvard University Press.

56. Seims, S.: Abortion availability in the United States, Family Planning Perspectives **12**(2):88-101, 1980.

57. Selik, R., Cates, W., and Tyler, C.: Effects of restricted public funding for legal abortions: a second look, American Journal of Public Health **71**(1):77-81, 1981.

58. Shain, R.: Abortion practices and attitudes in cross-cultural perspectives, American Journal of Obstetrics and Gynecology **142:**245-251, 1982.

59. Shusterman, L.: Predicting the psychological consequences of abortion, Social Science and Medicine **13A:**683-689, 1979.

60. Smith, E.: A follow-up study of women who request abortion, American Journal of Orthopsychiatry **43:**574-585, 1973.

61. Swigar, M., Quinlan, D., and Wexler, S.: Abortion applicants: characteristics distinguishing dropouts remaining pregnant and those having abortions, American Journal of Public Health **67:**142-146, 1977.

62. Tietze, C.: Induced abortion: a world view, 1981, ed. 4, New York, 1981, The Population Council.

63. Trussell, J., et al.: The impact of restricting Medicaid financing for abortion, Family Planning Perspectives **12:**120-130, 1980.

64. Wagner, N.: I am not that kind of girl, unpublished manuscript, Seattle, University of Washington.

65. Westoff, C., et al.: Abortions preventable by contraceptive practice, Family Planning Perspectives **13:**218-223, 1981.

66. World Health Organization: Induced abortion as public health problem: report on a working group, Copenhagen, April 1971, Regional Office for Europe, WHO.

67. Zabin, L., and Clark, S.: Why they delay: a study of teenage family planning clinic patients, Family Planning Perspectives **13:**205-217, 1981.

68. Zabin, L., Kantner, J., and Zelnik, M.: The risk of adolescent pregnancy in the first months of intercourse, Family Planning Perspectives **11:**215-222, 1979.

69. Zacharias, L., Wurtman, R., and Schatzoff, M.: Sexual maturation in contemporary American girls, American Journal of Obstetrics and Gynecology **108:**883-846, 1970.

70. Zelnik, M., and Kantner, J.: Reasons for nonuse of contraception by sexually active women aged 15-19, Family Planning Perspectives **11:**289-296, 1979.

71. Zelnick, M., and Kantner, J.: Sexual activity, contraceptive use and pregnancy among metropolitan-area teenagers: 1971-1979, Family Planning Perspectives **12:**230-237, 1980.

72. Zelnik, M., and Kim, Y.: Sex education and its association with teenage sexual activity, pregnancy and contraceptive use, Family Planning Perspectives **14:**117-126, 1982.

References for clients

Boston Women's Health Book Collective: Our bodies, ourselves, ed. 3, New York, 1979, Simon & Schuster, Inc.

Francke, L.B.: The ambivalence of abortion, New York, 1978, Random House, Inc.

Hongladarom, G., McCorkle, R., and Woods, N.: The complete book of women's health, Englewood Cliffs, N.J., 1982, Prentice-Hall, Inc.

Stewart, F., et al.: My body, my health: the concerned woman's book of gynecology, New York, 1981, John Wiley & Sons, Inc.

11

Sexuality and contraception

MARCIA KILLIEN

The potential for reproduction is one of the predominant characteristics of adulthood. The average woman in the United States begins menstruating at age 12½ and experiences menopause around age 50.[7,23] During the intervening years, at monthly intervals, she will ovulate over 450 times, barring interferences with her reproductive processes. The majority of men will produce mature sperm by age 16 and continue to do so for the remainder of their lives.[37] It is obviously not desirable for any man or woman to reproduce to their full capacity. Thus the concept of fertility control has meaning to all individuals.

Control of fertility may include postponing pregnancy, regulating the number of or spacing between pregnancies, or avoiding pregnancy entirely. In each situation fertility control also implies the modification of sexual behavior.

The management of reproductive potential has been a concern of individuals and societies for centuries. However, it is only recently that improvements in contraceptive knowledge and technology have allowed the majority of the population to separate the recreative and procreative aspects of sexual behavior.

The current availability of acceptable and effective contraceptive methods also means that individuals are faced with complex decisions about sexual behavior, contraceptive use, and having children. When contemplating these decisions, the individual considers several questions: Do I want to be sexually active? Do I want to use some method of birth control? If so, which method is acceptable to me? Do I want children? When do I want to have them? These are not easy questions to answer. Although individuals may be aware of their own values and motivations related to sexual behavior and procreation, they are also influenced in their decision making and behavior by societal values and the attitudes of significant others in their lives.

The purposes of this chapter follow:
1. To identify sociocultural, biologic, and psychosexual issues confronting persons who desire to control their fertility
2. To examine the impact of fertility control methods on sexuality and sexual behavior
3. To discuss the provision of health care services to individuals who wish to limit their fertility

Sociocultural influences

Historic and cross-cultural perspectives. Magic rituals, potions, and pessaries have been used since the days of the pharoahs to prevent pregnancy. Insertion of barriers into the vagina or uterus (e.g., dung, pebbles, lard, beeswax, silver balls) was common.[36] Similar approaches to prevent conception are used throughout the world currently. A cross-cultural survey by Ford[18] indicated that contraceptive methods include insertion of a pad of bark cloth or rag into the vagina before intercourse, consuming medicines derived from the bark, leaves, or roots of certain trees and plants, and respecting taboos on sexual intercourse at certain times.

The reproductive behavior of individuals, as reflected by coital behaviors, contraceptive use, and childbearing patterns, is influenced by the conditions of the societies in which they live. The economic structure of the society, availability of environmental resources, and birth and mortality patterns interact to influence societal and cultural norms about ideal family size, contraceptive use, and exposure to intercourse.[21] For example, in many nonindustrialized societies in which infant mortality rates are high and children are valued as a source of labor, there are few taboos on sexual intercourse, and contraception is not widely available or practiced.[18] In contrast, the People's Republic of China, the world's most populous country, has adopted strict policies and provided incentives to limit its population growth. These policies include waiving education and medical care fees for couples who have only one child, giving preference in housing assignments and employment to couples who have two or fewer children and those who marry late, and restricting government subsidies to couples who exceed the one-child limit. Nonmarital intercourse is rare, and contraceptive information is restricted to married couples. As a result of these measures, the birthrate was cut in half in 5 years.[11]

Similar effects of societal conditions have been evident throughout U.S. history. During the eighteenth and nineteenth centuries the environment appeared to be an infinite pool of resources. Mortality rates were high, and the survival of the family depended on increasing the odds by having large numbers of children. The social and economic structure was primarily agricultural, and large numbers of children were valued as laborers. Since the life span was relatively short and infant and maternal mortality rates were high, marriage and entry into intercourse occurred at an early age. Contraception was viewed as "illegal, illicit and improper."[36]

With the beginning of the twentieth century, several changes occurred that brought changes in attitudes and laws regarding contraception. The United States became more industrialized, and the number of women working outside the home increased dramatically. Women sought power through the suffragette movement, and clinics opened, offering birth control information and devices. Although such activity remained illegal, production of contraceptive devices flourished. The rubber condom was introduced at the Centennial Exposition in Philadelphia in 1876. The discovery of synthetic rubber in the early 1920s made the production of condoms and diaphragms a multimillion dollar industry. In 1930 the U.S. Court of Appeals ruled that the sale of contraceptives was not illegal in all cases.[36]

During the 1930s environmental resources no longer seemed as available, particularly because of an unstable economy. Contraceptive use was widespread. A survey of white married women born between 1901 and 1910 indicated that 71% practiced contraception.

The most popular methods were the condom, douche, and withdrawal. Women who used contraception tended to be well educated, non-Catholic, urban, and married to men in white-collar occupations.[10] Of the women in their prime childbearing years, 37% were childless. In 1936 the nation experienced its lowest birthrate (18.4) until the present day.[6,35,36] In 1935 a nurse, Margaret Sanger, and two physicians, Alan Guttmacher and Robert L. Dickinson, established the *Journal of Contraception,* which had as an objective the encouragement of research for "a simple, harmless and efficient chemical contraceptive."[27]

Although a 1936 survey indicated that 63% of the American people, including two thirds of Catholics, believed in "the teaching and practice of birth control,"[20,36] the legal status of contraceptive care remained controversial for many years. A Connecticut statute, making the *use* of contraceptives illegal, was upheld in 1961 by the U.S. Supreme Court.[36] However, in 1971 the U.S. Supreme Court ruled that a Massachusetts statute permitting married persons to obtain contraceptives but prohibiting distribution to single persons was unconstitutional, thus legalizing birth control for unmarried persons.[14]

Current sociocultural perspectives. In 1976 the national birthrate hit an all time low of 14.8/1000. Individuals are becoming acutely aware of the finite nature of natural resources, particularly food, water, and space. The democratic belief structure in the United States supports the view of childbearing as a matter of personal choice, yet there is pressure to have only as many children as the family and society can afford to support. In a period of inflation this pressure keeps the norm for family size a small one. Over 60% of women expect to have two or fewer children.[6] Increasing proportions of women are postponing childbearing until their later reproductive years or are remaining permanently childless. Between 1970 and 1975, childlessness among married white women aged 25 to 29 increased by 34.8% and increased 11.1% among women aged 30 to 34.[35]

The large percentage of women involved in the work force also operates to limit family size. Working women desire and have fewer children than their nonworking counterparts, and professional women tend to have smaller families than blue-collar workers.[45] Although there is increasing sexual freedom and entry into sexual relationships is occurring at increasingly earlier ages, contraceptives are also more available and acceptable than in the past. Data from 1978 indicated that about three fourths of sexually active, fecund females used some form of birth control at the time of their last intercourse.[13]

Group survey data indicated that the majority of white men and women in the United States believe that a couple should have a child 2 to 3 years after marriage and that subsequent pregnancies should be spaced every 2 to 3 years.[6] Thus it would appear that contraceptive use by married couples to achieve these family planning goals is supported by society. Societal attitudes toward contraceptive use by unmarried teenagers are less clear. By 1976 the majority of states had established, through state laws, the right of unmarried women aged 18 or older to obtain contraceptive services.[33] However, the rights of minors to obtain prescription contraceptives (such as "the pill" or intrauterine device [IUD] remained unclear. As of 1982, Utah was the only state with a statute specifically requiring parental consent for contraception. This Utah statute prohibits the use of any public funds to provide contraceptive information or services to minors without parental consent. Currently, this law conflicts with the federal statute related to Title X family planning programs under which minors are eligible for services without parental involvement. However, the U.S. Department of Health and Human Services has proposed new Title X regulations that would require family planning agencies receiving these funds to notify both parents within 10 days after prescribing contraceptives to minors.[12]

Sociocultural influences on the control of fertility can be better understood by examining the social meaning of parenthood. Veevers[43] proposed that the meaning of parenthood centers around six themes: morality, responsibility, naturalness, sex, marriage, and mental health. Parenthood as a mora obligation is the view supported by dominant religious groups in the United States, including Catholics and Mormons. Parenthood is seen as a civic responsibility linked to the continuation of society through reproduction of its members. Thus reproduction is one of the major responsibilities of the family. Parenthood is seen as natural in that the behavior is widely distributed throughout the society and is thus attributed to human nature. Parenthood can be seen as a measure of sexual identity and competence and as the meaning and purpose of marriage. Finally, wanting children is sesn as an attribute of normal mental health.

The association between sociocultural factors and sexual activity and contraceptive use has been examined in a number of studies. Zelnik and Kantner's 1976 survey[19,49] of a national probability sample of women aged 15 to 19 provides the best available data on adolescent sexual and contraceptive behavior. In 1976, 63% of black teenage women and 31% of white teenage women were sexually experienced.[49] Women whose parents or guardians had a relatively low level of education were more likely to be sexually active and to be nonusers or inconsistent users of contraception. Contraceptive use did not differ according to race; however, black women were more likely to use a medical method such as "the pill" or IUD. Age was found to be an important influence on contraceptive use. Regardless of socioeconomic status, unprotected intercourse was most common for the youngest teenagers. Older teenagers were more likely to use contraception at the time of first intercourse and to use a more effective method.[19,49]

Dryfoos[13] found similar effects of socioeconomic status on contraceptive use by older women. Low-income women were more likely to have unprotected intercourse or to use less effective contraceptive methods and, accordingly, had higher rates of unintended pregnancies. They were also more likely to report contraceptive method failure.

A final sociocultural variable influencing contraceptive use is religion. A number of religious groups, including Catholics and Mormons, advocate procreation as a major function of marriage. Fertility control, particularly use of medical methods, is discouraged by several religions. Although not all members of these groups follow their church's teaching about fertility control, religious background may influence contraceptive practice and feelings about fertility control.

Biologic considerations

Fertility. There are several factors influencing the fertility of a couple. These factors include the interactive effects of age and patterns of intercourse.

Age. A woman's fertility varies throughout her reproductive years. The mean age of menarche for girls in the United States is 12.5 years; however, there is considerable variation in the timing of menarche.[7,28] Fertility is low in the first months after menarche, reaches a peak in the mid-20s, and then declines until menopause, when the woman is again nonfertile.

It is commonly believed that young women are subfecund for a year or more after the onset of menses.[7,28] Early menstrual cycles tend to be irregular and short, indicative of the absence of a luteal phase and ovulation. This pattern has been attributed to an imbalance in the levels of estrogen and progesterone resulting from immature hypothalamic functioning. When estrogen production increases, cycles become more regular, the duration of menstruation increases, and cycles become ovulatory. Results of a study of pregnancy among young teenagers support the idea of a period of subfecundity.[53] Conceptions were rare among both black and white teenagers who had coitus during the first year after menarche. However, the rates of conception increased among teenagers who initiated coitus 2 or more years after menarche. Several studies[8,42,53] have found that women who begin to menstruate at early ages initiate intercourse at younger ages than those who have a late menarche. Udry[42] suggested that early menarche initiates a chain of events that place a woman at risk for pregnancy. He proposed that "(1) pubertal hormones lead to increased libido in adolescent females; (2) pubertal hormones lead to secondary sexual characteristics which attract males to the females who are physically developed; (3) those women with early puberty have more efficiently functioning reproductive systems, leading to higher fecundability independent of sexual behavior."[42]

Recent studies[16,23,32] suggest that female fertility declines abruptly from age 30 onward. Several factors may contribute to decreased fertility in older women, including an increasing proportion of abnormal menstrual cycles, increased exposure to infections, and a higher incidence of endometriosis and fibroid tumors.[9,23] As a woman nears menopause, the proportion of ovulatory cycles declines. This decline is believed to be the result of a diminished supply of oocytes and a decrease in estrogen production necessary for ovulation.[32]

Data on the age at which men produce mature sperm are less readily available. Richardson and Short[37] reported a mean age of 13.3 years; Katchadourian[28] reported 15 years as the mean age for spermaturia. In men, fertility also reaches its peak in the mid-20s and declines thereafter. Although fertility in men has been documented into the eighth and ninth decades of life, the quantity and quality of sperm deteriorate with age.[9]

Patterns of intercourse. The likelihood of pregnancy is related to both exposure to intercourse and the timing of coitus during the woman's menstrual cycle. Each of these factors is also influenced by age.

When age is held constant, the rate of conceptions rises with the frequency of intercourse. Frequent ejaculation appears to improve the degree and quality of sperm motility and thus enhance fertility. The frequency of intercourse is related to a variety of situational factors, including opportunity and availability of a sexual partner. Frequency of intercourse among young teenagers is quite low, often one to two times per month.[2] Teenagers may incorrectly assume they are not having coitus frequently enough to become pregnant. Zabin, Kantner, and Zelnik[53] reported that two thirds of teenagers who never used contraception became pregnant within 2 years afte beginning sexual activity; one fourth of these conceived within the first month. The frequency of intercourse also declines with age and duration of marriage.[23,41]

Couples who have daily unprotected intercourse for the week surrounding ovulation have about a 50% chance of conceiving.[38] There is evidence of a naturally occurring increase in sexual arousal and female-initiated coital frequency around the time of ovulation.[1,15,34] This increase appears to be associated with female plasma testosterone levels.[34]

Successful control of fertility, using many of the available contraceptive techniques, depends on knowing when conception is likely. Zelnik and Kantner[51] reported that of teenagers who had taken a sex education course including information about the menstrual cycle, only 36% could correctly identify when pregnancy risk was greatest. Such information is important: a major reason given by sexually active teenagers for nonuse of contraception is that coitus took place at a time in the month when they thought they could not conceive.

Health risks and benefits of fertility control. The various methods of fertility control have health benefits and risks associated with their use. All fertility control methods enable women to limit the number of children they bear and to regulate the spacing between children. Such control has benefits for the health of the woman and her family. Maternal morbidity and mortality increases with parity after the second birth. High parity is also associated with increased fetal wastage. When the interval between pregnancies is less than 12 months, the woman does not have time for physiologic restoration; the result may be a premature birth, delivery of a low birth weight infant, and maternal complications.[47]

Contraceptive risks for women are usually compared with the risks of morbidity and mortality associated with pregnancy and childbirth. It is commonly believed that use of any contraceptive method is safer than pregnancy, in terms of mortality rates. A comparison of risks should include consideration of the effectiveness of the contraceptive method and the age and health status of the individual. Table 11-1 illustrates such a comparison based on U.S. survey data from 1972 to 1978. Tietze[39] makes the following conclusions from these data:

1. Among women under age 30 (with the exception of women who smoke and take oral contraceptives), the risk of death associated with each major fertility control method is about equal and is lower than mortality associated with pregnancy and birth.
2. Beyond age 30 the risk to life increases for oral contraceptive users, especially for those who smoke. After age 30 the risk for pill users who smoke is higher than for women who become pregnant.
3. At all ages the lowest level of mortality is achieved by a combination of the use of barrier contraceptives with early abortion as a recourse in case of method failure.

Although mortality is a serious consequence, it is a relatively rare outcome of pregnancy or contraceptive use. Both alternatives are more often accompanied by side effects and sequelae that influence the woman and her health. Up to 40% of users report minor side effects associated with use of IUDs and oral contraceptives.[17]

Many women consider the risk of pregnancy to be the greatest negative outcome associated with contraceptive methods. The effectiveness of common methods is shown in Fig. 11-1.

Research is continuing on the health risks associated with contraceptive use, particularly prolonged use of oral contraceptives. Although the IUD and oral contraceptives are the most effective methods of fertility control, they also carry with them the greatest

Table 11-1. Comparison of contraceptive and childbearing risks (deaths per 100,000 women per year)

Regimen	Age in years					
	15-19	20-21	25-29	30-34	35-39	40-44
No control						
Birth related	4.7	5.3	6.5	10.7	19.3	23.2
Abortion only						
Method related	0.5	1.1	1.3	2.0	1.9	1.2
OCs only nonsmok-ers						
Birth related	0.1	0.2	0.2	0.3	0.6	0.5
Method related	0.6	1.1	1.6	3.0	9.1	17.7
Total deaths	0.7	1.3	1.8	3.3	9.7	18.2
OCs only smokers						
Birth related	0.1	0.2	0.2	0.3	0.6	0.5
Method related	2.1	4.2	6.1	11.8	31.3	60.9
Total deaths	2.2	4.4	6.3	12.1	31.9	61.4
IUDs only						
Birth related	0.1	0.2	0.2	0.3	0.6	0.5
Method related	0.8	0.8	1.0	1.0	1.4	1.4
Total deaths	0.9	1.0	1.2	1.3	2.0	1.9
Barrier methods only						
Birth related	1.1	1.5	1.9	3.3	5.0	4.0
Barrier methods, plus abortion						
Method related	0.1	0.2	0.2	0.3	0.3	0.2

From Tietze, C.: Induced abortions: a world view, 1981, ed. 4, New York, 1981, The Population Council.

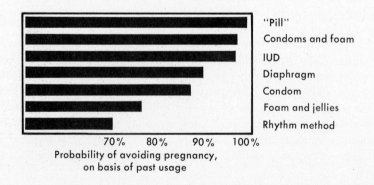

Fig. 11-1. Relative effectiveness of common contraceptive methods.

risks. In addition, problems with fertility may remain hidden in women who practice regular contraception and are only detected when these women attempt pregnancy at later ages.

Research on new methods of contraception is also continuing. Among these methods are the vaginal ring, cervical cap, injectable contraceptives, and an antipregnancy vaccine. The search for acceptable male contraceptive methods includes methods to stop sperm production, block sperm transport during coitus, and render sperm incapable of fertilization.[3,5]

Psychosexual issues

Contraceptive decision making. Women are becoming more aware of their need and right to control this aspect of their bodies. Consequently, they are making choices involving female-oriented contraceptives and are concerned with those methods healthiest for their bodies. First methods used are often those most easily accessible: foam and condoms, rhythm, and withdrawal. As sexual activity increases and concern about fertility becomes paramount, methods often change. It is no longer assumed that a couple will use the same method for a number of years; rather, they will alter methods to suit their life-style changes, desire for assured protection, and health. Thus decisions about fertility control are made, reexamined, and remade throughout one's reproductive life.

In 1978 there were 3.1 million unintended pregnancies in the United States; this number represents 55% of the pregnancies that occurred that year. Of these unintended conceptions, 58% occurred to women using some method of contraception.[13] These figures illustrate that all women are not achieving their fertility goals, despite wide availability of contraceptive methods. Failure to achieve fertility control is a result of nonuse of contraception, failure to use contraceptives correctly (''user failure''), and ineffectiveness of contraceptive methods themselves (''method failure'').

Nonuse of contraception. The high rate of unintended pregnancies reflects the many conflicting pressures influencing contraceptive use. Researchers repeatedly find that despite adequate knowledge of contraception, many women do not use contraceptives even though they do not want to become pregnant.*

The risk-taking behavior of these women is not as irrational as it may first appear. Luker's research[31] on 500 women, aged 15 to 45, seeking abortions documented that women have rational reasons for their decision not to use contraception or to use ineffective methods. She proposed that women used a cost/benefit approach to decision making, weighing the costs and benefits of effective contraceptive use against the costs and benefits of pregnancy. Women attempt to achieve many goals in their sexual lives; contraception will be used only if it does not interfere with major aims or if avoidance of pregnancy is a primary goal.

The following barriers to contraceptive use have been identified by Luker and others.

*References 13, 31, 48, 50, 52, and 54.

Acknowledgment costs. The psychosexual aspects of fertility control begin with the decision to be sexually active. To make this choice, both persons must acknowledge their sexual feelings and intended behavior, potential for fertility, and intent of using contraception. This acknowledgement requires some knowledge but most of all an awareness of oneself as a sexual being. For some this may occur at an early age and for others at a much later age, depending on progress with developmental tasks.

Some individuals find their sexual behavior so threatening that fertility control would only confirm their ''badness.'' By denying that they will be sexually active, these individuals can safeguard their self-esteem. For them, using a contraceptive method would be tantamount to admission of ''badness'' and would be seen as lowering their self-esteem.

Other women, particularly young teenagers who have not achieved adult cognitive development, believe themselves ''immune'' to pregnancy. These women seem to be living a ''personal fable'' in which they deny that pregnancy could happen to them.[7] Zelnik and Kantner[51] reported that 51% of sexually active teenagers did not use contraception because they believed they could not become pregnant.

Planning costs. Effective use of contraception requires preplanning. Nearly one third of the teenagers in Zelnik and Kantner's study[51] who had coitus more than once reported they had not used contraception because they did not expect to have intercourse or found themselves in situations where they could not use it. The psychic costs of planning ahead to have coitus may be disturbing to women if they are not in continuing, committed sexual relationships or if they believe it is wrong to take the initiative of planning for sex.[7,44]

Relationship costs. Attitudes of one's sexual partner toward contraceptive use can be very important. Use of some methods (e.g., condom, foam, rhythm) requires the cooperation of the male partner in altering sexual behavior. Interference with the spontaneity or pleasure of intercourse and objections by one's partner prevent some women from using contraception.[51] In a study comparing the knowledge and attitudes of 607 black male and female adolescents Freeman, Rickels, and Huggins[22] found that males were less likely to know when the risk of pregnancy was the greatest, had less information about contraceptives, and believed that sex without birth control showed love. Adolescent boys were also more likely to report that they did not respect girls who used birth control. In contrast, a supportive dyadic relationship can promote contraceptive use. Women who have regular intercourse with a single partner, who perceive power over sex and contraceptive matters, and who are satisfied with their ability to talk with their partner about their sexual relationship are more likely to use contraception.[26,30]

Fear of side effects. The potential health risks of contraceptive use were discussed earlier in this chapter. Unfortunately, the media have given more attention to contraceptive risks than to the comparable risks associated with childbearing. It is not surprising that some women believe contraceptive use is dangerous. Teenagers, who are very concerned about their bodies, often shy away from use of oral contraceptives, fearing weight gain and other side effects.[7,50] Between 1975 and 1978 the proportion of U.S. women aged 15 to 44 using oral contraceptives declined by 25%; IUD use similarly declined.[25,52]

Costs of obtaining contraceptives. The most effective methods of contraception are only available through the health care system. Unpleasant past experiences with this system, fear of medical examinations, and fear of family notification all may prevent a woman from seeking contraceptive services.[48]

• • •

These costs are weighed against the perceived benefits of a pregnancy, which include the following[29,31,40]:

1. Fulfilling traditional masculine and feminine roles
2. Providing a child to love
3. Proving fertility
4. Testing commitment to a relationship
5. Pleasing a spouse, lover, or family
6. Gaining attention from others
7. Experiencing parenthood
8. Replacing a loss

Characteristics of women who successfully use contraceptives. From these studies of contraceptive use and nonuse, a profile of the woman who is successful in achieving fertility control can be derived. She is a woman who values control over her body and believes she has the power, right, and responsibility to control her fertility. She is comfortable with her body, her sexuality, and her sexual partner. She has the knowledge and cognitive ability to plan ahead, select a contraceptive method, obtain necessary contraceptive services, and correctly use the method. She has the support and cooperation of her sexual partner in achieving her fertility goals.

Recent attention has focused on couples who have been successful at fertility control for many years and now are considering parenthood. Some couples have difficulty breaking the "contraceptive habit" and conceiving.[9,29] Often these individuals are highly educated, are successful in business professions, or value control over their lives. The loss of total control over their bodies and the timing and outcome of pregnancy lead to difficulty in making a decision about parenthood and may result in a unique psychosocial "fertility problem" among older couples.[9,29]

Impact of fertility control method on sexuality and sexual behavior. Whether individuals select mechanical, chemical, or behavioral fertility control methods, they are likely to find that the choice of a method is influenced by their sexuality and that, in turn, the method influences sexual behavior. The method itself can have a direct effect on sexual behavior. For example, the diaphragm and condom must be used at the time of sexual activity. In some instances the method can cause discomfort, as in the case of women who have uterine cramping with orgasm, which they attribute to their IUDs. In other instances methods require restraint of sexual behavior. In some instances the individual's perception of the meaning of using a contraceptive method or of being sterilized can affect sexual response. Some of the more important influences on sexual behavior associated with the more common methods of contraception are given in Table 11-2.

Table 11-2. Influence of contraceptive measures on sexual behavior

Method	Influence on sexual behavior
Mechanical	
Condom	Some men find that condoms reduce glans sensitivity. Others become annoyed at having to put the condom on during intercourse. Some men cannot maintain an erection while wearing a condom. Other men find that a condom helps them to maintain an erection; this is especially likely in older men or men who have had abdominal surgery. Putting the condom on can be integrated into sexual activity, that is, the woman may put the condom on her partner. Some condoms are available that allow more sensation to reach the glans. Condoms can be used in treating men who are premature ejaculators, since the condom reduces glans sensitivity. Condoms can help prevent sexually transmitted diseases such as gonorrhea, syphilis, trichomoniasis, herpes, and venereal warts. Condoms may also be used in treating some infertile couples in which the woman makes antibodies capable of agglutinizing her partner's sperm. Condoms are used for a period of months to prevent release of sperm antigens into the woman's vagina; after the woman's antibody titer decreases, condoms are used during the nonfertile part of the cycle. Condoms are useful for women who have an aversion to being touched by the man's penis and for men who are averse to having their penises touch the vagina.
Diaphragm	Women who are uncomfortable touching their genitals will probably not be comfortable using the diaphragm. Diaphragms require that women plan ahead by keeping their diaphragms with them so they can be inserted before intercourse. Inserting the diaphragm can be incorporated into sexual activity; for example, the partner can insert the diaphragm. During multiple acts of intercourse additional spermicidal jelly or cream should be inserted each time. After several acts of intercourse the jelly and/or cream and semen may feel "messy" to some people. The diaphragm is more likely to become dislodged during intercourse when the woman is astride (on top of) the man. The diaphragm can be worn during menstruation to hold back menstrual flow, thus making intercourse possible for those who find having intercourse during menstruation to be aesthetically objectionable. Some women report less cervical stimulation during intercourse. Some find this a positive, others a negative, effect of the diaphragm. Some men report feeling the diaphragm with deep penile penetration.
Intrauterine device (IUD)	Heavier menstrual flow may interfere with intercourse during the menses. Some women report having mild, moderate, or severe lower abdominal cramps with orgasm after having an IUD inserted. Some male partners report that they can feel the strings from the IUD during intercourse. The IUD requires no interruption of lovemaking and does not require one to "plan ahead." Infections with IUDs in place can be very serious and result in infertility if not treated.

Table 11-2. Influence of contraceptive measures on sexual behavior—cont'd

Method	Influence on sexual behavior
Chemical	
Spermicidal foam	Some persons have allergic reactions to foam, leading to problems such as vaginal or penile irritation. Persons having oral-genital sex note that foam has an unpleasant taste, but foam can be inserted after oral-genital sex and before intromission. Foam must be applied just before lovemaking. During sessions of multiple intromission two full applicators of foam should be used before each intromission. Some people object to this as messy. Foams can decrease the chance of contracting gonorrhea. Foam can be inserted as part of lovemaking; for example, the partner can insert the foam. For women who are uncomfortable about touching their genitals, foam will probably not be a comfortable choice of contraceptive method.
Hormonal contraceptives including "the pill," progestins, and morning-after pills	Use of "the pill," the progestin pill, progesterone injections, and postcoital progestins do not require use of a method at time of intercourse. Often women report enjoying sex more when they are using oral contraceptives, probably because they do not worry about becoming pregnant. Some women report a decreased sex drive and impaired orgasmic experience. For some women, fear of side effects interferes with sexual enjoyment while taking "the pill."
Behavioral	
Abstinence	It may be difficult to balance need for avoiding pregnancy with desire for intercourse, but can lead to discovery of new ways of giving and receiving sexual pleasure. Cooperation between partners can enhance understanding and closeness. It is impractical for someone not in a relationship with a committed and cooperative partner.
Temperature ovulation, symptothermic, and astrologic methods	This requires abstinence or the use of alternate method during fertile days. It can also lead to the exploration of new ways of giving and receiving sexual pleasure. Cooperation between partners can enhance understanding and closeness. It is impractical for someone not in a relationship with a committed and cooperative partner.
Coitus interruptus	Withdrawal requires self-control. Failure of this method can result from preejaculatory emission, the strong desire of the male partner for deeper penetration at time of impending orgasm, or deposition of semen on female's genitals. Interruption of the sexual response cycle by withdrawal may result in diminished sexual pleasure and cause the couple to focus on their performance rather than their pleasure.
Sterilization	
Vasectomy and tubal ligation	Sexual response may improve because of loss of fear of pregnancy after tubal ligation. There is no noticeable difference in ejaculate of vasectomized men. Despite the absence of direct effects of tubal ligation or vasectomy on sexual response, worries or fears about the procedures and the meanings of the procedures to persons involved *may* influence their response.

Provision of contraceptive services

The goal of family planning services is to make every pregnancy the result of an informed decision with the outcome being a wanted child. When contraceptive services are provided, the aim is to assist individuals and couples to find a method that they will be able to effectively use that is not detrimental to their individual health or their relationship. Family planning services are based on the following beliefs[24]:

1. Voluntary family planning has an important impact on the health of the individual, the family, the community, and the world.
2. Unless a specific method is contraindicated, clients have a right to make a voluntary, unpressured decision regarding birth control methods.
3. It is the responsibility of the family planning practitioner to provide thorough, accurate information to the client and encourage questions.
4. Clients have a right to be treated with dignity in a private setting and a right to complete confidentiality in medical records.
5. Each member of society has a right to family planning care regardless of ability to pay or social status.
6. Participation of male partners in family planning is an important dimension of care.
7. Family planning services include noncontraceptive services to clients that promote their general health and facilitate entry into other components of the health care system.

Family planning counseling includes assisting clients to examine their reproductive life plans and to select a contraceptive method that is congruous with those plans. Questions that can assist the individual to formulate reproductive life plans follow[4,24]:

1. Would I like to have children someday?
2. How old would I like to be when I have my first child? My last child?
3. How many children would I like to have? How far apart?
4. How sad would I be if I were not able to have any children?
5. How concerned would I be if I were to become pregnant outside of marriage?
6. If I were to become pregnant before I wanted to be pregnant, how would I approach this difficulty?
7. Would I want to be married before having sexual intercourse?
8. What are my educational and career goals?
9. Do I want to be married? If I do not marry, would I want to have children as a single or unmarried parent?
10. What are the advantages and disadvantages of having a baby? A toddler? A school-age child? An adolescent? An adult child?
11. Of all the things I could do in my life, the most important would be to be able to accomplish this: _____
12. This life goal would be affected by childbearing in the following ways: _____

It can be helpful to ask individuals to visualize what their lives would be like from the present until death if they were to have a child and also if they were not to have a child. These techniques assist individuals to consider contraception as part of their life plan, not just a short-term measure.

From this reproductive life plan, short-term and long-term fertility goals can be identified. Contraceptive methods can then be evaluated in terms of their compatibility with these goals. When assisting the client to select a contraceptive method, history taking and physical assessment are essential. Included in the history should be a detailed gynecologic and obstetric history, contraceptive history, a sexual history, and a general health history. Data gathered from this assessment can be used to identify which contraceptive methods are incompatible with the client's health status, life-style, sexual behavior patterns, or long-term fertility goals. Hatcher et al. developed a series of questions that can assist clients to determine which method would be a good choice for them*:

Am I afraid of using this method?	Yes	No
Would I really rather not use this method?	Yes	No
Will I have trouble remembering to use this method?	Yes	No
Have I ever become pregnant while using this method?	Yes	No
Will I have trouble using this method correctly?	Yes	No
Do I still have unanswered questions about this method?	Yes	No
Does this method make menstrual periods longer or more painful?	Yes	No
Does this method cost more than I can afford?	Yes	No
Is this method known to have serious complications?	Yes	No
Am I opposed to this method because of any religious beliefs?	Yes	No
Have I already experienced complications from this method?	Yes	No
Is my partner opposed to this method?	Yes	No
Am I using this method without my partner's knowledge?	Yes	No
Will use of this method embarrass my partner?	Yes	No
Will use of this method embarrass me?	Yes	No
Will I enjoy sexual intercourse less because of this method?	Yes	No
Will this method interrupt lovemaking?	Yes	No
Has a nurse or doctor ever told me not to use this method?	Yes	No
Is there anything about my personality which would cause me not to use this method correctly?	Yes	No

Total number of *yes* answers: ＿＿＿

Answering yes to any of these questions indicates factors that may interfere with optimal use of the method. Since all methods have some drawbacks associated with their use, these questions also illustrate the areas where making an informed choice is important.

Once the client has selected a method that seems best for him or her, the practitioner should make sure that information about correct use of the method is provided and understood. The use of written materials describing method use and possible side effects is helpful, so the client can refer to this material when questions or concerns arise. Some methods involve health teaching in other areas. For example, use of oral contraceptive reduces the body's ability to use certain nutrients. Therefore nutrition counseling is indicated for clients using birth control pills.[47] Finally, follow-up care is often indicated to provide support to the individual or couple as they implement their contraceptive plans,

From Hatcher R., et al.: Contraceptive technology, 1982-1983, ed. 11, 1982. Reprinted with permission of Irvington Publishers, Inc., New York.

to provide monitoring of the individual's health, and to aid in continuation of contraception. The satisfaction of the client with the initial family planning counseling session has a major impact on his or her return for continued follow-up.

Summary

This chapter has considered sexuality and its relationship to fertility control. Historic and contemporary sociocultural issues affecting contraceptive availability and use were discussed. The relationship of age and patterns of intercourse to fertility were examined, as well as the health benefits and risks of fertility control. Psychosexual issues related to contraceptive decision making were considered. The impact of common methods of contraception on sexuality and sexual behavior was reviewed. Suggestions for contraceptive counseling by health professionals were made, with emphasis on development of a reproductive life plan and selection of a contraceptive method.

Questions for review

1. How do values of the society and culture affect the availability and acceptability of contraception?
2. How does fertility change over the life span? What interrelated factors influence an individual's risk of pregnancy?
3. How do varying contraceptive methods influence the individual's sexual behavior? On the basis of the individual's feelings about sexuality, which of the contraceptive methods would be inappropriate?
4. What variables are likely to influence whether contraceptive methods are actually used?
5. How does each of the common methods of fertility control affect sexual behavior?
6. Maria, a 14-year-old girl, arrives at the family planning clinic seeking a prescription for "the pill." She indicates that she does not know much about other methods of contraception and that she is not yet having intercourse, but she is involved in an intimate relationship. Maria is knowledgeable about her body, feels comfortable touching her genitals, and has positive feelings about her sexuality. Outline your approach to counseling her. Does your personal sexual value system influence your approach to counseling her? Would your approach to Maria be different if she were 24 years old? In what way?
7. Patrick, a 20-year-old college student, arrives at the student health clinic asking questions about having a vasectomy and how reversible it would be. On further discussion, he confides that he has tried to use other methods of birth control, for example, condoms, but that he cannot seem to deal with the embarrassment he feels about using them, so he has not actually used any method of birth control. Does his acceptance of his sexual behavior have potential influence on a choice of contraceptive method? What other variables will you take into account when counseling him?
8. Jim and Claudia have always planned to have children but are now having difficulty deciding when to have a child. Claudia is 29, takes oral contra-

ceptives, and is at a strategic point in her career. She is concerned about the risks of postponing pregnancy several years. What do you discuss with her?

9. Arthur and Lillian had their fourth child last year and have three other children under age 5. Lillian tells you she does not want any more children, but Arthur does not believe in using contraception. How would you approach this situation? What information would you gather, and how would you counsel Lillian and Arthur?

References

1. Adams, D., Gold, A., and Burt, A.: Rise in female-initiated sexual activity at ovulation and its suppression by oral contraceptives, New England Journal of Medicine **299:**1145-1150, 1978.
2. Akpom, C.A., et al.: Teenage sexual behavior perceptive and behavioral outcomes associated with receipt of family planning services, Journal of Biosocial Science **11**(1):85-92, 1979.
3. Atkinson, L., et al.: Prospects for improved contraception, Family Planning Perspectives **12:**173-192, 1980.
4. Beach, L., Townes, B., and Campbell, F.: The optional parenthood questionnaire: a guide to decision making about parenthood, Baltimore, 1978, National Alliance for Optional Parenthood.
5. Benditt, J.: Current contraceptive research, Family Planning Perspectives **12:**149-155, 1980.
6. Blake, J.: Can we believe recent data on birth expectations in the United States? Demography **11:**25-44, Feb. 1974.
7. Chilman, C.: Adolescent sexuality in a changing American society: social and psychological perspectives, Department of Health, Education, and Welfare Pub. no. (NIH) 79-1426, 1979.
8. Cutler, W., Garcia, C., and Krieger, A.: Infertility and age at first coitus: a possible relationship, Journal of Biosocial Science **11:**425-432, 1979.
9. Daniels, P., and Weingarten, K.: A new look at the medical risks in late childbearing, Women and Health **4**(1):5-36, 1979.
10. Dawson, D., Meny, D., and Ridley, J.: Fertility control in the United States before the contraceptive revolution, Family Planning Perspectives **12**(2):76-86, 1980.
11. Djerassi, C.: The politics of contraception, New York, 1979, W.W. Norton & Co., Inc.
12. Donovan, P.: Fertility related state laws enacted in 1981, Family Planning Perspectives **14**(2):63-67, 1982.
13. Dryfoos, J.: Contraceptive use, pregnancy intentions and pregnancy outcomes among U.S. women, Family Planning Perspectives **14**(2):81-94, 1982.
14. *Eisenstadt v. Baird,* 92 S Ct. 1029, 1972.
15. Englander-Golden, P., et al.: Female sexual arousal and the menstrual cycle, Journal of Human Stress **6**(1):42-48, 1980.
16. Federation CECOS, Schwarts, D., and Mayaeux, M.: Female fecundity as a function of age, New England Journal of Medicine **306:**404-406, 1982.
17. Fogel, C., and Woods, N.: Health care of women: a nursing perspective, St. Louis, 1981, The C.V. Mosby Co.

18. Ford, C.: Control of conception in cross-cultural perspective, Annals of New York Academy of Sciences **54**:763-768, 1952.

19. Ford, K., Zelnik, M., and Kantner, J.F.: Sexual behavior and contraceptive use among socioeconomic groups of young women in the United States, Journal of Biosocial Science **13**(1):31-45, 1981.

20. Fortune: **11**(1):158, 1936.

21. Freedman, R.: Applications of the behavioral sciences to family planning programs, Studies in Family Planning **23**:5-9, 1967.

22. Freeman, E.W., et al.: Adolescent contraceptive use: comparisons of male and female attitudes and information, American Journal of Public Health **70**:790-797, 1980.

23. Gray, R.H.: Biological and social interactions in the determination of late fertility, Journal of Biosocial Science, Suppl. **(6)**:97-115, 1979.

24. Hatcher, R., et al.: Contraceptive technology, 1982-1983, ed. 11, New York, 1982, Irvington Publishers, Inc.

25. Henshaw, S., et al.: Abortion services in the United States, 1979 and 1980, Family Planning Perspectives **14**(1):5-15, 1982.

26. Jorgensen, S., King, S., and Torrey, B.: Dyadic and social network influences on adolescent exposure to pregnancy risk, Journal of Marriage and the Family **42**:141-155, 1980.

27. Journal of Contraception **1**(1):4, 1935.

28. Katchadourian, H.: The biology of adolescence, San Francisco, 1977, W.H. Freeman & Co., Publishers.

29. Killien, M.G.: Birth planning values and intentions of professional couples, doctoral dissertation, Seattle, 1982, University of Washington.

30. Litt, I.F., Cuskey, W.R., and Rudd, S.: Identifying adolescents at risk for noncompliance with contraceptive therapy, Journal of Pediatrics **96**:742-745, 1980.

31. Luker, K.: Taking chances: abortion and the decision not to contracept, Berkeley, 1975, University of California Press.

32. Metcalf, M.G.: Incidence of ovulatory cycles in women approaching the menopause, Journal of Biosocial Science **11**(1):39-48, 1979.

33. Paul, E., and Pilpel, H.: Teenager and pregnancy: the law in 1979, Family Planning Perspectives **11**:297-302, 1979.

34. Persky, H., et al.: Plasma testosterone level and sexual behavior of couples, Archives of Sexual Behavior **7**:157-173, 1978.

35. Poston, D., and Gotard, E.: Trends in childlessness in the United States, 1910-1975, Social Biology **24**:212-224, 1977.

36. Reich, P.: A historical understanding of contraception. In Notman, M., and Nadelson, C., editors: Sexual and reproductive aspects of women's health care, vol. 1, New York, 1978, Plenum Publishing Corp.

37. Richardson, D.W., and Short, R.V.: Time of onset of sperm production in boys, Journal of Biosocial Science Suppl. **5**:15-25, 1978.

38. Schwartz, D., MacDonald, P., and Heuchel, V.: Fecundability, coital frequency, and the viability of ova, Population Studies **34**:397, 1980.

39. Tietze, C.: Induced abortion: a world view, 1981, ed. 4, New York, 1981, The Population Council.

40. Townes, B., et al.: Birth planning values and decisions: the prediction of fertility, Journal of Applied Social Psychology **7**:73-88, 1977.

41. Trussell, J., and Westoff, C.F.: Contraceptive practice and trends in coital frequency, Family Planning Perspectives **12:**246-249, 1980.

42. Udry, R.: Age at menarche, at first intercourse, and at first pregnancy, Journal of Biosocial Science **11:**433-441, 1979.

43. Veevers, J.: The social meanings of parenthood, Psychiatry **36:**291-310, 1973.

44. Wagner, N.: I am not that kind of girl, unpublished manuscript, Seattle, University of Washington.

45. Wilkie, J.R.: The trend towards delayed childbearing, Journal of Marriage and the Family **43:**583-591, 1981.

46. Women who trust their method have fewer pregnancies: Family Planning Perspectives **13:**149-150, 1981.

47. Worthington-Roberts, B., Vermeersch, J., and Williams, S.: Nutrition in pregnancy and lactation, ed. 2, St. Louis, 1981, The C.V. Mosby Co.

48. Zabin, L., and Clark, S.: Why they delay: a study of teenage family planning clinic patients, Family Planning Perspectives **13:**205-217, 1981.

49. Zelnik, M., and Kantner, J.F.: Sexual and contraceptive experience of young unmarried women in the United States, 1976 and 1971, Family Planning Perspectives **9**(2):55, 1977.

50. Zelnik, M., and Kantner, J.F.: Contraceptive patterns and premarital pregnancy among women aged 15-19 in 1976, Family Planning Perspectives **10**(3):135-142, 1978.

51. Zelnik, M., and Kantner, J.F.: Reasons for nonuse of contraception by sexually active women aged 15-19, Family Planning Perspectives **11:**289-296, 1979.

52. Zelnik, M., and Kantner, J.F.: Sexual activity, contraceptive use and pregnancy among metropolitan-area teenagers: 1971-1979, Family Planning Perspectives **12:**230-231 + , 1980.

53. Zabin, L., Kantner, J.F., and Zelnik, M.: The risk of adolescent pregnancy in the first months of intercourse, Family Planning Perspectives **11:**215-222, 1979.

54. Zelnik, M., and Kim, Y.: Sex education and its association with teenage sexual activity, pregnancy and contraceptive use, Family Planning Perspectives **14**(3):117-126, 1982.

References for clients

Boston Women's Health Book Collective: Our bodies, ourselves, ed. 3, New York, 1979, Simon & Schuster, Inc.

Brewer, G.: The pregnancy after 30 workbook, Emmaus, Pa., 1978, Rodale Press, Inc.

Daniels, P., and Weingarten, K.: Sooner or later: the timing of parenthood in the life cycle, New York, 1982, W.W. Norton & Co., Inc.

Elvenstar, D.: Children: to have or have not? New York, 1982, G.P. Putnam's Sons.

Hongladarom, G., McCorkle, R., and Woods, N., editors: The complete book of women's health, Englewood Cliffs, N.J., 1982, Prentice-Hall, Inc.

Stewart, F., et al.: My body, my health: the concerned woman's book of gynecology, New York, 1981, John Wiley & Sons, Inc.

Whelan, E.M.: A baby . . . maybe, New York, 1975, The Bobbs-Merrill Co., Inc.

12

Sexuality and infertility

NANCY FUGATE WOODS and CYNTHIA LUKE

Although mechanisms for separating sexual behavior from reproduction have been known for centuries, it is only recently that technologies to separate the recreative from the procreative aspects of sex have been available to the majority of the population. This development has made it possible for a large segment of the population to choose not only whether or not to procreate but also when and how frequently to do so. The fact that reproduction can be accomplished at the control of the individuals involved has created a milieu that influences those persons whose concerns relate to fertility control and infertility.

Fertility is presumed until proven otherwise. By definition, fertility for women is the ability to conceive and give birth to a viable infant, and for men it is the ability to successfully impregnate. Thus fertility could be considered to be the residual category of infertility. One knows one is fertile by determining that one is not infertile. Infertility is considered to exist when, after a year or more of regular sexual intercourse without using a contraceptive method, a conception does not occur, or the pregnancy, if it occurs, cannot be carried to term. Infertility may be primary or secondary. In the former instance there is not a history of pregnancy; in the latter, infertility occurs after one or more successful pregnancies. The term *sterility* is reserved to describe permanent or incurable infertility.[4]

Menning[4] correctly points out that fertility is not a "life force" to be turned on at will, yet society's notion of "planned pregnancy" being available to nearly everyone is pervasive. Although much public attention has been devoted to issues and technology of population control, it is estimated that from 10% to 15% of American couples of child-bearing age are infertile. With this contradiction in mind, it is possible to better understand the different mind-sets of two groups of clients: those who are attempting to avoid pregnancy and those who are trying to achieve pregnancy.

Whether the individual's concern is limiting reproduction or fostering it, there will be common issues that may have rather pervasive effects on that person's sexuality. The purpose of this chapter is to outline some of the issues confronting persons who desire to achieve a pregnancy, determinants of infertility, and the sexual sequelae

222

of assessment and management of individuals seeking health services to achieve fertility.

Sexuality, fertility, and infertility: common issues

Whether an individual is concerned with limitation of reproduction or its facilitation, that person is confronted with issues related to the *control* of a process that is highly charged with emotion. Not only must the individual deal with "control issues" but that person must also confront his or her own *sexuality*. Because sexuality pervades many aspects of people's lives, it is often necessary for the person dealing with fertility control to address issues related to *self-image* and *self-esteem*.

The situation confronting infertile individuals is somewhat similar to that confronting persons pursuing the goal of fertility control: how to control their bodies and reproductive processes. Although there is much literature speaking to the relative effectiveness of fertility control measures, the area of infertility research is relatively new. Although some problems causing infertility are easily and readily treated, some are resistant to therapy, and in some instances no diagnosis can be made. It is estimated that 30% of infertile couples can be managed successfully with counseling, instruction, or minor medical treatment; another 20% require more significant therapy; and the remaining 50% will not achieve pregnancy. Thus it is not surprising that infertile persons may have and express feelings of loss of control during the course of their treatment.

Determinants of fertility and infertility

Factors that influence an individual's fertility and infertility are varied, some known and some unknown. For a female, fertility peaks at approximately 24 years of age, diminishing gradually from then to 30 years of age. After 30 it is thought to decline more rapidly, with pregnancy occurring rarely after 50 years of age. It is presumed that age factors relate to ovum composition, the body's hormonal changes, vaginal secretion alterations, and the woman's psychologic needs. Male fertility peaks at approximately 25 years of age and declines gradually after age 40, although it persists well into old age. The male's fertility is related to the sperm composition and activity, semen changes, the body's hormonal changes, and his needs. Another factor associated with fertility is the frequency of intercourse. It is believed that the greatest fertility potential of the male sperm occurs when sexual intercourse occurs four times per week; on the average this should produce a conception within a 6-month period for a couple. For the female, intercourse needs to occur within a 24-hour period around ovulation; time of ovulation therefore needs to be identified. Stress has been suspected to influence timing of ovulation, susceptibility to fertilization, and implantation. The effect of desires and ambivalences has been cited as an influencing factor; however, little research is available to support or disprove this speculation. Presently many other unknown variables account for the 10% of infertile couples for whom no cause can be determined.

When a couple decides to test fertility or desires to have a child, there is a period of "trying" before the state of infertility can be assumed. During this interim period there are fears and hopes and sometimes misinformation. Often it is a time when health professionals have no contact with the couple.

Sexuality and infertility

Infertility, self-image, and self-esteem. The infertile couple's initial response to their predicament may be one of surprise. This is especially likely among those who have vacillated in their decisions to parent or those who have delayed parenting for a time. It seems ironic that they have been using contraception for years and are now unable to become pregnant. Feelings of denial, isolation, anger, guilt or unworthiness, and depression may occur in response to the discovery of infertility. The couple eventually may grieve for the loss of their ability to conceive. However, their grief may be deterred for several reasons:

1. Their loss is a potential rather than a concrete one.
2. They may be unable to discuss their loss.
3. They may feel uncertainty about their fertility, so they do not grieve for its loss.
4. The loss may be negated or minimized by others who are unable to empathize with the infertile couple.
5. They may have no supportive persons to comfort them in their grief.

Resolution of feelings about infertility may involve the return of feelings of optimism or the channeling of energy into new directions.[4]

Infertility directly involves sexuality, since it is inherently linked to sexual and reproductive organs. Being infertile influences the way people think about themselves as sexual beings. Infertile women may feel unfeminine, and infertile men may feel impotent. These feelings, in part, can be attributed to the way in which sex roles are defined in society. For some women, being able to have a child is synonymous with or proof of being a woman. For some men, being able to father a child would be testimony to their masculinity. Thus people come to see themselves as successes or failures according to socially defined norms or expectations.

The infertility experience has the capacity to confirm an already negative self-image or cause individuals with positive self-images to feel less adequate or confident than they did previously. Loss of any parts of the reproductive system can compound feelings of inadequacy because of the profound influence of losing an organ symbolic of life or sexuality.

One's self-esteem can influence one's response to infertility. Those who have healthy levels of self-esteem will tend to see the situation as unfortunate and as external to them. Those who have poor self-esteem may see themselves as having caused the situation and feel guilty and unworthy.

Menning[4] suggests that the person who successfully resolves her or his feelings about infertility should regain feelings of being a "fully functioning sexual person" whose self-image is not made worse by the confrontation that he or she is infertile and who can focus on other areas of pride and worth as sources of self-esteem.

Effects of infertility on sexual behavior. Menning[4] describes the influence of infertility on sexual behavior and function. She notes that one of the sources of difficulty for infertile couples is the awareness of the temperature chart that they must keep as a record of ovulation. She comments that "a man, a woman, and a thermometer make strange bed fellows.'' Keeping track of each day's temperature and each sexual encounter can focus the couple's attention on their infertility and attempts at pregnancy, thus interfering with the pleasure they associate with sexual relations. After formal charting of the basal body temperature is no longer necessary for therapy the couple may continue to ''mentally chart'' the woman's cycle. Mental charting can be as troublesome as the written form of charting, inasmuch as both create demands for performance and remove spontaneity from the sexual relationship. Concerns may arise about the adequacy of a couple's frequency of sexual activity. Sometimes a partner may repress a desire for intercourse, saving it for the ''command performance'' around the time of ovulation. Lack of spontaneity in sexual behavior may lead to diminished sexual satisfaction.[1]

Although transient bouts with sexual dysfunction are extremely common among fertile and infertile men, the performance pressure associated with diagnosis and treatment of infertility can be severe. Inability to perform for diagnostic tests or at midcycle is common. Explanations given by men for midcycle sexual dysfunction include the ''this-is-the-night'' syndrome, changes in the purpose of sexual intercourse, stress of clinical testing by a third party, and self-doubt about adequate future performance after a single episode of sexual dysfunction.[2]

Some women may also experience a loss of sexual desire and interference with sexual arousal or orgasm. Although the nonorgasmic woman can still have intercourse, her feelings about herself and her relationship are likely to be compromised. Menning[4] indicates that following a final diagnosis of infertility, some couples may call a moratorium on sex. Some individuals may respond in the opposite way—by overcompensating.

Menning[4] suggests several ways of coping that eventually help the couple to again appreciate sex for its own sake. First, the individual involved needs to respect the wishes of the partner, particularly if one partner is not yet ready to resume sexual relations. Next, changes in time, place, and position may help, inasmuch as these changes can break up old associations with unpleasant memories. Some persons may need sexual counseling or therapy to facilitate change. Finally, Menning suggests that believing in sex for its own sake allows the couple to enjoy a loving way of communicating.

Assessment

The health care team's initial response to the client is an important variable in the relationships to follow. During the assessment process the practitioner gathers data from the client about the focus of concern, and the client gathers data about the interest, approach, and services offered by the practitioner. In some medical centers a team approach offers more comprehensive care for infertility and may include a gynecologist, endocrinologist, urologist, genetic counselor, psychiatrist, sexual therapist, nurse clinician, social worker, and counselor. This approach is aimed at a total assessment with cooperation and collaboration in the most effective and efficient way.

Many times the couple chooses to enter into the health care system together for an investigation and to provide each other with support. Although many clinicians see infertile couples together, at least on a single visit, it also is desirable to interview each partner in the relationship separately. This enables both individuals to share information with the professional that may not be appropriate or comfortable to share with the partner.

For couples or individuals whose concern is infertility, a sexual history is an integral part of the client history. This segment of the history assists the practitioner in understanding the relationship of sexuality to the client's health or illness; the facts about the client's relationships, living arrangements, life-styles, and sexual knowledge base; and the initiating of open communication in a sensitive area for discussion, teaching, counseling, and referring. It is helpful for the client in maintaining control and encouraging assertiveness to understand the practitioner's rationale for asking such intimate questions. A statement that understanding when a couple has intercourse in relationship to the woman's menstrual cycle is important to assessing the probability of conceiving assists the couple in revealing such information and may decrease their need to fabricate data for the health practitioner. Since there are many differing norms for sexual activity and feelings of sexual adequacy, the most open-ended questions will assist the practitioner in approaching data gathering in the least biased ways. Framing questions will assist the client to be more comfortable and enhance reliability, that is, assuming a range of behavior and avoiding assumptions. For the client it is helpful to know what course the sexual history will take and what information it will include (from general information to specific questions concerning the client's feelings and concerns), as well as the time involved. Confidentiality, privacy, and respect for the client's limitations or boundaries need to be assured. The client may wish to discuss some aspects at a later time in the interview and may wish to begin with the focus of concern.

It is helpful to use the language of the client and to clarify meanings; it is also important to share with the client terminology (e.g., uterus, vagina, clitoris, intercourse, menstruation) that enables the client to communicate more effectively with health care professionals. Sometimes using the language of the client may be uncomfortable for the practitioner, and language may need to be adapted so that both the client and practitioner are comfortable with and understand the terms being used. Labels the client may use, such as "I'm frigid" or "I'm impotent," should be clarified before the clinician assumes a diagnosis and perhaps introduces more positive labels. Encouraging self-knowledge, self-examination, and self-care questions and decision making aids the client in maintaining control. The interviewer attempts to make no assumptions about life-style or sexual relationships. If the client is sexually active, the practitioner uses the term "partner" until the client uses another term: boyfriend or girlfriend, wife or husband. The interviewer's awareness of her or his own feelings about various life-styles and sexual practices will help in being less judgmental in attitude, in focusing questions most appropriate to the client's needs, and in directing the interview.

The sexual history might begin with the client describing her or his sex education and attitudes, significant changes associated with development, and the effect of sexuality on present health and on relationships. The client's current attitudes toward sexuality and sexual activity may be important, such as what one feels about one's body and the activities that are most pleasurable, as well as practices (positions, use of vaginal creams, douching, means of maintaining erection) and concerns. General questions such as "Does the relationship meet your expectations?" "What would you want to change about yourself, your partner, the relationship?" "Can you ask for change?" may be helpful in guiding future interventions for the client or couple.

Sexual concerns arise during the assessment process for the client. These may be dealt with during history taking or may be identified for continued discussion. The health history helps to direct the practitioner in the physical examination to reaffirm normal functions and to identify problem areas for both the woman and man. Both the healthy components and problem areas need to be communicated to the client, as well as explanations for their possible development, further tests for assessment, implications of functioning and nonfunctioning states, and range of interventions with probable resolutions and risks. If the client is particularly anxious, a written summary, diagram, or readings may be suggested. A future discussion almost always is necessary after the client has time to process the initial information.

Those clients with infertility problems come to the practitioner with sexual concerns: "Am I (are we) doing something wrong?" "Am I fully a woman/man if I cannot reproduce?" Reproduction may become the only reason for sexual intercourse, and as with any long-term chronic problem, certain sequelae follow: lack of spontaneity, sexual desire, arousal, orgasm, and satisfaction accompanied by feelings of anger, guilt, unworthiness, depression, and grief.

The variety of tests that ensue for the infertile couple are numerous. Most often the hope is that at each step the cause of the infertility will be discovered. However, for some 10% of couples, finding a causative factor is not possible at present. *Infertility: A Guide for the Childless Couple*[4] reviews tests for women and men, as do nursing and medical texts. The primary issues during this continued assessment phase and ensuing treatment are presenting choices to the couple, ascertaining their values (importance of parenting, life-style changes, and effects of body image assaults), and emphasizing the controls that they perceive with their bodies and life decisions.

Self-help groups, such as the national group RESOLVE,[3] and group support and counseling are ways to decrease the isolated feelings couples may have. Monthly contacts with the nurse clinician provide an additional source of support and information for the couple. Each of these approaches can be most helpful by emphasizing the couple's coping mechanisms rather than focusing on pathology. When intervention is required for unsuccessful resolution, such as depression or long-term guilt, referrals may be indicated.

Summary

This chapter has considered sexuality and its relationship to infertility. Concerns of persons attempting to achieve fertility were discussed, with special emphasis on their desires to achieve control over their bodies' functions. The relationships of infertility to self-image and self-esteem were discussed, and the influence of infertility on sexuality and sexual behavior was considered. Implications for health professionals were outlined for assessment and intervention.

Some key considerations for professionals caring for individuals who seek to achieve fertility include the following:

1. The ability to reproduce is intimately tied to sexuality, self-image, and self-esteem. The extent to which this is important varies with cultural expectations and individuals.
2. Although 10% to 15% of couples are estimated to be infertile,

much more emphasis has been placed on population control measures than on the study of infertility.

3. The assessment and therapy for infertility may interfere with the couple's sexual pleasure by creating a demand for performance to coincide with ovulation or tests. This demand may have deleterious effects on the sexual pleasure of the woman and her partner.

4. Self-awareness on the part of the professional is essential for counseling individuals who wish to achieve fertility.

Questions for review

1. Compare and contrast the concerns of the person who is attempting to achieve a pregnancy with the person who is seeking a contraceptive method.
2. How can the mind-set and value system of the professional influence his or her ability to empathize with the individual seeking help with infertility?
3. At what point in the life cycle is fertility at its maximum? What sexual frequency is most compatible with achieving a pregnancy, and at what point should a couple expect to have conceived?
4. Describe how the infertility workup may affect the individual's sexuality and sexual behavior.
5. Marilyn and Rick have been married for 4 years, and during the last year they have used no contraceptive methods in hopes of having a pregnancy. They are both in their late thirties and have pursued professional careers before marriage and before deciding to have a child. Marilyn has had pelvic inflammatory disease associated with an IUD, and she decides to have tubal surgery. She expresses a great deal of guilt over her "selfishness"—"waiting too long to have a child so I could have a career." What influence is Marilyn's guilt likely to have on her sexuality? What types of sexual problems could occur for this couple in the course of their infertility therapy? What anticipatory guidance could you offer them?

References

1. Behrman, S.F., and Kistner, R.W.: Progress in infertility, Boston, 1975, Little, Brown & Co.
2. Dor, J., Homburg, R., and Rabau, E.: An evaluation of etiologic factors and therapy in 665 infertile couples, Fertility and Sterility 28:718-722, 1977.
3. Menning, B.E.: RESOLVE—a support group for infertile couples, American Journal of Nursing 76:258-259, 1976.
4. Menning, B.E.: Infertility: a guide for the childless couple, Englewood Cliffs, N.J., 1977, Prentice-Hall, Inc.

Suggested readings

Amelar, R., Dubin, L., and Walsh, P.: Male infertility, Philadelphia, 1977, W.B. Saunders Co.
Bell, J.S.: Psychological problems among patients attending an infertility clinic, Journal of Psychosomatic Research 25(1):1-3, 1981.

Boston Women's Health Book Collective: Our bodies, ourselves, ed. 3, New York, 1979, Simon & Schuster, Inc.

Cockett, A.T.K., and Urry, R.L., editors: Male infertility: workup, treatment, and research, New York, 1976, Grune & Stratton, Inc.

Drake, T., and Grunert, G.: A cyclic pattern of sexual dysfunction in the infertility investigation, Fertility and Sterility **32:**542-545, 1979.

Elstein, M.: Effects of infertility on psychosexual function, British Medical Journal **3:**296-299, 1975.

Hammons, C.: The adoptive family, American Journal of Nursing **76:**251-257, 1976.

Harrison, M.: Infertility: a couple's guide to its causes and treatments, Boston, 1977, Houghton Mifflin Co.

Huggins, G.R.: Contraceptive use and subsequent fertility, Fertility and Sterility **28:**603-612, 1977.

Hulka, J.: Current status of elective sterilization in the United States, Fertility and Sterility **28:**515-520, 1977.

Kistner, R.W.: The infertile woman, American Journal of Nursing **73:**1937-1943, 1973.

Lenton, E.A., Weston, G.A., and Cooke, I.D.: Long-term follow-up of the apparently normal couple with a complaint of infertility, Fertility and Sterility **28:**913-919, 1977.

Mitchell, C.: The infertile family. In Armstrong, M.E., et al., editors: Blakiston handbook of clinical nursing, New York, 1979, McGraw-Hill, Inc.

Platt, J., Ficher, I., and Silver, M.: Infertile couples: personality traits and self-ideal concept discrepancies, Fertility and Sterility **24:**972-976, 1973.

Speroff, L., Glass, R.H., and Kase, N.: Clinical gynecologic endocrinology and infertility, ed. 2, Baltimore, 1978, The Williams & Wilkins Co.

References for clients

Boston Women's Health Book Collective: Our bodies, ourselves, ed. 3, New York, 1979, Simon & Schuster, Inc.

Brody, J.E.: New hope for infertile couples, Woman's Day, p. 24, Feb. 3, 1978.

Kaufman, S.A.: You can have a baby, Nashville, 1978, Thomas Nelson, Inc.

Menning, B.: Infertility: a guide for the childless couple, Englewood Cliffs, N.J., 1977, Prentice-Hall, Inc.

Peck, E.: The baby trap, New York, 1971, Bernard Geis Associates, Inc.

Peck, E., and Senderowitz, J.: Pronatalism: the myth of mom and apple pie, New York, 1974, Thomas Y. Crowell Co., Publishers.

Silber, S.: How to get pregnant, New York, 1980, Charles Scribner's Sons.

Whelan, E.M.: A baby . . . maybe, New York, 1975, The Bobbs-Merrill Co., Inc.

13

Sexual assault*

CARMEN GERMAINE WARNER and CONSTANCE VAUGHT

Throughout the past decade there has been a marked increase in the number of sexual assault victims seeking individualized care from nurses, physicians, and counselors in health care and community-based settings. This trend has developed, in part, as a result of an increased level of consciousness raising resulting from broad-based professional and community education. Concomitant with greater awareness of the incidence of rape has been the alarming national increase in cases of reported rape.

In 1980 there were over 82,000 rapes reported in the United States, which is a rate of about *one reported rape every 6 minutes*. This rate converts to 71 reported rapes for every 100,000 females[1] (Table 13-1).

The number of reported rapes per 100,000 females has more than doubled throughout the past decade. It is not known, however, whether this increase in reported rapes is a result of a rise in the actual incidence of the crime, a change in the victim's willingness to report the assault, or a combination of both.

Historically, rape has been characterized as an underreported crime because most victims opt to remain silent and not seek care. Surveys conducted by the U.S. Census Bureau and the National Opinion Research Center, as well as FBI estimates, have indicated that the number of rapes actually committed is between 3.5 and 10 times the number of rapes reported.[1]

If there is no further increase in the rate at which rapes are committed, if a woman is at risk for a minimum of 35 years of her life, and if the conservative 4:1 estimate of the number of actual rapes is used, then the chance of a woman being raped sometime during her lifetime is about one in ten ($[71 \times 35 \times 4]/100,000 = 0.994$).

For many years much attention has been devoted to the rapist, his past problems, and the cause of the crime itself. Some investigators have studied the victim's characteristics to determine whether sexual assaults might be provoked by the person assaulted. In fact, this assumption, that the victim was not an innocent party to the rape, has permeated many articles on rape. Other studies have shown concern with the prevention of rape by

---

*In this chapter the terms *sexual assault* and *rape* are used interchangeably based on their common usage in a nonlegal sense.

Table 13-1. Numbers of rapes reported to police*

Year	Number reported	Rate per 100,000 inhabitants	Rate per 100,000 females
1965	23,330	12.1	—
1966	25,730	13.2	—
1967	27,530	13.9	—
1968	31,560	15.8	—
1969	37,050	18.4	—
1970	37,860	18.6	—
1971	42,120	20.4	—
1972	46,690	22.4	—
1973	51,230	24.4	—
1974	55,210	26.1	—
1975	56,090	26.3	51
1976	56,730	26.4	52
1977	63,020	29.1	57
1978	67,131	30.8	60
1979	75,989	34.5	67
1980	82,088	36.4	71

From Abarbanel, G., and Klein, S.: Statistical information about the crime of rape, Santa Monica, Calif., 1981, Rape Treatment Center, Santa Monica Hospital Medical Center.
*These statistics do not include unreported rapes or crimes involving other forms of sexual assault.

means of courses in self-defense. Until recently, however, the rape victim was a neglected entity, and little if any attention was devoted to her emotional response after the assault and its impact on her sexuality. Although there has recently been an increase in the literature concerning the emotional problems of rape victims, very little is known about the aftermath of sexual assault and the long-term effects of rape on the victim. Much more research in this area is greatly needed.

It is recognized that rapes of men, women, and children occur. The overwhelming majority of victims, however, are female, so this chapter addresses itself to the female rape victim.

Because the aftereffects of rape can be diverse, it is helpful to analyze them in a biopsychosocial framework. The purposes of this chapter then are to consider the following:

1. Biologic effects of rape as they interfere with a woman's sexual functioning
2. Psychologic responses that a woman experiences after rape
3. How society views a woman who has been raped
4. Possible interventions by health professionals to help a woman cope with the aftermath of sexual assault

Biologic consequences of rape

Sexual assault is a broad term applying to oral, genital, or manual contact with the genitals of a victim without the victim's consent. Rape is a crime of violence that is expressed in the sexual act.[17,25,35] Legally defined,[12,26] rape is carnal knowledge of a person by force and against that person's will. It is important to note that the slightest penetration or contact of the male's genitals with the female's labia majora constitutes carnal knowledge; neither laceration of the hymen nor evidence of ejaculation is a necessary element of the crime of rape.[6,40]

In addition to the legal definition of rape, there are a number of working definitions of rape and related assaults that may be identified and used by health care and counseling professionals during the initial assessment process. Some of these include the following:

- *Aggravated assault.* The perpetrator causes or attempts to cause serious physical and/or emotional injury to an individual, recognizing the seriousness of the act. This may be classified as a second-degree felony or a first-degree misdemeanor.
- *Attempted rape.* Actions are taken by the perpetrator toward completion of an act of rape. The perpetrator must have been exposed, attempted to subdue and penetrate the victim, either male or female, but was unable to complete the act.
- *Simple assault.* The perpetrator attempts to cause bodily harm or injury to a male or female. This is a third-degree misdemeanor.
- *Statutory rape.* Sexual intercourse takes place between an individual 18 years of age or older with a male or female under 14 years of age. This is a second-degree felony.

Many investigators have documented the physical consequences of rape, which include physical trauma to the genital area and to other parts of the body, pregnancy, and sexually transmitted disease. The first, genital trauma, is especially important, since its residual effects may interfere with a woman's future sexual functioning if not properly treated.

Genital injuries. In 1970 Masters and Johnson[23] discussed the consequences of rape for three of their clients. After a gang rape one woman required extensive reconstruction of the vagina, and she subsequently became vaginismic. Two women who were raped as young girls with the coercion of family members also became vaginismic as adults. Masters and Johnson noted that trauma initiating involuntary vaginal spasm can be either physical or psychic and that the consequences of forced sexual intercourse may be serious and enduring.

Masters and Johnson[23] also found that women who had been raped experienced dyspareunia. Three women who had been subjected to gang rape had scarring at the mucocutaneous junction of the vagina and perineal body, resulting in severe pain on intromission. It was also found that pelvic injury may cause traumatic tearing of soft tissues of the pelvis, such as the broad ligament. When the ligament providing uterine support becomes lacerated, a woman experiences feelings of chronic pelvic vasocongestion. Her uterus usually is in third-degree retroversion and is enlarged from chronic vascular congestion. In addition, a significant amount of serous fluid resulting from the torn ligament accumulates in the pelvis, and there may be bilateral tears of the broad ligament or sacrouterine ligament. Masters and Johnson pointed out that it was unfortunate that these women were told by their physicians that their symptoms were attributable to psychic trauma. Before they were treated surgically for the broad ligament damage, their marriages suffered severely because of sexually crippling dyspareunia.

To determine what types of injuries were sustained by rape victims, Robinson, Sherrod, and Malcorney[27] reviewed the medical records of ninety-four alleged cases of rape or child molestation at the Womack Army Hospital from 1957 to 1967. They found that genital injuries (present in 8.5% of individuals studied) were far less frequently documented than extragenital injuries (28.7%). In addition, only lacerations and abrasions of the hymen, labia, posterior fourchette, perineum, and vagina were documented. They suggested that since no ecchymoses were noted in the review of the genital lesions, it would have been advisable to reexamine the victim 24 hours after the assault, when they might be more likely to be visible.

Hayman and Lanza[16] investigated severe injuries connected with 2190 females brought to medical examination for alleged assault. Of the eighty-two women severely injured, twenty-four had to be hospitalized. Six children and one adult were hospitalized for vaginal or perineal lacerations and one child and sixteen adults for other injuries. Of the fifty-eight patients treated in the emergency department, eleven were children with vaginal or perineal lacerations. Hundreds of patients were treated for minor injuries. During Hayman and Lanza's investigation there were four proven murders from physical assault that included rape and three murders in which rape was suspected. The population studied by these authors ranged in age from 6 months to 91 years, with a peak age of 14 to 15 years, and was predominantly black.

At Boston City Hospital eighty rape victims were given counseling by a psychiatric nurse and sociologist.[8] In this group there were 147 signs of trauma evident on physical examination, most prevalent on the head, face, throat, arms, legs, and back of the women. In addition, there were lacerations to nearly every body part except the abdomen and back, with facial lacerations being the most prevalent. Gynecologic physical findings included bruises and lacerations to the perineum, hymen, vulva, vagina, cervix, and anus. The most predominant gynecologic finding in this sample was cervical, vulvar, and perineal bruising. One victim required immediate vaginal packing and hospitalization for copious vaginal bleeding. Women who were raped during their menstrual periods sometimes suffered additional trauma from having tampons pushed up into the cul-de-sac. The tampons were removed during a speculum examination.[8]

In Massey's 1971 study of 501 rape victims,[22] fifty-one showed external evidence of trauma ranging from small cuts to severe contusions and a facial fracture. Two of the victims had suffered from prolonged kidnapping and rape and had evidence of multiple episodes of physical trauma. Twenty-five victims had evidence of genital injuries, which ranged from laceration of the hymen to rupture of the cul-de-sac. Complete vaginal penetration in children frequently resulted in perineal lacerations.

Woodling, Evans, and Brodbury[40] examined data from five studies of rape victims in the following locations: Washington, D.C.; Dade County, Florida; Boston; San Francisco; and Ventura, California. Injuries in the form of large bruises, lacerations, minor fractures, or joint pain occurred in 10% to 46% of the reported cases. Major physical injuries, which included fractures, subdural hematomas, cerebral concussions, skull fractures, or intraabdominal injuries, all requiring hospitalization, occurred in 4% to 15% of the rapes reported. Many of the more seriously injured victims were noted to have sustained their injuries following the sexual assault rather than before or during the assault.

In 1974 Soules et al.[31] studied 110 alleged rape victims over a 4-month period in Denver, Colorado. They found extragenital trauma (e.g., bruises, lacerations, scratches) present in fifty-nine (45%) of the victims studied, three times as common as genital trauma. Signs of genital trauma such as hymenal tears, vaginal lacerations, and perineal ecchymoses were present in fourteen cases (13%). Many patients were reported to have both types of trauma. These statistics of the incidence of genital and extragenital trauma were much higher than reported in previous studies.

These studies verify the commonly held conclusion that there is a significantly high incidence of physical injury among victims of rape.

Sexually transmitted disease. Another unfortunate consequence of rape is acquisition of sexually transmitted disease from the assailant. In the sample studied by Hayman and Lanza[16] eighty-two new cases of sexually transmitted disease were diagnosed after assaults. There were seventy-six cases of gonorrhea, five cases of syphilis, one involving a 4-year-old child, and one case of lymphogranuloma venereum.

On the other hand, Voigt,[36] in his study in Copenhagen, found acquisition of sexually transmitted disease in only 0.8% of his total 650 cases of women and children. Of the 418 girls under 15 years of age, there were three cases of gonorrhea (0.07%) and no cases of syphilis.

Professionals must inform the victim about the possibility of having contracted a sexually transmitted disease. It is essential to explain that there is evidence that 1% to 3% of all victims will contract a sexually transmitted disease as a result of the assault and that up to 3% will prove to have an unrecognized, established sexually transmitted disease.[38] Individuals must be reminded that sexually transmitted disease can be transmitted through all mucous membranes (oral, genital, and anal) and that sexual relations are not safe until it has been determined whether or not a sexually transmitted disease was contracted or that prescribed treatment has been successful.

It is also important to reassure the victim with information regarding proven treatment and agencies available for follow-up care (see pp. 242 and 252 for specific intervention).

Pregnancy. Pregnancy is another potential sequela of rape. There is a 1% chance that a woman may become pregnant as a result of the attack.[4] According to Braen,[5] a careful gynecologic history should be obtained by the examiner, since 90% to 95% of conceptions that are the result of a single act of intercourse occur between 120 hours before ovulation and 10 hours after ovulation. If the time of ovulation can be estimated, the examiner may be able to advise the patient about the need for pregnancy prevention.

Specific assessment required to determine the victim's capacity to become pregnant can be established by determining the following:

1. Is she sterile?
2. Has she had a tubal ligation or hysterectomy?
3. Has she reached the age of menarche or passed menopause?

If pregnancy is possible, one must establish the following:

1. On what day of her cycle did the rape occur?
2. What is the length of her regular cycle?
3. What present methods of contraception, if any, are being used?

Specific intervention concerning the prevention of pregnancy is addressed on p. 251.

Discovery of pregnancy by the rape victim is usually an additional crisis that may lead to alterations in the woman's sexuality, as described in Chapter 9. Regardless of the prophylactic method used, the victim needs reassurance that pregnancy prevention or pregnancy interruption will be accomplished and that no victim need carry a pregnancy to term.

The biologic consequences of rape, which include trauma, sexually transmitted disease, and pregnancy, require that a thorough physical examination be done as soon as possible after the attack. It is important to keep in mind that each of these consequences has the potential to lead to sexual problems for the victim.

Psychologic responses to rape

During the last decade the psychologic consequences of rape have been studied by a few investigators. However, there are not many statistics describing how frequently the rape victim requires long-term psychiatric care or how frequently emotional problems directly attributable to the rape occur. Hayman and Lanza[16] documented that seventy-two of the 2190 women in their sample were subsequently placed under psychiatric treatment. Although these women are a small percentage of the sample, it is significant that nine of the women were still under treatment 4 years after the incident.

Weiss and Borges[39] conducted a study on females who attempt suicide, in which there seems to be a relationship between an earlier rape experience and suicide attempt. Clinical evidence of the silent rape reaction is noted by psychiatrists who uncover an earlier rape and find that the event is still unresolved in the mind of the victim.

Although it is extremely difficult at this point to predict all the long-term needs of the rape victim, Notman and Nadelson[25] have noted some psychologic issues that appear clinically in rape victims at a later date. These include mistrust of men, with resulting avoidance or hesitation; a variety of sexual disturbances, often presenting as sexual dysfunctions; persistent phobic reactions; anxiety and depression often precipitated by seemingly unrelated events, which cause the victim to reexperience the original trauma; persistent anxiety; and avoidance of gynecologic examinations or procedures.

Effects of victimization. Some of the emotional effects of victimization were described by Halleck,[14,15] who saw rape victims in his psychiatric practice. He points out that when a woman knows her attacker there is always a question in the minds of others about whether the force used in obtaining intercourse was indeed provoked. It is also possible that certain personality characteristics make a woman susceptible to attack, especially if she has had previous sexual contact with the attacker. Halleck further theorizes that if some women have indeed been involved with the attacker, it may minimize the trauma they experience after the assault. For other women previous involvement may only serve to intensify guilt feelings.

Women who do not know their attacker are faced with overwhelming anger that they cannot deal with at the time of the attack. It is not unusual for such a woman to search her own motives to determine whether there was some way she could have prevented the attack. She may blame herself for not having taken sufficient care or preventive steps. The rape may also influence the woman's concept of her sexual role. To her the female role may feel very helpless, and she may feel degraded as a woman. Often the woman wonders whether she will still be attractive to men and whether the attack will leave her disinterested in normal sexual relations.[14]

It is difficult to imagine that any woman would experience any form of sexual assault without an emotional reaction of some kind. Usually the person who has been raped has intense guilt feelings. Often they result from fear that she indeed provoked the attack. Intense self-accusation may lead to prolonged emotional problems requiring therapy.

Finally, Halleck[14] described a phenomenon often seen in rape victims: the person is unwilling to share the history of sexual assault with her family or husband. Halleck emphasized the health worker's role in supporting the woman's efforts to divulge her history, citing dramatic reversal of symptoms in some women who have done so.

Three phases of response. Eight years ago, the first clinical study of rape victims was reported by Sutherland and Scherl,[33] who conducted follow-up interviews with thirteen young victims. These victims, all social workers, ranging in age from 18 to 24 years, lived in low-income areas in which they were employed. Most of the women were seen within 48 hours of the assault in a community mental health facility. The psychologic healing process of each of the victims after the assault was observed by a therapist.

The investigators found that all the women experienced three distinct phases in their reaction to the rape: an acute reaction, outward adjustment, and integration and resolution. Phase 1, or the acute reaction, was characterized by signs of acute distress, including shock, disbelief, emotional breakdown, and disruption of normal behavior patterns. The women's behavior at this time was agitated, incoherent, and volatile. They found it difficult to discuss their experiences, and often any mention of the assault caused them to break down.

During the initial phase women who felt there was no seduction or willing compliance involved in the rape immediately phoned the police or went to a nearby medical facility. Five of the victims felt an inner sense of guilt regarding their involvement in the rape and delayed telling anyone about the rape or seeking legal assistance or medical care. One woman did not report her rape until 2 months after the episode, when she discovered that she was pregnant.

Notification of parents or family created great anxiety. Fear of divulging the episode to a woman's family was grounded in her feeling that her own lack of judgment might have led to the attack. During this phase the woman was also confronted with the decision of whether to press charges, the possibility of having to identify the assailant, the response of her friends, the nature of publicity, potential pregnancy, and the responses of significant others in her life.

Sutherland and Scherl[33] found that phase 1 lasted from a few days to a few weeks. As the phase progressed, the woman tended to be able to handle the realistic consequences of the assault and was less involved in nonspecific anxiety.

It is crucial that the health worker assist the rape victim in confronting her feelings during this phase rather than support some of her defenses, since the victim rarely has an opportunity to share her response with the other professionals involved in her medical care and legal proceedings. At this time the health professional also helps direct the woman's attention toward the future and how she might feel in a few weeks or months. The victim is told that fear and depression may arise and that she may feel uncomfortable in dating, engagement, or marriage. If necessary, the woman is encouraged to seek professional counseling.

Phase 2, outward adjustment, begins within several days to weeks after the rape. During this phase the woman usually returns to her normal life patterns. At this point she becomes outwardly composed and feels that she needs no further help. The investigators label this a period of "pseudoadjustment" and believe that it contains much denial and suppression. The personal impact of the rape is ignored in the interest of protecting self and others.

The victim also tends to set aside her doubts about her own role in the rape. She may deal with her feelings about the attacker by attributing the rape to chance or to a deeper social issue. At any rate the woman seems to have very little interest in gaining insight through professional help during this phase. The investigators suggest that the rationalizations offered by the victim during this phase are grounded in her fears about the rape.

Phase 3, that of integration and resolution, often goes unrecognized. This phase starts when the woman has a need to talk and feels depressed. It may take some time for the woman to integrate the event with her self-image and resolve her feelings about the rape and the rapist. "Her earlier attitude of understanding the man's problems gives way to anger toward him for having 'used her' and anger toward herself for in some way having permitted or tolerated this 'use.'"[33]

Sometimes a specific event triggers the third phase, such as diagnosis of pregnancy, a glimpse of the rapist, or a marriage proposal. Often, however, there is no single identifiable event that triggers this phase. Instead, the woman may find herself functioning less well and thinking more about the rape. During this period the woman may have obsessive thoughts about the assault, concerns about the influence of the rape on the rest of her life, and a real need to consult with a professional. If the client is told during the initial contact that she may experience this third phase, then she can actively seek assistance. With the help of a health professional, her emotions can be reduced to manageable intensities so that she is able to maintain control.

Psychologic processes. Burgess and Holmstrom[8-11] have conducted the most comprehensive clinical analysis to date on the crisis of rape. In their study of eighty rape victims in the Boston area they[8] were able to define certain psychologic processes operating during the initial period after the rape. The majority of women in their sample perceived the rape as a crisis. About half the women in the sample became verbal and talkative in the emergency area, to relieve their pressure, and the other half became quiet and guarded.

Another process occurred that influenced the women's emotional state immediately after the rape. Burgess and Holmstrom[8] stated that in view of the fact that an individual's emotional state tended to be exaggerated in response to stress, and because conversation about the rape was stressful, the victim's emotional response was exaggerated. Emotional responses fell into two major categories: an expressed style and a controlled style. In the expressed mode, anger, fear, or other feelings were vented in words or nonverbally, such as crying. The controlled victim was characterized by a composed or subdued affect. Some women were observed to have multiple responses during a single interview.

Anger was a predominant feeling, as were fear, humiliation, embarrassment, and feelings of abnormalcy, revenge, and self-blame. Often anger was expressed toward the rapist, police, hospital, and others by the victim after the rape. Many victims were terrorized by the assailant and were fearful that they would be murdered. Still others felt they were rendered abnormal, dirty, invaded, and undesirable. To some victims the pelvic examination in the emergency department caused them to feel they were reliving the invasiveness of rape. Some women were able to use the substitution process to handle their feelings. They literally laughed instead of cried.

Themes evident in the concerns of women who had been raped included shock, sexuality, loss, and their future sexual relationships. Many claimed they felt numb and that they only wanted to forget the event. Some women discussed their own sexuality, including loss of virginity during the rape, their previous sexual activity, and their attitudes toward sex. The theme of loss was often discussed in conjunction with previous relationships with men. Finally, many women were concerned about how their spouses or fiancés would respond to the rape.[8] Fear of sexual relations and of men in general may interfere with resumption of the woman's sexual activity. The woman who has had no sexual experience before the rape is especially vulnerable because her only sexual experience has been an unpleasant one.

Not all victims are successful in achieving full resolution of the rape experience. For many victims studied by Woodling, Evans, and Brodbury,[40] frightening dreams and nightmares were quite common and persisted for a long time. Many victims develop phobias, including fear of the indoors, fear of the outdoors, fear of being alone, fear of crowds, fear of people behind them, and sexual fears.

Woodling, Evans, and Brodbury[40] noted that their experience with rape victims shows that most victims have sexual problems after the assault, and about two thirds encounter serious interpersonal problems. According to Woodling, Evans, and Brodbury, the tendency for the victim to delay resumption of sexual activities for an indefinite period of time indicates serious underlying psychologic problems that require intensive counseling. In their study 30% of the victims developed problems adjusting to their job or school. Thus careful follow-up of rape victims is necessary to identify unresolved emotional problems.

The manner in which a victim emotionally responds to sexual assault varies with how the rape occurred, what the victim did, and how she felt during the rape, whether a suspect was apprehended and successfully prosecuted, and whether the victim had previous emotional problems.[28] According to Selkin,[28] emotionally healthy resisters—those women who were able to prevent all or part of the attack by screaming, escaping, or physically resisting—did not differ in age or socioeconomic status from those women who did not resist, but they did score higher on measures of dominance, sociability, social pressure, and communality on personality tests. Selkin found the more emotionally distraught victim had exhibited more compliant or passive behavior during the attack.

Woodling, Evans, and Brodbury's[40] study in Ventura showed that no matter how brutal or demeaning the attack, the single most important determinant of eventual emotional health was whether a suspect was identified and successfully prosecuted. Those victims in cases in which a suspect was not identified or prosecuted had more phobic reactions, were more fearful of male strangers, and had more sexual and interpersonal problems after the assault.

Burgess and Holmstrom[8] described a "silent reaction" that should alert the health worker to the possibility of an earlier and unresolved rape. In their sample the following cluster of signs suggested a previous rape experience: increased anxiety noted as the interview continues, history of a sudden increased irritability, avoidance of men and sexuality, reports of an acute onset of phobias and violent nightmares, and a loss of self-esteem.

In addition to the many stresses already discussed, there are also age-specific issues for the rape victim that vary with the woman's developmental phase. Notman and Na-delson,[25] and Burgess and Holmstrom[8] have given detailed accounts of these life stage considerations. The single young woman between the ages of 17 and 24 is the most frequently reported rape victim. If the rape is this woman's first sexual experience, she may become quite confused about the relationship between sexuality, violence, and humiliation. The rape incident may challenge her sense of adequacy, especially if she is involved in separating from her family and establishing an independent identity. The young woman who has an ongoing sexual relationship may choose not to tell her partner because of fear that this might disrupt their relationship. The divorced or separated woman is in an especially difficult position because her life-style, morality, and character are often frequently questioned by others. The rape may only serve to confirm her feelings of inadequacy about functioning in an independent and autonomous manner. The woman with children must decide what, how, and when to tell them about the incident. The middle-aged or older woman may already be in a crisis of reassessing her own life role in responding to changes in her relationship with her children and husband. Her husband may be in his own midlife crisis and may be less responsive and supportive of her emotional needs. At this time the overwhelming experience of rape can be particularly damaging. In counseling, the victim's previous adjustment should be assessed. She should be given support and reassurance, and specific considerations related to her life circumstances should be acknowledged and dealt with.

Nearly all the literature in this area supports Hilberman's description[17] of rape as "an act of violence and humiliation in which the victim experiences overwhelming fear for her very existence as well as a profound sense of powerlessness and helplessness which few other events in one's life can parallel." The rape victim may respond with any number of diverse emotions, and usually a period of months is necessary for her to completely resolve her feelings about the attack.

As a result of increased awareness of the psychologic processes, professionals will be better able to establish good communication and help the victim know they are caring and supportive.

There are several important points to be kept in mind during the initial contact with the rape victim:

- Help the victim get in touch with her feelings. She may feel angry, depressed, guilty, dazed, or numb, all of which are legitimate reactions. The expression of feelings at this time may be a healthy way for the victim to deal with rape.
- Assist the victim to accept her feelings concerning the incident.
- Be sensitive to nonverbal signals such as body position, fidgeting, shakiness, and incoherence in speech.
- Practice active listening by hearing what the victim has to say without judging.
- Take the victim's story seriously; help legitimize the experience.
- Communicate a sense of stability by remaining calm and empathic.
- Establish a common language, and "tune in" to the victim's terminology.

Society and the rape victim. As previously mentioned, society has been deeply concerned with the rapist but has neglected the victim. Many articles refer to the stigma of being raped, especially if the woman chooses to prosecute the alleged rapist.[8,12,29] However, not much is known about society's view of the rape victim.

Masters and Johnson[23] cite one client whose husband became impotent after his wife divulged to him that she had been raped. Burgess and Holmstrom[8] noted that a number of women in their sample feared the consequences of being rejected by husbands and fiancés if they divulged that they had been sexually assaulted. The woman's reluctance to share her crisis with significant others is probably based on how society views the woman who has been raped.

Unfortunately the belief that "nice girls don't get raped" is still widespread. Often there is a tendency to attribute fault to the victim, and her clothing, sexual history, and contraceptive status may all be explored in court in many states.

Symonds,[34] in his study of victims of violent crimes and society's attitudes toward victims, found a marked reluctance and resistance to accept the innocence or accidental nature of victim behavior as evidenced by community responses, police behavior, family reactions, and victims themselves. Many of the questions and early responses to victims after the initial shock response of the listener wears off show this reluctance to believe in total innocence of the victim. Some examples of commonly heard responses noted by Symonds were "Didn't you know this neighborhood is dangerous to walk in after dark?" "Did you have your door locked?" "Why didn't you scream?" All these questions tend to imply that the victims could have prevented or avoided their injuries.

Symonds[33] attributes this response pattern to a basic need for all individuals to find a rational explanation for violent behavior, especially brutal crimes. Exposure to irrational violent behavior causes one to feel vulnerable and helpless. Believing that the victim has done something to cause the attack or in some way contributed to the crime makes the individual feel less helpless and less vulnerable.

In further attempting to understand society's reactions to victims of violent crimes, Symonds[34] examined the etymology of the word *victim*. The term originally meant a beast selected for sacrifice and was intimately tied to the concept of scapegoat. Today it still carries unpleasant connotations. People generally feel uneasy when they are associated or identified in some way with victims. As a result, Symonds contends, individuals have developed a ritualistic defense against being a victim. People reason that if they are good, nothing bad will happen to them; if something bad happens, then obviously that person was not being good. This rationale would seem to explain the evidence that in general those victims who fight back or resist their attackers seem to have greater social acceptance than those who succumb to the demands of their assailants. Symonds[34,35] found this "double bind attitude of society to be particularly evident toward victims of rape."

Like the Symonds study,[34] a study by Jones and Aronson[19] focused on the "just-world hypothesis." Their study tested the hypothesis that a woman who is socially respectable is seen as being more at fault in a crime in which she was the victim. The investigators administered written case accounts of a rape to 234 male and female undergraduate students at the University of Texas. The students were required to study the account and to recommend a prison sentence for the convicted. They were also requested to describe how much they considered the crime to be the victim's fault. The description of the victim in the cases was varied as to whether she was a virgin, divorcée, or married woman. Another group of subjects was asked to rate the responsibility of a number of people in a variety of occupations, and they rated the virgin, the married woman, and the divorcée in that order.

The study was based on the assumption that the more respectable woman should be seen as more likely to have caused her own misfortune. Since there is the belief in a just world in which a victim gets what she deserves, people need to explain why a respectable woman was victimized.

The results supported the authors' hypothesis that when the victim of the rape was a divorcée, less fault was attributed to her than when the victim was a virgin or a married woman. When sentencing the rapist, the group assigned a significantly longer prison term to the person who had raped the married woman than the person who had raped the divorcée. The investigators believed that this result was understandable in view of the belief that injuring a highly respectable person is a more serious crime than harming someone who is considered to be less respectable.

The investigators[20] also suggested that as the consequences of a crime become more severe, there exists a greater need to attribute some blame to the victim. Since the rape of a married woman may have an ill effect on her family, there is a need to attribute more blame to her.

It is interesting that no significant difference was observed between the fault attributed to women who were raped and the fault attributed to those who experienced attempted rape. It appeared that the only variable strongly influencing the perception of how much fault the victim had in the crime was her character. The severity of her suffering, then, influenced the length of the prison sentence recommended for the rapist but did not determine how much fault was attributable to the victim.

Male victims of rape

As previously noted, all human beings are potential victims of rape, including men and boys.

Men who have been traumatized as a result of a rape assault are reluctant to seek professional, medical, and social service intervention. Consequently, accurate data identifying male rape victims are difficult to obtain. Should the injuries sustained during the rape attack require immediate emergency attention, the victim relates the injuries to some cause other than a rape attack.

Professionals must recognize that rape incidents involving males are extremely traumatic and frequently reflect violent acts of physical abuse. It is of the utmost importance that health care professionals interact with these victims in a sensitive and supportive manner.

The male victim experiences many of the same physical and emotional injuries as the female victim, and it is essential that these male victims *not* be viewed differently. In fact the commonalities of all rape victims should be stressed rather than the differences.

Specific points to acknowledge when caring for male victims include the following:
- Male rapes do not occur only to male prisoners or homosexuals. All males are vulnerable to the potential trauma of a rape incident.
- Male rapes are often extremely violent.
- The physical examination, medical and social history, and specific intervention should be the same as for a female victim, with special emphasis placed on rectal trauma, bleeding, or discharge; penile trauma, bleeding, or discharge; soreness,

infection of or trauma to the mouth or pharynx; and internal injuries, soreness, or pain.
- If the victim's anus is swollen and tender, an assessment can be made through the use of a rectal aspirate. This is performed by inserting 10 ml of normal saline into the rectum and aspirating the fluid after 5 to 10 minutes. This sample can be saved for acid phosphatase and/or sperm analysis.[5]

The elderly rape victim

Elderly persons who have experienced rape assaults are clearly victims who "did not ask to be raped." In fact it is their vulnerability to the attack that makes rape of the elderly so appalling.

Specific points of vulnerability characteristic of the elderly include the following:
- Age
- Skeletal and muscular changes
- Diminished sensory capacities
- Impaired ability for mobility and self-control
- Increased sensitivity of genitourinary organs
- Lack of transportation
- Living alone
- Well-established daily routines, obvious to the observer

These factors are valuable for health professionals to consider when they are caring for the elderly and wish to introduce appropriate preventive measures against rape attacks. This information is also helpful during postassault counseling sessions as a means of assessing the level of vulnerability and making appropriate changes.

Vital statistics are unavailable concerning rape attacks on the elderly primarily because of embarrassment, fear of reprisal, doubt about whether their complaint will be believed, and the feeling of being overwhelmed by the system.

Elderly victims who reported rape incidents have provided information such as the following that is helpful to the health professional caring for the elderly:
- The elderly rape victim lived alone.
- Physical force was applied to the victim, particularly to the genital region.
- The rape occurred in the home.
- The victim was raped by an individual who was a stranger to him or her, although the assailant had undoubtedly observed the victim on several occasions.
- The rape was associated with a theft.
- Aggression rather than exotic sexual behavior was more troublesome to the elderly.

In most cases the resulting loss of control over their lives has a permanent effect on these elderly victims. The resulting increased levels of fear frequently result in further isolation, with the increased risk of another potential assault.

Community rape crisis centers

Not all of society looks negatively at the rape victim. On the contrary, in recent years many women's groups throughout the country have taken the initiative in educating medical, social, and legal authorities regarding the large extent to which cultural biases and attitudes have affected the treatment of rape victims and have stimulated these institutions to make changes in this area. These organizations have attempted to provide support to rape victims and their families when few professional resources were available.

As part of a nationwide antirape movement during the past 10 years, rapidly growing numbers of community-based rape crisis centers have emerged in the United States.[13,17] These centers are largely staffed by volunteer nonprofessional and professional women, some of whom have been rape victims themselves or have had a close friend who was raped.

These organizations have several goals, one of which is to provide supportive services to victims.[13,17] This goal is accomplished in many centers by the use of 24-hour telephone "hotlines" that provide for immediate contact and support after a rape. Counseling services are limited to immediate support and short-term follow-up, with prolonged dependency on the center discouraged. The return of the rape victim's independent functioning and control is encouraged by the rape crisis center.

Professionals providing immediate telephone support service to the victim may choose to implement some of the following counseling approaches:

- Determine the exact location and correct name.
- Talk to the victim in a distinct, slow, calm voice.
- Try to assess the victim's physical and mental state.
- Reassure the victim that help is on the way, and encourage the victim not to leave.
- Inquire whether there is someone present to assist.
- Provide brief, clear instructions for some simple task that will help the victim gain control.
- Repeat over and over again, "I will help you" and "You will be okay."
- Practice active listening skills.
- Remind the victim that people care.

The initial response provided by this telephone contact is essential to establish the foundation for continued intervention. If the telephone counselor is supportive and comforting, the rape victim will be more willing to cooperate with other medical and law enforcement personnel.

It is imperative that both telephone counselors and personnel who provide immediate care to the victim be informed of the measures that must be taken to preserve the evidence. A list of "do nots" that are essential if prosecution is to be possible is provided on p. 244. If victims who have been informed of the purpose and validity of these requests insist that they must clean up, their wishes should be respected. The ultimate goal is to minimize the results of the rape, not intensify them.

The telephone counselor should continue talking to the rape victim until help arrives. Those who come to help should also be informed of the list of "do nots."

Another goal of rape crisis centers is education of their membership and the public on rape-related issues.[13,17] Information is disseminated on rape prevention, what to do if a rape occurs, and attitudinal changes. Programs for educating rape crisis counselors often involve professionals from both medical and legal areas. Many centers have collaborative relationships with medical centers and law enforcement agencies that allow the rape crisis counselor to remain with the victim throughout the required legal documentation pro-

For the preservation of evidence, do not:

Brush or floss teeth
Drink
Eat
Gargle
Shower
Take medication of any kind
Urinate
Defecate
Douche
Change clothes
Delay getting to the emergency department

From Bay Area Hospital Conference on Sexual Assault: Medical protocol for victims of sexual assault, San Francisco, 1976, Queen's Bench Foundation.

cedure. Rape crisis counselors often give additional support to the rape victim by attending the rape trial with the victim.

It would seem that overall treatment of rape victims would be greatly enhanced if health care workers were to become more aware of rape crisis centers and other community programs for rape victims and to collaborate with these organizations rather than to compete with them.[17]

Health care process
Assessment
Prehospital. Professionals who are the first to respond to the needs of a rape victim establish the foundation for the continued ease of intervention. If the individual is supportive and comforting and expresses a willingness to listen, the victim will be more able to develop an element of trust and will cooperate more fully with other medical and law enforcement personnel.

It is important to note that the initial reactions of the victim may vary greatly. Responses of both total hysteria and complete tranquility have been recorded as reactions to the rape incident. Personnel should refrain from interpreting the patient's response, since each individual will react differently.

There are several key points to be kept in mind during the prehospital assessment period:
- Attempt to comfort the victim.
- Secure the needed facts concerning the incident to determine appropriate support.
- Relate the importance of reporting the incident to law enforcement officials if they have not already been contacted.
- Inform law enforcement officials if need be.
- Activate all efforts to preserve the evidence. Therefore make certain that the victim follows the list of "do nots" listed above. (If the victim is informed of

the value of this request but insists on cleaning up, this request should be respected.)

- Assess physical injuries, and perform essential intervention.
- Assist patient in contacting family or friends if desired.
- Initiate the first stage of crisis intervention.
- Establish communication with the nearest emergency department.
- Accompany the victim to the medical facility if possible.
- Check with admitting personnel.
- Establish rapport with the emergency department nurse who will be coordinating ongoing care.

Professionals may choose to remain with the victim for a short period of time. This is recommended whenever possible as a means of facilitating a positive and comfortable transition, relating appropriate information concerning the victim and her condition, and ensuring that she will not be left alone in the examining room if at all possible.

Emergency department. Personnel working in an emergency department should conduct a total assessment of the victim and assign that person priority over all other admissions except life-threatening emergencies. Physical evidence should be collected to substantiate a possible charge of rape in court.[3]

Professionals must realize that all evidence collected in a criminal case is automatically the responsibility of the local law enforcement agency. Under normal circumstances, when law enforcement officials are present, emergency care personnel are to turn all evidence over to the responding agency. Should law enforcement officials be absent, evidence must be properly preserved until officials arrive. It is also important to explain and to instruct the victim concerning each procedure, its purpose, steps, and anticipated results.

As part of the general assessment process, it is essential that personnel consider some of the following functions:

- Admit the victim in a specially assigned rape examination room, removed from other emergency patients.
- Suggest that the victim may remain dressed in her own clothing until just before the examination begins, if desirable for the victim.
- Explain the entire assessment and intervention process, allowing ample time for questions and answers.
- Inquire whether or not the victim would like someone to accompany her during the examination.
- If the victim has children requiring care, assist in locating someone who will care for them.
- Assess if there is a need for counseling to be given individuals accompanying the victim.
- Assure the continued presence of a nurse throughout the assessment and intervention process if at all possible.
- Inquire about the victim's familiarity with pelvic and rectal examinations.
- Assess the victim's ability to tolerate the examination physically and psychologically.
- Observe, collect, and preserve the victim's clothing as noted on p. 246.

Preservation of rape victim's clothing

1. Note clothing, and record observations on chart.
2. Examine all clothing for soilage, tears, or presence of blood or semen.
3. Arrange for fresh clothing to be brought to the emergency department, should the patient's clothes need to be collected.
4. Collect patient's underwear. Do not crumple—place loosely in an ample-sized paper container.
5. Attempt to air dry wet evidence. Do not fan dry or use heat.
6. Circle wet marks with laundry marker to circumscribe the evidence.
7. Place clean paper over stain, and place in clean container. Do not allow stained areas to contact clean areas.
8. If female patient is menstruating, collect the tampon or sanitary napkin.
9. Place appropriate clothing in separate individual bags, seal properly, and mark with collector's initials and date.
10. Record on chart who collected the clothing and to whom it was given.
11. All clothing used as evidence should be forwarded to the appropriate scientific laboratory by law enforcement personnel.

From Warner, C.G., et al.: San Diego County protocol for the treatment of rape and sexual assault victims, San Diego, Fall 1978, City of San Diego. p. 14.

- Collect urine samples for possible future assessment of alcohol or drug use.
- Assist with any photographs that may be required.

Rape history. It is important that an accurate verbal recollection of the rape incident be obtained for both the legal aspects of the incident and for support of the victim's well-being and integrity.

It must be understood that recollection of the rape is similar to reliving the actual event, and the victim may be reluctant to complete the interview.

Professionals caring for the victim may consider these alternatives:

- Explain the rationale and value of the history in a clear and organized manner.
- Collect the rape history data following the physical examination and process of evidence collection.
- Have one individual collect and tabulate the history for all law enforcement, medical, and social service personnel so the victim does not have to repeat it several times.

The essential portions of the rape and general history that have to be obtained for either male or female victims are identified in Table 13-2.

Physical examination. Recognizing that the physical examination will involve contact with parts of the body that may be bruised, traumatized, and painful, the examining physician should take special care to avoid causing any pain or creating further humiliation.

It is not essential that the examining physician be female, as long as the individual is gentle, sensitive, and caring. In fact it is valuable for the female victim to experience this immediate interaction with a supportive, understanding man. This greatly aids in diminishing the "fear of men" these victims often develop.

Table 13-2. Rape and general history

Health history	Personal history: female	Personal history: male and female	Rape history	Postrape history
Current immunizations (primarily tetanus)	Reactions to estrogens	Present venereal disease	Time, day, and date	Recall of:
Recent illness, injury, or surface or internal trauma (past month)	Current practice of birth control	Past venereal disease	Physical surroundings (e.g., sand, grass, leaves, flowers, water)	Gargling
Prescribed medications	Previous or current sterilization	Present or past rectal bleeding or discharge	Physical forms of violence	Brushing teeth
History of sickle cell anemia	Early signs of pregnancy	Present or past lacerations or sores in the mouth	Weapon(s) used	Vomiting
Any medication, topical, or food allergies	Most recent consensual intercourse or sexual activity		Restraint(s) used	Douching (if female)
	Past pregnancies		Verbal forms of violence	Urinating
	Viable children		Threats of violence	Defecating
	Recent gynecologic injury or surgery		Blindfolds used	Taking an enema
	Last menstrual period		Number of perpetrators	Bathing
	Wishes regarding hormonal pregnancy prevention, abortion, or menstrual extraction		Forced use of alcohol and/or drugs	Changing clothes
	Present or recent vaginal infection		Loss of consciousness	Washing hair
			Fondling	Eating
			Vaginal entry or approach	Drinking
			Oral entry or approach	Taking medication
			Anal entry or approach	
			Forced to perform lewd acts	
			Ejaculation, urination, or defecation on body (be specific)	
			Use of condom or lubricant	
			Did perpetrator claim to be sterile?	

Reprinted from *Emergency Care* by T.C. Travis and C.G. Warner, editors, by permission of Aspen Systems Corporation, © 1982.

Each segment of the physical examination should be initiated with a step-by-step explanation of what the victim can expect. As noted earlier, it is important that the victim not be required to undress or be placed in stirrups until just before the examinations. Considerations of the physical examination for both male and female victims are identified in Table 13-3.

Collection and preservation of evidence. This portion of the assessment process is most critical. A court case can be made as a result of proper, careful, and accurate collection and documentation of facts obtained in medical tests, along with the collection and preservation of evidence. There are several medical tests that need to be processed throughout the assessment and intervention phases. These tests include the following:
- Gonorrheal cultures (Papanicolaou smear, oral and rectal specimens)
- Syphilis test (blood test)
- Evidence of sperm/semen
- Follow-up test for syphilis
- Follow-up test for gonorrhea
- Radiography for physical injuries
- Follow-up test for pregnancy
- Follow-up test for injuries
- Other tests to assess the existence of internal injuries

In addition, medication to prevent pregnancy may be prescribed.

The emergency clinician conducting the physical examination is responsible for the actual collection of evidence. Specific protocols[37] identify the exact procedures required for proper collection and preservation of the evidence, but professionals should be aware of the legal tests conducted on all victims and the extent of their thoroughness. This knowledge will be helpful when teaching the victim what is involved in the evidence collection process.

The areas of collection include the following:
- Foreign materials on the body or in hair
- Saliva
- Oral swab
- Nail scrapings
- Head hair
- Pubic hair combings
- Pubic hair trimmings or pluckings
- Perineal area (for foreign material)
- Vaginal swabs
- Vaginal aspirants
- Vaginal washings
- Anal swabs
- Clothing (handling and preparation—see p. 246)
- Photography

EVIDENCE COLLECTION KITS. Evidence collection kits may vary from facility to facility. The important thing to remember is that the kit be standardized throughout the facilities using them and that a forensic laboratory technician be involved in the design of the kit for each local community.

Table 13-3. Considerations of physical examination

General	Female genitals	Male genitals	Rectal
Note patient's general demeanor and emotional state. Record vital signs. Assess physical appearance. Examine skin (collect and label any foreign material such as seminal stains, botanical material, grass, plastic, paper, or blood). Assess upper trunk, noting breast trauma and sexual maturity. Examine lower trunk for signs of trauma, noting sexual maturity. Note extremities for bruises, fractures and sprains, and scratches. Record head and neck trauma including mouth, ears, and scalp. Collectible evidence may be secured from mouth, hair, or other orifices.	Carefully examine the vulva, noting signs of trauma or foreign matter, semen, dirt, grass, or pus. Gently examine introitus and hymen for signs of trauma. Very carefully assess vaginal area for trauma, signs of foreign objects, or internal lacerations and bleeding.* Gently inspect cervix for evidence of parity, signs of pregnancy, presence of menstruation, evidence of trauma, and signs of infection. Perform general pelvic assessment. Palpate uterus rectally. Utilizing a Wood's light (ultraviolet),† note signs of semen around the perineal area.	Examine penis for signs of trauma, foreign material, or infection. Examine scrotum for signs of trauma or foreign material.	Examine area for signs of trauma. Assess presence of lubricant, blood, semen, pus, or any foreign matter. Gently examine the rectum for possible trauma, placement of foreign objects, and internal lacerations and bleeding.

Reprinted from *Emergency Care* by T.C. Travis and C.G. Warner, editors, by permission of Aspen Systems Corporation, ©, 1982.

*It is critical that water be used to lubricate the speculum rather than a lubricant to prevent altering the results of the acid phosphatase test.
†Obtain photographs as necessary.

Table 13-4. Sample evidence collection kit

Examination item	Materials required
Record of rape and personal history	Appropriate forms
Collection of clothing	Paper bags, butcher paper, and labels
Physical examination	Appropriate forms
Urine for pregnancy test and drug test	Two containers and labels
Fingernail scrapings	Fingernail file, envelope, and label
Saliva sample	Paper disk or swabs, envelope, and label
Blood samples	Tourniquet, gauze pad (nonalcohol), syringe (20 ml), needle (21-gauge), gray-, red-, and lavender-top tubes; labels
Pubic hair combings	Plastic comb, towel, envelope, and label
Pelvic examination	Gloves, lubricant, speculum, cervical scraper (Ayre stick), two slides, and fixative
Vaginal swabs	Four cotton swabs, two plastic containers, saline, two glass slides, labels, and pencil
Vaginal washing	Normal saline (10 ml) and aspiration pipette and bulb
Microscopic examination for sperm motility	Microscope, slides, slide covers, vaginal swabs, and normal saline
Photography (optional)	Camera, film, and flashcube

A complete kit should be available at all times in the facilities conducting rape examinations. A sample of an evidence collection kit is noted in Table 13-4.

Intervention. Professionals caring for rape victims recognize that the assessment and intervention portions of the health care process frequently overlap. The assessment component is reintroduced with each new phase of care, and, in essence, the intervention phase may begin at any stage of the examination. When issues concerning physical injuries, sexually transmitted disease, possible pregnancy, or psychologic difficulties arise, all professionals caring for victims of rape must remember that before the institution of specific intervention measures, the following should be considered:

- Explain the concept of sexually transmitted disease and the importance of its treatment.
- Outline the value of pregnancy testing when appropriate.
- Identify and explain every phase of the examination process before initiating it.
- Assess the presence and severity of contusions, lacerations, abrasions, and internal injuries and the extent, degree, and location of pain.
- Identify acute anxiety reactions.

Sexually transmitted disease. The rape victim must be informed concerning the potential of having contracted a sexually transmitted disease and the existing alternatives of intervention. There is evidence that 1% to 3% of all rape victims will contract sexually transmitted disease as a result of the assault and that up to 3% will prove to have unrecognized, established sexually transmitted disease.[38]

The victim should be reassured that proper intervention and follow-up care are avail-

Table 13-5. Prophylactic intervention for syphilis and gonorrhea

Disease	Intervention	Special considerations
Syphilis	Benzathine penicillin 6, 2.4 million units IM If allergic to penicillin: tetracycline hydrochloride, 50 mg P.O. four times a day for 15 days or erythromycin, 500 mg P.O. four times a day for 15 days	Prophylactic treatment not recommended Advise the victim to have a repeat VDRL in 4 to 6 weeks
Gonorrhea	Ampicillin, 3.5 g P.O. with probenecid, 1 g P.O. Probenecid, 1 g P.O. followed in 30 min with aqueous procaine penicillin 6, 4.8 million U IM If allergic to penicillin: tetracycline hydrochloride, 1.5 g P.O. stat and 500 mg P.O. four times a day for 4 days Spectinomycin hydrochloride, 2 g IM	Advise victim to have a repeat examination in 7 to 10 days

able. If treatment is sought, the victim should be informed that antibiotic therapy may disrupt the normal balance of bacterial organisms in the vagina, resulting in a fungal infection. It must also be related that the assault may have produced genital tissue irritation or that the assailant may have transmitted something other than gonorrhea or syphilis (e.g., trichomoniasis, genital herpes, venereal warts, or lice). Urinary tract infections may result from irritation or injury, and sexual intercourse may be painful. If these concerns arise, the victim should be encouraged to seek professional attention. Specific intervention for sexually transmitted disease is noted in Table 13-5.

Pregnancy. If the victim is currently pregnant (2% to 3% of women who are raped will prove to already be pregnant at the time of the attack[38]), this needs to be clarified through a pregnancy test. Pregnancy can be determined through a urine sample (accurate only after 4 weeks of pregnancy) or through a newer serum test (β-HCG) that detects pregnancy after only 1 week of pregnancy.[4]

There are four alternatives that can be considered if the victim becomes pregnant:

1. β-HCG administered on the day of the physical assessment. It will take 2 weeks for the results to return, which will coincide with the time the victim is due for her return checkup. If, on return, the test is positive, it signifies the woman was already pregnant at the time of the rape. If the test returns negative, the β-HCG test should be repeated. After the second test, should the results return positive, the victim is probably pregnant as a result of the rape, and a suction curettage may be offered as an alternative.
2. Intravenous conjugated estrogen (Premarin), 25 mg, repeated once in 12 hours. Nausea and vomiting have been associated with this regimen, although considerably more compliance has been noted than with diethylstilbestrol (DES).
3. The morning-after pill (DES). This alternative has very little compliance, since 60% of the patients discontinue taking the medication following 2 to 3 days of nausea and vomiting.[16]
4. Abortions or a menstrual extraction.

Follow-up. Hayman and Lanza[16] conducted a unique follow-up program for rape victims in which a public health nurse visited women in their homes to provide early support and to evaluate the whole patient. Fifteen hundred referrals were made by the public health nurse for a group of 2089 patients. The nurse's interviews discovered many patients who needed referral for emotional disturbances after the assault. In most instances emotional support was provided by the public health nurse and secondarily by mental health professionals, especially in the first 90 days after the assault.

Another valuable follow-up service was provided by Burgess and Holmstrom,[8] who made themselves available for counseling on a weekly basis for a period of time long enough to permit the crisis to stabilize. A follow-up telephone call was made within 24 to 48 hours after the same professionals had seen the victim in the emergency department. The counselors determined whether the client needed advice, the knowledge that someone was concerned, a chance to ventilate, help in clarifying her thoughts, or no counseling. The most frequent requests were for confirmation of concern and ventilation.[6] If necessary, the counselors visited women at home and also accompanied them to court. Thus crisis intervention was provided by one or two consistent persons as long as necessary.

Kaufman et al.[21] noted that follow-up of victims increased markedly from 8% before a family practice health team began offering crisis counseling in the emergency department and follow-up care in the family practice clinic to 86% afterward. Family members of more than half the victims seen on follow-up received treatment for health-related problems. A wide range of health care needs of both victims and families was identified not in the emergency department but later on follow-up visits to the family practice clinic.

The traumatic impact of the rape incident often precludes the victim from remembering any recommendations concerning the need for follow-up care. However, a pamphlet covering common medical and psychologic concerns, placed in the victim's pocket, purse, or wallet, will be read once the patient is home. The following information represents a sample guide for follow-up care proven to be of value and support to many victims.

Guide to follow-up care

Medical care

Following the initial examination in the emergency department for collection of evidence and emergency medical treatment of sexual assault, the patient may still need basic medical care for general bodily injury, prevention of pregnancy, prevention of sexually transmitted disease, and psychologic reactions.

This section is designed to relate medical problems encountered by other victims of sexual assault, to describe methods of care, and to provide resources for ongoing care at various levels of cost, from low-cost clinics to private care.

Modified from Subcommittee on Sexual Assault and Intrafamily Violence, Advisory Board on Women: Taking care of yourself: a self-help guide, San Diego, 1979-1980, City of San Diego.

General bodily injury

Injuries sustained as a result of the sexual assault may require radiographs, laboratory work, dressing changes, minor surgical care, and/or medications. The patient should be informed about how to care for these injuries at home and when to return to the hospital or other community resource for follow-up care. The patient should be given an appointment card and written instructions before he or she leaves the hospital.

Prevention of pregnancy

There may be a chance that a female patient may have become pregnant as a result of the sexual assault. Emergency care personnel should discuss the probability of pregnancy with the patient. Two alternatives are available to avoid pregnancy if it is determined that the patient is at risk: (1) the morning-after pill (DES) and (2) abortion or menstrual extraction, which is early abortion.

DES involves a large dose of synthetic estrogen, which prevents implantation of the fertilized egg in the wall of the uterus. A full course of 25 mg taken two times a day for 5 days must be taken beginning within 24 hours of the sexual assault if it is to be effective. However, DES is known to be linked with a rare form of vaginal cancer in *daughters* of women who took DES from 1945 to 1970 as an antimiscarriage drug during their pregnancy with those daughters. (Should the patient become aware that she is a DES daughter, she should seek medical advice for thorough testing.) The choice to take DES is the patient's, and she should be made aware of the following facts before signing the consent form.

Possible side effects of DES include danger to the fetus if the patient is already pregnant at the time of the assault but was unaware of it and danger to the fetus if the patient remains pregnant as a result of the rape. (Counseling regarding abortion is recommended in the above two cases.) Nausea and vomiting, possible vaginal spotting, breast tenderness, insomnia, and/or rash during treatment may also be noted.

A pregnancy test done at the time of the sexual assault will show if the patient is already pregnant. If the patient should miss her menstrual period following the sexual assault, a second pregnancy test is advised approximately 6 weeks after the first day of her last period. Legal abortions and menstrual extractions are available in physicians' offices, clinics, and hospitals. Health facilities where pregnancy tests are done provide referrals for abortions.

Prevention of sexually transmitted disease

It is recommended that a gonorrhea culture be taken immediately and 7 to 10 days after the sexual assault and/or treatment. If oral or rectal penetration has occurred, swabs should be taken from those areas, as well as the vaginal swab. Gonorrhea is more difficult to detect in the female

Continued.

Guide to follow-up care—cont'd

than the male regardless of the testing used, and active cases can go unrecognized and untreated. It is therefore strongly recommended that preventive antibiotic therapy be undertaken. A blood test for syphilis (VDRL) should be taken immediately and repeated 4 to 6 weeks after the sexual assault.

Preventive antibiotic treatment may be given at the time of the sexual assault to prevent possible infection from the attacker. If the cost is prohibitive, there are many clinics where treatment and testing for sexually transmitted disease are available at low cost. If the patient chooses to be treated, he or she may not know for sure whether sexually transmitted disease has been contracted, but it is imperative that the patient have follow-up checks to ensure that the treatment has been effective.

If the patient chooses to be treated for sexually transmitted disease at the time of the sexual assault (and is female), such antibiotic therapy may disrupt the normal balance of bacterial organisms in the vagina. A fungal infection may develop but is readily treatable. In addition, the assault itself may also have an irritating effect on the genital tissues, or the attacker may have transmitted another kind of infection to the patient. These factors may lead to a female patient developing other sexually transmitted vaginal infections, such as trichomoniasis, genital herpes, venereal warts, or crab lice.

Urinary tract infections can result from irritation or injury, and intercourse may become painful. If the patient experiences an unusual or heavy discharge from the vagina, sores, burning on urination, vaginal itching, or painful intercourse, she should seek medical attention promptly. Again, low-cost care at clinics is available if the cost of private care is prohibitive.

Psychologic care

In most crisis situations people can become upset and may be faced with unexpected changes in their lives. Since sexual assault may present a serious threat to the patient's safety and well-being, it is understandable that he or she may experience mental or emotional stress as an aftereffect of such an assault. In addition, the patient's family and friends may also be affected by what has happened. The patient needs to be around people who can be supportive and sympathetic. Some women's antirape groups offer woman-to-woman support throughout the procedures following a sexual assault. They are available to assist the patient. The patient may also wish to seek short- or long-term counseling. Members of the patient's immediate family may also benefit from counseling assistance. Sexual problems arising as a result of sexual assault are also treatable. The patient should be aware that many victims experience nightmares, phobias, fear of going out alone, fear of the dark, and a general suspicion of men. All these symptoms can be alleviated with proper care and support from friends, family members, and/or counselors.

Evaluation

A model that permits both intervention and evaluation simultaneously is presented by Sutherland and Scherl,[33] who saw their clients in a community mental health center. They provided anticipatory guidance for the woman and intervened throughout each of the three phases of the victim's reaction to rape. Seeing these women over a period of time permitted the investigators to evaluate both the woman's emotional response and the effectiveness of management. In addition, the professional may have the opportunity to evaluate the spouse's and family's reactions to sexual assault, helping them to accept and support the victim.

Despite the careful assessment, planning, designing, and implementation of a medical rape management program, professionals may have developed a program that does not

---

Evaluation form for hospital examination, laboratory testing, and counseling

Our concern is that the best possible care be provided to you and other patients of sexual assault. To evaluate and improve this program, your suggestions are needed. Please take a few moments to answer these questions, and return the form at your convenience. Thank you for your cooperation.

1. Which hospital were you taken to?
   (List available hospitals)

2. Date of hospital examination _____
   Time of hospital examination _____
   Date this application was filled out _____

3. Were you left alone at the hospital? _____
   If so, for how long? _____
   Did this bother you? _____
   Was an explanation provided? _____

4. Please check any of the following areas that were explained to you before the procedure.

	Yes	No
• Reason for physical examination	_____	_____
• Collection of evidence process	_____	_____
• Steps in physical examination	_____	_____
• Reasons for asking personal questions	_____	_____
• Reasons for laboratory test(s)	_____	_____
• Possible treatment for disease or pregnancy	_____	_____
• Other:		
_____	_____	_____
_____	_____	_____

Continued.

Evaluation form for hospital examination, laboratory testing, and counseling—cont'd

5. Were the following counseling services satisfactory?

	Yes	No	Not given
• Advice on birth control measures	_____	_____	_____
• Advice on the prevention of sexually transmitted disease	_____	_____	_____
• Counseling on pregnancy prevention measures	_____	_____	_____
• Other:			
_____	_____	_____	_____
_____	_____	_____	_____

6. What type of social service counseling did you receive?
   _____ Were you counseled by the hospital social worker?
   _____ Were you referred to outside community resources?
   _____ Were family and friends involved in the counseling?
   Was the counseling satisfactory?   Yes _____   No _____

Comments

7. What type of follow-up recommendations were made?
   _____ Medical follow-up care was recommended
   _____ Signs and symptoms to watch for in case of complications were described
   _____ Psychologic follow-up care was recommended

8. Did you receive a follow-up call from the hospital? _____
   If yes, what did they recommend? _____
   _____
   _____

9. Were you pleased with your care and treatment? _____
   If not, what did you dislike? _____
   _____
   _____

10. What improvements would you suggest for the care of future patients of sexual assault?
    _____
    _____

11. How did you feel about your interview with the police officer? _____
    _____
    _____

    The plain clothes officer? _____
    _____
    _____

12. Other comments: _____
    _____
    _____

If you feel comfortable signing your name, it would be most helpful, but please recognize that this is not required.

_____

adequately meet the needs of these victims. Consequently, each health care social service and/or community crisis center should design and integrate an evaluation and feedback network to be used as a strengthening and reinforcement tool to coincide with the original goals and objectives of the program.

Victim-elicited response is an excellent method of obtaining specific recommendations for program modification. This type of evaluation should not be pursued before a 6-week follow-up visit. If social service personnel are used in a health care facility to maintain contact with these victims, the evaluation process can be easily implemented with their assistance.

An example of a victim evaluation form, used for feedback during the prehospital, emergency department, and social service phases of intervention, is noted on pp. 255-256.

Additional methods of evaluation should be integrated based on specific program design. Quality assurance and risk management personnel in each facility will be able to provide specific and appropriate direction in the design and implementation of a desired standard of excellence for the care of all rape victims.

Summary

This chapter has considered the biologic, psychologic, and social consequences of rape and a number of ways in which the health team can help a woman cope with the aftermath of sexual assault. Key considerations for health practice include the following:

1. Trauma to the genitals can be sufficiently severe to interfere with the woman's future sexual functioning if it is not properly diagnosed and treated.
2. Women who have sustained genital trauma have become vaginismic and may experience dyspareunia.
3. Rape victims may develop sexually transmitted disease or become pregnant after the assault.
4. Women who have been raped usually have intense guilt feelings. Sometimes these feelings are associated with a previous acquaintance with the attacker.
5. Victims of rape may experience three distinct phases in their emotional response: acute reaction, outward adjustment, and integration and resolution.
6. Some women become verbal and talkative immediately after the sexual assault, whereas others are quiet and guarded. Their emotional styles are intensified by stress.
7. Social response to the rape victim is influenced by unfounded beliefs and a desire to explain why a respectable person was victimized.
8. The health care process for the rape victim involves a thorough history and physical examination, both of which may seem invasive to the woman.

9. Crisis intervention with follow-up care may meet the woman's needs for emotional support until she is able to integrate her experience and resolve her feelings toward the rape.

Questions for review

1. What biologic effects of rape are most likely to interfere with the victim's future sexual functioning? How?
2. What preventive measures can be instituted for the rape victim to protect her from its biologic aftereffects?
3. Discuss the emotional impact of rape for the victim. In what respect is her response likely to differ if she is raped by a stranger? If she knows the rapist? If she has had previous sexual encounters with the rapist?
4. Discuss the three phases of response to rape as described by Sutherland and Scherl. In what way does the woman's future sexual functioning depend on resolution of the incident?
5. How is society likely to respond to the rape victim?
6. During assessment of the rape victim a pelvic examination is usually performed. Discuss the significance of the pelvic examination in light of the woman's recent trauma. How can health care providers decrease the trauma associated with the pelvic examination?
7. What aspects of rape counseling can be instituted by emergency department staff? By community health practitioners? By volunteer counseling services?
8. Which of the following rape victims is most likely to be at risk of negative aftereffects? Name the outcomes they are likely to experience.

   • Melissa Anderson, a 19-year-old coed, was raped in a parking lot at 2 AM on her way home from the library. She had dated the young man who raped her.
   • Mrs. Ruth Baldwin, a 45-year-old married woman, was walking home from work at 4 PM through a park in her neighborhood when she was raped.
   • Fran Johns, a 37-year-old divorcee and cocktail waitress, was raped in her apartment by a teenaged burglar.

References

1. Abarbanel, G., and Klein, S.: Statistical information about the crime of rape, Santa Monica, Calif., 1981, Rape Treatment Center, Santa Monica Hospital Medical Center.
2. Bard, M., and Ellison, K.: Crisis intervention and investigation of forcible rape, Police Chief 16(2):68-73, 1974.
3. Bay Area Hospital Conference on Sexual Assault: Medical protocol for victims of sexual assault, San Francisco, 1976, Queen's Bench Foundation.
4. Braen, G.R.: Physical assessment and emergency medical management of adult victims of sexual assault. In Warner, C.G., editor: Rape and sexual assault: management and intervention, Rockville, Md., 1980, Aspen Systems Corp.
5. Braen, G.R.: Management of the adult female rape victim. In Warner, C.G., and Braen, G.R., editors: Management of the physically and emotionally abused, Long Beach, Calif., 1983, Capistrano Press, Ltd.
6. Breen, L.L., Greenwald, E., and Gregor, C.A.: The molested young female: evaluation and therapy of alleged rapes, Pediatric Clinics of North America 19:717-725, 1972.

7. Brodsky, C.M.: Rape at work. In Walker, M.J. and Brodsky, S.J., editors: Sexual assault, Lexington, Mass., 1976, Lexington Books.

8. Burgess, A.W., and Holmstrom, L.L.: Rape: victims of crisis, Bowie, Md., 1974, Robert J. Brody Co.

9. Burgess, A.W., and Holmstrom, L.L.: Coping behavior of the rape victim, American Journal of Psychiatry **133:**413-417, 1976.

10. Burgess, A.W., and Holmstrom, L.L.: Rape: crisis and recovery, Bowie, Md., 1979, Robert J. Brody Co.

11. Burgess, A.W., and Holstrom, L.L.: Sexual disruption and recovery, American Journal of Orthopsychiatry **49:**648-657, 1979.

12. Evrard, J.R.: Rape: the medical, social and legal implications, American Journal of Obstetrics and Gynecology **111:**197, 1972.

13. Gager, N., and Schurr, C.: Sexual assault: confronting rape in America, New York, 1976, Grosset & Dunlap, Inc.

14. Halleck, S.L.: Emotional effects of victimization. In Slovenko, R., editor: Sexual behavior and the law, Springfield, Ill., 1965, Charles C Thomas, Publisher.

15. Halleck, S.L.: Treatment of the sex offender: the therapeutic encounter, International Psychiatry Clinic **8**(4):1-20, 1972.

16. Hayman, C.R., and Lanza, C.: Sexual assault on women and girls, American Journal of Obstetrics and Gynecology **109:**480-486, 1971.

17. Hilberman, E.: The rape victim, Washington, D.C., 1976, American Psychiatric Association.

18. Hilberman, E.: Rape: the ultimate violation of the self, American Journal of Psychiatry **133:**436-437, 1976.

19. Jaffe, A.C., Dynneson, L., and Bensel, R.W.: Sexual abuse of children, American Journal of Diseases and the Child **129:**689-692, 1975.

20. Jones, C., and Aronson, E.: Attribution of fault to a rape victim as a function of respectability of the victim, Journal of Personality and Social Psychology **26:**415-419, 1973.

21. Kaufman, A., et al.: Follow up of rape victims in a family practice setting, Southern Medical Journal **69:**1569-1571, 1976.

22. Massey, J.B., Garcia, C.R., and Emich, J.P., Jr.: Management of sexually assaulted females, Obstetrics and Gynecology **38:**29-36, 1971.

23. Masters, W., and Johnson, V.: Human sexual inadequacy, Boston, 1970, Little, Brown & Co.

24. Metzger, D.: It is always the woman who is raped, American Journal of Psychiatry **133:**405-408, 1976.

25. Notman, M.T., and Nadelson, C.C.: The rape victim: psychodynamic considerations, American Journal of Psychiatry **133:**408 + , 1976.

26. Report of the District of Columbia Task Force on Rape: Subcommittee of District of Columbia City Council, July 1973.

27. Robinson, H.A., Jr., Sherrod, D.B., and Malcorney, C.N.: Review of child molestation and alleged rape codes, American Journal of Obstetrics and Gynecology **110:**405-406, 1971.

28. Selkin, J.: Rape: when to fight back, Psychology Today **8:**70-76, May 1975.

29. Shaw, B.L.: When the problem is rape, RN **35:**27-29, 1972.

30. Silverman, D.: First do no more harm: female rape victims and the male counselor, American Journal of Orthopsychiatry **47:**691-696, 1977.

31. Soules, M.R., et al.: The spectrum of alleged rape, Journal of Reproductive Medicine **20**:33-39, 1978.
32. Subcommittee on Sexual Assault and Intrafamily Violence, Advisory Board on Women: Taking care of yourself: a self-help guide, San Diego, 1979-1980, City of San Diego.
33. Sutherland, S., and Scherl, D.: Patterns of response among victims of rape, American Journal of Orthopsychiatry **40**:503-510, 1970.
34. Symonds, M.: Victims of violence: psychological effects and aftereffects, American Journal of Psychoanalysis **35**:19-26, 1975.
35. Symonds, M.: The rape victim: psychological patterns of response, American Journal of Psychoanalysis **36**:27-34, 1976.
36. Voight, J.: Sexual offenses in Copenhagen: a medical study, Forensic Science **1**:67-76, 1972.
37. Warner, C.G.: Emergency management of rape and sexual assault. In Kravis, T.C., and Warner, C.G., editors: Aspen's comprehensive review of emergency care, Rockville, Md., 1982, Aspen Systems Corp.
38. Warner, C.G., et al.: San Diego County protocol for the treatment of rape and sexual assault victims, San Diego, Fall 1978, City of San Diego.
39. Weiss, K., and Borges, S.: Victimology and rape: the code of the legitimate victim, Issues in Criminology **8**:71-115, 1973.
40. Woodling, B.A., Evans, J.R., and Brodbury, M.D.: Sexual assault: rape and molestation, Clinical Obstetrics and Gynecology **20**:509-530, 1977.

References for clients

Arnold, P.: Lady beware, New York, 1976, Doubleday & Co., Inc.

Boston Women's Health Book Collective: Our bodies, ourselves, New York, 1973, Simon & Schuster, Inc.

Brodyaga, L., et al.: A prescriptive package: rape and its victims: a report for citizens, health facilities and criminal justice agencies, Pub. no. 1976-0-211-063/560, Washington, D.C., 1975, U.S. Department of Justice, Law Enforcement Assistance Administration, National Institute of Law Enforcement and Criminal Justice.

Brownmiller, S.: Against our will: men, women and rape, New York, 1975, Simon & Schuster, Inc.

Connell, N., and Wilson, C., editors: Rape: the first sourcebook for women, New York, 1974, The New American Library, Inc.

Csida, J.B., and Csida, J.: Rape: how to avoid it and what to do about it if you can't, Chatworth, Calif., 1974, Books for Better Living.

Gager, N., and Schurr, C.: Sexual assault: confronting rape in America, New York, 1976, Grosset & Dunlap, Inc.

Grimstead, K., and Rennie, S., editors: The new women's survival catalog, New York, 1973, Coward, McCann & Geoghegan, Inc.

Hopog, C.V.: Rape, New Canaan, Conn., 1974, Tobey Publishing Co.

Medea, A., and Thompson, K.: Against rape, New York, 1976, Farrar, Straus & Giroux, Inc.

Medical and legal aspects of rape: Women Organize Against Rape, P.O. Box 17374, Philadelphia, PA 19105.

National Center for the Prevention and Control of Rape: Regional directory: rape prevention and treatment resources, Washington, D.C., 1979, U.S.

Department of Health, Education and Welfare, National Institute of Mental Health.

Piercy, M.: Living in the open, New York, 1975, Alfred A. Knopf, Inc.

Rape prevention tactic: Rape Crisis Center, P.O. Box 21005, Kalorama Street Station, Washington, D.C. 20009.

Russell, D.E.H.: The politics of rape: the victim's perspective, New York, 1974, Stein & Day.

Selkin, J.: Rape: when to fight back, Psychology Today 8:70-76, Aug. 1975.

Stop rape: Women Against Rape, 2445 W. Mile, Detroit, MI 48203.

Walker, M.J., and Brodsky, S.L., editors: Sexual assault, Lexington, Mass., 1976, Lexington Books.

Weiss, K.: What the rape victim should know about the "morning after" pill, 1975, Advocates for Medical Information, 2120 Biggonnett, Houston, TX 77005.

14
Sexually transmitted diseases

THOMAS DeMARIA

Knowledge and awareness of sexually transmitted disease (STD) has grown substantially in the past 5 to 10 years. Before this time most health care practitioners used the term STD (or venereal disease) to refer to gonorrhea, syphilis, chancroid, granuloma inguinale, and lymphogranuloma venereum. Presently, however, the Centers for Disease Control recognize fourteen STDs. In addition to the five mentioned above, the following are officially recognized as STDs: nongonococcal urethritis, herpes simplex type 2 (genital herpes), condylomata acuminata (genital warts), trichomoniasis, candidiasis, scabies, pediculosis pubis (lice), *Gardnerella vaginalis* vaginitis, and hepatitis B.[15] Also considered significant problems are cervicitis and pelvic inflammatory disease caused by the *Chlamydia* organism and three intestinal diseases, giardiasis, amebiasis, and shigellosis.

STDs can be defined as "diseases that are *usually* or can be transmitted from one person to another during heterosexual or homosexual intercourse or intimate contact with the sex organs, mouth or rectum."[5] Many infectious diseases other than those mentioned above can be transmitted during sexual contact but are not primarily STDs and will not be considered in this discussion.

For the practitioner working with clients with STDs it is necessary to know more than the pathophysiology and antimicrobial treatment of specific microorganisms. Because of the psychologic, emotional, and sociocultural aspects of sexuality, a holistic approach to the study and treatment of STDs will be presented in this chapter.

The purposes of this chapter follow:
1. To review the historic development and recognition of STDs and current epidemiologic statistics
2. To describe a holistic approach to the study and treatment of STDs
3. To discuss specific clinical approaches for practitioners in the care of the client with an STD:
   a. A systems approach to assessment
   b. A syndrome approach to problem identification
   c. An organism-host-environment approach to diagnosis, treatment, and education
4. To identify and examine the major STDs and associated microorganisms

Epidemiologic history and statistical overview

In the study of the historic development and recognition of STDs syphilis has been the primary focus. One historic account suggests that syphilis was introduced to Europe in the late fifteenth century via Christopher Columbus' crew, who supposedly obtained the disease during explorations of North America.[1] Other theories indicate that syphilis was present much earlier than that time in Europe but was not recognized as such, the symptoms of late syphilis probably having been attributed to leprosy.[25] Some biblical passages describe what might be considered symptoms of syphilis. Whatever the early history, syphilis was first recognized in Europe as an STD in the late 1400s, and active treatment was being developed during that time. In addition, until 1838 gonorrhea and syphilis were considered the same disease, with gonorrhea presumably causing the "internal" symptoms (urethral discharge) and syphilis the "external" symptoms (genital lesions) of the disease.[1]

Until the latter part of the nineteenth century the treatment for syphilis consisted mainly of various mercury compounds. Various other preparations, such as potassium iodide and arsenic, were used from then until the 1920s, when bismuth was introduced as a fairly effective, much safer treatment.[1] In the middle to late 1940s penicillin became the treatment of choice for syphilis and gonorrhea.[25]

Very few records have been kept on the incidence of various STDs. Not until 1941 did the U.S. Public Health Service begin a compilation of STD statistics based on the required reporting (in most states) of cases of syphilis, gonorrhea, chancroid, granuloma inguinale, and lymphogranuloma venereum. It should be noted that even now a large percentage of cases of these STDs are not reported by private practitioners. Therefore most data on these and other STDs are collected through other medical care surveys.

From 1941 to 1977 there was a gradual decrease in reported cases of all stages of syphilis in the United States: from 485,560 to 64,621. The 3-year period from 1977 to 1979 showed a leveling off of this trend, with 67,049 cases reported in 1979.[22] The true incidence of syphilis is probably close to 100,000 new cases per year.[21]

Since 1967, the male/female ratio of reported syphilis cases has been steadily increasing, and in 1979, 77.1% of all reported cases were found in males.[22] This significantly higher incidence in males is probably reflective of a higher incidence of homosexual transmission of syphilis, especially in urban areas. Wiesner and Holmes[24] report that in Seattle in 1974, "sixty-eight percent of all reported primary and secondary syphilis, including 81% of all reported male syphilis, involved homosexual or bisexual men." It is uncertain whether this reflects a growing percentage of gay males contracting syphilis, a decreased percentage of heterosexuals contracting syphilis, an increased willingness of clients to reveal homosexual activity to clinicians, or some combination of all three.

Although the number of reported cases and case rates (number of cases per 100,000 population) of syphilis decreased from 1941 to 1977 and stabilized from 1977 to 1979, the number of reported cases and case rates of gonorrhea has increased since 1957. In 1957 the incidence of reported gonorrhea was at the lowest level since 1942: 214,496 cases. The number of reported cases climbed to over 1 million in 1976 (470/100,000 population) and has held fairly steadily at that point through 1979. The true incidence of gonorrhea is probably over 2 million cases per year.[22]

In 1956 females accounted for only about 30% of the reported gonorrhea cases, probably because of their higher level of asymptomatic gonorrhea. This proportion has grown to about 40% of the total in 1979 as a result of intensive screening and contact-tracing activities that were implemented in 1973.[22]

The three other reportable STDs (chancroid, lymphogranuloma venereum, and granuloma inguinale) have a much lower incidence in the United States than do gonorrhea and syphilis. In 1979, 840 cases of chancroid, 250 cases of lymphogranuloma venereum, and 76 cases of granuloma inguinale were reported.[22] These diseases are generally more common in tropical and semitropical areas of the world.

Genital herpes is a rapidly spreading STD, with approximately 300,000 to 500,000 new cases occurring each year.[21] In 1979 there were 260,890 consultations with private physicians for genital herpes, up from 29,560 in 1966—nearly a ninefold increase.[23] Genital herpes is of great concern because there is no known cure, it spontaneously recurs in individuals for many years, it can cause infant death if lesions are present during delivery, and it is associated with cervical cancer. It is clearly an epidemic that is estimated to affect 15% to 20% of all Americans.[21]

Nongonococcal urethritis (NGU) and nongonococcal cervicitis and their associated complications are frequently a result of infection caused by *Chlamydia trachomatis*. There are approximately 2 million new cases of NGU each year, 40% to 50% of which are caused by the *Chlamydia* organism, and approximately 1.2 million new cases of pelvic inflammatory disease (a possible complication of cervicitis) each year, at least 20% of which are caused by *C. trachomatis*.[21] In addition to *Chlamydia* species, causes of NGU include *Ureaplasma urealyticum* (about 40%), *Trichomonas vaginalis, Candida albicans,* and herpes simplex type 2. Nongonococcal cervicitis can be caused by *Chlamydia* species or herpes simplex. In total, 3 million chlamydial infections of various types affect Americans each year.[21]

T. vaginalis, C. albicans, and *Gardnerella vaginalis* are organisms that can cause vaginitis in females and urethral infections in males, although the infections usually produce few signs or symptoms in males. Because they produce symptoms primarily in females, the diseases often have not been acknowledged as sexually transmitted in the past, and sexual partners have not been routinely treated until recently. There are an estimated 3 million cases of trichomoniasis each year in the United States,[21] and physicians in private practice report that from 3% to 15% of female clients have trichomoniasis.[16] *C. albicans* can be transmitted sexually, but the organism often produces no symptoms and can be found in the vaginas of 25% to 50% of healthy females.[9] Candidal vaginitis (commonly called yeast infection) is thought to be several times more common than trichomoniasis[21] and is commonly found in females who have or have had other STDs.[16] Information regarding the incidence of infection with *G. vaginalis* is varied. Several different studies have indicated incidence rates of 23% to 96% of females with symptoms of vaginitis, mostly toward the lower end of that range.[16] Like candidiasis, *Gardnerella* vaginitis is often asymptomatic and is most frequently found in populations with a high incidence of other STDs.

Three other common and uncomfortable STDs are genital warts, scabies, and pediculosis pubis (crab lice). Approximately 500,000 new cases of genital warts occur each year.[21] Both scabies and crab lice are considered epidemic in the United States and are transmitted easily by nonsexual and sexual contact. Approximately 2% to 4% of new client visits to dermatologists result in a diagnosis of scabies.[21]

Both hepatitis A virus (HAV) and hepatitis B virus (HBV) produce STDs. The reported incidence of hepatitis in the United States is approximately 55,000 cases per year; about 27% are HBV, 55% are HAV, and the rest are unspecified. The true incidence of hepatitis is probably ten times the reported number of cases. Both types of hepatitis are more prevalent among the urban gay male communities than among the heterosexual population.[21]

Finally, in the past decade several enteric diseases have been recognized as sexually transmissible: amebiasis, giardiasis, and shigellosis. Although specific incidence rates are unknown, these diseases occur primarily in the gay male population in metropolitan areas.[21]

In summary it can be seen that recognition of STDs has grown tremendously in the past decade. Incidence rates are stabilizing for some STDs but growing rapidly for others because of increasing identification and increases in the actual occurrence of the diseases. As a result, the study and treatment of STDs has become a subspecialty for many health care practitioners.

A holistic approach to the study and treatment of STDs

Most health care practitioners focus on the microorganism in the study and treatment of communicable diseases. In fact a number of effective treatments involve the use of drugs designed to combat the disease at the level of the microorganism. To understand the full nature of disease, however, particularly STD, and to provide more complete treatment to the person as a whole, the practitioner needs to recognize the multidimensionality of the problem. Barrett-Connor addresses this concern[2]:

> In infectious disease, the etiologic microorganism is an essential cause, but by no means the only determinant of the outcome. Instead, the frequency with which exposure to an infectious agent results in disease is a function of the agent, the host, and the environment.

One of the purposes of this chapter, therefore, is to study the organism, host, and environment as they relate to STDs, especially in providing care and treatment to the client with an STD.

Organism. Almost all of the microorganisms associated with STDs have one common factor in relation to transmission, survival, and growth: the need for direct contact of the live organism with moist mucous membrane tissue. Most of these organisms die as soon as they become dried, with the exception of scabies and lice, which can live for comparatively longer periods in clothes and bed linen. (In fact scabies and lice infect the host on the drier, outer bodily surfaces and not the mucous membranes). The various STD organisms have different propensities for living in specific tissue areas, of which the following are of greatest concern: reproductive organ tissue (vagina, cervix, fallopian tubes), urethra, epididymis, mouth and pharynx, and rectum and lower bowel. Because of the great amount of information on microorganisms and therapy oriented toward their control or elimination, they are discussed in detail in later sections.

Host. The host for these organisms is, of course, the individual person. Using a holistic approach, one would want to consider the host as an individual whose physical, mental, and emotional condition and unique forms of sexual expression affect the manifestation of and response to STD.

The effect of physical structure on the manifestation of STDs is most clearly demonstrated when one considers asymptomatic disease. As previously discussed, females have a higher rate of asymptomatic disease caused by anatomic structures, that is, the fact that the vaginal canal, cervix, and other reproductive organs are internal. Infections in these areas produce less noticeable symptoms than do reproductive infections in males. Rectal infections in females and gay or bisexual males are also frequently asymptomatic.

There are three major concepts relative to the treatment of the physical being: good hygiene and primary prevention, frequent self-examination, and routine STD examination for the sexually active person. Primary prevention involves the avoidance of initial infection with the organism. The most obvious form of primary prevention is abstention from sexual contact—appropriate for some persons but often unrealistic and/or undesirable for most others. Use of a condom during sexual intercourse may also help prevent transmission of disease. Another form of primary prevention involves casual inspection of the sexual partner during the initial period of lovemaking. People who know something of the signs and symptoms of the major STDs can quite easily incorporate this small routine in an enjoyable and unobtrusive manner. Good physical hygiene before and/or after sexual contact may help prevent transmission of some STDs. Some STD organisms are easily killed by soap and water, although it should be noted that effectiveness of good hygiene is not thoroughly documented. Some people feel that urination immediately after sexual contact may help clear the urethra of some STD organisms. Routine douching for females is not recommended, since this may adversely alter the normal vaginal environment.

Frequent self-examination is recommended for sexually active people with more than one partner. These individuals can be taught to inspect their skin, mouth, genitals, and perianal areas for lesions and discharges, using a mirror as necessary. Frequent self-examination helps to establish knowledge and comfort with one's body.

For sexually active people who have more than one partner, or whose partner has other partners, the routine STD examination is of major importance. The routine STD examination is the best way to detect asymptomatic disease and should be done every 3 months, or even more frequently for very sexually active persons. The routine examination will be discussed more fully in a later section.

The individual's mental or intellectual awareness of sexuality and STDs can have an effect on the outcome of illness. There is a great amount of misinformation regarding sexuality and STDs, which can prevent early and adequate treatment and follow-up and may lead to complications. Client education during the examination process is often helpful in expanding that individual's awareness and should become routine with the clinician. It should also be recognized that high levels of anxiety during the examination may prevent the client from incorporating the educational information, and brochures should be given to the individual to take home. Teaching can involve the disease process, treatment, self-care, hygiene, and other areas regarding sexuality that are important to that individual.

The effect of a person's emotional condition on the expression of disease is not yet well defined. Most clinicians recognize that emotions can affect general physical health to some degree (as in some of the "life-style" disorders such as hypertension and cardiovascular disease), but it is less apparent in other problems, such as STDs. The one example that most practitioners recognize is the effect of emotional stress on genital herpes. It is felt that periods of high emotional stress in individuals who have had initial herpes infections may lead to recurrences of the lesions.[20] The teaching of stress reduction techniques then becomes part of the clinician's treatment.

Perhaps more clearly understood is the effect of emotions when the individual is confronted with the need to seek care for STDs. Fears and misconceptions about STDs and the resulting fears and anxieties about individual sexuality can prevent timely care seeking, adequate follow-up, and resolution of the problem. To treat the whole person, as well as to ensure adequate resolution of the particular STD, the clinician needs to be sensitive to these emotional issues. Good listening and communication skills become the treatment tools of the practitioner at this point. Allowing persons to ventilate fears and anxieties, dispelling misconceptions, and showing acceptance of a person's unique form of sexual expression will contribute to treatment of the whole person. Assisting individuals to achieve comfort with and enjoyment of their sexuality will also enable them to seek help for STD when necessary. In addition, those people who become more comfortable with their sexuality will be more able to accept responsibility for the health and well-being of their sexual partners.

Persons seeking help for STDs may also have other problems relating to sexuality. One study[6] showed that about 21% of all males and 29% of all females attending an STD clinic had sexual dysfunction problems. These problems included erectile impotence, premature ejaculation, coital orgasmic dysfunction, vaginismus, dyspareunia, and loss of libido. The clinician can assist the client to express these concerns and can provide referral to sexual counselors as necessary.

Different forms of sexual expression affect the ways that STDs are manifested, and the practitioner should be aware of this variation to ensure thorough examination and treatment. A clinician who is uncomfortable with or unknowledgeable about different forms of sexual behavior may transmit these feelings to the client, who may then avoid giving an accurate history.

The rise in incidence of many STDs is often attributed to three social changes in recent years: permissiveness, promiscuity, and "the pill" (the "three P's").[7] Permissiveness is an attitude whose direct effect on the incidence of STD is difficult to evaluate.

If there has been a fundamental change in attitudes toward sexuality, then one would want to examine the behavioral changes resulting from permissiveness that may lead to an increase in STDs.[7] Similarly, it has been said that the substantial rise in the use of oral contraceptives ("the pill") in the 1970s may have had an effect on the incidence of STDs.[3,7] Again, one would want to examine specific behavioral changes resulting from the use of "the pill" that would have this effect. The major behavioral change that one would want to examine is promiscuity (defined as having more than one sexual partner).

The rise in availability and use of oral contraceptives may have resulted in an increase of persons with multiple partners, and having multiple sexual partners seems likely to increase the risk of contracting an STD, particularly if those partners also have more than one sexual partner. In one study[7] the percentage of persons diagnosed with gonorrhea at a clinic was highest at a level of four different partners within the 30 days before examination and declined with either fewer or more partners.

A less significant behavioral change that may have occurred with increased use of "the pill" is decreased use of other contraceptives, notably condoms, that may have prevented some disease transmission.[7] Some studies have shown that condoms are effective in reducing the transmission of STDs, but the extent to which people use them regularly is unclear. One investigator[7] found that only 2% of the sample always used condoms during sexual intercourse.

If the increase in promiscuity *has* had a large effect on the incidence of STDs, the practitioner is still left with the question of what advice to give individual clients. It would not be appropriate to suggest that persons limit themselves to one partner, since the clinician cannot presume to know what benefits any client receives from having different sexual partners. Perhaps the best advice to give a client in these circumstances is to "know your partners." Knowing one's partners, and especially having names and phone numbers for contact tracing (discussed later), could lead to more comfort with mutual questions about possible STDs and could create a greater sense of responsibility for one another's health and well-being.

Other components of sexual expression to consider are specific kinds of sexual activity and also sexual orientation (heterosexual, homosexual, or bisexual). Very few STDs are transmitted only through kissing, although it is known to happen (e.g., when syphilis lesions are present on the lips). Genital-genital contact and genital-rectal contact are the most frequent modes of STD transmission. With oral-genital contact, the most likely mode of transmission is from the genitals to the mouth or pharynx. Clear documentation is lacking on the likelihood of transmitting pharyngeal infections (notably gonorrhea) to a partner's genitals. Oral-anal contact increases the risk of acquiring intestinal diseases (giardiasis, amebiasis, and shigellosis) and hepatitis A. In addition to diseases caused by organisms, sexual injuries (such as rectal damage) may occur with overzealous use of sexual paraphernalia.

Knowing a person's sexual orientation can be important information for the clinician.

Lesbians seem to have a very low incidence of most STDs, although there has been little research in this area. One study of 148 sexually active lesbians revealed no cases of four major STDs.[17] Possible explanations include decreased transmissibility of genital and rectal infections with sexual contact between females and/or a higher level of monogamous relationships in the lesbian community.

Gay males, as a population, are at comparatively high risk for contracting many of the STDs. Several studies have supported this concept and suggest that explanations for this higher risk include more frequent sexual activity with multiple partners and a wider variety of sexual behaviors than heterosexuals.[8,26] Even though lesbians seem to be at comparatively low risk for STDs and gay males seem to be at comparatively high risk, the clinician should consider the individuality of each client, since sexual orientation does not prescribe individual forms of sexual expression.

Environment. The environment in which the organisms and hosts function is extremely important in the study and treatment of communicable disease. Environmental factors that one examines in relation to STDs include the disease reservoirs (where the organism lives in the environment), the modes of transmission, and also the accessibility to treatment and education.

The term sexually transmitted disease is actually a reflection of the mode of transmission of the pathogenic organism (i.e., a disease that is transmitted primarily through sexual contact). The disease reservoir consists mainly of sexually active persons who have more than one partner or whose partner has more than one partner. Therefore the major approaches to environmental control of STDs are really measures aimed at the individual on a massive scale.

The most well-known intervention on this scale is contact tracing, in which the clinician or epidemiologist attempts to identify, locate, evaluate, and treat the sexual partners (and their respective partners) of each client. Contact tracing requires considerable knowledge of STDs, excellent communication skills, and the ability to establish trust and confidentiality with the client. Having clients contact their own partners has worked well for some persons who are reluctant to give names to staff epidemiologists.[14]

Mass screening for high-risk groups is another large-scale intervention.[14] This technique has been used with some success at gay steambaths and bars but requires considerable trust to be developed between client and clinician so as not to be an invasion of privacy. A number of large metropolitan areas have gay STD clinics staffed by gay health professionals, and screening programs are emphasized. Prostitutes, as a group, do not seem to be as high risk as they were thought to be before World War II.[4] For example, prostitutes now account for less than 5% of syphilis cases.[4] Young people (age 15 to 24) are at high risk for development of STDs because of their comparatively high level of sexual activity.[4] Mass screening, however, would be an even more difficult task for adolescents than gays.

Mass education for high-risk groups, if done well, may help increase knowledge and awareness, eliminate misconceptions, and establish greater comfort in seeking treatment. This can be provided in the school system for adolescents and through various community groups established for gay people.

The final environmental factor to consider in relation to STDs is the accessibility to STD treatment services. Accessibility includes characteristics of the care received, as well as actual presence and location of the facility. Factors indicative of highly accessible services include nonjudgmental staff who are sincerely interested in the client, short waiting periods, smooth flow of services, convenient hours of operation, and availability of educational materials.[10]

Clinical examination of the STD client*

It is apparent from the previous discussion that clinical evaluation of the STD client consists of more than an examination of the genitals. Information obtained through a verbal history includes behavioral aspects of sexuality, physical symptoms,

*Much of the clinically related information presented here was obtained through the STD Training Program sponsored by the Seattle STD Training Center, Harborview STD Clinic, 325 9th Ave., Seattle, Washington. The purpose of this section is to provide an outline of an effective clinical approach to the patient with an STD and does not include detailed information necessary for advanced clinical diagnosis.

knowledge of sexual health, and individual emotional responses to the STD problem. The routine physical examination should include a thorough evaluation of several body systems and includes routine laboratory tests. It is important to perform a standardized evaluation to detect asymptomatic disease and because of the many STD problems that patients do not recognize as such. The goal of the clinical evaluation is to identify the STD syndromes that apply to the client and then determine the associated microorganisms. Identification of the organism will lead, in most cases, to antimicrobial therapy used in conjunction with treatment of the whole person, as described previously.

Routine history. Information that is gathered during the routine history begins with establishing the reason for the visit, whether it is a routine examination, the client is experiencing symptoms, and/or the client is a contact of someone who has recently had an STD. The client should be questioned regarding prior STD illness and the kinds of treatment that were provided. It is important to know if the patient takes any medications, particularly antibiotics that may interfere with clinical manifestations of STD but that do not completely eradicate the organism. Allergies to penicillin and other medications should be noted.

As previously mentioned, it is important to know the client's sexual orientation—exclusively heterosexual or homosexual or bisexual. Some people are threatened by this question, and the clinician should display sensitivity in the manner in which the question is asked. One nonthreatening way to phrase the question is, "Have you been having sex with men, women, or both?" Other important information to obtain is the date of the last sexual contact and the number of partners the client has had in the 2 months before the examination. The first is important because length of onset and duration of symptoms vary with different STDs. The number of partners in the prior 2 months will suggest the client's relative risk of having an STD, the amount of contact tracing that will have to be done, and how often the client should receive a routine STD examination. Some clinicians prefer to directly ask clients what kinds of sexual contact they have had: genital-genital, genital-rectal, oral-genital, and oral-anal. If this information is asked for, it should be done with language appropriate to the client's language, using slang when needed. Other clinicians tell the client they plan to examine his or her mouth, genitals, and rectum unless there has been absolutely no sexual contact with that area of the body. The method used to elicit this information should be tailored to the individual client.

Information gathered about disease symptomatology will vary with the sex and sexual orientation of the client. Any affirmative answers should be explored concerning onset, duration, and special characteristics (such as color and consistency of a discharge). Females should be questioned about vaginal discharge, vulvar itching, dysuria, urinary urgency, lower abdominal pain, rectal symptoms, sore throat, genital lesions, any skin rashes or itching, and abnormal menstrual periods. Exclusively heterosexual males (who have had no rectal contact) should be questioned about urethral discharge, dysuria, genital lesions, skin rashes or itching, testicular pain, and sore throat. In addition to the questions routinely asked of heterosexual males, gay or bisexual males should be asked about rectal symptoms such as pain, bleeding, discharge, and diarrhea. If hepatitis is suspected, questions should be asked about dark urine, clay-colored stools, fatigue, and jaundice.

Throughout the history taking the clinician should be assessing the knowledge level of the client and offering information about the purpose of the questions being asked, especially with those questions regarding sexual behavior. The sensitive clinician will also note any anxiety that the client is showing, try to explore the reasons for the anxiety, and help to alleviate it.

Physical examination. The routine STD physical examination uses inspection and palpation of the integumentary system, reproductive system, oropharynx, and anorectal area. The physical examination for females includes the following[19]:

1. Inspection of the skin of the lower abdomen, inguinal areas, hands, palms, and forearms
2. Inspection of the pubic hair for lice and nits
3. Inspection and palpation of the external genitals, including inspection of the perineum and anus
4. Speculum examination of the vagina and cervix
5. Bimanual pelvic examination
6. Palpation for inguinal and femoral lymphadenopathy
7. Inspection of the mouth and throat, including tonsils

The speculum and bimanual examination can be embarrassing and uncomfortable for the client and should be done carefully. The clinician should explain each step of the examination and inform the client of normal sensations she may experience. Warming the speculum in warm water will help to ease some of the discomfort and provide a lubricating effect to ease insertion. The clinician should establish eye contact frequently and request feedback from the client about her feelings and sensations.[12]

The physical examination for heterosexual males includes the following[19]:

1. Inspection of the skin of the genitals, inguinal areas, lower abdomen, hands, palms, and forearms
2. Inspection of the pubic hair for lice and nits
3. Inspection of the penis, including the meatus, with retraction of the foreskin and "milking" of the urethra
4. Palpation of the scrotal contents
5. Palpation for inguinal and femoral lymphadenopathy

"Milking" of the urethra is done in a succession of three gentle squeezes from the base to the tip of the penis to express any discharge from the urethra.

The physical examination for gay or bisexual males should include the items listed for heterosexual males plus an inspection of the mouth, throat (including tonsils), and anorectal area. If the client complains of rectal symptoms, an anoscopic examination should be performed.

Routine laboratory tests. Every client with an STD should receive a serologic test for syphilis if it has not been done within the preceding 2 months. All clients should also have routine cultures for gonorrhea. The culture sites depend on the sexual contact the client has had but generally include urethral cultures for heterosexual males; cervical and possibly pharyngeal and rectal cultures for females; and pharyngeal, urethral, and rectal cultures for gay and bisexual males.

A Gram stain of the smear is used to identify the presence of gonococci and/or polymorphonuclear leukocytes (PMNs) that are indicative of infection. Gram stains of smears are appropriate for urethral, cervical, and rectal discharges but not for identification of pharyngeal gonorrhea because of the normal presence of similar bacteria in the oropharynx.

Other routine laboratory tests include the wet prep and KOH prep for examination of vaginal secretions. In addition, some STD clinics provide chlamydial and herpes tissue cultures, although these can be expensive and often have to be paid for directly by the client. There are several other laboratory tests not routinely used that will be discussed in later sections.

Major STD syndromes

After the history, physical examination, and appropriate laboratory tests have been performed, the clinician should classify findings into one or more STDs. The major STD syndromes are vaginitis, cervicitis, lower abdominal pain, urethritis, epididymitis, pharyngitis, proctitis, and skin or mucous membrane lesions.

Vaginitis. Vaginitis, or inflammation of the vagina, is usually marked by mild-to-moderate discomfort, pruritus, and/or discharge. The normal vaginal environment usually includes small amounts of viscous secretions with abnormal discharge being more copious, yellow-green or thick white, and sometimes malodorous. Vaginitis can be caused by *T. vaginalis, C. albicans,* or *G. vaginalis.*[19]

Cervicitis. Cervicitis is asymptomatic for many females, but others may experience pelvic pain and dyspareunia, as well as a vaginal discharge. Inspection of the cervix may reveal a viscous, yellow or turbid discharge from the cervical os, cervical edema, and bleeding on contact with a swab. Causes of cervicitis include *Neisseria gonorrhoeae, C. trachomatis,* or herpes simplex. In addition, candidiasis and trichomoniasis may involve the cervix, as well as the vagina.[19]

Lower abdominal pain. All females complaining of lower abdominal pain should be evaluated for pelvic inflammatory disease (PID) by a bimanual pelvic examination. Symptoms of PID include bilateral tenderness on palpation of the ovaries and tubes, tenderness when the cervix is moved, pain on fundal pressure, vaginal discharge, fever, dysuria, and/or menometrorrhagia. PID is usually caused by *C. trachomatis* or *N. gonorrhoeae,* or both concurrently. PID can be serious and may require hospitalization for treatment.[19] Complications include sterility and ectopic pregnancy.[21]

Urethritis. Urethritis is the most common complaint of males coming to STD clinics. At least 90% of males with a urethral infection have symptoms—over 95% when the infection is caused by gonococci. Symptoms of urethritis may include urinary frequency, pain, or burning and purulent white, yellow, or green discharge. Urethritis is usually classified as gonococcal or nongonococcal urethritis, with *C. trachomatis, U. urealyticum,* and possibly some other organisms as the cause of NGU. In addition, trichomonal, candidal, or herpes infections may occasionally cause urethritis in males.

Females may also experience dysuria caused by urethritis or cystitis. Urethritis or cystitis in females should be clearly differentiated from dysuria caused by passing the stream of urine over the labia in the presence of vaginitis. More than one half of the cases of lower genitourinary tract infections in females are caused by gram-negative organisms. The rest may have infections with *N. gonorrhoeae* or *C. trachomatis.*[19]

Epididymitis. The most common complication of male urethritis is epididymitis, which causes unilateral scrotal pain and swelling, often very tender on palpation. When a client seeks help for these symptoms, torsion caused by trauma should be ruled out before establishing a tentative diagnosis of epididymitis. The most common cause of epididymitis is a gonorrheal or chlamydial infection. Epididymitis may also be caused by gram-negative organisms in males who have some form of genitourinary disease.[19]

Pharyngitis. Pharyngitis is marked by sore throat, enlarged lymph glands in the neck, and/or exudate in the pharynx or on the tonsils. Pharyngitis has many possible causes, both viral and bacterial, and is frequently not caused by an STD organism. In cases of pharyngitis associated with STD the only organism known to be an etiologic agent is *N. gonorrhoeae* and, as stated previously, can only be diagnosed by culture. It is unlikely that the client with gonococcal pharyngitis will transmit the organism to other persons through sexual contact.[19]

Proctitis. As previously mentioned, rectal infections are frequently asymptomatic, thus creating a necessity for routine examination and culture of the ano-rectal area in clients who have rectal sex. With symptomatic proctitis, persons may experience rectal pain, itching, discharge, bleeding, or coating of the stool with discharge. On anoscopy the clinician often will observe rectal irritation, lesions, or discharge. The major causes of proctitis are gonorrhea and/or herpes infections. STD organisms causing acute diarrhea include *Giardia lamblia, Entamoeba histolytica,* and *Shigella sonnei.*

Skin or mucous membrane lesions. Many different lesions are seen in patients with STD that may or may not be related to STD organisms. Generally STD skin lesions can be divided into two groups: ulcerative and nonulcerative. Lesions differ in their location, appearance, distribution, duration, and general symptoms according to the causal organism and will be elaborated on in the next section. Ulcerative lesions can be caused by herpes, syphilis, lymphogranuloma venereum, and granuloma inguinale. Nonulcerative lesions are most commonly caused by scabies and warts. There are also generalized skin rashes caused by secondary syphilis and disseminated gonococcal infections.

Major organisms associated with STD

After the clinician has established the syndrome or syndromes applicable to the STD client, a differential diagnosis of the associated microorganism is made with the assistance of laboratory data. Antibiotics are used to treat nearly all of the STDs, in addition to the other interventions described previously. In this section the major organisms associated with STD are identified, clinical signs and symptoms are discussed, and various interventions, especially antimicrobial therapy, are presented.

Gonorrhea. Gonorrhea, often called "GC," the "clap," and the "drip," is caused by a gram-negative diplococcus, *N. gonorrhoeae*. It most commonly infects the urethra, epididymis, cervix, fallopian tubes, rectum, and pharynx.

Urethral gonorrhea in males produces symptoms in over 95% of all cases. Onset of symptoms after infection is rapid (usually within 2 to 8 days) and usually includes severe dysuria and large amounts of mucopurulent discharge, often yellow or green in color. Diagnosis is made with either a Gram stain of the smear or urethral culture grown on Thayer-Martin culture media. Because the severity and frequency of symptoms in males usually cause them to seek treatment quickly, complications such as epididymitis are infrequent.

Cervical gonorrhea, in contrast to male urethral gonorrhea, is frequently asymptomatic, and it is not uncommon for females with cervical gonorrhea to seek treatment only after experiencing symptoms of PID (signs and symptoms of cervicitis and PID were discussed in the previous section). A Gram stain of the smear may confirm diagnosis of gonorrheal cervicitis, but has a sensitivity of only 50%. Diagnosis is usually made with a cervical culture. If gonorrheal PID goes untreated for too long, it may cause infertility because of scarring of the fallopian tubes.

Rectal gonorrhea, most common in gay or bisexual males, is frequently asymptomatic and is usually discovered with a routine rectal culture. When the client experiences symptoms of proctitis, a Gram stain of the smear from the rectum may result in a diagnosis of gonorrhea but, like the cervical smear, is only sensitive about 50% of the time. Examination and culture with the aid of an anoscope increases the likelihood of an accurate diagnosis.

Pharyngeal gonorrhea is asymptomatic most of the time, only rarely causing mild pharyngitis. Diagnosis cannot be made from a Gram stain of the smear; only a pharyngeal culture can confirm gonococcal pharyngitis.

For uncomplicated genital gonorrhea in males and females, tetracycline is the treatment of choice because it is also effective against chlamydial infections (and other NGU organisms) that may occur concomitantly with gonorrhea. If the client seems unreliable to take several days' worth of oral medications, then one-dose treatment with either injectable procaine penicillin G or oral ampicillin is preferable. For rectal infections, procaine penicillin is the treatment of choice, and in the case of penicillin allergy spectinomycin is effective. Pharyngeal infections should be treated with either procaine penicillin or tetracycline; ampicillin and spectinomycin are not effective. For persons who are at risk for multiple-site infections, procaine penicillin is the treatment of choice. In situations of treatment failure caused by penicillin-resistant gonorrhea, spectinomycin should be given.

When administering intramuscular procaine penicillin, there are two possible medication reactions of which the clinician should be aware. The first is an allergic reaction to penicillin, which may result in urticaria and/or anaphylactic shock. Although a rare occurrence, an allergic reaction is potentially life threatening. Second, there may be a temporary reaction to the procaine, during which the client may become disoriented, combative, and fearful and suffer from hallucinations. This is more common than penicillin allergy but is not life threatening. The client may need to be restrained by two or more people to prevent injury until the reaction is over in several minutes.

The client should return for reculturing of the positive sites 4 to 7 days after completion of antibiotic treatment. Clients should be urged to abstain from sexual activity until after treatment and posttreatment cultures have been completed. All sexual partners within the past 2 months should receive an STD examination, and all contacts within the past month should routinely be given treatment.

In addition to epididymitis and PID, disseminated gonococcal infection (DGI) is a possible complication of gonorrhea. In contrast to the local complications, which occur most frequently in males with symptomatic urethritis, DGI occurs most frequently in males with asymptomatic urethritis. Symptoms of DGI include skin rash with lesions, primarily on the extremities (usually few in number), and acute, transitory arthritis, which can occur in any joint. Treatment of DGI may include hospitalization for intravenous antibiotic therapy.

Chlamydial infections and other causes of NGU. *C. trachomatis* is a major cause of NGU, epididymitis, and PID. Other organisms associated with NGU include *U. urealyticum, T. vaginalis, C. albicans,* and herpes simplex, with 80% to 90% of NGU caused by *C. trachomatis* and *U. urealyticum.*

Symptoms of NGU usually differ from symptoms of gonococcal urethritis in several ways. The incubation period for NGU is usually longer (7 to 14 days), onset is more gradual, dysuria is milder and often absent, and there is usually less discharge.[19] Diagnosis is made by documenting urethritis on the basis of the discharge and/or on the presence of many PMNs on a Gram stain of the smear from the urethra and by the ruling out of gonococcal infection. Diagnosis of cervical and pelvic chlamydial infections is based on symptoms of cervicitis, PID, the ruling out of gonorrhea, and the diagnosis of the sexual partner. Tissue cultures for identification of *C. trachomatis* are available in some metropolitan clinics but are often expensive.

Treatment for NGU and cervicitis is a 7-day course of tetracycline. In cases of epididymitis and PID that can be treated without hospitalization the tetracycline regimen is lengthened to 10 days. Follow-up for clients with epididymitis and PID should include examinations by the clinic physician. Females with PID may need bed rest for several days and should abstain from sexual contact for at least 2 weeks.

Syphilis. Syphilis is caused by the organism *Treponema pallidum,* a spirochete that usually infects the mucous membranes of the genitals, rectum, or mouth. It can also gain entry directly through the skin, usually in the perineal area. If untreated, syphilis passes through a series of stages and over a number of years can cause pathologic damage to several body systems. Because of the potential for great damage, routine serologic testing for syphilis is strongly recommended for sexually active persons with multiple partners.

Primary syphilis. A painless, ulcerative lesion (chancre) appears at the site of entry 10 days to 3 months after exposure to *T. pallidum.* The classic chancre is well demarcated and drains a serous fluid that is highly contagious. However, the chancre can have differing appearances, and any painless lesion on the client with STD should be considered suspect. The chancre heals within 2 to 8 weeks and usually leaves no scar. For this reason, and because it is painless, it is often overlooked. Diagnosis at this stage is based on examination of the chancre fluid under a dark-field microscope to identify the spirochete. Serologic tests for syphilis are often negative the first several weeks after appearance of the chancre, and the client may need a repeat test in following weeks.

Secondary syphilis. Signs and symptoms of secondary syphilis may begin to appear as early as 2 to 4 weeks after the appearance of the chancre, and this stage usually lasts for several years before becoming latent. Signs and symptoms will vary among individuals and include a generalized rash over the body (often including the palms of the hands and soles of the feet), low-grade fever, myalgia, and headache. Fluid from any of the skin lesions is highly contagious. Serologic tests at this point are 97% positive.

Latent syphilis. Early latent syphilis may last up to 20 years when there are no clinical signs of illness, and the only method of diagnosis is through serologic testing. The disease may arrest at this stage, or it may continue to late latent syphilis and involve the cardiovascular system or spinal cord and brain (neurosyphilis). Tumorlike tissues may scar different organs, the heart may be damaged, or neurologic problems such as paralysis, paresis, confusion, and delusions may occur.

There are two types of serologic tests for syphilis: nontreponemal antigen tests and treponemal antigen tests. The Venereal Disease Research Laboratory test (VDRL) is a nontreponemal test that is usually performed first. If the VDRL is positive, a treponemal test, usually the fluorescent treponemal antibody-absorption (FTA-ABS) test, is performed to confirm the diagnosis of syphilis. The FTA-ABS is performed because there are occasional false-positive VDRLs as a result of acute mononucleosis, chickenpox, measles, typhus, pregnancy, or smallpox vaccination. Once a person has been treated successfully for syphilis, the VDRL titer will fall to nonreactive or slightly reactive levels over several months' time. The FTA-ABS, however, will always remain positive.

Treatment for syphilis is usually with intramuscular injection of benzathine penicillin, using different doses and schedules depending on the stage of the disease. In persons allergic to penicillin the use of tetracycline for 15 to 30 days is recommended. It is also interesting to note that treatment of gonorrhea with procaine penicillin may arrest a case of incubating syphilis. Persons receiving treatment for syphilis may experience a Herxheimer reaction the evening or day following the treatment. This reaction is characterized by fever, malaise, chills, headache, and myalgias and usually subsides within 24 to 36 hours.[19]

Persons diagnosed with syphilis should abstain from sexual contact until treatment is completed, and contacts within the past 3 months should be routinely examined and treated. Because of the potential severity of syphilis, contact tracing should be done by an experienced epidemiology counselor. Emotional counseling may be especially necessary for the syphilis client because of the strong social stigma associated with syphilis.

Genital herpes. Genital herpes is generally caused by *Herpesvirus hominis* type 2 (HVH-2), although it can also be caused by the type 1 virus associated with oral infections. The virus can infect the external genitals, urethra, vaginal canal, cervix, rectum, and mouth.

The incubation period for herpes is usually 3 to 7 days and often begins with a prodromal period of tingling sensations or a feeling of fullness in the pelvic area. The signs and symptoms include the presence of painful, grouped, fluid-filled lesions that, with the initial infection, usually last from 14 to 28 days before forming a scab and healing. Other symptoms include voiding difficulties, proctitis, fever, and inflammation of lymph glands. Recurrences of the lesions occur in most people and can happen one to many times a year for an unpredictable number of years. The lesions during recurrences are usually less severe than during the primary infection and often appear during periods of emotional stress or menstruation or in the presence of fever or sunlight.[20] Recurrences are also often preceded by the prodromal symptoms of tingling and fullness. Diagnosis is usually made by history and physical examination, although only tissue cultures or serologic tests confirm the diagnosis.

Until very recently no specific treatment for herpes has been available except for supportive measures, which include washing the lesions with soap and water frequently, drying with a hair dryer, using cornstarch or talc to keep the area dry, avoiding occlusive undergarments, and using systemic analgesics as necessary. Persons with herpes infections should avoid sexual contact when lesions are present, both in the initial period and during recurrences.

The Food and Drug Administration (FDA) has recently approved the use of Acyclovir ointment for treatment of genital herpes. This medication inhibits the growth of the virus and shortens the duration of initial herpes infections. Systemic Acyclovir, not yet approved by the FDA, may prevent active herpes infections in persons previously exposed to the virus, although it is not a cure.[18]

A serious complication of herpes infections in females is transmission of the virus to the neonate if active lesions are present during delivery. If the baby is delivered during an active infection, there is a 40% to 50% chance of the infant becoming infected. There is a 50% mortality rate of neonates infected with herpes simplex. If lesions are present at time of delivery, a cesarean section is performed. There is also a possible correlation between herpes infections and cervical cancer, and females with herpes are encouraged to have annual Pap smears.[20]

Because of the chronicity and severity of the problem, patients with herpes infections may need tremendous psychologic support. Education regarding the disease, transmission, and treatment is essential, and many cities have herpes support groups.

Chancroid. Chancroid, caused by the gram-negative bacillus *Haemophilus ducreyi,* is rare in the United States but more common in tropical and semitropical areas. After an incubation period of up to 10 days lesions usually appear on the genitals or perineum at the site of entry. The ulcerated lesions are typically irregular, friable, ragged, and covered with purulent exudate.[13] They are clearly differentiated from the syphilis chancre because the chancroid ulcer is painful. Swollen inguinal lymph glands occur in about half the cases.[13] Diagnosis is usually confirmed by Gram stain of the exudate, and cultures may also be grown. Treatment usually consists of oral sulfonamides or tetracycline.

Granuloma inguinale. Granuloma inguinale, often called donovanosis, is caused by the bacterium *Calymmatobacterium granulomatis* and is rare in the United States.[16] After an undetermined incubation period a papule appears that develops into a granulomatous ulcer.[13] Lesions may spread from the initial ulcer. Diagnosis is made by examination of lesion tissue from biopsy. Tetracycline, gentamycin (Garamycin), and chloramphenicol have been used to treat this STD.[13]

Lymphogranuloma venereum. Lymphogranuloma venereum (LGV) is caused by chlamydial organisms. After an incubation period of usually less than 3 weeks a primary lesion appears that is a small, painless, nonindurated papule, vesicle, or ulcer.[13] It generally heals quickly after several days and is followed in 2 to 8 weeks by painful lymphadenitis. Other symptoms such as malaise, fever, and headache may develop. Lymph glands may suppurate, scar, and become blocked, producing edema and ulceration.[13] Complications such as proctocolitis and stricture formation may occur.[13] Diagnosis of LGV is based on history, physical examination, and aspiration of lymphatic fluid for the LGV complement-fixation test. Drug therapy used to treat LGV includes tetracycline and erythromycin.

Trichomoniasis. Trichomoniasis, caused by the protozoan *T. vaginalis,* is a common STD that infects the cervix in females and urethra in males. Even though trichomoniasis is limited to the urogenital tract, it is an important STD to consider because of several factors. Postpartal women who have trichomoniasis experience a twice normal rate of persistent fever, prolonged vaginal discharge, and endometritis.[11] In addition, the client may be at higher risk for cervical malignancy because of a high rate of cervical erosion caused by trichomoniasis.[11]

Trichomoniasis in females is symptomatic about 75% of the time.[16] Signs and symptoms in females include vulvovaginal pruritus, inflammation of the labia, dysuria, dyspareunia, and a copious, frothy, malodorous, green-yellow discharge. A speculum examination of the cervix often shows an excoriated surface having a "strawberry" appearance. In males a urethral discharge with itching, burning, and inflammation may be seen.

Diagnosis of trichomoniasis is made by examination of the discharge on a wet saline mount. Microscopic examination of motile trichomonads confirms the diagnosis.

Trichomoniasis is usually treated with metronidazole (Flagyl), and sexual partners should be treated concomitantly. Persons taking metronidazole should be warned against alcohol consumption because of the disulfiram-like effect of the drug. Metronidazole is contraindicated for use in pregnant women.

Candidiasis. Candidiasis, often called a yeast infection, is caused by *C. albicans.* As previously mentioned, a substantial number of females carry this organism in small numbers without experiencing symptoms.

Symptoms of candidiasis appear more often with diabetes and hypoparathyroidism or in women who are pregnant or have received antibiotic treatment for other problems.[16] Vaginal candidal infections are most frequently characterized by vulvar pruritus, and on speculum examination the clinician usually observes a thick, white, tenacious discharge adherent to the vaginal wall. Only about 10% of male sexual partners experience symptoms of urethritis and balanitis, but the organism can be frequently cultured from the urethra of the male contact.[16] Diagnosis of candidiasis is based on microscopic examination of the discharge on a saline wet mount or with a 10% KOH preparation.

Treatment for candidiasis consists of nystatin vaginal tablets twice a day for 7 days. Male sexual partners are not routinely treated, but those complaining of balanitis may be treated with nystatin cream. Gentian violet is also effective for treatment of vaginal candidiasis but stains clothing and has low patient acceptance.

***Gardnerella vaginalis* vaginitis.** Another type of vaginitis may be caused by *G. vaginalis,* also called nonspecific or *Haemophilus* vaginitis, and is usually not accompanied by severe symptoms. Symptomatic infection with *G. vaginalis* is characterized by a small-to-moderate amount of malodorous, thin, gray discharge and occasional mild vaginal pruritus. On examination with a speculum the clinician may observe slightly irritated vaginal walls. Diagnosis is usually made by microscopic examination of the discharge on a wet mount and by a characteristic amine odor when the slide is treated with 10% KOH.[19]

Antibiotic treatment consists of oral ampicillin for 7 days. Regular sexual partners are usually treated also.

Giardiasis, amebiasis, and shigellosis. In the past several years these three intestinal problems have been recognized as being sexually transmissible through oral-anal contact. Primarily seen in gay males, these illnesses usually cause a syndrome of acute diarrhea.

Giardiasis, caused by the organism *G. lamblia,* is characterized by watery diarrhea, nausea, abdominal pain, and flatus. Diagnosis is made from stool cultures, and serial cultures over several days may be necessary. Antibiotic treatment of giardiasis is with metronidazole for 10 days. Amebiasis, caused by *E. histolytica,* has a more insidious onset, with intermittent, malodorous diarrhea that is occasionally bloody. In addition, 50% of the clients have high fevers. Diagnosis is made by stool culture, and treatment for amebiasis is metronidazole also. Shigellosis has a more abrupt onset with liquid green diarrhea. In addition, fever, abdominal pain, nausea, and myalgias may also be present. Shigellosis is usually a self-limiting disease that will last about 1 week, although it can be treated with sulfamethoxazole (Septra). The use of antidiarrheal medications is contraindicated.

Pediculosis pubis and scabies. Pediculosis pubis (crab lice) is caused by the louse *Pthirus pubis* and can be transmitted during close bodily contact or through clothes and bedsheets. Pediculosis pubis causes mild to intense pruritus, and the organisms are usually found in the hair around the pubic area, perineum, abdomen, and thighs. Diagnosis is made by observation of the organism or its nits attached to the hair shaft. Treatment is with one application of gamma benzene hexachloride lotion (Kwell) to be washed off after 24 hours. All clothes and bedsheets should be laundered in hot water, and sexual contacts within the past month should be examined and treated.

Scabies is caused by the mite *Sarcoptes scabiei* and is also acquired through close bodily contact. Symptoms usually appear about 1 month after infestation and include erythematous skin eruptions that are pruritic and most often in the finger webs, wrists, and belt line. Diagnosis is made by microscopic observation of the organism scraped from a skin lesion. Treatment is with one application of Kwell, which is left on for about 24 hours. As with pediculosis, all clothes and sheets should be laundered, and close personal contacts should be treated.

Genital warts. Genital warts, medically termed condylomata acuminata, are associated with a papovavirus.[16] They appear as cauliflower-like lesions on the external genitals, perineum, or perianal or rectal areas. Anyone with perianal warts should receive anoscopic examination; often, internal warts are not seen or treated and can keep spreading. Genital warts are usually treated with podophyllin resin (25%) in tincture of benzoin, applied weekly until the problem is resolved. Podophyllin is very corrosive and should be washed off several hours after application, increasing the length of time with each treatment up to 24 hours. Small warts may need to be treated with liqiud nitrogen or electrocautery, and extensive warts may need to be surgically removed by a dermatologist or proctologist.

Summary

This chapter has focused on sexually transmitted disease in the context of an organism-host-environment model. To effectively understand and treat the client with an STD, the health care practitioner must be knowledgeable about human sexuality, intellect, and emotion, as well as the pathophysiologic processes of disease. The following are *key* considerations for the practitioner:

1. The STD microorganism is an agent that needs a mode of transmission and a hospitable host for survival.
2. Most STD organisms quickly die outside the human body.
3. Asymptomatic disease is a major problem in the control of STDs.
4. Sexually active persons with multiple sexual partners are at high risk for acquisition of STDs.
5. Frequent self-examination, routine STD examination and cultures, and knowing one's sexual partners are important factors leading to good sexual health.
6. The clinician is most effective when she or he incorporates good listening, communication, and sensitivity into the examination and treatment process.
7. The clinical examination should consist of a systems approach to assessment and a syndrome approach to problem identification before attempting to identify the microorganism.
8. Treatment of the STD client involves the prescription of antibiotics; education in the areas of disease pathology and transmission, use of medications, personal hygiene, and self-care; and identification of sexual problems and referral to other services as necessary.
9. Environmental control is achieved mainly through contact tracing and public education.

Questions for review

1. Consider the populations currently served by the clinical facility in which you are employed or studying. Given the age range and other health characteristics of the populations, what STDs are likely to be most prevalent? What topics should be addressed in educational materials for the staff and clients in the facility?
2. Which of the STDs can be transmitted by nonsexual contact? What precautions are essential to protect nursing personnel and clients from acquiring these STDs?
3. What aspects of the social environment affect the incidence of STDs? What host characteristics make clients vulnerable to STDs? What host/environmental combinations place clients at highest risk for STDs?

References

1. Barlow, D.: Sexually transmitted diseases: the facts, Oxford, 1979, Oxford University Press.
2. Barrett-Connor, E.: Epidemiology of infectious diseases. In Barrett-Connor, E., et al.: Epidemiology for the infection control nurse, St. Louis, 1978, The C.V. Mosby Co.
3. Bauman, K.E., and Wilson, R.R.: Contraceptive practices of white unmarried university students: the significance of four years at one university, American Journal of Obstetrics and Gynecology **118:**190-194, 1974.
4. Blount, J.H., Darrow, W.W., and Johnson, R.E.: Venereal disease in adolescents, Pediatric Clinics of North America **20:**1021-1033, 1973.
5. Campbell, C.E., and Herten, R.J.: V.D. to S.T.D.: redefining venereal disease, American Journal of Nursing **81:**1629-1635, 1981.
6. Catalan, J., et al.: Sexual dysfunction and psychiatric morbidity in patients attending a clinic for sexually transmitted diseases, British Journal of Psychiatry **138:**292-296, 1981.
7. Darrow, W.W.: Changes in sexual behavior and venereal diseases, Clinical Obstetrics and Gynecology **18:**255-267, 1975.
8. Darrow, W.W.: The gay report on sexually transmitted disease, American Journal of Public Health **71:**1004-1011, 1981.
9. Drake, T.E., and Maibach, H.I.: Candida and candidiasis. I and II, Postgraduate Medicine **53:**83-120+, Feb.-March 1973.
10. Hacker, S., Palchik-Allen, N., and Rosey, C.: Factors influencing the success of a community VD program held in a university facility, Public Health Reports **95:**247-252, 1980.
11. Jirovec, O., and Petru, M.: Trichomonas vaginalis and trichomoniasis, Advances in Parasitology **6:**117-188 1968.
12. Magee, J.: The pelvic examination: a view from the other end of the table, Annals of Internal Medicine **83:**563-564, 1975.
13. McCormack, W.: Sexually transmissible conditions other than gonorrhea and syphilis. In Spittell, J.A., editor: Practice of medicine, vol. 3, New York, 1974, Harper & Row, Publishers, Inc.
14. Meheus, A.: Surveillance, prevention, and control of sexually transmitted disease, American Journal of Obstetrics and Gynecology **138:**1064-1070, 1980.
15. Miles, P.A.: Sexually transmissible diseases, Journal of Emergency Nursing **6:**6-12, May-June 1980.
16. Rein, M.F., and Chapel, T.A.: Trichomoniasis, candidiasis, and the minor venereal diseases, Clinical Obstetrics and Gynecology **18**(1):73-88, 1975.
17. Robertson, P., and Schachter, J.: Failure to identify venereal disease in a lesbian population, Sexually Transmitted Diseases **8**(2):75-76, 1981.
18. Saral, R., et al.: Acyclovir prophylaxis of herpes-simplex-virus infections: a randomized, double-blind, controlled trial in bone-marrow-transplant recipients, New England Journal of Medicine **305**(2):63-67, 1981.
19. Seattle STD Training Center: Unpublished manual from STD Training Program, Harborview STD Clinic, Seattle, 1979, The Center.

20. U.S. Department of Health, Education, and Welfare; Public Health Service; NIH: Herpes genital infection, Pub. no. 00-2939, Atlanta, Centers for Disease Control.

21. U.S. Department of Health, Education, and Welfare; Public Health Service; NIH: Summary and recommendations of the National Institute of Allergy and Infectious Disease Study Group on sexually transmitted diseases, Bethesda, 1980, National Institute of Allergy and Infectious Diseases, NIH.

22. U.S. Department of Health and Human Services; Public Health Service: STD fact sheet, ed. 35, HHS Pub. no. (CDC) 81-8195, Atlanta, 1981, Centers for Disease Control.

23. U.S. Department of Health and Human Services; Public Health Service: Morbidity and Mortality Weekly Report, **31**(11): March 26, 1982, HHS Pub. no. (CDC) 82-8017, Atlanta, 1982, Centers for Disease Control.

24. Wiesner, P.J., and Holmes, K.K.: Current view of the epidemiology of sexually transmitted diseases in the United States. In Danielsson, D., Juhlin, L., and Mardh, P.A., editors: Genital infections and their complications, Stockholm, 1975, Almqvist and Wikcell International.

25. Willcox, R.R.: The treponemal evolution. In Nicholas, L., editor: Sexually transmitted diseases, Springfield, Ill. 1973, Charles C Thomas, Publisher.

26. Willcox, R.R.: Sexual behavior and sexually transmitted disease patterns in male homosexuals, British Journal of Venereal Disease **57**:167-169, 1981.

15

Adaptation to hospitalization and illness

The frequency with which people entering the health care system are hospitalized demands that the health professional consider the consequences of removing individuals from their community, families, and homes at a time of stress.

The purposes of this chapter follow:

1. To review the process of becoming a patient and the inherent sexual adaptation
2. To document experiences of the patient that may compromise his or her image of self as a sexual being and precipitate feelings of shame
3. To discuss some cultural implications for behavior in clinical settings
4. To examine some of the motivating forces for patients sexually ''acting out'' when hospitalized
5. To review interventions designed to prevent shaming experiences, maintain privacy, and promote sexual integrity of the hospitalized patient

Becoming a patient

Admission. From the moment of admission to a hospital until the time of discharge, people are subjected to a wide variety of intrusive experiences that have the capacity to minimize sexual integrity and human dignity. There are several aspects of the admission process that have the potential to challenge a person's sexuality and self-image. These include intrusive questions about social status, removal of personal effects that convey to others who the person is, and transportation in a wheelchair.

The final assault of the admitting process takes place on the ward. It is at this point that the person is asked to undress or is undressed. Any remaining signs of position and prestige are removed, and substituted in their place is a short, shapeless hospital gown with a split up the back. Hospital attire is usually distinctly neuter, lacking any resemblance to clothing usually worn by men and women.

Further intrusions arise during the course of diagnosis and treatment.

Assessment and therapy. Once the person is officially a ''patient,'' he or she becomes subject to an array of procedures designed to diagnose and treat the problem for which she or he was admitted. Many of these procedures involve further intrusion into physical and psychologic aspects of sexual privacy.

Initially, a nurse sees the patient to collect basic data. Often this process entails numerous questions that, at face value, may be innocuous. However, patients may find them intrusive. It is usually best to proceed from "safe" topics to those that are more emotion laden.

Next, one or a number of physicians may obtain a detailed medical history. Although designed to collect biologic, psychologic, and sociologic data for diagnostic purposes, the history may also be a potentially embarrassing experience. The patient's surrender of intimate information to the physician can be anxiety provoking. The patient may later regret having divulged information about sexuality and sexual problems, fearing alienation from and labeling by medical personnel.[39]

Once data are obtained by means of the history, they are supplemented by methods that require direct contact between practitioner and patient and removal of clothing. Adequate examination of the chest in women by means of inspection, palpation, percussion, and auscultation requires removal of her clothing. Inspection and palpation of the genitals in both sexes require that the examiner's eyes and hands come in contact with areas of the body traditionally reserved for sexual intimacy. These processes may evoke anxiety, since touching of the genitals may be a long-standing taboo established by parents during childhood and may also be sexually arousing.

In addition to routine physical examinations, a patient is subjected to a number of additional potentially intrusive procedures. The rectal examination for the male may be embarrassing, particularly when prostatic stimulation precipitates emission of semen. Procedures such as catheterization or enemas may be compromising simply because they invade body territory in the vicinity of the genitals.

Sexual expression and institutionally enforced limits. The process of role socialization as a patient in a health care institution may be an experience that has potentially "neutering" effects. Separation from a partner, lack of privacy, and the hospital structure require changes in the person's usual sexual behavior.

Separation from a spouse or sexual partner demands that the patient abstain from sex or make a substitution in sexual outlet. Substitution may entail autoerotic behavior, such as masturbation. Complete abstinence requires that the patient deny an integral part of his or her personality. However, hospital staff do not always comprehend the nature of autoerotic behavior. Hence "labeling" may occur. As a result, patients may inhibit sexual feelings because of fear of censure by medical personnel.

Behavior may be greatly inhibited by lack of privacy. Patients frequently blush or apologize if they are seen holding hands, kissing or hugging, or engaging in other sexual contact. The patient who acts in a more overt sexual fashion may encounter disapproval.

The presence of a strange roommate in the hospital setting may greatly inhibit the patient's usual sexual behavior patterns. Territory is shared, and a roommate's right to privacy also needs to be respected. Even if the patient has a private room, it is not truly "private," since most hospital doors do not have locks.

The sick role and sexuality

Lederer[22] describes three stages of the experience of illness: the transition period from health to illness, the period of accepted illness, and convalescence. From this framework one can view a number of adjustments the "sick" person must make that directly influence sexuality.

Transition phase. During the period of transition from health to illness a patient may exhibit a number of reactions that range from denial to aggression. If a man who is becoming ill equates masculinity with activity and the refusal to acknowledge physical discomfort, then he may find being ill an emasculating process. If a woman equates femininity with being passive and intolerant of pain, then she is apt to perform in this fashion when she is ill. These attitudes may provoke denial of illness, anxiety, and an attempt to overcompensate for the physical assault.

Great apprehension may be associated with dysfunction of any part of the body, particularly those parts linked to gender identity and sexual functioning. The genitals and breasts are intensely valued, particularly in American society. A person who has pathology involving the face, skin, breasts, or genitals may be fearful of disfigurement and loss of sexual attractiveness. He or she may have fantasies of rejection and feelings of anxiety, guilt, and shame.

Some sexually related health problems may provoke intense guilt feelings. For example, people who have sexually transmitted diseases or single women who become pregnant may deny these problems because shame is so intense. Fear of submission to the control of others may also prompt denial, especially for those who view themselves as "controllers" of others.

In contrast, some people may feel relieved by the act of being hospitalized. Illness is one of the few acceptable reasons for not meeting social responsibilities; the sick role has the advantage of permitting one to escape social expectations without incurring disapproval.[28]

Illness, then, may legitimize an otherwise deviant state. Under strictly regulated conditions, people are able to indulge dependency needs. The element of exemption from ordinary role obligations may be readily welcomed.

Unfortunately, the price of this indulgence is often steep, especially when one views the adaptations it necessitates. Not only is the individual's sex role performance altered but also others' perceptions of those male or female characteristics so germane to that role. In addition, certain proscriptions pertain to sexual behavior in the hospital. The transition to illness, then, requires changed patterns of sexual behavior.

Accepted illness. The second stage in the process that Lederer[22] describes is acceptance of the illness. It is at this point that concerns related to the illness are actually substituted for those of mature life. Patients' reactions may range from infantile regression to blatant tyranny.

Physical weakness often underlies the dependency on others. Parsons[31] thinks that American society views dependence as a primary threat to achievement. Thus the American pattern of illness is shaped by achievement-oriented goals: getting well becomes a job.

During the acceptance phase egocentricity is common. There is great concern about body function, which may include sexual performance. At this point testing may be obvious. Flirtatious behavior may be used to elicit attention from staff members of the opposite sex. These behaviors may be directed at answering questions such as: "Am I still sexually attractive?" "Can I still function sexually?" Loss of power or control over life situations during this phase of illness may be equated with or may occur concurrently with a decrease in sexual desire or impotence.

Convalescence. During the convalescence stage the job of getting well is nearly completed. It is at this time that dependencies must be relinquished. Lederer[22] believes that this phase is somewhat analogous to adolescence, with medical and nursing personnel assuming parentlike roles. Just as the adolescent experiences confusion related to sexual identity and has concerns regarding sexual behavior, so may the convalescing patient. The patient's gratitude and appreciation may be interpreted as sexual attraction by the nurse; the nurse's attentiveness may be interpreted as being sexually provocative by the patient. Misunderstanding of spoken and body language may lead to unpleasant experiences for the patient if avoidance and withdrawal behaviors on the part of the nurse or other health professionals result.

Effects of illness on sexuality

Illness may influence one's sexuality in many ways. Certain disease processes may interfere with sexual function as a result of physiologic changes or tissue damage (see Chapters 16, 17, and 18). Others may create changes in body image that are viewed as incompatible with maintaining a sexual relationship (see Chapter 19). Pharmacologic agents or therapies used to treat disease states may interfere with sexual functioning (see Chapter 23). Physical symptoms such as fatigue may render a patient unable to perform sexually. Anxiety related to illness may interfere with sexual response. Depression or grief may be associated with impaired libido or sex drive. Finally, illness may necessitate physical separation from a partner.

Cultural variables and sexual behavior in clinical settings

In certain cultures there are proscriptions that may modify the individual's response to hospitalization and treatment. As an example, the response of Mexican Americans to white health professionals will be explored.

For some Mexican-American men, illness is a manifestation of weakness; they may have a tendency to conceal illness. Loss of blood, even for laboratory tests, is thought to impair their sexual vigor. Some Spanish-speaking men are reluctant to submit to physical examination even with male physicians. The situation is potentially much more embarrassing for them when the health care provider is female.[34] Mexican-American men may find it distasteful to relate to female nurses. Giving a urine sample is especially threatening to their masculinity and self-esteem. Some patients preserve their dignity by refusing to comply. They may also be reluctant to participate in tests for sexually transmitted diseases.[25]

Mexican-American men may also be reluctant to leave the examining room during the time their wives are having obstetric or urogenital examinations. This behavior is prompted by the belief that the role of the ''good husband'' is to protect his wife's modesty.[25] The physician or nurse may see his attitude as stubbornness or stupidity and therefore respond inappropriately.

For a Mexican-American woman, the physical examination may be very unpleasant, particularly if the examiner is male. Fear of being examined may be sufficient to keep her away from medical practitioners. (It is interesting that many of the healing personnel in the Spanish-American culture are women.[35]) The need to undress may cause intense embarrassment. Lurie and Lawrence[25] found that their Mexican-American female patients were more satisfied when a female nurse initiated this action during the physical examination. This is only one example of how awareness of patients' cultural backgrounds is crucial to nurses' understanding of the roles they should assume in helping a patient and/ or family cope with situations that have sexual overtones.

Acting out sexually

Why do patients act out sexually? In some instances patients are testing the response of others to themselves as sexual beings. Several men were found to act out sexually after myocardial infarction. Their behavior pattern included touching the breasts of nursing staff and using sexual terminology inappropriately during the course of treatment. Analysis of this behavior led the health providers to conclude that these men, whose feelings of masculinity were threatened by the heart attack, were seeking a reaction to themselves as sexual beings.[10]

In other situations suggestive remarks and exposure of the genitals may be used as a means of gaining control of a situation. Meyer[29] describes a situation in which an adolescent male used seductive language and indulged in petting with his girlfriend, to the chagrin of the nursing staff. The young man was attempting to exert control over a situation in which he felt totally helpless.

Edwards[16] described a case study of a man who was hospitalized for 24 years because he "couldn't keep his hands off women." His maladaptive behavior was sufficiently incapacitating to keep him institutionalized. However, the undesirable behavior of touching nurses attracted their attention, and even though the attention was disapproval, it reinforced the touching behavior. This man learned to control his impulses as the result of a behavior modification program.

Patients may make sexual overtures to obtain validation of their sexuality, to gain control of a situation in which they are dependent, or to attract attention. Patients may also be expressing the effects of sexual deprivation.

One successful approach in helping staff deal with such encounters involves behavioral rehearsal.[40] Situations in which a patient attempts to involve the staff in sexual activity are role played with health professionals. Four kinds of behaviors are suggested as a result of the role plays. First, it is recommended that the professional be aware of patients' needs to discuss sexual matters and to address this need promptly. It is also recommended that the professional convey empathy for the person who has been hospitalized for a long period and express understanding that this would produce frustration in meeting sexual needs. The nature of the professional-patient relationship must be clearly defined. While some professionals feel comfortable acknowledging that patient's verbal overtures are complimentary, all would appropriately stress that the professional does not intend to act on the patient's suggestions and establish limits. An example of this occurred as a young man with a spinal cord injury wheeled up behind a young nurse and slapped her derriere.

She turned to him and quipped, ''You know that's very flattering, but next time ask my permission first.'' Finally, professionals who cannot comfortably discuss sexual issues would do well to inform the patient that someone better prepared will be found to talk with her or him.

Interventions

Preventing shaming experiences.[21] Shame is a feeling synonymous with embarrassment, and it usually occurs as the result of social discomfort. Feelings of shame result from tension between the ego and the ego ideal when a goal or an ideal is not met. It is interesting to note that the German word from which *shame* is derived relates to the genitals.

Shame reactions are denoted by withdrawal from visual contact, sudden change in skin color such as blushing, nervous physical gestures, or difficulty with speech. Shame implies admitting to oneself that part or all of the self is unacceptable.

Hospitalized patients are extremely vulnerable to shaming experiences: they are subject to physical exposure, and the most private rituals are performed among strangers. Men who view themselves as invulnerable to pain may experience shame if they yield to painful stimuli and cry out or request pain medication. Disfigurement and lack of sexual prowess often produce shame. Hospitalized patients are constantly forced to deal with the threat of social disapproval at a time when they are not well equipped to do so.

Some patients deal with shaming experiences by projecting them onto the health care provider. It is not unusual for a male patient to say to a female nurse, ''You must be embarrassed,'' during a procedure that involves his physical exposure. It is more likely than not that the patient is embarrassed and is indirectly conveying this fact to the nurse.

Lange[21] suggests two means by which to approach shaming situations. First, one can avoid these situations by avoiding discussion of loaded topics and preventing physical exposure. These strategies are not always possible. Second, one can correct the shaming situation by acknowledging or challenging the shamer. For example, when performing an intrusive procedure, the practitioner can indicate that the person's embarrassment is typical.

Shaming situations can be prevented by providing both physical and psychologic privacy, avoiding ''touchy'' areas, and explaining that the situation does not, of necessity, need to be shaming. In addition, health providers can anticipate shaming situations (such as exposure of the genitals during catheterization or during obstetric experiences). Regressive role behavior in response to stress, such as loss of control, may engender shame. Finally, staff reactions to critical situations such as disfigurement may evoke embarrassment. Once this feeling is hypothesized, the health professional can help a patient to acknowledge shame and deal with it. The ego ideal may require reality testing, and the person's goals may need to be revised.

Maintaining privacy. Privacy is the individual's right to exclude others from knowledge about self.[5] Privacy permits emotional release, personal autonomy, and self-evaluation and provides for limited and protected information. During hospitalization, personal autonomy and the limitation and protection of information are probably most easily jeopardized.

As previously mentioned, lack of physical privacy requires major adjustments in sexual behavior. Patients frequently share a room with others, are constantly barraged by strangers, and have limited choices regarding the management of their life situations. These factors modify relations to and with a sexual partner. Health professionals have virtually unlimited access to the patient's body and personal history.

Patients' disclosure of intimate information to health professionals is anxiety laden because each change in self-disclosure patterns changes individuals' areas of essential privacy.[38] Eliciting personal information is often essential for providing adequate health care. Since the persons eliciting information are often imposed on patients, the patients' sense of invasion of privacy increases. When health providers are unaware that they are invading patients' privacy, the patients' sense of violation is multiplied. Disclosing personal information, then, may cause intense anxieties, particularly if patients fear that they may later regret their disclosures.

Pointing out that information is assembled to permit health workers to provide better health care may allay some anxieties. Telling patients that their disclosures will be treated confidentially will probably further their trust in the care providers. Acknowledging that it is sometimes difficult to divulge information about oneself, particularly if it is sex related, appears to enhance the person's comfort; the patient is then aware that the health professional is in tune with his or her feelings. The health professional can seek out the "real" person in the patient and react as a "real" person.

Providing some dimension of physical privacy for hospitalized patients is indeed a challenge. However, allowing patients predictable times during which they can enjoy solitude or be alone with a partner is not impossible. Drawing curtains, closing doors, and respecting sexuality and sexual behavior as a natural aspect of living are all simple acts but meaningful contributions to physical and psychologic privacy.

Promoting sexual integrity. Promoting sexual integrity for hospitalized patients is a complex task. To implement this goal, it is necessary to determine how patients perceive themselves sexually.

Assessment of patients' self-concept as sexual beings can be ascertained as early as admission to the hospital. Usually a capsule summary of the initial interactions with patients contains some reference to sex roles.

Eliciting information related to usual sexual practices is a fairly simple activity, yet many health care providers find it difficult to obtain an accurate sexual history (see Chapter 5). Several nursing history models have included information about sexuality as relevant data on which to base a nursing diagnosis. On the basis of this information the health provider gains further insight into sexual behavior before illness and the variety of sexual expression meaningful to patients. Does the woman who has had a hysterectomy see herself as "neuter"? Does the man who has had a heart attack see himself as "half a man"?

Embarrassment of the health provider is perhaps the most frequent reaction to invading a patient's privacy. However, it is rarely acknowledged. Entering the room of a patient who is involved in sexual activity is usually an unanticipated event. It is not unusual for both the patient and the health provider to avoid one another's feelings at that time and during later encounters. However, acknowledging that the person's privacy has been invaded would imply to the patient that she or he indeed has a right to privacy, that the health professional has infringed on this right, and that the infringement was unintentional. Respecting the person's need for physical privacy and viewing sexuality as a normal and integral part of the person can help health personnel to manipulate environmental variables to maintain patients' sexual integrity.

Promoting usual sexual behavior during hospitalization is often difficult, if not inappropriate, because of physical restrictions of place and distance from significant others. Providing for privacy during visiting hours or giving evening or weekend passes is often a solution in those institutions geared toward rehabilitation and long-term care. Professionals in those institutions caring for patients who are not of legal age or who are unable to exercise adult judgment regarding their sexual behavior and its consequences are obligated to protect the rights of all patients in the institution and could be held accountable for controlling patients' sexual behavior. Often patients adapt by means of autoerotic behavior or by keeping their sexual encounters secret from staff. "Free spaces," areas ignored by staff, may become havens for sexual activity. Although staff may be aware of the free spaces, neither they nor the patients acknowledge this awareness. In some European long-term care facilities, attendants may actually physically assist disabled persons to have intercourse by transferring and positioning them.

Often physical contact from a significant other has healing properties. Persons who are isolated for infectious diseases or for protection from microorganisms have reported that being held or caressed by a significant other or spouse provided the impetus to want to survive the disease and the treatment. Health professionals might do well to foster this sort of healing.

In summary, shaming experiences can be avoided or their effect minimized. A potentially shaming experience may be made more acceptable to the patient by explaining the nature and purpose of a procedure and by having a health professional of the same sex present. A female patient who is given an accurate explanation of a pelvic examination and accompanied by a female nurse or examined by a female physician is probably less likely to view this experience as shameful than a female who is placed in stirrups and examined with little or no understanding of the purpose. A male patient who must be catheterized by a female nurse will probably feel much less shameful when presented with the rationale and when his feelings of shame are acknowledged. Conveying acceptance of the patient's sexuality in the many ways previously mentioned does much to support the patient's self-image as a sexual being and acknowledges the importance of this dimension of being human.

Sexuality and the health professional

Sexism in the hospital family. It has been suggested that the members of the hospital family can be compared to the traditional American family: the physician is seen as father, the nurse as mother, and the patient as child (and therefore asexual). In addition to being aware of the neutering effects of hospitalization on patients, health professionals would do well to correct the sexism in their own interactions. The "doctor-nurse game" is probably the best example. The cardinal rule of the "doctor-nurse game" is that open disagreement between physicians and nurses must be avoided at all costs.[37] Nurses are allowed to influence patient care but not directly. They influence physicians toward a course of action by convincing them that it was "the physician's" idea. The subordination of women and the former sex segregation between the two professions probably contributed to the development of these strong interactional patterns, which in turn have been reinforced by hospital training, administration, and restrictive state licensure laws.[8]

Not only does sexism interfere with relationships among professionals but there is also some evidence that sexist bias influences diagnosis and therapy. Mental health professionals' concepts of a healthy adult corresponded more closely to concepts of a healthy man than concepts of a healthy woman.[6] One publication suggests that this bias may be disappearing.[1] Images of women in medical advertisements[27] and textbooks[24,36] reinforce sex-role stereotypic expectations of patients and plant not-so-subtle bias in treatment. Sex bias can be detected and corrected by means of consciousness-raising efforts on the part of the staff.

The health professional: a sexual being. Although the primary emphasis of this chapter has been on patients' sexuality, it is important to keep in mind that health professionals are sexual beings as well. Acknowledging this is a first step toward self-awareness. Professional ethics forbid sexual involvement of health professionals with patients in their care, particularly in situations in which the patient is extremely vulnerable (e.g., very young or unable to make a rational decision). One survey revealed that female physicians were more likely than males to use nonerotic touch in their encounters with patients but were less likely to use erotic touch with patients than male physicians. Female physicians denied having sexual intercourse with their patients, although a small minority of male physicians in a comparable survey said they had done so.[32] No similar surveys have been done with a population of nurses.

It would be foolhardy to imagine that health professionals can "turn off" their sexuality by virtue of entering a clinical setting. Discussions with students and practicing health professionals reveal that this is not the case. Men and women alike report having been sexually aroused by patients. In some instances this could be attributed to seductive behavior on the part of the patient. More commonly it is attributable to the fact that health professionals are also human and have access, by virtue of their profession, to intimate contact with patients.

Coping with one's sexuality is sometimes difficult. In some instances health professionals need to acknowledge that their sexual feelings are interfering with their practice. This awareness may be fostered through clinical supervision, and the professional may need to acknowledge inability to be therapeutic with a specific patient. In some instances the health professional will need to confront the person whose behavior seems purposefully seductive or intended to embarrass the professional. Recognizing such behavior as a maneuver to gain control is helpful, since on an intellectual level the professional can see the behavior as separate from a purely sexual issue. On an emotional level the professional may feel sexually aroused and have physical manifestations of sexual arousal, erotic fantasies, and desire for sexual relationships with patients. An important ethical distinction exists between experiencing such feelings and acting on them. Peer support and supervision can be valuable resources to help professionals acknowledge and share these feelings and put them in perspective.

Summary

This chapter has presented a review of the process of becoming a patient and the influence of hospitalization and illness on sexual self-concept and behavior. The motivations to act out sexually were examined in the context of hospitalization. The concepts of shame and privacy were explored, and strategies designed to promote sexual integrity of the hospitalized patient were suggested. Following are key considerations for health practice:

1. Hospitalization can modify one's customary sexual behavior.
2. Becoming a patient can have "neutering" effects.
3. Attitudes toward sexuality and sexual behavior vary between and among cultures and influence individuals' responses to health care.
4. Hospitalized patients may act out sexually to test the response of others to their sexuality, to gain control in a situation that makes them feel helpless, or to attract attention.
5. Shame, or embarrassment, is a feeling that occurs in a social context when one's goal or ego ideal is not met.
6. Privacy is the individual's right to exclude others from certain knowledge about self, and its boundaries are defined by the individual.
7. Promotion of sexual integrity encompasses interventions designed to maintain one's optimal self-concept as a sexual being and to promote usual sexual behavior.
8. Health professionals, as well as patients, need to deal with conflicts between their personal sexual feelings and professional ethics.

Questions for review

1. Mr. Ford, a 42-year-old real estate broker, is admitted to the hospital after myocardial infarction. He reaches out to touch female nurses, uses sexual language inappropriately during conversation, and displays his genitals during his bath. What inferences can be made regarding the meaning of this behavior? How could you cope with his behavior in a way that validated his sexuality but maintained your professional relationship?
2. Alice Jones, an 18-year-old single woman is admitted for pelvic inflammatory disease. She has never before had a pelvic examination. How can you help her to see the examination as a positive part of her hospitalization?
3. John Williams, a 21-year-old newly married man, is hospitalized in traction after multiple fractures. How can you assist him to maintain his normal sex role behavior pattern? What avenues are available to help him cope with the separation from his partner?

4. Catherine Norton, a 32-year-old woman, has been hospitalized for a terminal illness. Her husband has been visiting every evening. She may not leave her bed because of the severity of her illness, but she indicates that she highly values her husband's visits and wishes that they could have more intimate contact. How can you provide them with essential privacy?

5. Mrs. Ramona Chavez, a Mexican-American migrant worker, refuses to take off her clothing for the pelvic examination unless her husband is present. What information will help you to intervene on her behalf? How might you structure the situation so that the values of her culture are respected?

6. Martin Smythe, a 75-year-old man, must be catheterized during the middle of the night. You are female and the only professional nurse available, and there are no trained orderlies or male physicians available. How can you help him to minimize his feelings of shame?

7. You find that you are sexually aroused by a patient. How might you cope with these feelings? What resources are available to help you deal with your feelings? In your situation, can you change the nature of the interactions you have with patients (e.g., change assignments)?

References

1. Abramowitz, S., et al.: Sex bias in psychotherapy: a failure to confirm, American Journal of Psychiatry **133:**706-709, 1976.

2. Aletky, P.: Sexuality of the nursing home resident, Topics in Clinical Nursing **1**(4):53-60, 1980.

3. Barton, D.: Sexually deprived individuals, Medical Aspects of Human Sexuality **6:**88-97, Feb. 1972.

4. Beyers, M.L.: The hospitalized adolescent, Nursing Outlook **15**(8):32-34, 1967.

5. Bloch, D.: Privacy. In Carlson, C., editor: Behavioral concepts and nursing intervention, Philadelphia, 1970, J.B. Lippincott Co.

6. Broverman, I.: Sex role stereotypes and clinical judgments of mental health, Journal of Consulting and Clinical Psychology **34**(1):1-7, 1970.

7. Brown, E.L.: Newer dimensions of patient care, patients as people, part 3, New York, 1964, Russell Sage Foundation.

8. Bullough, B.: Barriers to the nurse practitioner movement: problems of women in a women's field, International Journal of Health Services **5:**225-233, 1975.

9. Carey, P.: Temporary sexual dysfunction in reversible health limitations, Nursing Clinics of North America **10:**575-586, 1975.

10. Cassem, N.H., and Hackett, T.P.: Psychiatric consultation in a coronary care unit, Annals of Internal Medicine **75**(1):9-14, 1971.

11. Chenevert, M.: Special techniques in assertiveness training for women in the health professions, St. Louis, 1978, The C.V. Mosby Co.

12. Comfort, A.: Sexuality in the institutionalized patient. In Comfort, A., editor: Sexual consequences of disability, Philadelphia, 1978, George F. Stickley Co.

13. de la Cruz, F., and La Veck, G.: Human sexuality and the mentally retarded, New York, 1974, Penguin Books.

14. Dougherty, M.C.: A cultural approach to the nurse's role in health care planning, Nursing Forum **11:**311-322, 1972.

15. Duff, R., and Hollingshead, A.B.: Sickness and society, New York, 1968, Harper & Row, Publishers.

16. Edwards, J.: If I touch, will you tell? American Nurses' Association Regional Clinical Conferences of 1967, New York, 1968, Appleton-Century-Crofts.

17. Hall, J.: Sexuality and the mentally retarded. In Green, R., editor: Human sexuality: a health practitioner's text, Baltimore, 1975, The Williams & Wilkins Co.

18. Heslinga, K., Schellen, A., and Verkuyl, A.: Not made of stone: the sexual problems of handicapped people, Springfield, Ill., 1974, Charles C Thomas, Publisher.

19. Kaplan, H.: The new sex therapy, New York, 1974, Brunner/Mazel Inc.

20. Kassebaum, G., and Baumann, B.: Dimensions of the sick role in chronic illness. In Jaco, G.E., editor: Patients, physicians, and illness, New York, 1972, The Free Press.

21. Lange, S.: Shame. In Carlson, C., editor: Behavioral concepts and nursing intervention, Philadelphia, 1970, J.B. Lippincott Co.

22. Lederer, H.D.: How the sick view their world. In Skipper, J., and Leonard, R.C., editors: Social interaction and patient care, Philadelphia, 1965, J.B. Lippincott Co.

23. Leininger, M.: Nursing and anthropology: two worlds to blend, New York, 1970, John Wiley & Sons, Inc.

24. Lennane, K.J., and Lennane, R.J.: Alleged psychogenic disorders in women—a possible manifestation of sexual prejudice, New England Journal of Medicine **288:**288-292, 1973.

25. Lurie, H.J., and Lawrence, G.L.: Communication problems between rural Mexican-American patients and their physicians: description of a solution, American Journal of Orthopsychiatry **42:**777-783, 1972.

26. Major, L.: Human sexuality and the mentally retarded: an annotated bibliography, Health Education Monographs, pp. 278-285, Sept. 1974.

27. Mant, A., and Davoch, D.: Media images and medical images, Social Science and Medicine **9:**613-618, 1975.

28. Mechanic, D.: Response factors in illness: the study of illness behavior. In Jaco, G.E., editor: Patients, physicians, and illness, New York, 1972, The Free Press.

29. Meyer, H.L.: Predictable problems of hospitalized adolescents, American Journal of Nursing **69:**525-528, 1969.

30. Muff, J., editor: Socialization, sexism and stereotyping: women's issues in nursing, St. Louis, 1982, The C.V. Mosby Co.

31. Parsons, T.: Definitions of health and illness in the light of American values and social structure. In Jaco, G.E., editor: Patients, physicians, and illness, New York, 1972, The Free Press.

32. Perry, J.A.: Physicians' erotic and non-erotic physical involvement with patients, American Journal of Psychiatry **133:**838-840, 1976.

33. Samora, J., Saunders, L., and Larson, R.F.: Medical vocabulary knowledge among hospital patients. In Skipper, J., and Leonard, R.C., editors: Social interaction and patient care, Philadelphia, 1965, J.B. Lippincott Co.

34. Saunders, L.: Healing ways in the Spanish southwest. In Jaco, G.E., editor: Patients, physicians, and illness, New York, 1972, The Free Press.

35. Schwartz, L.H., and Schwartz, J.L.: The psychodynamics of patient care, Englewood Cliffs, N.J., 1972, Prentice-Hall, Inc.
36. Scully, D., and Bart, P.: A funny thing happened on the way to the orifice: women in gynecology textbooks, American Journal of Sociology **78:**1045-1050, 1970.
37. Stein, L.: The doctor-nurse game, Archives of General Psychiatry **16:**699-703, 1967.
38. Tagliacozzo, D.: The nurse from the patient's point of view. In Skipper, J., and Leonard, R.C., editors: Social interaction and patient care, Philadelphia, 1965, J.B. Lippincott Co.
39. Taylor, C.: In horizontal orbit: hospitals and the cult of efficiency, New York, 1970, Holt, Rinehart, & Winston, Inc.
40. Withersty, D.: Sexual attitudes of hospital personnel: a model for continuing education, American Journal of Psychiatry **133:**573-575, 1976.

Media

"Sex and the professional," Texture Films, New York.
"Sexual behavior: nursing reactions," "Sexuality: a nursing concern," "When the topic is sex," Sexuality and nursing concerns, Concept Media, 1500 Adams Avenue, Costa Mesa, CA 92626.

16

Sexuality and cardiovascular disease

Cardiovascular diseases account for a large proportion of chronic illness in Western society. Like many other forms of chronic illness, heart disease has the capacity to affect most aspects of daily living, including sexuality. This chapter will consider the effects of cardiovascular disease on the individual's self-concept and self-esteem, sexual functioning, and sexual relationships. In addition, it will explore the influence of sexual activity on the health of people who have had a myocardial infarction (MI) and the effects of exercise training programs on sexual health.

Effects of sexual activity on the cardiovascular system in healthy persons

Intercourse. As early as the 1950s investigators were studying cardiovascular change during intercourse. Bartlett[1] studied the heart rate and pulmonary ventilation of three couples (22 to 30 years old) before, during, and after intercourse. During orgasm the heart rate approached 170 in both sexes, although the heart rate was greater in men. Female responses were more variable than male responses, both among and between subjects. However, the heart rate rapidly returned to normal after orgasm in both sexes.

Respiratory rates were recorded in excess of 60 breaths per minute. Minute volumes were recorded that were compatible with markedly severe exertion. Again, respiratory rates and minute volumes decreased quickly after orgasm.

Masters and Johnson[19] studied cardiovascular changes during the human sexual response cycle in the laboratory. During excitement they found a gradual increase in the respiratory rate, a slow increase in the heart rate, and a mild elevation of the blood pressure. During plateau, recorded heart rates averaged from 100 to 175 beats per minute. The blood pressure increased 20 to 80 mm Hg (systolic) and 10 to 40 mm Hg (diastolic). Hyperventilation also preceded orgasm. At orgasm maximal physiologic changes were noted. The pulse increased to as high as 180 beats per minute in some individuals, and the blood pressure increased as much as 30 to 100 mm Hg (systolic) and 20 to 50 mm

Hg (diastolic). The respiratory rate accelerated as high as 40 breaths per minute. These physiologic parameters quickly returned to baseline rates during the resolution phase.

Masturbation. Although Masters and Johnson found that in general the physiologic responses were more pronounced with masturbation than with sexual intercourse, other findings are worthy of mention here. Wagner[36] studied ten young men, three trials each, in the laboratory setting. He found that orgasm with masturbation led to heart rates of only 110 to 130 beats per minute. This is in contrast to the coital cost of 180 beats per minute in a sample of men of comparable age and health state. Naughton[21] suggests, however, that if masturbation is associated with feelings of guilt or anxiety, the energy cost may be increased.

Anal stimulation. Although there are no data on the effects of anal intercourse on cardiac function, rectal stimulation may innervate the vagus nerve. Anal stimulation may have the following parasympathetic effects on cardiac function: decreased rate and rhythmicity of the sinoatrial node, decreased force of contraction of the cardiac muscle (especially the atria), decreased rate conduction of impulses through the heart, and decreased blood flow through the coronary vessels.

Coital position. Some investigators have suggested that because of the detrimental effect of isometric contractions of arm and shoulder muscles during intercourse, the supine position during sexual activity is less stressful and therefore advantageous for postcoronary individuals.[9] Nemec, Mansfield, and Kennedy[22] explored the effect of position for intercourse on eight healthy male volunteers (mean age 29.25 years) in the privacy of their homes with their partners of at least 6 months. Heart rate and blood pressure data were collected during rest, intromission, orgasm, and at 1 and 2 minutes each after orgasm. Mean maximal heart rate for the male-astride position was 114, compared to 117 for the female-astride position. Mean maximal blood pressure at orgasm was 163/81 with the male-astride position, compared to 161/77 with the female-astride position. These differences do not support the recommendation of the supine position.

Some investigators believe that the age at which an MI is likely to occur is also the age of diminishing sexual behavior. The psychologic reaction to the threat of an MI may then evoke feelings of loss of manhood. These feelings may in turn cause compensatory efforts to prove this false, which generate greater anxiety to perform. This can contribute to a vicious cycle potentially leading to sexual dysfunction. Soloff[30] suggests that anxiety over futile attempts at intercourse may be a significant contributing factor to increased energy costs.

Myocardial infarction and sexual activity

Sexuality and self-concept. Concerns about sexual behavior are evident among individuals even during their stay on the coronary care unit. Cassem and Hackett[3] reported that several men on a coronary care unit whom they studied were greatly concerned about impotence. Furthermore, three of the 100 men in the sample acted out sexually toward female nurses. Themes related to sexual prowess and functioning were found in the men's conversations. Once the threat of death was no longer present, the men's behavior in many instances became sexually provocative. Perhaps this behavior reflected their change in focus from being concerned with death to being concerned about the quality of remaining life. It also might be inferred that acting out sexually was a means of validating their sexuality. This type of testing might be used to reinforce feelings of masculinity or femininity if a health care provider of the opposite sex responded to flirtatious behavior. This behavior underscores the concern patients have for their sexuality, particularly their adequacy as men and women.

Sexual behavior. Hellerstein and Friedman[10] monitored forty-eight subjects with cardiac disease by telemetry for 24 to 48 hours. The men were instructed to carry on their normal activities and to keep a diary of events in this period. Fourteen of these men engaged in sexual intercourse during the time they were monitored. The investigators found that with orgasm the mean heart rate reached 117.4 beats per minute, with a range in all subjects from 90 to 144. The mean heart rate decreased to 97 and 85, respectively, during the first and second minutes after orgasm.

Blood pressure measurements were estimated by comparing heart rates achieved with sexual activity with heart rates achieved by the same subjects in laboratory testing during ergometric exercise with bicycles. With this comparison, blood pressures averaged 162/89 mm Hg with orgasm and averaged 145/88 mm Hg in the 2-minute period before and after orgasm. Hellerstein and Friedman concluded that the oxygen cost was less than that required by Master's two-step exercise test. However, they did not control for body position of the subjects.

Electrocardiographic changes during coitus were compared to those during work activities. It was noted that four men developed ST-T depression associated with ischemia and angina. Of three men who developed ectopic beats, two had ventricular beats, and one developed both atrial and ventricular beats. Two of the three men with ectopic beats also developed ischemic ST-T depression. Of the four who experienced ST-T depression and angina during work, three had similar symptoms during coitus. The investigators concluded that cardiovascular responses occurring during coitus and those occurring during the activities associated with the individual's occupation were comparable in frequency and severity.

Hellerstein and Friedman concluded that conjugal sex with a partner of 20 years or more in the privacy of the couple's bedroom demanded only modest physical requirements (in the absence of congestive heart failure) and was similar to walking up one flight of stairs, walking briskly, or performing ordinary tasks in many occupations.

Larson et al.[17] demonstrated that the effects of climbing two flights of stairs and having intercourse are similar. They found that for eight men with coronary artery disease (CAD) (average age 50) the mean maximal heart rate was 115 ± 7/min during sexual activity and 118 ± 6/min during stair climbing. Mean maximal heart rates for nine healthy subjects (average age 49) were also similar: 123 ± 8 and 122 ± 5/min for sexual activity and stair climbing, respectively (Fig. 16-1). Mean maximal systolic blood pressure (SBP) for the CAD group was 144 ± 6 mm Hg at orgasm but 164 ± 7 mm Hg at the end of stair climbing. In healthy subjects mean maximal SBP was 146 ± 2 mm Hg for stair climbing and 146 ± 4 mm Hg for orgasm (Fig. 16-2). There were no significant differences in the pressure rate product across groups or activities. Four of the CAD patients demonstrated electrocardiogram (ECG) changes, ST segment changes, or premature atrial or ventricular contractions.

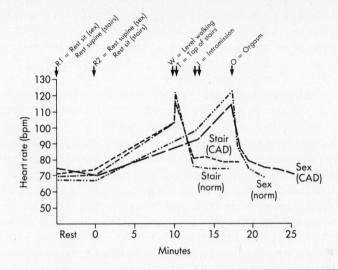

Fig. 16-1. Mean heart rate during stair climbing test and sexual activity.
(Modified from Larson, J., et al.: Heart rate and blood pressure: responses of
coronary artery disease patients during sexual activity and a 2-flight stair climbing test, masters thesis, Seattle, 1978, University of Washington.)

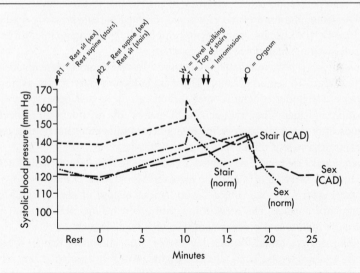

**Fig. 16-2. Mean systolic blood pressure during stair climbing test and
sexual activity.** (Modified from Larson, J., et al.: Heart rate and blood pressure: responses of coronary artery disease patients during sexual activity and a
2-flight stair climbing test, masters thesis, Seattle, 1978, University of Washington.)

Stein[31] asked six men who had MIs 4 to 6 months previously to wear Holter monitors during sexual activity in their own homes on four occasions. He found no significant differences in the mean maximal heart rate or blood pressure between the male- and female-astride positions. He suggests that the restriction of designated coital positions for CAD individuals is not necessary.

      Sudden death danger with sexual activity. How likely is it that a person with CAD will have an MI during intercourse? No one knows for certain; probably because of social propriety, these deaths are not always reported as such. Ueno,[34] a Japanese pathologist, performed autopsies on thirty-four individuals (twenty-eight men and six women) who died suddenly during coitus. These deaths represented 0.6% of all endogenous sudden deaths over a 4½-year period. The deaths of eighteen of the men and two of the women were determined to be of cardiac origin. In addition, 25% (nine) of the deaths occurred in hotel rooms; 15% (five) more occurred outside the home. In most cases (70%) the sexual relations were extramarital, and men were with partners who were on the average 20 years younger than they. The women who died were with men 3 years their senior. Three sudden deaths occurred after masturbation. Inebriation was noticed in twelve cases. Malek's work[18] also suggests that both the physical and emotional responses to sexual activity under unusual circumstances (e.g., with a partner much younger, in an unsafe place, when inebriated) factors associated with sudden death.

      Effects on sexual functioning. As early as 1964 Tuttle, Cook, and Fitch[33] evaluated thirty-nine men (30 to 69 years of age) 1 year after their MIs and found that one third of the men had reduced their sexual frequency by 50% (Table 16-1). Another third of the men had reduced the frequency of intercourse to less than 25% of their pre-MI level. The remaining third of the group had returned to their previous sexual patterns. Four of the men (10%) became permanently impotent. The average interval between the MI and resumption of intercourse was 3 months.

The investigators also found that two thirds of the sample were given no advice regarding the return to sexual activity. The remainder were given nonspecific or vague advice. The investigators concluded that the change in sexual behavior was based on misinformation and fear. They recommended that health providers give specific advice to individuals after coronary attacks regarding return to sexual functioning to minimize this sociologic response of diminished sexual behavior.

Hellerstein and Friedman[10] conducted a comprehensive study of sexual activity after MI. They studied forty-eight men who had an MI at least 3 months previously and compared them with forty-one subjects who had no history of cardiac disease but were prone to coronary attacks. The men in the study were white, middle-aged, middle- to upper-class individuals, and predominantly Jewish businessmen.

These investigators found through the use of a questionnaire that of the forty-eight persons with arteriosclerotic heart disease, eighteen (42%) developed one or more cardiovascular symptoms during coitus. Thirteen (30%) experienced tachycardia, four of whom also had anginal pain. Nine men (21%) experienced angina, and five needed to interrupt intercourse, one because of tachycardia and four because of anginal pain.

In all subjects the interval between the coronary event and the resumption of sexual activity was significantly influenced by symptoms. This interval was 16.4 ± 2.6 weeks in the group of men who were experiencing symptoms, in contrast to 11.7 ± 2.4 weeks

Table 16-1. Sexual functioning in postcoronary patients

Investigator and year	Sample	Change in sexual frequency (%)		
		Increase	No change	Decrease
Tuttle, Cook, and Fitch (1964)	39 men 1 year after MI	0	33	67
Hellerstein and Friedman (1970)	48 men 3 months after MI	—	42	48
Bloch, Maeder, and Haissley (1975)	88 men and 12 women 11 months after MI	—	—	73
Kushnir et al. (1975)	80 men 4 months and 10 months after MI	—	—	47

in the asymptomatic group. Resumption of sexual activity also occurred earlier in those who were more sexually active before the MI. The impact of the coronary event on sexual activity usually decreased to the precoronary level by the end of the first postcoronary year.

Twenty (41.7%) of the forty-eight subjects indicated no change in frequency of orgasm after their MI. However, in the other twenty-eight men orgasmic frequency did decrease from 2.1 times per week 1 year before the attack to 1.6 times per week 6 months after the MI. Many factors were cited to account for these changes in these twenty-eight men, including change in sexual desire (eleven men), the woman's decision not to have sexual intercourse (seven), feelings of depression (six), fears (five), and symptoms of CAD (six). Not one of the subjects attributed the decrease in orgasmic frequency to impotence. Quality of the sexual experience did not change for twenty-three men (52%), improved for ten (23%), and deteriorated for eleven (25%).

Cohen, Wallston, and Wallston[5] reported an investigation of seventeen men 3 to 4 months after hospitalization for MI. They found that questions and concerns regarding sexual activity had resolved themselves, either because the couples sought advice or because the couples had arrived at an unspoken agreement. They therefore emphasized the need for sexual counseling as part of the cardiac rehabilitation during the hopsital phase or immediately afterward.

In Switzerland Bloch, Maeder, and Haissley[2] reported an evaluation of eighty-eight men and twelve women (age range of 28 to 71) seen 11 months after an acute MI. They found that the mean frequency of sexual intercourse before MI was 5.2 times per month, as compared to 2.7 times per month 11 months after MI. Of the eighty-five individuals who engaged in pre-MI sexual activity, sixty-two (73%) experienced diminished frequency of intercourse after the coronary event. Main reasons given for decreasing sexual frequency were decrease in desire, depression, anxiety, partner's decision, fear of sudden death, fatigue, angina, and impotence. The investigators concluded that the most prevalent reasons for decreased sexual activity were the psychologic aspects. No comparisons were made between male and female subjects.

In 1975 Kushnir et al.[16] reported the resumption of work, driving, and sexual activity in thirty-two men (mean age 53) who had experienced ventricular fibrillation after MI.

They also studied a control group of ninety-five men (mean age 52) whose MI was not complicated by ventricular fibrillation.

Data were available for comparison of sexual activity for ten men in the ventricular fibrillation group and seventy men in the control group. The investigators found that 4 months after discharge 47% (thirty-three) of all men had decreased sexual activity as compared to their precoronary level. In addition, there was a significant difference between the two groups. Fewer individuals in the fibrillation group had resumed full sexual activity. At 10 months this difference had disappeared; resumption of sexual activity was comparable in the two groups. As at 4 months, overall reduction in frequency of sexual activity was experienced by 46% of the men at 10 months. The authors concluded that in terms of short-range rehabilitation (4 months) individuals who experienced ventricular fibrillation in conjunction with MI probably harbored more fears of sudden death than those with uncomplicated courses. Therefore resumption of sexual activity was pursued more cautiously. They proposed that these effects did not persist in the long-term rehabilitation.

Effects of exercise training on sexual functioning. Stein[31] exposed sixteen men, ages 46 to 54, to a 16-week bicycle ergometer training program 3 to 4 months after their first MI. Each man used a portable ECG tape recorder to record an ECG twice before and after the training program. A control group of 6 MI patients who were not trained completed the same testing protocol. Exercise training led to an average decrease in the peak coital heart rate of 5.5% (127/min to 120/min) and an increase in VO_2 max (measured during bicycle ergometer ECGs) of 11.5%. The control group showed no change in peak coital heart rate and an increase of only 2% in VO_2 max.

Johnston et al.[13] found that a greater decrease in coital frequency occurred for MI patients than for those who had experienced myocardial revascularization, despite the fact that both groups participated in an exercise training program. The decrease in coital frequency for trained MI patients, however, was less than that seen in nontrained patients in other studies.

An additional study was reported by Kavanagh and Shepard[15] in 1977 regarding resumption of sexual activity. The sample included 161 men 3 years after MI who were attending an exercise-centered rehabilitation program. Half of the men (eighty out of 161) reported no change or an increase (number distinguishing these groups not reported) in sexual activity after the MI. The other eighty-one subjects reported reduced sexual activity, compared with the period before the MI. Reasons given for diminished frequency were apprehension by either member of the couple (thirty-six), loss of desire (thirty), or a combination of these factors (fifteen). Seventy-five percent of the men had made no change in patterns of foreplay or the position adopted during coitus. Eighty-four percent (139) of the subjects indicated that sexual intercourse was as enjoyable as before the MI.

Sexual concerns of the MI patient's spouse. Recognition of the stress experienced by wives of MI patients is not new,[29] yet the sexual concerns of these women have been largely ignored. Papadopoulos et al.[23] studied 100 women whose husbands had experienced an MI. Only forty-five of these women had received any sexual information before their spouse's discharge from the hospital, yet seventy-six couples resumed sexual activity. Examples of the sexual instructions women received are shown in Table 16-2.

Table 16-2. Sexual instructions given before and/or after husband's discharge from the hospital (as reported by wives)

Sexual instructions	Number of wives receiving instructions
Take it easy	22
It is all right to resume sexual activity as long as it is not strenuous; it should be in moderation	20
Resume and have sexual activity in relaxed atmosphere, comfortable temperature, and normal surroundings	18
If husband has chest pain during intercourse, he should stop and rest, then resume	17
Do not have intercourse after patient eats a big meal; wait several hours	16
Husband should use his own judgment and common sense	13
Resume sexual activities when husband feels like it	11
Resume sex in 6 to 8 weeks	7
Side-lying position should be used	6
If husband has persistent chest pain after intercourse, call physician the next day	5
Patient should take nitroglycerin before starting sexual activity	5
During sexual activity, if he has chest pain, he should stop and take nitroglycerin, rest, and then resume	5
Use position normally used	5

From Papadopoulos, C., et al.: Archives of Internal Medicine **140**:38-41, Copyright 1980, American Medical Association.

Couples who resumed sexual activity tended to be younger, were married fewer years, had a higher frequency of sexual activity before the MI, were able to talk about sex with one another, and had received instructions regarding sexual activity after the MI. Fear of sexual activity was, however, greater among women who had received sexual information than among their counterparts. Fears included recurrent chest pain, MI, or coital death. Forty-three women reported they would have liked to have received instruction from both a nurse and a physician, nine from a nurse, and forty-five from a physician. Ninety-two expressed a desire to receive instructions together with their husbands.

Questions these women had are listed below in decreasing order of frequency:

- Is it unusual for a man to lose his desire for sex after he has a heart attack?
- Do men have the same ability to become excited sexually after they have a heart attack?
- Why does my husband have more difficulty getting an erection since his heart attack?
- Why can't my husband maintain an erection?
- Will my husband ever be able to get an erection again?
- Is it unusual for a man not to have a desire for sex after the age of 50 years? Does age have anything to do with his lack of interest?
- If my husband has symptoms during intercourse, what is the best thing to do?
- What is the safest position?

- When is the best time? Is one time of the day safer than another to have sex?
- How much energy is used during intercourse? Does the heart work harder?

Women who did not resume sexual activity or who had unsuccessful attempts at intercourse reported sexual anxiety and frustration.

Hypertensive vascular disease and sexual activity

There have been no studies conducted specifically with hypertensive individuals to document their cardiovascular responses to sexual activity. Hypertension increases left ventricular work, eventually causing left ventricular hypertrophy and reduced cardiac output. Howard[12] therefore indicates that the sustained exertion and rapid heart rate accompanying sexual activity, in the presence of decreased cardiac output, may result in rapid backward pressure and acute pulmonary edema. He advocates that hypertensive persons with blood pressures of 180/110 or with target organ involvement must be cautioned to play a less aggressive role in sexual activity.

Alternatively, some investigators stress the importance of aggressive treatment in hypertension to return blood pressure to as normal readings as possible. After this is accomplished no restriction need be placed on physical exercise, including sexual activity. Persons experiencing dyspnea (from congestive heart failure) will limit their own sexual activity when necessary. Others also suggest resumption of sexual activity no sooner than 6 weeks after an episode of acute intracranial bleeding (subarachnoid or intracranial). In addition, several antihypertensive medications have been shown to interfere with sexual functioning (see Chapter 23).

What is the risk of having a cerebrovascular accident (stroke) during sexual activity? There is no published evidence that sexual activity will precipitate cerebrovascular accidents. However, the incidence of cerebrovascular accidents has been shown to increase with a corresponding increase in systolic blood pressure levels.[12] The only documented deaths from cerebrovascular accidents during sexual activity have been reported by Ueno.[34] He found that of thirty-four individuals, four women died during coitus as a result of cerebrovascular accident. There is currently one study available that provides information regarding the sexual activity of individuals after cerebrovascular accident. Kalliomaki, Markkonen, and Mustonen[14] studied fifty-six men and forty-nine women between the ages of 20 and 60 years. They found that for individuals with right-sided paralysis there was a significant decrease in libido, as compared to subjects with left-sided paralysis. The side of paralysis had no effect on coital frequency. Thirty-four of the men (61%) and eleven of the women (22%) experienced a decrease in coital frequency after cerebrovascular accident (see pp. 377-380).

Health care for clients with cardiovascular disease

Assessment. Assessment of the person with cardiovascular disease includes a thorough history, a physical examination, and laboratory data. Scalzi and Dracup[27] recommend considering previous patterns of sexual activity, including availability of a partner, usual frequency and duration of sexual activity, time of day, and preferred positions. These data provide information about patterns of sexual activity that may be stressful and also provide a basis for individualizing teaching or counseling. Data about past experience with angina during sexual stimulation or intercourse may suggest ways of coping that the patient and/or partner have employed and may also suggest fears that the patient and/or partner may experience.

Scalzi and Dracup also recommend exploring a history of sexual problems that have occurred 1 to 3 months before MI. In particular the type of sexual problem, surrounding circumstances, medication regimen, and other health problems involved may provide clues about the patient's fears of permanent sexual dysfunction and factors responsible for the problem and its persistence. Finally, the patient and partner's understanding of when to resume sexual activity is an important discussion item. These data may indicate misconceptions, lack of information, or expectations that may not be met. Anxiety among newly discharged individuals may interfere with sexual functioning. Of what importance is the sexual problem to the individual? Of what importance is the sexual problem to the couple? Is there evidence of performance anxiety?

Another approach to assessment involves determining the patient's readiness to resume sexual activity. Larson et al.[17] has shown that the two-flight stair climbing test, which includes 10 minutes of rapid walking (120 paces per minute), followed by a climb of two flights of stairs in 10 seconds, provides an adequate cardiovascular challenge with responses similar to those of sexual intercourse with a long-term partner.

Assessment of the relationship is also important. Can the postcoronary individual currently fulfill his or her previous role expectations? Does each member of the couple understand the constraints placed on the sexual relationship by the disease if applicable? Is the well member overprotective of the other? Is the individual with cardiac disease overly dependent on the other? Is hostility apparent in the relationship? Is the mate supportive of the limits the cardiac member may perceive that his or her disease warrants? Is the couple well informed about the possibilities for sexual functioning? Is the relationship stable? Is it marital or nonmarital?

For the person with hypertension, assessment of previous patterns of sexual activity, experience with symptoms during sexual activity, and sexual difficulties before diagnosis will assist the nurse in establishing information similar to that discussed for MI patients. In addition, it is particularly important to assess whether the individual's blood pressure is currently controlled. Certain antihypertensives, such as reserpine, methyldopa (Aldomet), and guanethidine (Ismelin), are associated with decreased sexual desire and sexual dysfunction (see Chapter 23). Use of these medications may have changed the patient's sexual frequency and/or functioning. Finally, it is important to determine whether intracranial bleeding has occurred previously and if so, how recently. People may have experienced bleeding during sexual activity, although hypertension was not controlled, and may fear recurrent bleeding. Fear may lead to sexual dysfunction. The hypertensive person may have been warned against overexertion in the past and may fear sexual activity. Effects of the disease and treatment on self-image are important. The person may feel inadequate or less masculine or feminine because of changes in sexual desire or fears about sexual activity. Finally, the individual may have difficulty in performing roles other than lover, either because of the disease or its treatment.

Sexual activity program for patient with uncomplicated myocardial infarction

Convalescent phase: in hospital—week 3

Activity level
General
    Walk hall 2 to 3 times/day at normal walking pace; receive family visitors; shave
Sexual
    Masturbation to partial erection
Education
Cardiac
    Heart rate should not exceed base-line 20 bpm
    Contradictions to above activities—faintness, dyspnea, diaphoresis, tachycardia
    Teach patient to take pulse and pace himself
Sexual counseling
    Interview patient, spouse, and couple prior to discharge

Convalescent phase: post-hospital—weeks 4 to 6

Activity level
General
    Maintenance of hospital activity program
    Begin slowly, daily walks on level surface
Sexual
    Self-stimulation to partial erection
    Couple begin sensate pleasure for one another with quiet nondemanding stroking of back, face, arms, legs; focus on self-pleasure; exclude genital areas (do not attempt sexual intercourse or stimulation to ejaculation despite occurrence of erection)
    Both partners must be well rested prior to exercises
Education
    Contraindications to above activities include dyspnea, faintness, rapid pulse, fatigue, emotional upset
    Take pulse prior to, during, and after stroking episodes
    Sessions 3 times/week for 20 minutes
    Telephone contact with nurse clinician regarding problems or progress; office visit with physician

Convalescent phase—weeks 7 to 9

Activity level
General
    Continue all previous activities; physician may order treadmill test
Sexual
    Masturbation to full erection
    Husband and wife on alternate occasions stroke the other's pelvic area, under the direction of the other; focus attention on each other

From Watts, R.G.: Nursing Clinics of North America 2:349-359, June 1976.

Sexual activity program for patient with uncomplicated myocardial infarction—cont'd

Education
> Note previous complications; sessions three times/week for 20 minutes each; contact with nurse clinician for support and guidance

Convalescent phase—weeks 10 to 12

Activity level
General
> Continue daily walks and moderate exercises; climb two flights of stairs; work to tolerance

Sexual
> Masturbation to ejaculation
> Couple engage in manipulative play
> Oral-genital sex if accepted as norm
> Sexual intercourse in position comfortable for couple (avoid isometrics)

Education
> Adequate pacing of activities; check pulse
> Avoid sudden exercise or competitive efforts
> Note unusual symptomatology
> Avoid clustering of other physical activities with coital activity (e.g., eating, drinking, fatigue, emotional upsets)
> Suggest couples read: *Sound Sex and the Aging Heart*
> Telephone contact with physician or nurse clinician

Intervention. Perhaps the most important intervention designed to promote sexual health in the individual with cardiac disease is sharing of information. Individuals frequently ask questions such as "Is it safe to resume intercourse? When? How often?"

The postcoronary individual can be evaluated to determine fitness level. Heart rate response to exercise can be used as a reflection of oxygen capacity. Each individual must be evaluated in terms of his or her own activity response. A plan for resumption of sexual activity has been proposed by Watts[37] (p. 306 and above).

Hazardous conditions, such as extremes of temperature, having intercourse sooner than 3 hours after a meal, and having intercourse within 3 hours of alcoholic consumption (alcohol increases the heart rate and dilates vessels), are best avoided. Since rest is an essential component of care, coitus is probably best enjoyed in the morning, after a good night's sleep, and then followed by a rest period.[9]

Coitus under conditions other than those of gentle relaxation may be hazardous. Secretive, anxiety-provoking conditions with time limitations and coitus with a resented partner (such as with a prostitute) are best avoided.

The individual with cardiac disease who experiences angina during or after intercourse, prolonged palpitations after intercourse, or sleeplessness or marked fatigue after intercourse should be referred for medical evaluation.[9] Modification of his or her sexual activity may be necessary to permit optimal cardiac functioning.

Some cardiologists recommend that patients take nitroglycerin prophylactically before intercourse or other sexual activity likely to precipitate pain. Patients with congestive heart failure or general debilitation are usually cautioned against strenuous physical activity, including sexual activity.

Physical conditioning programs specifically designed for people who have had MIs may improve the individual's sexual functioning. Participation in such a program may also enhance self-esteem.

Finally, education and counseling of patients is not sufficient. As seen in the studies of spouses of MI patients, sexual misinformation or lack of information may be responsible for needless anxiety or even denial of an important aspect of living.

Guidelines for resumption of sexual activity after cerebrovascular accident are not well established. Alterations in libido and coital frequency have been documented.[14] However, couples may be encouraged to know that sexual functioning may not be altered after cerebrovascular accident and that each couple must be evaluated individually. The topic of sexuality in relation to hypertension is discussed infrequently. Health care providers can make available current data and let individuals make use of the information as desired. Awareness of effects of sexual activity on blood pressure may serve as an incentive for blood pressure regulation. If blood pressure is adequately controlled, there is probably no need to advise any specific coital positions or precautions. Interventions aimed at considering sexual side effects of antihypertensive medications may be very helpful to couples. If sexual dysfunction is occurring, exploring flexibility in medication regimens may be of great help in promoting sexual health.

Summary

This chapter has focused on sexuality and sexual adaptations necessitated by cardiovascular diseases.

Key considerations for clinical practice include the following:

1. Adaptation in the area of sexual functioning is one of many aspects to be included in promotion of "normalizing" strategies for persons with cardiovascular disease.
2. Assessment of biologic, psychologic, and sociologic variables that influence sexual functioning provides a holistic basis for assisting the person with cardiovascular disease to experience optimal sexual adaptation.
3. During the human sexual response cycle the cardiac rate, blood pressure, and respiratory rate increase rapidly but not markedly in comparison with other modes of exercise.
4. Doubts about the sexual self-image may occur in the immediate period after MI and may surface in sexually provocative behavior.
5. Sexual dysfunction after MI might be attributable to diminished feelings of masculinity.

6. Restrictions on sexual activity after MI are best created on an individual basis. In view of the demands of intercourse in a conjugal relationship, most middle-aged men with arteriosclerotic heart disease, who do not have congestive failure, may safely resume intercourse.

7. A graduated activity level may be used to promote optimal sexual adaptation in postcoronary individuals.

8. Overprotective partners and lack of information about when to resume intercourse after an MI may prevent resumption of the precoronary sexual pattern.

9. Restriction of sexual activity need not be advised for hypertensive persons if the blood pressure is adequately regulated.

10. Loss of sexual functioning is not a necessary consequence after cerebrovascular accident.

Questions for review

1. Discuss the implications of waiting until the client with cardiovascular disease asks about the sexual aspect of his or her chronic illness.

2. James Wilson, a 45-year-old executive, is currently in the coronary care unit where you are working. Today is the fourth day after his MI. During his bath he displays his genitals and constantly uses sexually provocative language. What inferences can you make about the reasons for his behavior?

3. How can you help him to maintain his dignity and image of himself as a man and yet eliminate the undesirable behavior simultaneously?

4. Mr. Wilson is almost ready to go home. What information will you make available to him regarding resumption of his preillness sexual activity (provided he is not in congestive failure)? What information should be shared with his wife?

5. Mr. Wilson returns to the cardiology clinic for a checkup 2 months after hospital discharge. How will you know whether he is physically able to tolerate sexual activity?

6. Mrs. Wilson seems constantly anxious about her husband's status. She makes certain that he has a chair in the clinic waiting room even though she must stand. At 6 months after discharge she will not let him drive and insists on taking him to work each day. What inferences might you make about the effects of this behavior on Mr. Wilson's self-concept? On their sexual activity?

7. William Jackson, a 45-year-old black man, comes to the hypertension clinic for a 6-month maintenance visit. He tells you he has had several episodes of impotence in the past month and attributes it to his age. What biologic variables will you need to assess? Which psychologic and sociologic variables?

8. Marion Lacy, a 40-year-old woman, tells you her antihypertensive medications are getting too expensive and that the medicine "doesn't make me feel differently." How do you proceed?

9. Mary Walker confides to you that her husband, who is in the hospital re-

covering from a stroke, would not ever mention it but will feel "less than a man" now. What further data do you need for assessment purposes? What information could you share with her about the sexual aspect of his rehabilitation? What could you share with both of them?

References

1. Barlett, R.G., Jr.: Physiologic responses during coitus, Journal of Applied Physiology **9:**469-472, 1956.
2. Bloch, A., Maeder, J.P., and Haissly, J.E.: Sexual problems after myocardial infarction, American Heart Journal **90:**536-537, 1975.
3. Cassem, N.H., and Hackett, T.P.: Psychiatric consultation in a coronary care unit, Annals of Internal Medicine **75:**9-14, July 1971.
4. Clausen, J.P., and Trap-Jensen, J.: Heart rate and arterial blood pressure during exercise in patients with angina pectoris: effects of training and nitroglycerine, Circulation **53:**436-442, 1976.
5. Cohen, B.D., Wallston, B.S., and Wallston, K.A.: Sex counseling in cardiac rehabilitation, Archives of Physical Medicine and Rehabilitation **57:**463-464, 1976.
6. Dawber, T.R., et al.: Risk factors: comparison of the biological data in myocardial and brain infarctions. In Zulch, K.J., et al., editors: Brain and heart infarct, New York, 1977, Springer-Verlag, New York, Inc.
7. Friedman, J.M.: Sexual adjustment of the post-coronary male. In Lo Piccolo, J., and Lo Piccolo, L., editors: Handbook of sex therapy, New York, 1978, Plenum Publishing Corp.
8. Goldbarg, A.N.: Energy cost of sexual activity, Archives of Internal Medicine, **126:**526, 1970.
9. Griffith, C.: Sexuality and the cardiac patient, Heart and Lung **2**(1):70-73, 1973.
10. Hellerstein, H.K., and Friedman, E.H.: Sexual activity of the postcoronary patient, Archives of Internal Medicine **125:**987-999, 1970.
11. Hott, J.: Sex and the heart patient: a nursing view, Topics in Clinical Nursing **1**(4):75-84, 1980.
12. Howard, E.J.: Sexual expenditure in patients with hypertensive disease, Medical Aspects of Human Sexuality **7:**82-92, Oct. 1973.
13. Johnston, B., et al.: Sexual activity in exercising patients after myocardial infarction and revascularization, Heart and Lung **7:**1026-1031, 1978.
14. Kalliomaki, J.L., Markkanen, T.K., and Mustonen, V.A.: Sexual behavior after CVA: a study on patients below the age of sixty years, Fertility and Sterility **12:**156-158, 1961.
15. Kavanagh, T., and Shepard, R.J.: Sexual activity after myocardial infarction, Canadian Medical Association Journal **116:**1250-1253, 1977.
16. Kushnir, B., et al.: Primary ventricular fibrillation and resumption of work, sexual activity, and driving after first acute myocardial infarction, British Medical Journal **4:**609-611, 1975.
17. Larson, J., et al.: Heart rate and blood pressure: responses of coronary artery disease patients during sexual activity and a two-flight stair climbing test, master's thesis, Seattle, 1978, University of Washington.
18. Malek, M.: Sudden coronary deaths associated with sexual activity, Journal of Forensic Sciences **24:**216-220, 1979.

19. Masters, W., and Johnson, V.: Human sexual response, Boston, 1966, Little, Brown & Co.
20. Masters, W., and Johnson, V.: Human sexual inadequacy, Boston, 1970, Little, Brown & Co.
21. Naughton, J.: Stress involved in masturbation vs. coitus, Medical Aspects of Human Sexuality 8:94, 1976.
22. Nemec, E., Mansfield, L., and Kennedy, J.: Heart rate and blood pressure responses during sexual activity in normal males, American Heart Journal 92:274-277, 1976.
23. Papadopoulos, C., et al.: Sexual concerns and needs of the post coronary patient's wife, Archives of Internal Medicine 140(1):38-41, 1980.
24. Reichgott, M.: Problems of sexual function in patients with hypertension, Cardiovascular Medicine 4(2):149-156, 1979.
25. Renshaw, D.: Stroke and sex. In Comfort, A.: Sexual consequences of disability, Philadelphia, 1978, George F. Stickley Co.
26. Satterfield, S.: Sexual rehabilitation for the postcoronary patient, Topics In Clinical Nursing 1(4):85-89, 1980.
27. Scalzi, C., and Dracup, C.: Sexual counseling of coronary patients, Heart and Lung 7:840-845, 1978.
28. Scheingold, L.D., and Wagner, N.: Sound sex and the aging heart, New York, 1974, Human Sciences Press, Inc.
29. Skelton, M., and Dominian, J.: Psychological stress in wives of patients with myocardial infarctions, British Medical Journal 2:101-103, April 1973.
30. Soloff, L.A.: Sexual activity in the heart patient, Psychosomatics 18(4):23-38, 1977.
31. Stein, R.A.: Coital positions for coronary patients, Medical Aspects of Human Sexuality 9:71-75, 1975.
32. Stein, R.A.: The effect of exercise training on heart rate during coitus, in the post myocardial infarction patient, Circulation 55:738-740, 1977.
33. Tuttle, W.B., Cook, W.L., and Fitch, E.: Sexual behavior in postmyocardial infarction patients, American Journal of Cardiology 13:140, 1964.
34. Ueno, M.: The so-called coition death, Japanese Journal of Legal Medicine 17:330-, 1963.
35. VanBree, N.: Sexuality, nursing practice and the person with cardiac disease, Nursing Forum 14:4, 1975.
36. Wagner, N., and Sivarajan, E.: Sexual activity and the cardiac patient. In Green, R., editor: Human sexuality: a health practitioner's text, ed. 2, New York, 1979, The Williams & Wilkins Co.
37. Watts, R.J.: Sexuality and the middle-aged cardiac patient, Nursing Clinics of North America 2:349-359, 1976.

Media

Sexuality and nursing concerns, Concept Media, 1500 Adams Avenue, Costa Mesa, CA 92626

- Sexual behavior: nursing reactions. *Discusses specific sexual behavior with which the nurse might be confronted in hospital setting.*
- Medical conditions: impact on sexuality. *Discusses how heart attack and diabetes can affect sexual functioning.*

17
Sexuality and renal disease

ROSA M. JOHNSON

As with any acute illness episode, acute renal failure undoubtedly affects sexual functioning; however, survival and treatment are the primary concerns with acute renal failure. In chronic renal failure, psychosocial concerns, including sexual functioning, become paramount and are the major causes of disability.[18,29,58] This discussion will therefore focus on sexual functioning concerns associated with chronic renal failure.

Eighty persons per 1 million population come to hospitals each year with chronic renal failure.[13] Chronic renal failure exists when the kidney is permanently diseased to the extent that it is unable to remove adequate amounts of the end products of metabolism, resulting in a toxic internal environment. This toxic state is called *uremia*. In the earlier stages of this broad, general disease category, dietary restrictions and medications may provide adequate management. As chronic renal failure progresses to the later, more severe stages, usually referred to as an end-stage renal disease (ESRD), death results from uremia and its complications unless dialysis or renal transplantation intervenes.[35]

In 1978, 35,000 clients with chronic renal failure were treated by maintenance dialysis, and by 1984 this number is predicted to be almost 60,000. Of these patients, 8% to 10% go on to have renal transplantation.[44,54]

The etiology of chronic renal failure includes may disorders, the most common of which are acute or rapidly progressive glomerulonephritis, pyelonephritis, polycystic kidney disease, diabetic glomerulosclerosis, severe hypertension, gout, lower urinary tract obstruction that results in hydronephrosis, nephrotoxic reactions, neoplasm, and congenital anomaly.[18,53]

Effects of chronic renal failure: an overview

Chronic renal failure produces a wide spectrum of stressors affecting the entire person, both in ways that are common to other chronic illness and in ways unique to chronic renal failure.[27] The stressors affect the physiologic, psychologic, social, financial, and sexual realms of the person's existence and functioning.

All body systems are affected by chronic renal failure. Carbohydrate, protein, and fat metabolism are interfered with, resulting in glucose intolerance, amino acid level abnormalities, and increased serum triglyceride levels.[18,53] Electrolyte imbalances occur, resulting in life-threatening states such as acidosis and hyperkalemia. Calcium-phosphorus imbalances may result in calcification of soft tissue or pathologic bone fractures. Anemia, coagulation defects, and hypertension inevitably occur. The uremia syndrome itself causes many symptoms within various systems. These symptoms include anorexia, vomiting, hiccups, hallucinations, irritability, inability to concentrate, muscle cramping, deafness, amenorrhea, electroencephalogram changes, prolongation of nerve conduction time, peripheral neuropathy, pericarditis, and pleuritis.[18,53] In addition, the person has weakness, lethargy, headache, confusion, restlessness, itching, drowsiness, and loss of libido.[11,47]

Sources of psychologic stressors for the person with chronic renal failure include both those that are inherent in any chronic illness and those that are more unique to this situation. A major source of psychologic stress is the change in body image. Body image can be defined as the mental picture one has of his or her body's appearance and functioning.[43] Even though the changes in the body and its functioning may not be as manifest in chronic renal failure as in situations such as limb amputation, the person with chronic renal failure perceives definite, permanent loss of functioning. When this person becomes involved in dialysis, as almost always occurs, an arteriovenous shunt or fistula is present, external bleeding occurs, weight fluctuates, frequently there is severe edema, skin color changes, and the body depends on a machine for its survival. These changes necessitate body image changes that frequently produce much anxiety.[4] Changing body image also affects the total self-image. Any alteration in the body is a disturbance of one's integrity and a threat to the self. Thus to lose a body part or its function is to be threatened with loss of self.[25] In a discussion of adaptation to dialysis and body image, Basch[8] states the following:

> The changes in external appearance, internal organs, and physiology are usually so profound and apparent that they intrude themselves on the patient's conscious life, forcing him to acknowledge to himself the physical alterations. The sudden or marked metabolic shifts from a previously familiar body state to an unknown and unpredictable physiological predicament also create not only a physical, but a psychological disequilibrium.

Other sources of psychologic stressors are the threat of the progressive course of this disease along with a fear of imminent death, the frequent hospitalization experiences with accompanying feelings of dehumanization and isolation, guilt over behavior imagined to be the cause of kidney disease, anger about having the illness, loss of the feelings of control and independence, and feelings of depression.[43]

The dietary restrictions that all clients with chronic renal failure encounter frequently limit oral gratification. Eating usually is a very positive experience emotionally, and its restriction causes much oral frustration.[6,16,32,42] Some clients find relief from dietary restrictions by occasionally eating prohibited food just before dialysis and/or by dialyzing for a longer time period.

Social stressors also result from chronic renal failure. Job loss or change, loss of mobility, changes in interpersonal relationships and social roles including changes within the family or significant others, loss of recreational activity, and status losses frequently occur and are stressful. In addition, the sick role for clients with chronic renal failure is different from that for many other illnesses in that clients must become knowledgeable about and participate actively in their own treatment, especially when they become involved in home dialysis. This contrasts with the usual sick role of the client being the passive, unquestioning recipient of the health team's care.[42]

Financial stressors are encountered by most clients with chronic renal failure. Strauss[51] states that chronic renal failure inevitably involves its victims in a dual crisis: physical and financial. The treatment regimen frequently involves hospitalization and leads eventually to dialysis and/or transplantation, with the majority of clients remaining on dialysis. The dialysis machine, supplies, and personnel necessary to sustain life cost from $15,000 to $25,000 per year.[53] Even though medicare and other health insurance programs now pay for the major costs of dialysis, additional uncovered expenses remain. In addition to the expenses of treatment, loss of pay from absenteeism, job change or loss caused by the inability to meet job requirements, and generally fewer hours in which the person can work add economic stress.[6]

Chronic renal failure and sexuality. Many clients with chronic illness experience a threat to sexual functioning. This is especially true for those clients with progressively deteriorating and debilitating diseases, since these diseases are likely to abolish sexual desire.[52] Chronic renal failure is one of these illnesses. Chronic or recurrent uremia with the lethargy, listlessness, and peripheral neuropathy accompanying it can produce a state of gross emotional maladjustment with depression and decrease or loss of libido.[25] Clients frequently experience a marked decrease in sexual drive and/or performance.[4]

Bailey's report of unpublished clinical studies suggests that the severity of uremia is associated with lower sexual desire and activity in clients with chronic renal failure. Both sexes seem equally affected even though the deficiency is more obvious in men because of requirements for performance and psychologic adjustment. In women ovulation and menstruation frequently cease, libido diminishes, and sex may become repulsive. In men testicles become soft and atrophic, spermatogenesis decreases, and plasma testosterone levels fall to those of castrate levels.[7] Men may become impotent.[19] Abram, who studied thirty-two male dialysis and kidney transplant clients, found that the frequency of intercourse for all clients before the onset of renal disease was 10.4 times per month, compared with 5.7 after the onset of renal disease. Fourteen clients (44%) reported a decrease in frequency of intercourse of 50% or more.[2] However, 20% reported no reduction in frequency of intercourse. Levy's questionnaire study[26] of 519 dialysis and transplant clients revealed that 40% of the men and 26% of the women noted worsening of sexual problems with progressive uremia before dialysis treatment.

Effects of maintenance dialysis

Chronic renal failure, or more specifically ESRD, leads to maintenance dialysis and/or kidney transplantation as treatment, with the majority of these clients remaining on maintenance dialysis because of the many difficulties involved in obtaining a suitable kidney donor and complications of the transplant surgery, including the problem of rejection. Dialysis refers to the use of an artificial kidney to separate soluble crystalline particles in a solution by diffusion through a semipermeable membrane. This process mimics the kidney's function of removal of waste products from the blood.[55] Since the artificial kidney cannot be used constantly, it is usually used three times per week for several hours at a time.[18]

Dialysis can be accomplished by either the peritoneal route or by direct access to the bloodstream through an arteriovenous shunt or fistula. Hemodialysis is usually the preferred method, since peritoneal dialysis is much less efficient and may have a higher rate of complications.[55] In this discussion maintenance dialysis refers to a program of regular hemodialysis.

Maintenance dialysis affects every body system and the total person in much the same way that chronic renal failure does, and although the artificial kidney in the dialysis process mimics the kidney, it in no way approximates normal kidney function. Dialysis only makes these clients feel better; it does not make them well, since the client undergoing maintenance dialysis is only in a state of controlled uremia.[4,18] Therefore many of the physiologic stressors outlined for the client with chronic renal failure continue. The extent to which they continue depends on many variables, including the degree of kidney failure, other body system(s) pathology, the frequency of dialysis, and adherence to the medical regimen.

The most common physiologic problems encountered are anemia and complications of the transfusions necessary to treat the anemia, including hepatitis, abnormal calcium and phosphorus metabolism resulting in osteodystrophy and its associated problems, neuropathy, elevated uric acid levels, peptic ulcer, constipation, ascites, insomnia, menstrual dysfunction, and infertility.[18] In addition, the dialysis process itself can produce physiologic stressors. Headache, weakness, fatigue, apathy, nausea, and emesis commonly occur during dialysis. Hypertension or hypotension may occur. Other cardiovascular problems that are frequent are congestive heart failure, arrhythmias, and chest pain. Muscle cramping and febrile reactions frequently accompany the dialysis process along with itching, restlessness, and mood changes.[18] In spite of the continuing physiologic problems with maintenance dialysis, life is extended; the laboratory blood values are more nearly normal, there is less physiologic disequilibrium, and the client does feel much better more of the time than when untreated.

The psychologic stressors as delineated for chronic renal failure continue for the client undergoing maintenance dialysis, with dialysis bringing more stressors. Initially there is the need to make a decision about which if any treatment modality is desired and acceptable to all concerned. In the past this process included careful scrutiny of clients by the health care team to see if they were acceptable for the treatment method chosen. If clients were accepted, they were usually elated, but they also frequently experienced guilt, since they may have been keeping someone else from living.[4] With the advent of medicare coverage for all those who need dialysis, along with adequate facilities for dialysis or transplantation, this stressor is now minimized or eliminated entirely. If clients choose to remain untreated and thereby choose death, conflict for all involved with the situation can result.

The ''machine'' (artificial kidney) usually is an additional source of stress. First, the client must learn how it works. Then there is the fear of malfunction with the threat of injury or death as a result.[6] Regardless of what is going on in the client's life, the machine must be used to sustain life. An ambivalent relationship often develops with the machine.

Clients have commented that it takes on its own personality, since it makes noises, has blinking lights, and seems to function differently on different days. Dialysis, in many ways, recreates a situation that is analogous to the early mother-child dependency in that the client must rely on "an external life support system, placenta-like, to clean the blood. It, at once, deprives the patient of independence but saves his or her life."[42]

This forced dependence on the artificial kidney brings to the fore dependence-independence conflicts. If the person is already dependent, placement in this position encourages regression and further dependency. However there are many expectations by the health care team and family members that the client be as independent as possible by continuing to work, take responsibility for home dialysis, and continue in usual social roles.[32,57]

The social and financial stressors already stated for the client with chronic renal failure usually remain and may even be intensified while the client is on a program of maintenance dialysis, or at least until adaptation occurs.

The stressors of chronic renal failure and maintenance dialysis enumerated thus far would seemingly tax clients beyond their ability to adjust or adapt.[4] In spite of these stressors 90% of long-term dialysis clients have a reasonably productive life.[23] Many clients describe their life as worthwhile and satisfying, and families feel they have had their relationships strengthened.[34] To deal with these stressors, clients use such psychologic defenses as denial, along with projection, displacement, isolation of affect, and reaction formation.[18,29,58]

Some maintenance dialysis clients do not adapt effectively. Anxiety, depression, and hostility are frequently observed continuing reactions along with the behaviors of "food kleptomania," excess water ingestion, and shunt or fistula neglect. Each of these can lead to death. Death caused by these reactions and behaviors is sometimes seen as "passive suicide."[18] A study involving 3478 renal dialysis clients demonstrated that the incidence of active suicide (obvious) direct actions by clients, such as overdosages and "binges" in which large amounts of restricted foods and fluids are ingested, is 100 times that of the general population.[2]

Buchanan and Abram[12] have categorized clients' adaptation as occurring in two phases: acute adaptation and chronic adaptation. Time periods for these phases are not delineated. In acute adaptation initial hope and confidence soon give way to anxiety and fear as the client realizes that real wellness will not occur. Social withdrawal and isolation commonly accompany this realization. Panic reactions are observed at times. The chronic adaptation phase begins as anxiety changes to realization of dialysis as a way of life. The primary psychologic reactions observed at this time are variations of depression and/or regression.[12] Levy[28] sees long-term adaptation being characterized by some degree of acceptance of the situation with all its stressors. Transition to this period is gradual and usually occurs in association with doing some meaningful work or acceptance of doing little or no work at all.

Dialysis and sexuality. Although there is disagreement about the cause of sexual dysfunction when clients are undergoing maintenance dialysis, there is agreement about the existence of sexual dysfunction. Table 17-1 summarizes the data available on sexual functioning in the presence of renal disease, including during uremic states without treatment, during maintenance dialysis, and after transplantation.

Abram[1] found that 78% of male dialysis and transplant clients had significantly diminished sexual functioning while undergoing maintenance dialysis. Levy[26] interviewed ten men and eight women. Six of the ten men reported a decrease in the frequency of sexual intercourse and impotence. Only one man reported little to no change in sexual activity. The women reported fewer sexual problems, although three had sexual intercourse less frequently and experienced fewer orgasms. Three of the women could not be evaluated because of the lack of an available partner. In his later study Levy found that maintenance dialysis clients of both sexes reported substantial deterioration of sexual functioning in comparison to their preuremic states. Men reported a decrease in frequency of intercourse and increased prevalence of impotence. Women reported a decrease in both frequency of intercourse and orgasm during sexual intercourse. It is of special significance that initiation and continuation of maintenance dialysis was associated with worsening of sexual functioning in 35% of the men and 24% of the women, as measured by frequency of intercourse, incidence of impotence, and/or orgasm during intercourse. Only 9% of the men and 6% of the women experienced improvement in sexual functioning while undergoing maintenance dialysis. Since sexual problems are caused by either physical and/or emotional factors, and overall physical improvement occurs with maintenance dialysis, Levy hypothesized that it is likely that emotional factors are of primary importance in the cause of sexual dysfunction in these clients.

In a recent study of maintenance dialysis clients Milne found that in comparison with the preuremic state, overall sexual satisfaction had decreased for four of the seven male and five of the eleven female clients. One man and three women reported an increase in their overall sexual satisfaction, whereas the remainder reported no change. Frequency of intercourse declined in ten clients, including five of the eleven women in the study. Sexual dysfunction, including erectile and ejaculation difficulties, decreased lubrication, a low level of arousal during sexual activity, and less frequent or absent orgasm, occurred for five of the seven men and seven of the eleven women. Four of the men experienced a decreased libido, one reported no change, and two reported an increased libido. Of the eleven women, six reported a decreased libido, and five experienced no change. Analysis of physical factors, medication, and depression showed no clear association with sexual dysfunction. Thus this study again suggests the importance of psychosocial factors in the sexual functioning of maintenance dialysis clients.[17,46]

Finkelstein and Steele[15] confirmed the high prevalence of sexual problems among dialysis clients. These problems included reduced frequency of intercourse and specific dysfunctional symptoms. Most of the men and nearly half of the women reported difficulty obtaining or maintaining excitement and difficulty achieving orgasm. After correlating sexual difficulties with duration of dialysis, depression, organicity and physical symptoms, they concluded that the cause of sexual dysfunction among dialysis clients is very difficult, if not impossible, to determine.

Eight women undergoing maintenance dialysis reported no significant difference in the frequency of sexual activity when comparing frequency after being on a program of maintenance dialysis with sexual frequency before chronic renal failure.[21] Four of the eight participants, however, reported a decrease in frequency of sexual activity, libido, and physical sensation during intercourse. The participants also reported psychosocial factors, rather than the effects of maintenance dialysis, as the important variables in the cause of change in sexual functioning.

Sherman's study[47] of impotence suggested that impotence is more frequent in the

Table 17-1. Sexual functioning in renal failure: effects of dialysis

Investigator	Year	Sample	Results
Levy	1973	515 individuals, total of 91% white, varied occupations represented; 343 men—and 287 on hemodialysis (3 modalities) and 56 transplant recipients; 172 women—142 on hemodialysis (3 modalities) and 30 transplant recipients	*Men* Overall decrease in intercourse frequency, compared to preillness levels; 55% (160) on dialysis considered themselves partially or totally impotent, compared to 15% (44) before uremia; 43% (24) transplant recipients considered themselves partially or totally impotent, compared to 13% (7) before uremia *Women* Overall decrease in intercourse frequency for women on dialysis as compared to preillness levels; overall decrease in orgasmic frequency for women on dialysis: 33% (47) orgasmic, compared to 63% (90) preillness; modality of hemodialysis had no effect on sexuality functioning; no consistent changes were noted in intercourse or orgasmic frequency for transplant recipients from preillness to current functioning
Abram	1975	32 men, mean age 41.5 years; average dialysis duration of 15.4 months	For all men, frequency of intercourse was 10.4 times per month before illness, 5.7 times per month after illness onset, 4.0 times per month during dialysis, and 7.5 times per month after transplant; 44% (14) reported reduced sexual activity after onset of illness; 34% (11) reported reduced sexual activity only after dialysis was instituted; 22% (7) reported no change in sexual activity during disease or dialysis; reasons given for decreased intercourse frequency

Author	Year	Sample	Findings
Sherman	1975	14 men, 23 to 53 years of age; average dialysis duration of 2 years	were decreased libido and difficulty with erection; 22% (3) maintained sexual activity as before illness onset; 39% (5) had decreased intercourse frequency during dialysis and remained unchanged after transplant; 39% (5) had decreased intercourse frequency during dialysis and reported increased intercourse frequency after transplant; 39% (5) were impotent and had been so for more than 1 year 50% were impotent
Karacan	1978	6 men with ESRD but without dialysis (group I); 5 men receiving dialysis (group II); 4 men after renal transplantation (group III)	Significant reduction in penile erectile capacity in groups I and II; no significant reduction in group III
Milne, Golden, and Fibus	1978	7 men and 11 women on dialysis	In comparison with preuremic state: 50% (9) sexual satisfaction decreased; 22% (4) sexual satisfaction increased; 28% (5) sexual satisfaction unchanged; 67% (12) dysfunction of sexual response; erectile and ejaculation difficulty for men; decreased orgasm, lubrication, and arousal for women; analysis of physical factors, medication, and depression showed no definitive etiology for sexual dysfunctions
Finkelstein and Steele	1978	54 men and 23 women receiving dialysis	65% (35) of men and 43% (10) of women had difficulty obtaining and maintaining sexual excitement; 39% (20) of men and 43% (10) of women had difficulty achieving orgasm; duration of dialysis, depression, organicity, and physical symptoms showed no clear correlation with sexual dysfunction difficulties

chronic dialysis group than in the general population. Half of the men in the study were impotent. All seven had prolonged nerve conduction and absent bulbocavernosus reflexes. Several of them exhibited clinical depression and low plasma testosterone levels.

Karacan[22] assessed nocturnal penile tumescence activity in men undergoing maintenance dialysis. In comparison to their control group there was a significant decrease in total tumescence time.

It has been noted by Hampers et al. that a period of adequate dialysis may restore ovulation and menstruation in women. However, there are only five reported cases of successful pregnancies in women undergoing maintenance dialysis.[19,36] In men testosterone levels tend to rise to the normal range, and potency may return. Atrophied testes and impaired spermatogenesis remain. There are, however, numerous reports of fertility in men undergoing maintenance dialysis.[19] Bailey[7] noted that within 30 to 60 days after the beginning of maintenance dialysis, true gynecomastia may develop in men. This condition is accompanied by a resurgence of sexual desire and potency.[7]

Lim et al.[33] investigated the role of gonadal dysfunction in the etiology of sexual dysfunction in male and female clients with chronic renal failure. They documented evidence of testicular and ovarian damage. Spermatogenesis was poor, and testosterone production was impaired in men; all the women were anovulatory. Dialysis did not improve either testicular or ovarian functioning. Despite abundant evidence of gonadal function deficiencies, it was not clear to what extent these aberrations were responsible for the prevalence of sexual dysfunction.

The role of other biologic etiologic factors is being explored. Antoniou and Shalhoul[5] have studied zinc deficiency, and Massry et al.[37] have investigated secondary hyperthyroidism.

Fears and misconceptions about the effects of dialysis on sexual functioning abound. Hickman[20] reported that one man believed his impotence occurred because his "sex hormones were dialyzed off." A woman thought she could discontinue all birth control measures, since she was indefinitely infertile. Renshaw[47] noted frequent concerns about transmission of renal disease through coitus, obtaining infection through coitus, sperm being unsafe or different, the occurrence of pregnancy, the normalcy of the baby if conception occurred, the effect of pregnancy on the female maintenance dialysis client, coitus being dangerous, fears that the indwelling cannula would come apart during sexual activity, and fears about the ability to perform sexually.

Although clients undergoing maintenance dialysis experience improvement in their overall physiologic condition as compared with their untreated state, many physiologic, psychologic, social, financial, and sexual stressors remain. As a result of these anxiety-producing stressors, there is much use of the adjustment technique of denial. Depression, which may lead to suicide, regression, and hostility, is a common psychologic reaction. In spite of the stressors, however, many maintenance dialysis clients are able to eventually reach an effective level of adaptation.

Effects of renal transplantation

In the last 20 years renal transplantation has become an accepted treatment for clients with ESRD. Renal transplantation, when successful, frees the client from dialysis, is less expensive, and can return the client to an essentially normal life. When the kidney functions well, the recipient experiences rapid recovery and initially experiences euphoria, some of which may be a result of corticosteroids.[10]

Renal transplantation presents yet another set of stressors. Clients awaiting transplant from cadavers often have difficulty waiting for a suitable match. Those receiving a kidney from a relative may have much conflict about accepting such a gift.[10] While waiting for the transplant, they are receiving maintenance dialysis and are experiencing the stressors already delineated. After transplantation, conflicts in relation to the donor may continue. Time is needed for incorporation of the new kidney into the body image.[10]

Most transplant recipients experience major stress related to fear of acute and chronic rejection, complications of corticosteroid therapy, and the adjustment of becoming independent. Fear of rejection is probably never completely eradicated. Rejection means pain and more hospitalization along with a return to dialysis, a previously rejected treatment. Corticosteroids in large doses over long time periods to prevent rejection may first cause euphoria and then depression and/or other emotional and mental problems. In addition, corticosteroids cause cosmetic problems and vulnerability to infections, neoplastic diseases, and bony avascular necrosis.[10,13,31] Successful transplantation results in the expectation that the individual give up the sick role and become independent. This adjustment may be difficult in any situation. Clients who have undergone transplants frequently encounter the additional complication of having to give up the governmental health care benefits that they have undoubtedly become eligible for as their resources were depleted with uremia and dialysis. Since they still need frequent medical supervision, they may find that their income from employment does not make up for the benefits lost. Thus, for many, the sick role is more profitable financially.[10,13]

As with maintenance dialysis clients, denial is a commonly used mechanism to cope with the stressors of transplantation. Excessive use of denial may result in exaggerated reports of well-being with failure to describe significant symptoms. Those with unrealistic expectations who become disillusioned tend to give up and die from failure to comply with the treatment regimen.[10,13]

Many do adapt successfully. Sophie and Powers' study[49] of satisfaction with life after transplantation showed that the twenty-four subjects in the study felt significantly more satisfaction with life than during the dialysis period, expected even more satisfaction in the future, and were as satisfied as before chronic renal failure occurred.

Renal transplantation and sexuality. Even though successful renal transplantation leads to much improvement in the client's well-being, sexual dysfunction problems continue for many (Table 17-2). A small percentage of men and women experience improvement in sexual functioning after transplantation,[1,29,46] and a few return to their preillness level of sexual activity.[48] Some actually experience a deterioration in sexual functioning.[29] One investigation revealed gender differences. Whereas men experienced a significant increase in the frequency of intercourse, sexual interest, and satisfaction with sexual performance, women found a decline in the frequency of intercourse and no change in sexual interest. There was actually an increase in the number of women who identified themselves as having a sexual problem.[46] After transplantation all nine men in a study of gonadal dysfunction by Lim et al.[33] had an improvement in testicular function as plasma testosterone levels were normalized, but sperm counts moved toward normal in only five of the men. In contrast to the previous findings, Karacan's investigation[22] of the involvement of erectile function of four males after transplantation

Table 17-2. Incidence of impaired sexual functioning in renal failure: effects of transplantation

Investigator	Year	Sample	Results
O'Brien et al.	1975	20 male transplant recipients, mean age 42.5 years	75% (15) still had nocturnal or early morning erections; 25% (5) reported no change in sexual activity at any time since illness onset; 75% (15) noted decreased intercourse frequency during dialysis; 56% (11) noted improvement in sexual functioning after transplantation
Salvatierra et al.	1975	94 men, age range 20 to 60 years	Significant decrease in frequency of intercourse after onset of renal failure, with additional significant increase to near preillness level after transplantation; 66% had intercourse one or more per week preillness; 22% had intercourse once or more per week during renal failure; 47% had intercourse once or more per week after transplantation
Levy	1977	69 men after renal transplantation	In comparison with sexual functioning on dialysis: 35% (24) experienced improved sexual functioning after transplantation; 13% (9) experienced worsened sexual functioning after transplantation; 29% (20) experienced no change after transplantation; 22% (16) not sure
		31 women after renal transplantation	26% (8) experienced improved sexual functioning after transplantation; 16% (5) experienced worsened sexual functioning after transplantation; 36% (11) experienced no change; 22% (7) not sure
Procci	1978	20 men and 17 women with renal transplantation	In comparison to dialytic state: *Men:* significant increase in frequency of sexual intercourse, sexual interest, and satisfaction with sexual performance; *Women:* no significant difference between dialytic and posttransplantation state but significant decline in frequency of intercourse when compared with preuremic state; 35% nonorgasmic during intercourse at least 50% of the time

showed no significant difference in the total nocturnal penile tumescence time between these clients and groups of men with ESRD with and without dialysis.

Overall, the general effect of transplantation on sexual functioning tends to be positive, especially for men. A significant number, however, do not experience alleviation of sexual dysfunction, and in some there is continued deterioration. A number of etiologic factors are probably involved. Antihypertensive agents that are commonly used to control blood pressure are suspect in contributing to sexual dysfunction. Alpha-methyldopa and guanethidine are associated wtih erectile failure and retrograde ejaculation, respectively.[13,24,46] Psychosocial stressors associated with maintenance dialysis are also thought to contribute extensively to sexual functioning problems after transplantation.*

Assessment and intervention

Assessment of the sexual health of the client with chronic renal failure should proceed generally in the same manner as for any sexual health assessment.

Because a methodology to determine definitive causes of sexual dysfunction secondary to the complications of chronic renal failure has not been established, even the most thorough assessment will only narrow the field of probable etiologic variables that need to be addressed in the intervention plan. However, an accurate assessment for clients with chronic renal failure must include knowledge of deviations in the physiologic status consequent to the renal failure. Measurement of nocturnal penile tumescence can help to diagnose organic versus psychologic causes. In addition, assessment of current and historic sexual self-concept, genital sexual functioning, sexual activity, sex drive, sexual satisfaction, sexual relationships, emotional adjustment, and mental status must be included in the data base.[9,22,40,56]

At present there are no effective medical treatment measures for sexual dysfunction in clients with chronic renal failure, since there are no definitive causes known. Based on gonadal endocrinologic studies, therapeutic measures used on a trial basis have included clomiphene citrate, bromocriptine, and zinc supplementation. All have improved endogenous gonadal hormonal production, but the effect on spermatogenesis and ovulation has not been established.[5] Until further investigation confirms etiologic factors, related treatment strategies cannot be recommended.[13,24]

The most effective intervention strategy at this time probably is the multidisciplinary treatment team, who can integrate the requisite physiologic deviation information with psychosocial skills and provide sex education, sex counseling, and sex therapy with a strong rehabilitation focus. The rehabilitation focus recognizes that functional losses may be permanent and deals with these by capitalizing on the remaining strengths.†

In one of the few programs reported in the literature McKevitt[40] has provided a model of such an approach. This program demonstrated an assessment and intervention process using the framework of Masters and Johnson.[38,39] The assessment phase included a series of interviews with the client and sexual partner. Areas assessed were those just outlined. A final assessment session was held with the couple to share conclusions and suggest

*References 9, 10, 13, 22, 24, 30, 31, 33, 40, and 46.
†References 9, 17, 24, 28, 40, and 41.

treatment approaches. Intervention approaches frequently included further nephrologist consultation to review antihypertensive medications and overall physiologic status, consultation with a psychiatrist when marked psychiatric symptoms were present, and a behavior modification program to deal with the most common problems of orgasmic dysfunction and secondary impotence.[40] A systematic evaluation of such an approach has not been reported.

Golden and Milne[17] suggest that counseling about sexuality be provided within the context of an ongoing, routine, educationally oriented counseling program in which a variety of issues with less emotional impact are discussed. Many clients will benefit a great deal from realizing the incidence of sexual dysfunction in clients with chronic renal failure and from understanding the potential causes of sexual dysfunction. This may reduce their perceptions of themselves as inadequate.

Studies have shown that many clients with chronic renal failure experience depression. Since sexual dysfunction frequently accompanies depression, appropriate psychotherapy and/or antidepressant medication should be obtained when depression is diagnosed. A trial of antidepressant medication is definitely indicated when the depressive syndrome is initially diagnosed as a primary depressive illness. Tricyclic antidepressants are metabolized in the liver and thus can be safely administered to these clients.[13]

Until further information is available on both the etiology of and interventions for sexual dysfunction in these clients, sex counseling, sex education, and commonly accepted sex therapy methods may increase communication between client and partner, decrease anxiety, lessen depression, raise self-esteem, and introduce or reinforce options to obtain sexual satisfactions. These changes will improve the overall quality of life.

Summary

1. Chronic renal failure produces a wide spectrum of stressors affecting every body system and the entire person, including sexual functioning.

2. Whether defined as reduced frequency of sexual activity or as specific dysfunction symptoms, there is a high incidence of sexual dysfunction in clients with chronic renal failure. This high incidence occurs in clients with untreated uremia, those undergoing maintenance dialysis, and those who have had transplants.

3. To date, research has identified only a few biologic factors that may be implicated and a greater number of psychologic and social factors that probably are implicated in the cause of sexual dysfunction in chronic renal failure.

4. No intervention(s) has been identified that will return the majority of these clients to their preillness level of sexual functioning.

5. After thorough assessment and manipulation of biologic variables when possible, a counseling approach by a multidisciplinary team that integrates sex education, sex counseling, and sex therapy as appropriate for the individual client and partner is probably the

most used and effective way to deal with the sexual dysfunction
problems experienced by clients with chronic renal failure.

Questions for review

1. Harold Brown, a 35-year-old father of three, has come to the satellite center
   for his maintenance dialysis. He has not been able to go back to his job
   because of the time required for dialysis. What other variables could you
   assess to discover if he is experiencing other role changes? What implications
   might this have on his concept of himself as a man?
2. When you next see Angela, Harold's wife, she says that Harold is rarely
   interested in her sexually. How can you assess the effect of Harold's behavior
   on her self-image? What information would you be able to give her?
3. What further information would you need from Harold to assess organic
   dysfunction?
4. Angela mentions that she is relieved not to worry about birth control. How
   will you respond?

References

1. Abram, H.S.: Sexual activity and renal failure. In Villarreal, H., editor:
   Proceedings of the Fifth International Congress of Nephrology, Mexico,
   vol. 3, Basel, Switz., 1974, Karger.
2. Abram, H.S., Moore, G.L., and Westervelt, F.B.: Suicidal behavior in
   chronic dialysis patients, American Journal of Psychiatry **127:**1199-1204,
   1971.
3. Abram, H.S., et al.: Sexual functioning with chronic renal failure, Journal
   of Nervous and Mental Disease **160:**220-226, 1975.
4. Anger, D.: The psychologic stress of chronic renal failure and long-term
   hemodialysis, Nursing Clinics of North America **10:**449-460, 1975.
5. Antoniou, L.D., and Shalhoub, R.J.: Zinc in the treatment of impotence
   in renal failure, Dialysis and Transplantation **7:**912-915, 1978.
6. Bahn, M.A.: Maslow's hierarchy of needs as a framework for care of the
   end stage renal disease client, Journal of American Association of Nephrology Nurses and Technicians **3:**163-168, 1976.
7. Bailey, G.L.: The sick kidney and sex, New England Journal of Medicine
   296:1289-1299, 1977.
8. Basch, S.: Adaptation to dialysis and body image. In Villarreal, H., editor:
   Proceedings of the Fifth International Congress of Nephrology, Mexico,
   vol. 3, Basel, Switz., 1974, Karger.
9. Berkman, A.H.: Sex counseling with hemodialysis patients, Dialysis and
   Transplantation **7:**924-927+, 1978.
10. Brundage, D.J.: Nursing management of renal problems, ed. 2, St. Louis,
    1980, The C.V. Mosby Co.
11. Brunner, L.S., and Suddarth, D.S.: The Lippincott manual of nursing
    practice, ed. 3, Philadelphia, 1982, J.B. Lippincott Co.
12. Buchanan, D.C., and Abram, H.S.: Psychological adaptation to hemodi-
    alysis, Dialysis and Transplantation **5**(2):36-42, 1976.
13. Chatterjee, S.N., editor: Renal transplantation: an interdisciplinary ap-
    proach, New York, 1980, Raven Press.

14. Finkelstein, F.O., and Steele, T.E.: First Japanese baby delivered of mother in dialysis, Medical Tribune **19**(5):2, 1978.

15. Finkelstein, F.O., and Steele, T.E.: Sexual dysfunction and chronic renal failure: a psychosocial study of 77 patients, Dialysis and Transplantation **7**:877-878 + , 1978.

16. Garron, M.S.: The adjustment period: coping with the diet, Journal of American Association of Nephrology Nurses and Technicians **3**(1):42-45, 1976.

17. Golden, J.S., and Milne, J.F.: Somatopsychic sexual problems of renal failure, Dialysis and Transplantation **7**:879-890, 1978.

18. Gutch, C.F., and Stoner, M.: Review of Hemodialysis for Nurses and Dialysis Personnel, ed. 4, St. Louis, 1983, The C.V. Mosby Co.

19. Hampers, C., et al.: Long-term hemodialysis, ed. 2, New York, 1973, Grune & Stratton, Inc.

20. Hickman, B.W.: All about sex . . . despite dialysis, American Journal of Nursing **77**:606-607, 1977.

21. Johnson, R.M.: Sexual function of adult females with chronic renal failure on maintenance dialysis, unpublished master's thesis, Seattle, 1979, University of Washington.

22. Karacan, I.: Assessment of nocturnal penile tumescence as on objective method for evaluating sexual functioning in ESRD patients, Dialysis and Transplantation **7**:872-876, 1978.

23. Kintzel, K.C.: Advanced concepts in clinical nursing, ed. 2, New York, 1977, J.B. Lippincott Co.

24. Kolodny, R.C., et al.: Textbook of human sexuality for nurses, Boston, 1979, Little, Brown & Co.

25. Leonard, B.J.: Body image changes in chronic illness, Nursing Clinics of North America **7**:687-695, 1975.

26. Levy, N., editor: Living or dying: adaptation to hemodialysis, Springfield, Ill., 1974, Charles C Thomas, Publisher.

27. Levy, N.: The problem of being a patient on maintenance hemodialysis. In Villarreal, H., editor: Proceedings of the Fifth International Congress of Nephrology, Mexico, vol. 3, Basel, Switz., 1974, Karger.

28. Levy, N.: Psychological studies at the Downstate Medical Center of patients on hemodialysis, Medical Clinics of North America **61**:759-769, 1977.

29. Levy, N.: Letter to the editor, New England Journal of Medicine **297**:725-726, 1977.

30. Levy, N.: Sexual factors and rehabilitation, Dialysis and Transplantation **7**:591-594, 1978.

31. Levy, N.: The effects of psychosocial factors in the rehabilitation of "The Artificial Man," Dialysis and Transplantation **8**:213-216, 1979.

32. Levy, N.B., and Wynbrandt, G.D.: The quality of life on maintenance hemodialysis, Lancet **1**:1328-1330, 1975.

33. Lim, V.S., et al.: Gonadal dysfunction in chronic renal failure: an endocrinologic review, Dialysis and Transplantation **7**:901-907, 1978.

34. MacElveen, P.M., Hoover, P., and Alexander, R.A.: Patient outcome success related to cooperation among patient, partner, and physician, Journal of the American Association of Nephrology Nurses and Technicians **2**:148-156, 1974.

35. Marshall, J.R.: Problems of a chronic renal failure patient on peritoneal dialysis: a systems approach, unpublished master's thesis, Seattle, 1972, University of Washington.
36. Marwood, R.P., et al.: Plasma estrogens in a pregnancy associated with chronic hemodialysis, British Journal of Obstetrics and Gynecology **84:**613-617, 1977.
37. Massry, S.G., et al.: Impotence in patients with uremia: a possible role for parathyroid hormone, Dialysis and Transplantation **7:**916-923, 1978.
38. Masters, W.H., and Johnson, V.E.: Human sexual response, Boston, 1966, Little, Brown & Co.
39. Masters, W.H., and Johnson, V.E.: Human sexual inadequacy, Boston, 1970, Little, Brown & Co.
40. McKevitt, P.M.: Role of the nephrology social worker in treating sexual dysfunction, Dialysis and Transplantation **7:**928-937 +, 1978.
41. Milne, J.F., Golden, J.S., and Fibus, L.: Sexual dysfunction in renal failure: a survey of chronic hemodialysis patients, International Journal of Psychiatry in Medicine **8:**335-344, 1977.
42. Moore, G.L.: Psychiatric aspects of chronic renal disease, Postgraduate Medicine **60:**140-146, 1976.
43. Murray, R.L.E.: Foreword: symposium on the concept of body image, Nursing Clinics of North America **7:**593-594, 1972.
44. Najarian, J.S., and Ascher, N.L.: Renal transplantation: current trends in high risk patients, Dialysis and Transplantation **8:**164-166, 1979.
45. O'Brien, K.M., et al.: Sexual dysfunction in uremia, Proceedings of the Dialysis Transplant Forum **5:**98-101, 1975.
46. Procci, W.R.: Persistent sexual dysfunction following renal transplantation, Dialysis and Transplantation **7:**891-894, 1978.
47. Renshaw, D.C.: Sexual function and renal dialysis, Journal of Sex Education and Therapy **2**(1):47-50, 1976.
48. Salvatierra, O., et al.: Sexual function in males before and after renal transplantation, Urology **5:**64-66, 1975.
49. Sherman, F.P.: Impotence in patients with chronic renal failure on dialysis: its frequency and etiology, Fertility and Sterility **26:**221-223, 1975.
50. Sophie, L.R., and Powers, M.J.: Life satisfaction and social function: post transplant self-evaluation, Dialysis and Transplantation **8:**1198-1202, 1979.
51. Strauss, A.L.: Chronic illness and the quality of life, St. Louis, 1975, The C.V. Mosby Co.
52. Wahl, C.W., editor: Sexual problems, New York, The Free Press.
53. What happens in kidney failure. Nursing '77 **7**(10):51-52, 1977.
54. Wineman, R.J.: End stage renal disease: 1978, Dialysis and Transplantation **7:**1034-1037 +, 1978.
55. Wing, A.J., and Magowan, M.: The renal unit, Philadelphia, 1975, J.B. Lippincott Co.
56. Woods, N.F.: Human sexuality in health and illness, ed. 2, St. Louis, 1979, The C.V. Mosby Co.
57. Wright, L.F.: Maintenance hemodialysis, Boston, 1981, G.K. Hall & Co.
58. Wright, R.G., Sand, P., and Livingston, G.: Psychological stress during hemodialysis for chronic renal failure, Annals of Internal Medicine **64:**611-621, 1966.

18

Sexuality and diabetes

MARILYN WHITLEY and PATRICIA BERKE

Sexual dysfunction in diabetic men

Impotence

Incidence. In 1958 Rubin and Babbott[35] reported the first major investigation concerning the incidence of erectile dysfunction in diabetic men. In the process of interviewing women in the gynecologic clinic they found some women who reported that their husbands were impotent. Further inquiry revealed that many of the men had diabetes mellitus. This study revealed a surprisingly high incidence of impotence associated with diabetes. Among 198 diabetic men (from 16 to 92 years of age), impotence occurred at an earlier age and more frequently than it did among the 4108 nondiabetic men studied by Kinsey during the 1940s.[21] From the age of 35 years onward, the cumulative incidence of impotence among the diabetic population was two to five times higher than among the Kinsey male population.

Of the men with diabetes of less than 1 year's duration, 70% suffered from erectile dysfunction (mean age 50.7 years). Of those who had had diabetes of 1 to 5 years' duration, 43% were impotent (mean age 57.8 years). It was postulated that the high incidence of impotence among the men who were diagnosed less than a year earlier might be attributed to the possibility that their disease was not yet under control. Many of the men reported that their impotence disappeared when their diabetes stabilized. However, those who became impotent while their disease was well controlled found that it persisted, usually permanently. Of all those who became impotent, 30% did so within 1 year of the clinical diagnosis of diabetes; 60% developed impotence within 5 years of the onset of their diabetes.

In the Rubin and Babbott study[35] no relationship was disclosed between the age at onset of diabetes or the severity of the disease and the incidence of impotence. Other complications of diabetes were no more frequent among impotent diabetic men than among those who were not impotent. However, poor control of diabetes was associated with transient periods of impotence. In addition, there appeared to be no higher incidence of impotence among these men before the clinical onset of their diabetes than among the

Kinsey population. Most of the impotent men stated that libido persisted for some time after they were unable to have coitus. However, 53% had no morning erections after they became impotent.

Klebanow and MacLeod[22] postulated in their 1960 investigation that ejaculatory dysfunction resulting from a failure of ejaculatory process was often a progressive phenomenon among diabetic men. By analyzing the semen quality of nineteen men, they found nine men who produced no seminal fluid externally in spite of normal orgasmic sensation. Spermatozoa were found in the urine of six men but not in the quantity usually associated with retrograde ejaculation. The duration of diabetes in all the men studied was more than 12 years.

In 1963 Schoffling et al.[40] reported that 51% (160 diabetic men) of a sample of 314 men had observed disturbances in sexual functioning. The predominant complaint was erectile dysfunction. Of the men experiencing impotence, 48% reported no decrease in libido. The known mean duration of diabetes was 9.3 years among the impotent group, compared to 4.3 years among the nonimpotent group.

In 1963 Greene, Panayotis, and Weeks[15] reported cases of ejaculatory dysfunction. They reported case studies of four men with diabetes, with a duration since onset ranging from 6 months to 29 years, who were plagued with retrograde ejaculation of semen into the bladder. All four of these men had neuropathy associated with diabetes. Two of the men also experienced erectile dysfunction.

In 1977 Whitehouse[46] reported a case study that demonstrated a gradual progression to the ejaculatory dysfunction of retrograde ejaculation. Potency remained intact, but absence of semen in ejaculate with intercourse or masturbation indicated a probable loss of semen via the bladder. The man studied had a 7-year duration of diabetes. All of these research studies continue to affirm the early studies that diabetic men have a higher rate of sexual dysfunction than their healthier nondiabetic counterparts.

      Etiology. The mechanism for impotence in diabetes becomes clearer over time. Two main mechanisms have been suggested: decreased androgenic function and diabetic neuropathy with pelvic involvement. Belief in endocrine theories is waning as more evidence of neurologic dysfunction is obtained through postmortem and other tissue study.[36]

Previous theories about the cause of diabetic impotence have included testicular atrophy and poor nutrition. Calcification in the walls of the vas deferens has been associated with diabetes and has been implicated, since the entire smooth muscle of the reproductive tract was involved and therefore responsible for both the progressive erectile and ejaculatory dysfunction. Schoffling et al.[40] reported findings of impairment of pituitary gonadotropic function in their study, in which 51% of the 314 men studied complained of erectile dysfunction. However, Faerman et al.[10] reported normal androgenic function in their study of seven impotent diabetic men.

In 1974 Faerman et al.[9] reported the first study of the autonomic nervous system in the penile corpora cavernosa of five impotent diabetic men. The men had a mean age of 51 and a diabetes duration of 9.6 years. Although the sample size was small, the study of the nerve fibers during autopsy revealed morphologic alterations in four of the five men. On this basis Faerman et al. drew support for the thesis that impotence in diabetic men is caused by diabetic neuropathy.

This thesis is supported repeatedly in the literature. McCulloch et al.[31] surveyed 541 diabetic men attending an Edinburgh outpatient department, representing 61% of the male clinic population aged 20 to 59 years. Data were collected by means of a detailed questionnaire, and retinopathy and neuropathy were documented through physical and laboratory analysis. Diabetic control was assessed by averaging the 2-hour postprandial glucose estimates from the previous clinic visits. Presence of impotence was assessed by self-report of erectile difficulties in the last 6 months. McCulloch et al. showed that 35% of the 541 diabetic men studied were impotent. They demonstrated that diabetic impotence was associated with age, treatment with insulin, retinopathy, peripheral neuropathy, and autonomic neuropathy. Furthermore, they found that impotence was associated with duration of diabetes, ischemic heart disease, nephropathy, and poor diabetic control. This is the first study that compared nonimpotent diabetic men with impotent diabetic men in an attempt to ascertain the prevalence of diabetic impotence in a diabetic clinic population.

The more recent laboratory studies in the vascular and neurologic areas seem most helpful in understanding the cause of diabetic impotence. The recently developed techniques of measuring penile tumescence and blood pressure have allowed researchers to report more exact findings. Abelson[1] used Doppler ultrasound to demonstrate the pressure of penile hypotension in three of the fifteen impotent diabetic men he studied. Through the use of spectroscopic techniques, Gaskell[14] was able to reveal vascular obstruction in seven of the eight impotent diabetic men known to have peripheral vascular disease. Postmortem studies, such as that done by Ruzbarsky and Michal,[36] allow the use of microscopic techniques to study the arterial tree of the penis. Their studies showed accelerated fibrotic changes in the Ebner pads (thought to act as valves during erection) in the fifteen diabetic men in their sample of thirty men over 38 years of age.

The 1979 study by Meiman[32] of insulin-dependent men demonstrated a marked reduction of norepinephrine present in the study group's erectile tissue. He hypothesized that these findings suggest impairment of the sympathetic nerves of the penis. Finally, Karacan[18] monitored nocturnal tumescence in thirteen diabetic men and demonstrated the presence of some erectile ability. Although he was able to demonstrate abnormally low nocturnal penile tumescence and penile blood pressure in the diabetic group, only one had no nocturnal penile tumescence. His studies suggested that nine of the thirteen clients studied had a neural impairment and five a vascular impairment, although in four clients both may have been operant.

Treatment. Since the ability to be sexually potent is so closely connected to the male ego, the importance of good differential history cannot be underestimated when assessing and proposing treatment for impotence in men. The history may reveal the presence of erections with masturbation or early morning awakening, indicating a psychologic component to the dysfunction. Waxberg[43] reports two case studies showing the importance of assessing the presence of even a small amount of tumescence. Both cases showed long-standing impotence in diabetic men related to the lack of attraction to their wives. These men were greatly defended by psychologic mechanisms yet had some nocturnal tumescence. Treatment using sex therapy methods reversed what was thought to be permanent impotence.

Diabetic men suffering from other chronic or acute diseases may also be taking medication that impairs sexual functioning. Overuse of alcohol may also interfere with potency (see Chapter 22). Before final assessment is made, offensive drugs need to be eliminated, the diabetes controlled through diet and insulin or oral hypoglycemic drugs, excessive drinking of alcohol reduced, reasonable exercise begun, and sexual counseling instituted. The counseling needs to include sexual information, information about the aging process, and also content about the human need for intimacy and noncoital ways it can be achieved.[25]

Diabetic men who do not achieve potency by any means and who have markedly reduced penile blood pressure and tumescence may be candidates for a penile prosthesis. There are two kinds of prostheses: inflatable or a more rigid, permanently erect silicone rod. Clients need to be carefully selected and advantages and disadvantages of each kind considered before attempting implantation.[13,25,33]

One type of semirigid prosthesis is a device by which a pair of silicone rods are inserted into the crus of the corpus cavernosum of the penis (Small-Carrion). There are two other adjustable semirigid implants. The Finney prosthesis is hinged, and the Jones prosthesis is a device containing flexible silver rods. These can be implanted with the client under local anesthesia, require that the client stay only a short time in the hospital, and are not considered an expensive form of treatment.

There are a few disadvantages to these types of prostheses. They are always semierect, and therefore some adjustment in clothing is necessary to hide the device. Semirigid prostheses also do not expand in width or fullness during intercourse. Occasionally the flexible type has "buckled" during intercourse. Semirigid prostheses do present an added difficulty when treating urinary infections and prostatic dysfunctions. However, only 1% of the semirigid devices cause damage to the penis and must be removed.[45]

The inflatable device has the advantage of being totally undetectable in an ordinarily clothed man. Fluid is stored in a container in the abdomen and is propelled via a pump implanted in the scrotum as a third testicle into plastic storage tubes installed in the penis. This allows the penis a natural appearing change from limp to rigid.

The disadvantage of this prosthesis is that it sometimes has mechanical failures. The mechanical problems are usually easy to repair, and although annoying, they happen in only about 10% of men with implants. The procedure for installing this prosthesis is more costly and complicated and requires a 5- to 7-day hospital stay. Overall, however, couples report an 89% satisfaction rate with the inflatable penis implant.[13]

The need for careful assessment of clients before implantation is of utmost importance. Clients with severe physical and mental illnesses, as well as those with complicated marital discord, are not good candidates for this surgery. People with antisocial and borderline personality disorders are also not recommended for this form of treatment. Depression and grief reactions need to be fully treated before the implantation is attempted.

Clients need educational and psychologic preparation before surgery. This is best accomplished with both members of the sexual dyad. Clinics such as the Mayo Clinic that install a number of penile prostheses a year recommend careful sexual history taking for the screening out of other common treatable sexual dysfunctions. They also recommend the correction of misinformation about sexual functioning and the nature of impotence before the surgery. Postoperative care includes demonstration of the device installed both to the client and his partner within 2 to 3 postoperative days. Follow-up is necessary to assure the client and the health team that everything is working properly.[13]

Sterility and fertility. Although there are no known effects of diabetes on the ovaries and testes, certain complications of the disease appear to interfere with reproduction. Babbott, Rubin, and Ginsburg[2] interviewed 167 randomly selected diabetic men and compared them with a control group of nondiabetic men. The populations were similar with respect to number of conceptions, premature births, stillbirths, livebirths, sex ratio of offspring, and birth weights. Although the wives of diabetic men had a significantly greater incidence of spontaneous abortions than the wives of the control group, the authors concluded that there was no evidence to support the theory that children of diabetic men differed discernibly at birth from those of other men.

Klebanow and MacLeod[22] considered the potential fertility of 28 men between 20 and 57 years of age who had been clinically supervised for diabetes mellitus between 1 and 22 years. They found that semen quality in diabetic men controlled with insulin did not indicate serious disturbances in spermatogenesis when ejaculation was present. In half the subjects somewhat diminished sperm motility was noted. Ejaculatory dysfunction was documented; one third of the group was under good diabetic control but had completely lost ejaculatory function. Some men reported a gradual decrease in ejaculatory volume during the years in which they were being treated for diabetes. The average duration of recognized diabetes in this group was 18 years.

Schoffling et al.[40] studied endocrine changes in diabetic men with erectile impotence. Two thirds of these men had decreased urinary levels of gonadotropin. Urinary levels of 17-ketosteroids were elevated, but the fraction containing metabolites of testosterone was decreased (one third of the men in this series had low sperm counts; one half had low amounts of fructose in the semen, which indicated androgen deficiency). Testicular biopsies in 24 men demonstrated thickening of the basement membrane in the tubules and abnormal spermatogenesis. Some of the men under 40 years of age who were treated with a combination of chorionic gonadotropin and testosterone later fathered a child.

Sexual dysfunction in diabetic women

Until 1971 there were no studies that described sexual dysfunction in diabetic women. At that time Kolodny[24] reported a study of 125 hospitalized women between the ages of 18 and 42 with previously diagnosed diabetes mellitus. A control group of 100 nondiabetic women was also studied. All the women were white and were hospitalized at the time of the study. Only women who had had coitus during the previous year were included in the sample. A modified version of Masters and Johnson's sexual history was used to collect data. Orgasmic dysfunction was defined as absence of orgasm from any source within the preceding 12 months.

Orgasmic dysfunction was significantly more prevalent among the diabetic women than among the control group. Forty-four (35.2%) of the diabetic women and six (6%) of the nondiabetic women were nonorgasmic. None of the nonorgasmic women in the control group had ever experienced orgasm. Forty of the forty-four nonorgasmic diabetic women, however, previously had been orgasmic. The diabetic women gradually became nonorgasmic over the course of 6 months to 1 year. In all women orgasmic dysfunction followed the onset of diabetes. There was no significant relationship between sexual dysfunction and other complications of diabetes.

Six of the forty-four nonorgasmic diabetic women and all of the nonorgasmic women in the control group reported difficulty with vaginal lubrication. Two of the diabetic women became orgasmic after use of an artificial lubricant and instruction to the couple. Chronic candidal vaginitis caused pain and interfered with orgasm in two diabetic women. One of the women returned to orgasmic functioning after appropriate therapy for candidal infection. Of the four diabetic women who had never been orgasmic, rigid antisexual attitudes developed during childhood were variables for two. The other two women expressed strong negative feelings about their marital partners.

Kolodny[24] concluded that increased incidence of sexual dysfunction among diabetic women was not surprising. He further suggested that a variety of etiologic factors might be involved, including neuropathy, susceptibility to infection, microvascular changes, and the attendant psychosocial adaptation to the chronicity of the disease.

Ellenberg[5] tested the hypothesis that diabetic neuropathy was responsible for impairment of sexual functioning in women. He studied sexual functioning in fifty-four diabetic women with clinically demonstrable neuropathy, compared to a control group of forty-six diabetic women without clinically demonstrable neuropathy. The ages (range of 24 to 73 years) and duration of diabetes (range of 1 to 53 years) were comparable for both groups. The presence of neuropathy was established by absent deep reflexes (particularly ankle) and sensory impairment of the toes and feet. Forty-four (81%) of the fifty-four women with neuropathy and thirty-eight (79%) of the forty-six women without neuropathy reported the presence of libido and orgasmic reaction. Only seven of the fifty-four women (13%) with neuropathy experienced diminution of both libido and orgasm. Three of the women (7%) reported absence of both libido and orgasm. None of the women reported retention of libido with loss of orgasmic attainment. These findings related to orgasm are comparable to the nondiabetic female population as reported in Kinsey's data,[21] although Hite's more recent study[15] revealed orgasmic attainment in 88%.

The women Ellenberg studied were from the same medical practice in which a 60% occurrence of erectile dysfunction was reported in diabetic men. He therefore held that his sample was representative of the diabetic population. Ellenberg concluded that there was no basis to explain the observed sexual differences between diabetic men and women on anatomic, neurologic, or physiologic bases. However, the difference in findings between men and women was significant. Lack of deep reflexes and sensory impairment may not be the best measures of neuropathy.

We conducted a case control study[47] of seventy-three diabetic persons and fifty-five controls based on a different synthesis of the literature about human sexual functioning. Throughout the professional community studying human sexuality, male and female sexual responses have been considered analogous. Erection in men and lubrication in women are considered the initial physiologic indicators of the psychophysiologic sexual response stage usually labeled excitement.[27] The male reflexogenic erection is produced by stimulation of the nervi erigentes, which promotes dilation of the penile arteries, increases blood flow, and produces tumescence in the corpus cavernosum and the corpus spongiosum.

Homologous nervous structure and vasculature in women are found in and under the labia and outer one third of the vagina. It is thought that with sexual stimuli an increased vascular load results and a "sweating" phenomenon occurs. A transudate-like material is the result of marked dilation of the venous plexus. This transudate coalesces in the form of a fluid, known as vaginal lubrication. Lubrication occurs within seconds after the woman has become aroused.

The vagina is actually only a potential space and with stimulation expands to accommodate the hypothetical penis. It then adjusts to the actual size of the penis inserted. A symptom of the excitement phase recognized less often is ballooning of the vagina. Women are apt to recognize the absence of ballooning, since it is correlated with pain or discomfort on insertion of the penis or with vigorous thrusting. Masters and Johnson[30] report that a woman who has some failure with the ballooning process might experience itching, aching, burning with insertion of the penis, or even pain with continued thrusting.[12] Based on this information, it seemed logical to us that a combination of lack of lubrication and decrease in the ballooning process would lead to discomfort rather than pleasure with the insertion of the penis and the usual thrusting occurring during sexual intercourse.

Finally, given the analogous nature of the sexual response cycle in both men and women and the equal prevalence of diabetic neuropathy in both sexes, it was hypothesized that women with diabetes would experience malfunction in their initial response to sexual stimuli during the excitement phase rather than the orgasmic phase, as studied by both Kolodny and Ellenberg.

Two groups of diabetic subjects and controls participated in our study. The first group (volunteers) consisted of twenty-eight diabetic subjects and twenty-two control subjects. The second group was drawn from a regional diabetic research center's registry and consisted of forty-five diabetic subjects and thirty-three control subjects.

A mailout questionnaire was sent to diabetic subjects and their control subjects. The data collection tool included a group of questions about both lifetime prevalence and point prevalence of first-stage sexual disorder. The epidemiologic method of measuring risk of disease given the presence of a particular factor (diabetes) was used. Diabetic subjects and control subjects were compared and relative odds assessed.

Although it was tempting to combine the two groups in computing the results, they seemed sufficiently different to contraindicate such a move (Table 18-1). Persons in the registry sample were about 5 years older than the volunteers. Both groups had had diabetes a similar number of years. The registry group had experienced intercourse a little less frequently in the preceding 30 days and masturbated slightly less often. The registry subjects were less highly interested in sexual activity and were more likely to have experienced orgasm than were the volunteers. The groups had similar frequencies of experience with retinopathy, neuropathy, and nephropathy. Considering sexual interest and frequency of intercourse, we felt that the volunteers seemed to be more comfortable with their sexuality and more sexually active.

Results from the questionnaire were variable (Table 18-2). Neither group reported a clear difference from their controls in response to the lifetime prevalence question, *Have you ever experienced pain or discomfort during foreplay or intercourse?* The sixty-four registry participants who answered the question, *Are you currently experiencing pain or discomfort?* reported a 3.71 times greater prevalence than control subjects, and the volunteer group reported 1.4 greater prevalence than control subjects. To the lifetime prevalence question, *Have you ever felt your vagina was dry during foreplay or intercourse?* the volunteers replied "yes" 3.5 times more often than control subjects. The registry

Table 18-1. Characteristics of women in Whitley and Berke's study

Study groups	Age in years	Duration of diabetes (years)	Frequency of intercourse in preceding 30 days	Currently masturbating	Current high interest in sexual activity	Never experienced orgasm	Evidence of retinopathy	Evidence of neuropathy	Evidence of nephropathy
Volunteers									
Diabetic subjects	$\bar{x}$ = 33.9 Range = 22 to 59	$\bar{x}$ = 13 Range = 1 to 26	10.9 times	18 (64%)	21 (75%)	0	7 (25%)	19 (68%)	2 (25%)
Controls	$\bar{x}$ = 33.9 Range = 22.50		10.6 times	12 (55%)	15 (68%)	0			
Registry									
Diabetic subjects	$\bar{x}$ = 39 Range = 20 to 60	$\bar{x}$ = 12.2 Range = 1 to 36	9.3 times	24 (53%)	23 (51%)	6 (13%)	12 (27%)	20 (41%)	15 (33%)
Controls	$\bar{x}$ = 35.7 Range = 22 to 60		7.1 times	13 (39%)	15 (45%)	6 (18%)			

Table 18-2. Experiences with pain and dryness during sexual activity: diabetic subjects and control subjects

Study groups	Current pain with intercourse		Ever dry with intercourse		Currently dry with intercourse		Ever dry with intercourse		Currently dry with masturbation	
	Yes	*No*	*Yes*	*No*	*Yes*	*No*	*Yes*	*No*	*Yes*	*No*
Volunteers										
Diabetic subjects	4	21	23	4	21.	7	11	11	10	8
Controls	2	14	13	8	14	8	4	13	4	8
Relative odds	1.4		3.5		1.7		3.25		2.5	
Registry										
Diabetic subjects	8	28	29	16	27	18	12	20	15	30
Controls	2	26	18	15	13	20	8	16	8	25
Relative odds	3.7		1.5		2.31		1.2		1.04	

participants replied "yes" 1.5 times more often than the control subjects, again showing a directional trend. To the point prevalence question, *Has your vagina been dry during the last ten episodes of sexual intercourse?* the registry subjects answered "yes" 2.3 times more often than control subjects. The volunteers replied "yes" 1.7 times more often. In response to the lifetime prevalence question, *Has your vagina ever been dry during masturbation?* the volunteers answered "yes" 3.25 times more often than control subjects. The directional trend for the registry was the same, with a "yes" answer occurring 1.2 times more often than for control subjects. In response to the point prevalence question, *Has your vagina been dry during the last ten episodes of masturbation?* the directional trend continued with relative odds of 2.5 for volunteers and 1.04 for the registry group.

These results led us to believe that there may be first-stage difference in sexual response between diabetic and nondiabetic women. These data indicate that the registry group perceives the difficulty as current pain and dryness, whereas the more sexually aware volunteers rightly recognize that they have had difficulties with lubrication over time. They did not experience it at the current rate during intercourse that the registry subjects reported but did note a higher current rate with masturbating activity.

To test the concern that progressive experience with diabetes reduced sexual functioning, we grouped years since diagnosis dichotomously and cross-tabulated this category with the question, *Has your vagina ever been dry with intercourse or foreplay?* Since men report difficulty with impotence at a higher rate after 6 years' duration of diabetes, the groups were separated into women having diabetes less than 6 years and those having diabetes more than 6 years. Those having 6 years' or more experience answered "yes" 5.8 times more often than the group with less than six years' experience with diabetes. Only 18.5% of the sample, however, had had diabetes less than 6 years (Table 18-3).

All diabetic subjects were then grouped according to use of insulin or not. There was no significant difference between those currently using and not using insulin with regard to any of the questions about pain or lubrication.

Finally, the responses to the questions designed to identify retinopathy, neuropathy, and nephropathy were compared with the prevalence questions. Neuropathy appears to be associated with both the lifetime and point prevalence of a dry vagina (Table 18-4).

The question of female sexual response and diabetes is not yet settled. In this study diabetic women do report a higher rate of dryness and pain during intercourse and masturbation than do nondiabetic women. Those who have had diabetes for 6 years or longer report lifetime difficulty with lubrication more often than their controls do. Neuropathy appears to be associated with dryness for diabetic women. These questions will most likely be answered by carefully conducted laboratory research that employs insertable, electronic instruments to have a closer look at the lubrication process for diabetic women. The answers may be related to degree of neuropathy and/or length of experience with diabetes.

Diabetes appears to affect the first-stage arousal process in women, as it does with men. Orgasmic response does not seem to be the relevant issue.

Treatment. Treatment for diabetic women is similar to that for men. Good history taking, sexual counseling, regulation of the diabetes, and elimination of inhibitory drugs are essential features.

Although medical science is actively installing devices to effect potency for men, the

Table 18-3. Association between duration of diabetes and dryness with intercourse for all diabetic women

Duration of diabetes	Ever dry with intercourse	
	Yes	*No*
Duration ≤5 yr	12	1
Duration ≥6 yr	39	19
Relative odds	5.8	

Table 18-4. Association between neuropathy and dryness with intercourse for all diabetic women

Neuropathy	Ever dry with intercourse		Currently dry with intercourse	
	Yes	*No*	*Yes*	*No*
Yes	35	6	32	9
No	17	14	16	16
Relative odds	4.8		3.56	
χ^2	6.75		5.095	
Significance	$p \le .01$		$p \le .02$	

only additives available for women are good lubricants. These are sold under various names in sex shops. They are colorless, odorless, tasteless, and effective. These additions to the human body are no substitute for each client's understanding of the chronic illness to which she must adjust her life, nor are they a substitute for a thorough knowledge of human sexuality. There is no reported protocol for helping people adjust to sexual dysfunction induced by diabetes. However, sex therapists are taking time to collect careful histories from diabetic clients seeking their help to begin to reverse the common dysfunctions present before the onset of diabetes. Health care practitioners are becoming more careful about listening to the client's concerns about the chronic illness to use those concerns to promote adjustment to the altered health state prompted by diabetes. Still others are more exacting in educating their diabetic clients about human sexuality. A woman must understand the roles that diet, insulin, exercise, rest, excessive weight, and body attractiveness play in her sexuality. The more she strives to form an attitude of openness to melding body needs with desired life-style, the more often she should be able to achieve the sexual satisfaction she desires even though she may be suffering from a chronic illness.

Summary

Sexual concerns and problems accompany many chronic illnesses, including diabetes; however, organic causes for sexual dysfunction should not automatically be assumed to exist in all clients with diabetes. The incidence of sexual dysfunction among diabetic persons tends to increase with the duration of the disease. Diabetic men may experience transient episodes of erection dysfunction when their diabetes is well controlled. Difficulty with arousal and vaginal lubrication contributes to sexual problems in diabetic women. These problems may be complicated by vaginitis.

Questions for review

1. Compare and contrast the sexual problems seen in diabetic women and men.
2. Martin Wienberg, a 28-year-old diabetic man comments that he has recently experienced difficulty getting an erection. What factors related to his diabetes might explain his erectile problems? What nonorganic factors should you consider? What information do you need to counsel Mr. Wienberg?
3. Discuss the advantages and disadvantages of initiating a discussion of sexual dysfunction and diabetes with diabetic clients. How might you approach the discussion?
4. Julia Mason, a 35-year-old diabetic woman, comes to the women's clinic for vaginal itching. She is also experiencing vaginal dryness. She has had two stillborn infants and recently had a successful delivery. What needs for education and counseling will you explore with her?

References

1. Abelson, D.: Diagnostic value of the penile pulse and blood pressure: a Doppler study of impotence in diabetics, Journal of Urology **113:** 636-639, 1975.
2. Babbott, D., Rubin, A., and Ginsburg, S.J.: Reproductive characteristics of diabetic men, Diabetes **7**(1)33-35, 1958.
3. Campbell, I.W.: Diabetic autonomic neuropathy, British Journal of Clinical Practice **30**(8):153-156, Aug. 1976.
4. Christiansen, J.S., and Nerup, J.: Smoking and diabetic neuropathy, Lancet **1:**605, 1978.
5. Ellenberg, M.: Impotence in diabetes: the neurologic factor, Annals of Internal Medicine **75:**213-219, 1971.
6. Ellenberg, M.: Sexual aspects of the female diabetic, Mount Sinai Journal of Medicine **44**(4):495-500 1977.
7. Ellenberg, M.: Sex and diabetes: a comparison between men and women, Diabetes Care **2**(1):4-8 1979.
8. Ellenberg, M.: Sexual function in diabetic patients, Annals of Internal Medicine **92**(Part 2):331-333, 1980.
9. Faerman, I., et al.: Impotence and diabetes, Diabetes **21:**23-30, Jan. 1972.
10. Faerman, I., et al.: Impotence and diabetes, Diabetes **23:**971-976, 1974.
11. Fairburn, C.: The sexual problems of diabetic men, British Journal of Hospital Medicine **25:**484-491, 1981.
12. Finney, R.P.: New hinged silicone penile implant, Journal of Urology **118:**585-587, 1977.
13. Furlow, W.L., editor: Male sexual dysfunction, Urologic Clinics of North America **8**(1):1981.
14. Gaskell, P.: The importance of penile blood pressure in cases of impotence, Canadian Medical Association Journal **105:**1047-1051, 1971.

15. Greene, L.F., Panayotis, P.K., and Weeks, R.E.: Retrograde ejaculation of semen due to diabetic neuropathy, Fertility and Sterility **14:**617-625, 1963.

16. Hite, S.: The Hite report: a nationwide survey on female sexuality, New York, 1976, Dell Publishing Co., Inc.

17. Hosking, D.J., et al.: Diabetic impotence: studies of nocturnal erection during REM sleep, British Medical Journal **2:**1394-1396, 1979.

18. Karacan, I.: Diagnosis of erectile impotence in diabetes mellitus, Annals of Internal Medicine **92**(Part 2):334-337, 1980.

19. Karacan, I., et al.: Nocturnal penile tumescence and diagnosis in diabetic impotence, American Journal of Psychiatry **135:**191-197, 1978.

20. Katchardourian, H.A., and Lunde, D.T.: Fundamentals of human sexuality, New York, 1972, Holt, Rinehart & Winston.

21. Kinsey, A.C., Pomeroy, W., and Martin, C.: Sexual behavior in the human male, Philadelphia, 1948, W.B. Saunders Co.

22. Klebanow, D., and MacLeod, J.: Semen quality and certain disturbances of reproduction in diabetic men, Fertility and Sterility **11:**255-261, 1960.

23. Kline-Grabner, G., and Grabner, B.: Woman's orgasm: a guide to sexual satisfaction, Indianapolis, 1975, The Bobbs-Merril Co., Inc.

24. Kolodny, R.C.: Sexual dysfunction in diabetic females, Diabetes **20:**557-559, 1971.

25. Krosnick, A., and Podolsky, S.: Diabetes and sexual dysfunction: restoring normal ability, Geriatrics **36**(3):92-100, 1981.

26. Lawrence, A.M., and Abraira, C.: Diabetic neuropathy: a review of clinical manifestations, Annals of Clinical and Laboratory Science **6**(1):78-83, 1976.

27. Marble, A., et al.: Joslin's diabetes mellitus, ed. 11, Philadelphia, 1971, Lea & Febiger.

28. Martin, L.: Impotence in diabetes: an overview, Psychosomatics **22:**318-329, 1981.

29. Masters, W.H., and Johnson, V.E.: Human sexual response, Boston, 1966, Little, Brown & Co.

30. Masters, W.H., and Johnson, V.E.: Human sexual inadequacy, Boston, 1970, Little, Brown & Co.

31. McCulloch, D.K., et al.: The prevalence of diabetic impotence, Diabetologia **18:**279-283, 1980.

32. Meiman, A., and Henry, D.: The possible role of the catecholamines of the corpora in penile erection, Journal of Urology **121:**419-421, 1979.

33. Montenero, P., and Donatone, E.: Diabete et activite sexuelle chez l'homme, Le Diabete **8:**327-332, 1962.

34. Narayan, P., and Lange, P.H.: Semirigid penile prostheses in the management of erectile impotence. In Furlow, W.L., editor: Male sexual dysfunction, Urologic Clinics of North America **8**(1):169-179, Feb. 1981.

35. Rubin, A., and Babbott, D.: Impotence and diabetes mellitus, Journal of the American Medical Association **168:**498-500, 1958.

36. Ruzbarsky, V., and Michal, V.: Morphologic changes in the arterial bed of the penis with aging, Investigative Urology **15:**194-199, 1977.

37. Salway, J.G., et al.: Effects of myoinositol on peripheral-nerve function in diabetes, Lancet **2:**1282-1284, 1978.

38. Schiavi, R.C., and Hogan, B.: Sexual problems in diabetes mellitus: psychological aspects, Diabetes Care 2(1):9-17, 1979.
39. Schione, R.C.: Psychological treatment of erectile disorders in diabetic patients, Annals of Internal Medicine 92(Part 2):337-339, 1980.
40. Schoffling, K., et al.: Disorders of sexual function in male diabetics, Diabetes 12:519-527, 1963.
41. Small, M.S.: Small-Carrior penile prosthesis: a new implant for management of impotence, Mayo Clinic Proceedings 51:336-338, 1976.
42. Wabrek, A.J.: Sexual dysfunction associated with diabetes mellitus, Journal of Family Practice 8:735-740, 1979.
43. Waxberg, J.D.: Sexual therapy of diabetic impotence, Connecticut Medicine 42:555-556, 1978.
44. West, K.M.: Epidemiology of diabetes and its vascular lesions, New York, 1978, Elsevier North-Holland, Inc.
45. Whitehead, E.D.: Impotence, Diabetes Forecast 35(4):July-Aug. 1982.
46. Whitehouse, F.: Two minutes with diabetes, Medical Times 105(1):61-63, 1977.
47. Whitley, M.P., and Berke, P.: Sexual response in diabetic women, submitted for publication, 1982.

19

Sexuality and selected cancer therapies

CANDACE WALTERS KIRCHNER

Historically, cancer and sexuality have been seen as incongruous concepts. Whereas sexuality implied life and energy, a cancer diagnosis meant clients were dying from their disease. Since the therapeutic goal was to keep the client alive, it was difficult to give high priority in the treatment plan to the client's sexual concerns. Stereotypes which suggested that aging and disability were significant deterrents to sexual interest or enhancement compounded the problem of recognizing and intervening to promote sexual health for the client with cancer.

Knowledge about sexuality in disability and in normal aging has helped to change this picture. In addition, with creative combinations of different forms of therapy, the challenge of cancer is being met. The therapeutic goal for many clients with cancer is no longer only survival. Indeed, the focus of helping the individual cope with both the diagnosis and treatment of cancer is changing. Most recently the therapeutic goal focuses on living with cancer. Issues about quality of life are increasingly prominent in the treatment plan. If sexuality is one important component of quality in the lives of cancer clients and current cancer therapies can profoundly affect sexuality, then health care workers need to incorporate sexual issues in the treatment plan.

There are many ways that cancer therapy can negatively affect the client's sexuality. The ability of professionals in the oncology field to assist clients in living with alterations in sexuality necessitates an understanding of sexual health, the influence of cancer therapy on sexuality, the client's perception of that influence, and principles for intervening to promote sexual health.

The purposes of this chapter follow:
1. To review the concept of sexuality
2. To consider the sexual consequences of specific cancer therapies
3. To explore the therapeutic roles of health professionals as they assist the client with cancer toward sexual health

Concept of sexuality

Human sexuality is a complex concept reflecting who people are and how they live their lives. Sexual self-concept, sexual relationships, and sexual functioning are important aspects of sexuality.

Sexual self-concept has been conceptualized as a mental image of oneself as a man or woman—the way the body appears to the self and the individual's sense of adequacy about that image—implying a personal investment of conscious and unconscious feelings in various parts of the body. Sexual self-concept is dynamic, being subject to change in response to influences on the body itself or the person's perceptual apparatus. People develop a total perception of their bodies through multiple sensory experiences; this process begins as infants discover their body parts. The concepts of the body are also formed in response to attitudes and emotional overtones that individuals experience within the family and from evaluations of their physique by parents and, later, peers.

Disturbances in sexual self-concept may occur when there is a discrepancy between the way in which the individual had mentally pictured the body and the way the body is currently perceived by the individual. This conflict invariably arouses anxiety because distortion of the customary body image is seen, in essence, as a distortion of self. Perception of body distortion may create additional anxiety by resulting in fear of rejection. Childhood conditioning may cause certain parts of the body, particularly those with sexual significance, to be equated with "badness" and "dirtiness." Thus the loss of sexual organs or their function may carry special significance or be interpreted as punishment. Loss of reproductive or sexual organs may precipitate doubts about one's sexuality even though the organs removed may not be essential to the human sexual response. Although not all surgical intervention is visible to others, persons who are recovering from surgery may see themselves as different and may feel less than whole.

Sexual relationships are those interpersonal interactions that people establish in social situations. The role as man or woman is expressed in an interpersonal relationship by the way a person behaves, for example, in a work situation versus a home situation. Style of dress chosen, hobbies, or recreational activities exhibit these roles.

Sexual functioning involves the ability of the individual to engage in and experience pleasure from sexual activities. Intact genitals with adequate circulation, innervation, sensation, reflexes, and hormonal milieu are physiologically necessary for sexual functioning. Psychologic factors, the ability to relax, and freedom from pain are also necessary to be able to give and receive pleasure or satisfaction. In addition, sexual functioning involves the preferences for different types of sexual activity.

Sexual self-concept, sexual relationships, and sexual functioning are interrelated aspects of sexuality. Disturbances of one aspect may threaten another. A person's concept of self influences interaction with others. The response of loved ones to a disfiguring injury or loss of an organ has been thought to exert a significant influence on the injured person's ability to reintegrate his or her sexual self-concept. Clients who feel that they are not attractive or lovable will shun social situations and may feel inadequate in a sexual relationship. They may seek privacy and isolation from those who may potentially be shocked or disgusted by their appearances. Feelings of emasculation or loss of femininity may be reinforced by a change in or loss of sexual functioning, such as impotence or orgasmic dysfunction.

Models of cancer surgery that will be explored in terms of their impact on sexuality include radical neck dissection with laryngectomy, mastectomy, hysterectomy, and enterostomal surgery. Whenever possible, less radical surgery is done. However, the surgical procedures considered in this chapter may be performed when cancer is diagnosed in particular organs, and the surgeries can have a serious impact on sexuality. Cancer chemotherapy may also have a negative impact on sexuality. Much research needs to be done in this area.

Radical neck dissection with laryngectomy

Alterations in sexual self-concept. Much of a person's self-concept is derived from the acceptability of the physical appearance both to the individual and to others. The face is immediately visible in an encounter and is one aspect of attractiveness. Advertisers exploit facial beauty by employing beautiful or handsome models to promote products. In general the media and literature portray heroes and heroines as facially beautiful, whereas villains and others are not. St. Jerome said that ''the face is the mirror of the mind,'' and even today people tend to accept this.

The voice is important in making a positive impression on the listener. Pitch and vocal intonation are important communication cues. Voices are often described as sexy. Physical appearance that is not congruous with vocalization is distinctive but not necessarily attractive.

With this in mind it is not difficult to see how radical neck dissection with laryngectomy can detract from the person's self-concept. Initial limited neck mobility, loss of the voice, and scarring are readily apparent to others. Functional changes that can occur as complications of surgery, such as increased secretions and diminished range of motion of the affected shoulder, can further compromise the individual's sense of self-control. Concerns about maintaining the patency of the altered airway may compromise the individual's sense of personal safety and promote feelings of vulnerability. Anxiety about the inability to signal for help in an emergency can heighten the person's sense of powerlessness and helplessness.

Alterations in sexual relationships. After radical neck dissection and laryngectomy, individuals may try to cope with a negative self-concept by withdrawing from relationships, seeking privacy, and shunning social situations. The tendency to isolate themselves from others because of concerns about the degree of difficulty of care or concerns about physical appearance may be reinforced by the initial reaction of family, friends, and the public to their altered appearance and voice.

The literature contains anecdotal information about individuals who believed that their voices were so important to the success of their business contacts or teaching professions that they voluntarily retired or quit their jobs after laryngectomy.[8] For these individuals difficulty producing sounds or the quality of the resulting voice was unacceptable and interfered with effectiveness in work relationships.

In other instances conditions of employment, for example, working in areas with exposure to environmental pollutants or temperature extremes, may be harmful for an individual with a laryngectomy.[5] Job positions that require lifting heavy objects may be difficult for an individual after laryngectomy or with altered shoulder mobility and strength or both. Noise pollution in the work environment may be partially countered by the use of amplifiers.

Alterations in sexual functioning. There are few research reports in the literature that are concerned with sexual functioning after laryngectomy. In one study forty-eight individuals out of the 200 members of a Lost Cord club returned a brief mailed questionnaire dealing with sexual functioning. Few of these people reported that their physicians had discussed the effect of laryngectomy on their sex lives, but, paradoxically, most felt the physician should not discuss this.

Almost all of the respondents felt they were less attractive, and most reported a change in their sexual relationships. Most also wished that things could be different with regard to their postoperative sexual relationships.[44]

After radical neck dissection with laryngectomy, control of secretions can interfere with sexual functioning by making the person more reticent about engaging in intercourse or even sharing the same bed with the partner. Using a disposable pad on the pillow case and having tissues and a disposal bag near the bed can aid in managing secretions.

An alteration in sexual position can help those who have limited mobility in the arm on the affected side or who have excessive secretions from the laryngectomy stoma. The typical male-astride position may be unacceptable for a man with a weakened arm and uncomfortable if neck mobility is limited. Other sexual positions could be explored with the couple according to their openness to alternatives. When the amount of secretions is the major deterrent, changing the relative position of the partners from face-to-face to face-to-shoulder will position the partner's face away from the secretions.[37] Coughing in private to clear secretions before intercourse and covering the stoma with a porous cover will also help.[37] Rapid shallow breathing accompanying orgasm can produce coughing, which interferes with enjoyment of orgasm. The individual may compensate for the inability to hold his breath at climax by exaggerating pelvic tilt and pelvic thrust.[36] Masturbation or oral sex are other alternatives that can be explored if both partners are receptive.[37]

Finally, when walls are not thick, the intensity of sound from the electrolarynx may penetrate adjoining rooms. Those with a laryngectomy may become reticent about verbalizing sexual feelings while in bed. Touching and other physical signaling have added importance in lieu of speech.[36]

Living with a radical neck dissection and laryngectomy. Psychologic adjustment and incorporation of subsequent feelings into a resumption of former life-style may be facilitated by a variety of means. The Lost Cord Club of the American Cancer Society is composed of members who have had a laryngectomy. These individuals can serve as role models in that they have learned to communicate and have resumed their former life-styles. However, their sexual adjustment may vary.

Client education materials dealing with self-care activities and resumption of speech are available from the American Cancer Society and other sources and should be made available to the client postoperatively.[4]

The speech therapist is an important member of the health care team who can demonstrate methods of speech postoperatively and provide other counseling that speeds postoperative psychologic adjustment and positive involvement in self-care.

Mastectomy

Alterations in sexual self-concept. Understanding the sexual significance of the breasts is facilitated by a brief exploration of the meanings associated with the breasts. The breasts may form the primary source of female sexual identity. The advertising media frequently use the breasts as the symbol of a woman's femininity. Many men's magazines use breast size and shape as criteria for sexual desirability. The breasts have a physiologic role in lactation and therefore may symbolize potential for motherhood and nurturance. In addition, female breast tissue undergoes distinct physiologic changes paralleling the intensity of sexual excitement. Some women may find that stimulation of their breasts is essential in foreplay and sexual arousal.[6]

The value assigned to a lost breast is probably influenced by the extent to which the woman bases her sexual self-concept on her general appearance and the appearance of her breasts in particular. If she has less emotional investment in the appearance of her breasts, she may find loss of a breast less threatening than if her body image and self-esteem are founded on her breasts.

A woman who has a radical mastectomy for breast cancer experiences several changes in her body. The excision of breast tissue, pectoral musculature, and axillary lymphatic tissue is a visible loss of a sexually associated organ that can also contribute to restricted strength and mobility of the affected arm. Compensation for the weight of the excised tissue can change posture and carriage. In some women lymphedema is a further change in body appearance. The swollen arm can be cumbersome and painful.

With these considerations in mind, it is not difficult to imagine how women can experience profound anxiety when contemplating loss of a breast. In a Gallup poll conducted for the American Cancer Society 1007 women 18 years and older were polled with regard to their attitudes toward breast cancer and breast surgery.[79] Worry about cancer, as opposed to disfigurement from mastectomy, caused conflicting fears and anxieties. Women were evenly divided in terms of their response to having a breast removed: 36% said they would wonder if the cancer was completely removed, and 32% were concerned with the emotional adjustment to mastectomy. Among younger, outgoing middle-class women, breast loss seemed to assume greater significance. Of the women interviewed, 51% felt they would lose their sense of femininity after mastectomy. Single women 18 to 34 years of age and women who were tense, highly sociable, and more concerned about their physical appearance than the average woman were most likely to feel that mastectomy impaired their sense of femininity.

Sexual adaptation after mastectomy probably depends on the age of the woman and the extent of physical change. Sanger and Reznikoff[58] found that breast-saving surgical techniques provided better cosmesis and significantly less disturbance in body satisfaction. They implied that the women in their study who had a modified radical mastectomy indicated a decrease in satisfaction with their breasts, energy level, health, weight, sleep, arms, and hands. Some women who undergo mastectomy and adjuvant chemotherapy are more concerned with weight change than with physical changes associated with the surgery.[65]

It is probable that a woman's response to a mastectomy reflects the following factors: the value that she assigns to the lost breast, the response of others to her surgery, the positive reinforcement she obtains from health professionals regarding her body and her rehabilitation, the role models or positive identification models to which she is exposed (such as a Reach to Recovery volunteer), and coping principles that she can learn in an environment of interpersonal acceptance.[6] Family, friends, and others with a mastectomy can be a great support system for the woman who has had a mastectomy.

Alterations in sexual relationships. The woman who perceives herself as mutilated by surgery may perceive herself as less acceptable to society and withdraw from social engagements and work. Silberfarb, Maurer, and Crouthamel[65] found that half of the women employed before mastectomy remained employed after surgery, but many took a leave of absence, and a few quit their employment.

Change in the homemaker role is not uncommon after mastectomy. Postoperatively many women desire assistance with heavy housecleaning,[81] shopping, laundry, and food preparation.[65]

Most women believe a single woman's chances of being happily married are decreased after mastectomy. However, they do not believe that an already happy marriage will be endangered by a mastectomy.[79] After mastectomy, married women who were satisfied with their sexual relationships reported that they felt they could confide in their husbands, and they did perceive their husbands as understanding.[81] Schoenberg and Carr[62] contend that if the marital relationship is supportive and there is a good sexual adjustment preoperatively, the postoperative adjustment will be less difficult. Conversely, if the preoperative sexual relationship is unstable, the postoperative course may be very difficult.

A woman who feels defective or undesirable may withdraw from a sexual relationship. She may consciously or unconsciously prompt rejection by her partner through nonverbal communication. Still, she may be able to cope with a sexual relationship if she can be helped to openly communicate her concerns with her partner.

A woman may believe that since her breasts are important in her own sexual gratification, her partner will find her less gratifying after surgery. Indeed, some women in Bard and Sutherland's sample[6] feared that their sexual feelings and drives would be depressed by removal of a source of sexual stimulation. Before surgery some of the women had dreams of the husband's love being given to another highly sexual woman. Some women projected their own feelings of unacceptability to men whom they felt judged women on the basis of their breasts.

Indeed, some men are initially shocked by the surgical changes in the woman's body and may unintentionally convey their feelings to the woman. A man who is revulsed by the appearance of the woman's body may find his sexual satisfaction threatened. To prevent extreme guilt over such thoughts, he needs help to express his feelings. While trying to disguise his feelings, he may convey a less than genuine enthusiasm for sex to his partner and subsequently cause her to question her femininity.

The operative site may stimulate anxieties about mutilation in men, as well as women. If these feelings become too intense, the partner may unconsciously withdraw from the sexual relationship, reinforcing the woman's feeling of rejection. Careful preoperative assessment may highlight these feelings and help determine interventions to minimize strain on the sexual relationship.

Husbands may be reluctant to resume intercourse if they fear they will hurt their wives. The husband's fear of hurting his wife may reinforce her fears of injury and her view of herself as an invalid. If the husband cannot discuss these fears with his wife, she may interpret them to mean "rejection" rather than protection. If the man can be helped to discuss his feelings, misconceptions and groundless fears will probably be less likely to disrupt the marital relationship.[6]

Alterations in sexual functioning. Few literature reports deal with sexual functioning in married heterosexual women after mastectomy. More information is needed in that area and in the area of sexual functioning in single women or lesbians after mastectomy.

After mastectomy, women may experience many fears about sexual functioning. Many women in the Bard and Sutherland sample[6] continued to fear rejection, and some coped with their feelings of disfigurement by wearing clothing such as a brassiere during sexual intercourse or by having sex only in the dark. A number of women expressed the fear that resumption of intercourse would cause injury to the surgical wound. For those couples who prefer the male-astride position the placement of a small pillow over the operative incision may diffuse the pressure caused by the partner's weight and thereby minimize discomfort and fear. Other positions for intercourse may be used if both partners are willing. The female-astride position removes pressure from the operative site.[60] Initially the female-astride position may be uncomfortable for the woman to support her weight with the affected arm, and this position puts the operative site in direct line with the partner's gaze. Alternatively, a side-by-side approach may be comfortable for both partners. When the woman turns toward her operative side to face her partner, she presents the unaffected breast to the man for fondling with his free hand. Creative use of supportive pillows is necessary in this position to prevent undue pressure on the affected arm and thus minimize the risk of lymphedema.

The sparse literature regarding actual change in desire, frequency of intercourse, or orgasmic response after mastectomy may reflect the societal view of women who have lost a breast as "too fragile to interview" or even more likely the hesitancy to consider sexual functioning in the face of a life-threatening illness.

A survey[81] of thirty-four married women who had survived for 4 years after mastectomy revealed that most experienced no change in sexual frequency, with the minority reporting a decrease in frequency following surgery. Most were satisfied with their sexual relationships. In comparison with those whose sexual activity had decreased since their surgery, those women whose sexual activity remained the same were slightly better prepared for their surgeries, were twice as likely to be premenopausal (under 46 years of age), reported more interest in sex, were much more satisfied with their current sexual relationships, were less likely to have had radical surgical procedures, had fewer persisting complications and fewer symptoms of depression, and were more satisfied with their husband's companionship. Of these, only sexual satisfaction and satisfaction with the husband's companionship differed significantly between groups.

Another study of forty-one married women following mastectomy revealed that half demonstrated sexual desires following surgery.[26] This represented a slight decrease in the amount of desire expressed preoperatively. Women were also queried about their comfort when undressing in front of their husbands. Of these women, 43% felt comfortable undressing in the presence of their spouses. The types of sexual activities in which the women engaged were also studied. The most significant preoperative-to-postoperative change involved touching of the breast. Before surgery 46% of the women reported stimulation by touching of the breast, whereas only 33% reported such stimulation postoperatively. In general, frequency of intercourse decreased following mastectomy, but this might have been attributable to age.

Living with a mastectomy. Occasionally, sexual counseling or sexual therapy may be necessary for couples adjusting to mastectomy. One approach described in the literature advocates assisting the couple to confront and integrate the experience of the mastectomy.[78] The therapist discourages the use of a prosthesis during intercourse, believing that it delays confrontation. Sex therapy exercises designed to help the couple assess the strengths of the woman's body and the obvious loss are stressed, as are exercises that help the couple determine which parts of the body can be stimulated in a pleasing way. It is suggested that intercourse be resumed as soon as possible and that if weakness or fear intervenes, the caring of the spouse should be expressed in any case. This approach rejects the assumption that mastectomy is always grounds for psychotherapy and that the spouse should simply deny what has happened to the woman. Instead, emphasis is placed on honest sharing of emotions.

Reach to Recovery. Reach to Recovery is a program of the American Cancer Society. The Reach to Recovery volunteer is a woman who has had a mastectomy and whose successful adaptation has, in part, prepared her to help other women facing the experiences of the same surgery. These volunteers from Reach to Recovery can function as positive role models for the woman with a mastectomy. They demonstrate successful resumption of life-style after surgery, share personal coping methods, and show the woman ways to emphasize an attractive personal appearance.

Manuals published by the Reach to Recovery program address practical information relating to self-concept, relationships, and sexual functioning. The Reach to Recovery manual encourages women to believe that mature love is based on more than physical attributes and that the total relationship can be very rewarding. A portion of the manual deals with sexual functioning. The woman is reassured that as she recovers from her surgery and begins to feel better, her desires for sexual relations will return. The woman is cautioned that pain in the incisional area may initially cause some physical discomfort during sexual intercourse. Women are encouraged to share their feelings about sex with their partners. If the woman was in the habit of undressing in front of her husband before surgery, she is encouraged to behave the same way postoperatively. One portion of the literature deals with attractive clothing styles and fabrics that emphasize appearance but do not put pressure on the affected arm and shoulder. Information about breast prostheses is shared so that women are aware of the range of products available, as well as some characteristics of prostheses. Fullness, size, and weight of the prosthesis are important in promotion of good posture and carriage. Range of motion exercises for the affected shoulder and arm that help prevent lymphedema and contractures are illustrated, with a cautionary note to consult the woman's individual surgeon about applicability.

Elsewhere in the Reach to Recovery literature, practical information about relationships and sexual functioning is discussed for the married and the single woman. The woman who is not involved in a long-term relationship is encouraged not to discuss her surgery with a man she dates until she feels comfortable talking about it. The unmarried woman is encouraged to give her male friend time to adjust to the news—just as she required time to make an adjustment to her surgery.

Adoption of positive health habits. After mastectomy a woman needs to incorporate positive health habits into her life-style. Those women who are not familiar with the technique of breast self-examination should be taught. After mastectomy a woman should be encouraged to continue monthly self-examination of the remaining breast to assure herself of the continued health of the remaining breast. The woman should also be taught to incorporate practices into her life-style that will minimize her risk of lymphedema. She should take precautions to prevent burns, scratches, and pressure on the affected arm.[57] In one study those women who developed lymphedema after mastectomy were not taught methods of prevention.[81] Finally, birth control methods must be assessed for premenopausal women after mastectomy. The use of birth control pills for these women is generally discouraged.

The option of breast reconstruction. Some women cannot accept the loss of a breast and are not satisfied with external breast prostheses. Breast reconstruction may be an option for these women. During surgery a Silastic implant is placed below the pectoral muscles, which results in a breast mound that has a more normal contour and a consistency that is similar to breast tissue. An areola and a nipple may be reconstructed from a skin graft, graft of the remaining nipple, or a graft from the mucous membrane of the labia. The resulting physical appearance may be more satisfactory to the woman and help in psychologic adaptation to the effects of losing the breast. Some volunteers of the Reach to Recovery Program have had breast reconstruction.

Hysterectomy

Alterations in sexual self-concept. Perhaps the most crucial factor in a woman's response to hysterectomy is the manner in which she perceives herself after surgery. Although hysterectomy is not readily apparent to others, concomitant changes in physiologic functions, such as cessation of menses, appear to alter a woman's concept of herself and her body. Drellich and Bieber[20] studied a group of twenty-three premenopausal women who had had hysterectomies. Their findings indicated that the uterus is an important symbol of femininity and that its removal influences a woman's perception of her effectiveness. Among the functions attributed to the uterus were reproduction, excretion, regulation of bodily processes, expression of sexuality, maintenance of strength and vitality, and maintenance of youth and attractiveness. Each of these functions was valued differently by each woman.

It is apparent that women who face hysterectomy may be concerned about the anticipated inevitable loss of childbearing ability. Although some clients have denied apprehension over the loss of their reproductive organs, investigators attribute this response to intolerable feelings of impending loss. To those women who no longer desired pregnancy, hysterectomy came as a relief and often freed them of the burden of contraception. The ability to bear and raise children appeared to serve a variety of needs and functions for women. Even women who desired no more children felt that the knowledge that they were fertile made them feel complete and feminine.

For the majority of the women who were studied, cessation of the menstrual periods was viewed with regret. This was true even for those women who expressed strong negative feelings toward symptoms accompanying their periods. Menstruation was viewed by some as cleansing, a type of excretory function. Some women saw their periods as "the rhythm of life," and they even planned social events around them. The uterus was seen as a bodily time clock that helped regulate other body functions.

Lessening of sexual desire and disappearance of the ability to respond sexually were among the fears mentioned preoperatively by some women. Some feared that their surgery would mean loss of sexual attractiveness and a subsequent loss of their husbands' interest and perhaps their fidelity. Others anticipated an improvement in sexual functioning.[20]

Another major concern of women who were about to have a hysterectomy was inability to carry out housework and other daily duties. Many expected the surgery to have a deleterious effect on their strength. Some believed the uterus to be the source of their ability to function.[20]

In addition to the functions already mentioned, women also believed that the uterus prevented aging. A few women were anxious about postoperative pain. Some were fearful of loss of excretory control.[20] Several women viewed their surgery as punishment for guilt-laden activities involving the sexual organs.[20] Themes in their conversations included sexual relations outside of marriage.

A comparative study of Mexican-American and Anglo-American women who had undergone hysterectomy revealed that hysterectomy threatened their being a satisfactory sexual partner, heightened fears that others would view them as less than a "whole woman" because of not being able to bear children, and resulted in some long delays in having the necessary surgery. Some women also reported intense anxiety at the prospect of the operation. This type of response was especially noted among the Mexican-American women and is attributed by the investigator to the cultural pattern of the feminine role. Thus it would seem especially important to ascertain the meaning of such surgery to the woman involved, as well as to her spouse, within the context of cultural beliefs.[76,77] A more recent study of forty inner-city women (60% black) revealed that hysterectomy did not change feelings of femininity or sexual attitudes toward their partners.[15]

Alterations in sexual relationships. The literature emphasizes the importance of the spouse's reaction to surgery. Some men have difficulty in continuing the sexual relationship. A few become unable to have intercourse with their spouses, based on their fears of injury to their penises or their negative attitudes toward a woman without a uterus. Often these changes may be attributable to misinformation or myth.[42]

Alterations in sexual functioning. In one study[64] of predominantly black women after vaginal hysterectomy with or without partial vaginectomy for carcinoma in situ no significant postoperative decrease in sexual functioning or sexual desire was found. The authors propose several reasons for the lack of change. All of these women had at least one child and were delighted to no longer need birth control. Many women expressed relief that their cancer had been removed. In no instance were ovaries removed. Finally, the vaginal hysterectomy left no visible scar.

Some physicians think that irrational fears and beliefs about the loss of a valued organ are responsible for the sexual disturbances that occur after surgery. However, Morgan[45] points out that there are several reasons to believe that hysterectomy changes the sexual sensations of women whose uteruses have active roles in their sexual response. During arousal there may be less vasocongestive change in the pelvis because of the absence of the uterus, there would be no elevation of the uterus with sexual excitement, and the ballooning of the vagina with sexual arousal would be limited by the inelasticity of the surgical scar. Morgan also notes that absence of the uterus could be noticed during the plateau phase, during which the extra increment of sexual tension might not be felt by the woman who has had a hysterectomy. Finally, some women perceive contractions of the uterus with orgasm; women who have had hysterectomies would be without this sensation. Morgan further points out that placement of the surgical scar may make intercourse uncomfortable if the scarred area is struck by the penis during penetration. Morgan cautions that there are several reasons for reconsidering studies that have found no change in sex after hysterectomy. First, satisfaction with sex may have been interpreted as satisfaction of a male partner. Next, positive outcomes of the surgery, such as feeling better, may overshadow the sexual changes. Finally, women may have trouble verbalizing the subtlety of their changed feelings.

Certainly the removal of the ovaries and thus the ovarian hormones may lead to thinning of the vaginal wall and a decrease in lubrication, which may be responsible for discomfort during intercourse. However, an oophorectomy is not always done concurrently with a hysterectomy. Estrogen replacement therapy may be considered in some cases to reverse vaginal changes.

Enterostomal surgery

Alterations in sexual self-concept. The initial sight of a colostomy was usually shocking and frequently precipitated transient to chronic depression in twenty-nine men and twenty-eight women studied by Sutherland et al.[68] Depression was thought to be triggered by the perception of the colostomy as mutilation or disfigurement. Several clients described such severe weakness after surgery that they occasionally required periods of prolonged bed rest. The sensation of weakness was attributed to the person's perception of the body as being rendered fragile and vulnerable by the surgery. Marked invalidism was manifest in those who demonstrated both weakness and depression.

Loss of self-esteem was seen in both male and female ostomates.[22] Feelings of unacceptability were reflected in the woman's desire to conceal the colostomy. Some individuals reported a loss of esteem despite favorable family situations. However, strong preoperative relationships were usually capable of surviving in spite of strong negative feelings of disgust or revulsion at the colostomy.[21]

Perhaps the strongest fear expressed by the ostomate was fear of spillage. Severe humiliation and even suicidal ideation occurred in response to fecal spilling. Ostomates also tended to be anxious concerning the noise or odor from flatus.[68]

The interference with body image often led to social restrictions. Concepts of body worth, integrity, and autonomy were often severely compromised by enterostomal surgery. The creation of the stoma removed the control of feces that was established in early childhood. The cultural demand for cleanliness, initially mediated by parents during toilet training, causes children who soil themselves to risk loss of acceptance and love. Failure of sphincter control elicits criticism and even punishment in childhood.[29] It is therefore not surprising that some adults who had ostomies described themselves as infantile or childlike.

Some clients were concerned with the fact that the artificial anus was in the front of the body.[49] Some ostomates attached sexual significance to the stoma. Handling the stoma became an erotic experience and possibly a masturbatory equivalent.[10]

A majority of men and women described an unpleasant initial reaction on seeing the stoma: "After I saw it, I avoided looking at it for days." Another client stated, "It is a terrible thing to find this change in one's anatomy.'' Others reacted by denying any feelings: ''I can't remember.'' Clients voiced reluctance to discuss their colostomy with others for fear of being viewed as a ''freak.''[22] Some men reacted to this surgery as if it represented castration. Some unconsciously equated the initial bleeding of the stoma with menstruation and hence feminization. Some women equated the mutilation with being sexually violated.[49]

Alterations in sexual relationships. Fear of social rejection prevented many of the clients in the sample of Sutherland et al. from socializing outside their homes. Isolation was a common consequence of the perceived odor and the fear of fecal spillage after creation of a colostomy.

Dyk and Sutherland[22] sought to better understand the family's adaptation to the client with a colostomy on the premise that the emotional response of the family becomes an important factor in the person's efforts to restore self-esteem and social function. Clients with colostomies who believe that surgery has reduced their value and acceptability, then, are in a precarious position as they make their transition back into the community.

Often demands are made of the spouse for participation in the client's care. In some instances these demands create conflicts inasmuch as some individuals cannot integrate the role of caretaker with that of lover. Spouses may find that they are unable to feel sexual desire or experience physical arousal because of their involvement in personal care.

Male ostomates. The results of the study by Dyk and Sutherland[22] indicated that some wives expressed lowered esteem for their husbands by making derogatory statements about the colostomy. Some of the wives complained about reduced income and the need for them to help support the family. A few refused to assist with colostomy care or complained about the large amount of time the bathroom was in use. Some of the men withdrew from intercourse; others were embarrassed in social situations by flatus or the threat of spillage and so retreated from social engagements.

In marriages in which esteem was maintained wives attempted to make their husbands feel wanted, provided physical care without complaint, made provision for use of bathroom facilities, and sometimes encouraged their husbands to reduce their workload. Sexual intercourse was sometimes continued, although frequently a mutual decision was made to stop having intercourse in an attempt to maintain husbands' self-esteem. Concealment of the colostomy and denial of the need for care were means by which husbands lessened their fears of rejection.[22]

Female ostomates. Most women with a colostomy did not believe that they had lost the esteem of their husbands. Husbands generally did not terminate intercourse or complain about their wives' lessened housework, but husbands were sometimes annoyed by their wives' self-enforced social isolation.[22]

Husbands were not in situations in which they were expected to assist with ostomy care. They were not repelled by the sight of the colostomy as were wives of male ostomates. A more tolerant attitude toward weakness was found for the female ostomates than for the men, which probably reflects societal expectations for the sexes in the mid-1950s.[22]

Alterations in sexual functioning. The literature dealing with adaptation to a stoma is largely based on studies of married heterosexuals. Little is known about the adaptation of single or homosexual individuals.

The findings of several investigations of sexual functioning after ileostomy and colostomy are summarized in Table 19-1. Desire, arousal, intercourse, and orgasm are slightly to moderately depressed after creation of the stoma. There appears to be less interference with sexual functioning among those having an ileostomy, compared with those having a colostomy. Extent, area of surgical dissection, type of surgery, and age differences between those having a colostomy and those having an ileostomy have been advanced as variables affecting sexual functioning. Interruption of autonomic nervous system pathways near the rectum during colostomy and abdominoperineal resection has been advanced as a cause of sexual dysfunction.[52,73,75] Dissection that spares as much peritoneum as possible near the sacral promontory and rectum is believed to prevent damage to these nerves. However, the extent of malignancy dictates the extent of dissection of tissue and nerves.

The frequency of impotence in men as a result of surgery varied according to age of the man and the operative technique chosen (Table 19-1). Most men with sexual dysfunction expressed dissatisfaction, felt degraded, and attributed a deterioration in rapport with their spouses to absence of sexual relations. Men who experienced transient impotence expressed feelings of personal inadequacy. In some instances the partners of men who had sexual dysfunction encouraged them not to continue having intercourse. Some men coped by never showing their stoma to their partner.

When reasons for cessation of intercourse were given, they were frequently attributable to the woman with a stoma or to a female partner. In general the older women in one study[73] did not resume intercourse after enterostomal surgery. Death of the spouse or physical separation from a husband who was in a nursing home was postulated as contributing to this finding. The older men in this study did resume intercourse. One wonders if these findings reflect societal mores about suitable age differences in sexual partners.

Brouillette, Pryor, and Fox[9] isolated concerns about trauma to the stoma and fears about fecal spillage during intercourse, which interfered with enjoyment of sexual experiences in women. Prolonged drainage from perineal wounds also hindered sexual functioning.

Women who were studied in the 1950s and 1960s reported more dysfunction attributable to ostomy surgeries than did women who were surveyed in the 1970s and 1980s. This may reflect changing sexual norms for women, as well as more careful surgical dissection.

The aging ostomate. In one study[18] 160 ostomates over 50 years of age responded to a questionnaire about their surgery and preoperative and postoperative sexual behavior. Most of these individuals maintained an active and interested sex life after surgery. The frequency of intercourse per month did decrease after surgery, as did interest in sex and the ability to attain orgasm. However, Dlin and Perlman concluded that the high interest in sex in a population over age 50 years who have experienced radical surgical alteration speaks well of the fact that aging people still have a significant investment in life.

In contrast, Weinstein and Roberts[73] reported a study of 24 elderly men and 20 elderly

Text continued on p. 358.

Table 19-1. Sexual functioning after colostomy and ileostomy

Study	Sample	Results
Persons with colostomies or ileostomies		
Dlin, Perlman, and Ringold (1969)	211 men and 198 women (from 17 to 87 years of age) who had ileostomies or colostomies and were members of various ostomy associations	78% said surgery had not interfered with their established sexual practices; frequency of intercourse did not decrease postoperatively; 92.6% of men had erections preoperatively, but only 75.8% did postoperatively; 87% of total sample were able to experience orgasm postoperatively, only 3% less than preoperatively; frequency of extramarital affairs and multiple orgasms decreased postoperatively; 89% had enjoyed intercourse preoperatively, and 85% did postoperatively; 90.5% rated their marital adjustment excellent to average preoperatively, and 85% did postoperatively; 21% reported decreased interest in sex, and 22% increased interest
Persons with colostomies		
Sutherland et al. (1952)	29 men with a colostomy (from 28 to 69 years of age), 5 to 15 years postoperatively	14 men were impotent; 5 had impaired erectile strength; 7 had only slight or no changes in potency
	28 women who had a colostomy (from 21 to 76 years of age), 5 to 15 years postoperatively	14 women would not discuss sexual matters; 3 had terminated intercourse preoperatively, 4 postoperatively; 2 had intercourse after surgery but under protest; 2 were able to maintain sexual relations and experience orgasm
Dyk and Sutherland (1956)	22 men (from 28 to 72 years of age) at time of operation who had a colostomy with abdominoperineal resection for cancer	Only 3 men noted little change in sexual functioning after surgery; 12 were totally impotent; 7 had impaired erectile strength and frequency postoperatively
	15 women (from 38 to 69 years of age) at time of operation who had a colostomy with abdominoperineal resection for cancer	5 women discontinued intercourse preoperatively; 7 had intercourse less frequently after surgery and expressed decreased interest; 3 were fearful that having intercourse would cause them injury; 1 experienced dyspareunia

Table 19-1. Sexual functioning after colostomy and ileostomy—cont'd

Study	Sample	Results
Persons with colostomies—cont'd		
Druss, O'Connor, and Stern (1969)	22 men studied after abdominoperineal resection and colostomy for cancer of the large intestine (average age at surgery was 56.5 years; average age at time of interview was 61 years)	32% of the men reported loss of sexual desire after surgery; 41% of the men were less active after surgery; 4 had sexual relations less frequently after surgery
	14 women who had abdominoperineal resection and colostomy for cancer of the large intestine (average age at surgery was 56.5 years; average age at time of interview was 61 years)	28% of the women described decreased sexual desire after surgery; 3 described either pain or lack of sensation with intercourse
Weinstein and Roberts (1977)	11 men and 13 women who had a colostomy and anterior resection for rectal carcinoma (average age of the sample at follow-up was 73 years)	*Anterior resection* 8 men (average age 66 years old) had successful intercourse; 1 made no attempt at intercourse; 2 were impotent (they both had a prostatectomy); 4 women had successful intercourse; 9 others made no attempt at intercourse
	13 men and 7 women who had a colostomy and abdominoperineal resection for rectal carcinoma; (average age of the sample at follow-up was 73 years)	*Abdominoperineal resection* 12 of the men were impotent; 1 made no attempt at intercourse; 3 of the women had successful intercourse; 4 made no attempt at intercourse
Fazio, Fletcher, and Montague (1980)	9 men (mean age 29 years) underwent proctocolectomy for inflammatory bowel disease	1 man reported decreased frequency of erection after proctocolectomy; 8 others reported no change in sexual functioning
	7 men who had abdominoperineal resection for carcinoma and 5 men who had anterior resection with low colorectal anastomosis (mean age 60.2 years)	3 of the 7 men who had an abdominoperineal resection reported sexual dysfunction: 1 was impotent; 2 others reported decreased frequency of erection; 1 of these also reported pelvic pain on ejaculation; the other reported absence of antegrade ejaculation; after anterior resection with low colorectal anastomosis, 2 men reported decreased frequency of erections, one of whom also reported decreased ability to sustain an erection; the other noted absence of antegrade ejaculation

Continued.

Table 19-1. Sexual functioning after colostomy and ileostomy—cont'd

Study	Sample	Results
Persons with colostomies—cont'd		
Williams and Slack (1980)	19 men and 9 women with rectal cancer and 3 men and 1 woman with ulcerative colitis	10 of 19 men with rectal carcinoma were sexually active before surgery (mean age 65.4 years); 5 of these sexually active men underwent anterior resection; other 5 underwent abdominoperineal resection; after anterior resection, 2 men were sexually active 3 months after operation; 2 were potent but unable to ejaculate; 1 was temporarily impotent but recovered potency by 3 months after surgery; after abdominoperineal resection, 1 man had satisfactory erection; another reported very poor erection; 1 was impotent; 1 recovered potency 3 months after surgery; 3 of the 9 women with rectal carcinoma were sexually active before surgery (mean age 65.1 years); after anterior resection 1 woman reported satisfactory sexual activity; after abdominoperineal resection and removal of posterior vaginal wall, 1 woman had normal sexual intercourse and orgasm; the other lost her sexual partner because vaginal stenosis prevented penetration; all 4 clients with ulcerative colitis who underwent panproctocolectomy reported satisfactory sexual activity
Persons with ileostomies		
Roy et al. (1970)	298 of 497 ileostomy clients were polled, some of whom had cancer (all were adults, with the oldest over 60 years)	260 of 298 noted no change in sexual activities; some said their sexual functioning had improved; of those persons whose sexual habits were affected, 4 women had dyspareunia from scarring or poor wound healing; 2 were impaired by the ileostomy itself; 4 men became totally impotent; 3 were unable to ejaculate; 8 claimed that their sexual frequency decreased
Burnham, Lennard-Jones, and Brooke (1977)	376 of 540 members of the Ileostomy Association of Great Britain and Ireland (316 complete responses) who had ileostomy for ulcerative	24 men and 21 women married after creation of the colostomy; 37 men and 19 women had children; of 42 men who did not have rectal ex-

Table 19-1. Sexual functioning after colostomy and ileostomy—cont'd

Study	Sample	Results
Persons with ileostomies—cont'd	colitis; results reported for only 175 married women and 128 married men (ages ranging from 18 to over 65 years of age)	cision, none reported sexual dysfunction; of 118 men who had rectal excision, 6 were unable to have erections; 12 could have only partial erections; 21 found it difficult to maintain an erection; 9 could no longer ejaculate; of 57 women who did not have rectal excision, 15% experienced new discomfort during intercourse; of 165 women with rectal excision, 41 experienced some discomfort with intercourse before removal of the rectum, and 54 experienced new discomfort after surgery; a greater proportion of women experienced orgasm and pleasurable sensation after surgery than reported in previous studies
Yeager and Van Heerden (1980)	25 men (from 16 to 48 years of age) who had proctocolectomy for benign disease	22 of 25 men who had proctocolectomy reported no sexual difficulties; 2 reported improved sexual function; 1 was impotent; 2 others had trouble maintaining an erection
	20 men (from 30 to 49 years of age) who had abdominoperineal resection mainly for rectal cancer	17 of 20 men who had abdominoperineal resection were able to have and sustain an erection; 2 were potent but could not ejaculate; 3 were impotent
Nilsson et al. (1981)	29 women (20 to 63 years old) and 13 men (25 to 65 years old) studied after conversion of an ileostomy (primarily done for ulcerative colitis) to a continent ileostomy	After conversion 5 reported occasional leakage; 37 reported ileostomy completely continent; 98% reported occasional embarrassment and uncertainty or inhibition by ileostomy; after conversion to continent ileostomy, 24% reported a similar reaction; 4 men and 15 women reported decreased or absent sex life after ileostomy; 1 man and 1 woman felt sex life was not normal after conversion; one third claimed partner was embarrassed by ileostomy; after conversion to continent ileostomy, all claimed that no partner had a negative reaction toward the continent ileostomy

women who underwent stomal surgery for rectal carcinoma. The majority of the men who had an anterior resection were able to have intercourse successfully; the majority of women made no attempt at intercourse. On the other hand, the majority of men who had an abdominoperineal resection could not have erections. More of the women who had an abdominoperineal resection made no attempt at intercourse, but those who did all reported pleasurable intercourse. The ostomates reported that lack of marital partners and lack of interest in sex resulted in forgoing intercourse.

Living with a stoma. Living with a stoma involves making psychologic adaptations, as well as learning problem-solving techniques and incorporating care of the stoma into the life-style of the individual. Many persons do register embarrassment by the ostomy or feel less attractive sexually. When asked to describe their stomas, a small percentage of persons indicated that the stoma was "repulsive or unpleasant," a slightly larger proportion responded "unsightly," and the majority called it a "natural opening." Men tended to have slightly more positive responses than women, probably reflecting the differential value placed on appearance for men and women.[10]

Studies of married heterosexuals reveal that persons with a stoma are comfortable discussing sexual concerns and problems with their partners. However, single ostomates who have not known their partner can have more concerns in this area.

Psychologic acceptance of the stoma is fostered by the health care provider who explores the meaning of the stoma with the individual and encourages a strong self-concept. Autonomy, impulse control, and cleanliness are a partial list of areas of possible concern. Preoperative discussion of the appearance of the stoma can shape the individual's expectations. Incremental postoperative involvement of the individual in the physical care of the stoma facilitates acceptance of the stoma and confidence in the ability to cope with unexpected occurrences. Although a small number of men and women indicate that a stoma physically makes intercourse difficult, men and women fear damage to the stoma, leakage, odor, noise, and displacement of the appliance during intercourse. Men find the appliance a physical hindrance. Some men and women recommend concealing the appliance during intercourse with a garment or appliance cover or draping the abdomen with a towel. Most suggest emptying and cleansing the appliance before intercourse, and some prefer changing the appliance some time before intercourse to ensure adhesion. Some restrict dietary intake somewhat before having sex.[11] An enterostomal therapist is invaluable in discussing current improvements in equipment to counter fears about spillage and odor and demonstrating methods of coping with the stoma. For some individuals a visit by a member of the American Cancer Society's Ostomy Club may be beneficial in reinforcing positive self-concept and promoting incorporation of the care of the stoma into the life-style.

Resumption of the life-style of the individual is facilitated by a sense of humor, advance preparation for unexpected exigencies, and integration of stoma care routine into other normal daily routines. Anecdotal literature reports demonstrate that those individuals with a strong self-concept are able to counter embarrassing situations with a sense of humor and a graceful temporary exit. Many find it helpful to ensure appliance adhesion before intercourse and before attending work or social functions. Keeping an extra appliance in the purse, briefcase, or car glove compartment is a frequently useful precaution. Incorporating stomal care into the routine of daily life instead of incorporating daily life into the routine of appliance change and stoma irrigation is necessary for ultimate resumption of the life-style of the individual.

Cancer chemotherapy

The effect of cancer chemotherapeutic agents on fertility has been summarized in a recent review[28] (Table 19-2). As a result of treatment with alkylating agents, hormonal and germinal epithelial changes occur that may result in temporary or permanent ovarian or testicular gonadal suppression in females or males. For those with temporary gonadal suppression the resulting effects are oligospermia or azoospermia in men and decreased numbers of ova and irregular menses or amenorrhea in women. These effects may last a variable period of time. Total drug dosage, duration of treatment, intermittent or continuous treatment,[72] and age of the client receiving cancer chemotherapy are important variables. Adolescents may experience gonadal suppression that differs from that in adults. Women who are premenopausal at the initiation of cancer chemotherapy may experience temporary ovarian failure, and those who are perimenopausal may be more likely to experience permanent ovarian failure.[69a]

Many cancer chemotherapeutic agents may be teratogens. Some men, oligospermic as a result of cancer chemotherapy, have fathered children.[14] Therefore those individuals who are sexually active may be counseled to use a reliable contraceptive method while undergoing chemotherapy. Individuals who want children may be counseled to explore sperm banks before initiation of chemotherapy, artificial insemination either by client or by donor, or adoption. Stereotypes about cancer may be a liability in adoption proceedings. Surrogate mothers may be another option for some in the future.

Chapman, Sutcliffe, and Malpas[13] found that ovarian dysfunction as a result of cancer chemotherapy for Hodgkin's disease can result in loss of a woman's self-confidence in her sexuality and alienation from significant relationships. Chapman et al.[14] reported that

Table 19-2. Cancer chemotherapy: effects on sexuality

Effect on sexual self-concept	Effect on sexual relationships	Effect on sexual functioning
Alopecia induced by cancer chemotherapy has a significant negative impact on body image only for those individuals who rate their hair as important to them.[71] The influence of other side effects needs to be reported in the research literature.	Symptoms of ovarian failure secondary to certain cancer chemotherapy agents were associated with disruption in sexual relationships (e.g., separation or divorce) in 10 of 33 couples. In 8 of these cases women were 31 years or younger. These women also reported arguments with other family members and disruption of friendships and work relationships.[13]	Libido decreases in some women after ovarian failure induced by cancer chemotherapy. Some women may have difficulty achieving arousal during foreplay. Vaginal dryness can produce painful intercourse.[13] Libido and sexual performance may decrease in men during and after certain cancer chemotherapy.[14]

the men with Hodgkin's disease in their study did not report alteration in aggressiveness despite direct questioning. However, three partners volunteered information that the men had been irritable and physically violent toward wives and families. Counseling the client and partner about the possibility of irritability and its effect on the relationship may assist them to anticipate these changes and determine alternative coping mechanisms.

Chapman et al.[14] found few men with Hodgkin's disease treated with nitrogen mustard, vinblastine, procarbazine, and prednisolone (MVPP) who had diminished libido and abnormally decreased hormone levels. However, low hormonal levels from induced ovarian failure are associated in women with Hodgkin's disease treated with MVPP.[13] Hormonal therapy may be an option for some of these women. Women may counter any associated problems with vaginal dryness and painful intercourse by sparing use of a water-soluble lubricant, use of the woman's or her partner's saliva as a lubricant, or increasing the length of foreplay. Topical estrogen cream may be appropriate for some women with some cancers. It is important that the advice of the physician be sought, since some tumor types are hormonally dependent. Impotence related to inadequate testosterone was very uncommon in the study by Chapman et al.[14] Discussing this possible change with the man and his partner will help them anticipate this change and discuss alternatives for communcating affection.

Other side effects of cancer chemotherapy may alter the expression of sexuality. It seems reasonable to expect that mouth pain associated with stomatitis could limit oral verbalization and expression of affection. Acne, weight gain, or gynecomastia could adversely affect sexual self-concept. Cardiac toxicity, pulmonary toxicity, or malaise could limit the individual's ability to engage in and experience pleasure from intercourse. Leukopenia could restrict the individual's ability to participate in intercourse based on the risk of overwhelming infection. Wagner and Bye[71] found that alopecia had a significant negative impact on body image only for those individuals who rate their hair as important to them. The influence of side effects of cancer chemotherapeutic agents on sexuality needs to be specifically researched and reported in the literature.

The health care process and the person after cancer therapy

Living with the effects of cancer therapy can affect the component parts of sexuality for both the individual and the partner, but the impact of cancer therapy on sexuality varies with the individual. Cancer therapy may enhance sexuality, interfere with sexuality, or have no effect on sexuality.[35] Not all individuals are affected in a similar manner by the same therapy; not all effects are perceived in a similar manner by the individual and partner. To ascertain the effect of cancer therapy, a sexual assessment must be performed. Data obtained should be interpreted in light of the individual's and the partner's cultural background, religion, age, sexual preference, and life-style.

Sexual assessment. Sexual assessment should include data about the individual's sexual self-concept, sexual relationships, and sexual functioning before cancer therapy. The individual's feelings associated with appearance or body integrity should be determined, as well as his or her definition of femininity or masculinity and how it is expressed in relationships. The health care worker should determine the individual's satisfaction with frequency and desire for sexual functioning, and consider how the cancer therapy might influence physical appearance and physiologic function. The extent and visibility of change in appearance should be determined, as well as which physiologic functions may be compromised and whether the change will be permanent or temporary. It is important to learn the individual's comprehension of the effects of therapy. The client might have misunderstandings or unfounded fears that could interfere with ultimate acceptance of the effects of therapy. The health care worker should discern the value the individual has assigned the altered body structure or function in terms of self-concept, relationships, and sexual functioning. The practitioner should then note preoperatively those modes of adaptation that the client used in the past, which problem-solving techniques the client uses, and whether the client is dependent or independent.

Since the sexual partner may have a profound effect on the individual's recovery and resumption of normal sexual functioning, it is important to assess the relationship and the concerns and fears of the partner. The stability and security of the relationship should be determined, and the partner's comprehension of the person's body and the partner's understandings and fears about the consequences of therapy should be assessed.

It is also important to recognize various sexual life-styles and determine the individual life-style of the client. The health care worker can ask whether the individual is currently involved in a relationship and whether the partner is of the same or opposite sex. This information individualizes the effects of therapy on self-concept, relationships, and sexual functioning. Sensitivity to the individual involves not applying stereotypes.

To ensure that the health care worker proceeds at the client's pace, a brief sexual assessment technique proposed by McPhetridge[41] considers the components of sexuality and the progression of focus from less to more sensitive issues. For example, a married male colostomate might be asked the following, in order of least sensitive to most sensitive:

- Has having a colostomy interfered with your being a husband and father?
- Has the colostomy changed the way you see yourself as a man?
- Has the colostomy affected your ability to have and enjoy sexual relations?

The technique of diffusing the impact of the sexual assessment questions encourages discussion by reinforcing that there is a wide range of normal answers and no wrong answer. For example, an individual might be asked the following:

- Some men have found that having a colostomy has little or no effect on their ability to provide for their families. Other men find that stoma care routines and concern about the stoma interferes with their involvement in work. Have you found that a colostomy interferes with your role as a provider?

It is important to emphasize that the sexual assessment is not meant to illuminate nonexistent problems. In addition, the client is not forced to confront problems for which he or she cannot discern solutions; rather, the assessment is conducted so that the client has permission and encouragement to discuss sexually related issues when he or she is ready for the discussion. By introducing the subject, the client is made aware that sexual concerns are legitimate concerns and that discussion with the health care worker is appropriate whenever the client is ready for the discussion.

Intervention. The PLISSIT model, developed by Annon, is one method that can be used to provide sustained support for the individual with sexual concerns or difficulties after cancer therapy.[3] This model presumes that different sexual concerns and difficulties require different levels of intervention.

Some sexual concerns may be alleviated by giving permission (P) for the client or partner or both to express feelings and concerns in their own words. For example, after mastectomy a woman may benefit from encouragement to explore or discuss her fears about injury to the surgical site during intercourse.

By giving limited information (LI) about sexual concerns and difficulties commonly encountered after cancer therapy, the health care worker can help the client to realize the range of concerns of individuals who are maintaining their life-styles after cancer therapy.

Specific suggestions (SS) for dealing with sexual concerns or sexual difficulties are within the capability of the professional health care worker. Clients may welcome these specific suggestions on how to deal with changes in their self-concept, relationships, and sexual functioning. After mastectomy some women prefer to wear a brassiere to bed. Some women tend to be fearful about resuming sex after hysterectomy for fear of "damaging themselves." Reassurance to the contrary may facilitate resumption of their usual sexual patterns. Female ostomates report wearing lacy covers over ostomy bags for aesthetic purposes. Both male and female ostomates recommend emptying the ostomy bag before coitus or wearing a small protective pouch such as a stoma seal if appropriate. If erection is impaired in the male ostomate, alternative forms of sexual satisfaction, such as manual or oral stimulation, may be practiced if acceptable to both partners.

By intervening with permission, limited information, and specific suggestions, the health care worker can help the client deal with some common sexual concerns and difficulties.[74] Misinformation can be clarified. Conflicting values can be explored. Difficulty in communicating about sexual issues between partners can be facilitated. Anxiety or guilt about sex can be explored. In addition, the health care worker can discuss methods of relaxation so that sexual activity can be enjoyed. Diminished interest in sexual activity or outright sexual dissatisfaction, as well as difficulty in pleasing or being pleased by the partner during sexual activity, can be explored.

Individuals who have been helped to discuss their sexuality openly may volunteer information regarding their needs and progress. When difficulties in sexual adaptation become apparent, the health care worker must evaluate the client's progress.

At times the expertise of the experienced health care worker is insufficient to help the client or partner work through sexual concerns or difficulties. Referral to a sex therapist, sex counselor, or psychotherapist may be necessary. Intensive therapy (IT) in the PLISSIT model is within the realm of these professionals.

Since the spouse's or partner's influence is crucial with regard to promotion of the client's ability to accept and live with alternatives in sexuality, it is imperative that the partner be involved in teaching and counseling sessions. Discussion of appropriate expectations after therapy can open communication channels and help prevent any self-imposed restrictions after hospital discharge.

After therapy the person may not be ready to immediately resume sexual relations. A temporary reluctance is not uncommon, or necessarily a sign of sexual dysfunction. Again, the partner needs to be apprised of this reluctance so that he or she can better understand what the client is experiencing.

Evaluation. It may be difficult to measure the effect of methods aimed at promoting psychologic acceptance of physical and functional change. Psychologic adaptation, as well as knowledge and application of coping techniques promoting independence in self-care and resumption of former life-style, should be assessed.

By shifting the emphasis from sexual concerns toward using the strengths remaining in the individual's mind and body, sexual health may be promoted. Viewing a function (e.g., communication) as an asset in and of itself and not negatively comparing that function with an ideal can also help an individual live with the effects of cancer therapy on sexuality.

Outpatient assessment of sexuality over an extended period of time after hospitalization will yield information about sexual adjustment. However, asking the client specific questions about his or her adaptation is probably the most fruitful approach. In one study 63% of women indicated they would have liked to discuss their feelings about sexuality after mastectomy with a nurse, but their perception of the nurse's negative attitudes about such a discussion served as a deterrent.[26]

Summary

This chapter has presented basic concepts related to sexual self-concept, relationships, sexual functioning and their alteration by selected cancer therapies. Concerns of the individual and partner were explored. Methods of promotion of living with the alterations in sexuality were discussed. The health care process was used to relate methods to promote living with alterations in sexuality for the client who has undergone cancer therapy.

Key considerations for health care include the following:
1. Body image is the way that people view their bodies. It is a dynamic concept subject to the influence of one's own perceptual apparatus and the reactions of others.
2. The perceived value of an organ or a change in body function or structure will vary for each individual. Not all individuals experience the same effects or degree of effects from therapy.
3. Body image distortion may elicit feelings of unacceptability, thus negatively influencing the person's perception of self as a sexual being and in turn influencing sexual functioning.
4. Sexual relationships may be adversely affected by cancer therapy.
5. The ability to engage in pleasurable sexual activity can be threatened, strengthened, or unaffected by cancer therapies.
6. Loss of a body function, such as that experienced by a client with an ostomy or laryngectomy, generates anxieties about independence, control, and social interactions.
7. Creation of an ileostomy or colostomy with accompanying colectomy may sometimes result in impotence if the pelvic autonomic outflow is traumatized; however, the person's feelings

about self-worth and integrity probably have equal, if not greater, influence on sexual functioning.

8. Loss of fertility after hysterectomy or other cancer therapy may create intense anxieties about sexual attractiveness and sexual identification even though no visible change occurs in the body.

9. Removal of the uterus or a breast does not usually constitute an organic cause of sexual dysfunction and should not physically interfere with intercourse. There may, however, be diminution of sexual sensations in some women who have had a hysterectomy or a mastectomy.

10. Some cancer chemotherapeutic agents can adversely affect fertility. The effect of cancer chemotherapy on sexual self-concept, sexual relationships, and sexual functioning needs to be more fully explored.

11. Adaptation of a partner to an alteration in the structure or function of the other, such as mastectomy, is a crucial factor influencing the future sexual relationship.

12. Education and counseling related to a change in the body image that has the potential to affect sexual relationships ideally include both client and partner.

Questions for review

1. Henry Wilson, a 35-year-old businessman, recently had a colostomy because of rectal carcinoma. He is believed to have been surgically cured. As he prepares for discharge from the hospital, what concerns might he have about sexual roles and relationships?

2. At his 6-month checkup Henry reports that he has been able to have an erection through masturbation but has not attempted to have an erection with his female partner since the time his appliance leaked during intercourse 1 week ago. What inferences might you make about his behavior?

3. Lilian Radke is a 28-year-old model who was admitted for a modified radical mastectomy for breast cancer. What emotional responses might you expect to the resultant change in her body?

4. William Radke, a 34-year-old businessman, is waiting for his wife to have her 3-month checkup after her mastectomy before he feels comfortable resuming sexual intercourse. What may motivate him to delay resuming intercourse?

5. What effects might this have on his wife?

6. Michael Webber, a 65-year-old man, recently underwent a laryngectomy and radical neck dissection. Although he was active in visiting his friends preoperatively, postoperatively he stays in his home and watches television. What inferences might you make about his behavior?

7. At his 6-week checkup Mr. Webber tells you that his wife has begun to sleep in an adjacent bedroom. What inferences might be made about their sexual adaptation? How would you assess the validity of your inferences?

8. Winifred Madison is a 27-year-old woman who was admitted yesterday for a hysterectomy for cancer of the cervix. Ms. Madison reveals to you

that she is going to be married soon and wonders if intercourse will be possible after surgery. How would you respond?

9. Ms. Madison says her fiancé has not had intercourse with her since before her diagnosis of cervical cancer. What fears might he have about sexual activity?

10. Gloria Carr, a 28-year-old married woman, is receiving adjuvant chemotherapy, including an alkylating agent, for breast cancer. She tells you that she and her husband want children in the near future but that she is concerned that she may be becoming sterile. How would you handle this situation? What advice about contraceptives would you share with Mrs. Carr?

References

1. Abitbol, M.M., and Davenport, J.H.: Sexual dysfunction after therapy for cervical carcinoma, American Journal of Obstetrics and Gynecology **119:**181-189, 1974.

2. Adams, G.K.: The sex-counseling role of the cancer clinician. In Vaeth, J.M., Blomberg, R.C., and Adler, L., editors: Frontiers of radiation therapy and oncology, vol. 14, Body image, self-esteem, and sexuality in cancer patients, New York, 1980, S. Karger.

3. Annon, J.S.: The behavioral treatment of sexual problems. Brief therapy, New York, 1976, Harper & Row, Publishers, Inc.

4. Baker, B.M., and Cunningham, C.A.: Vocal rehabilitation of the patient with a laryngectomy. I. Pre- and postoperative counseling, Oncology Nursing Forum **7**(4):23-27, 1980.

5. Baker, B.M., and Cunningham, C.A.: Vocal rehabilitation of the patient with a laryngectomy. III. Specific techniques in laryngectomy vocal rehabilitation, Oncology Nursing Forum **7**(4):33-36, 1980.

6. Bard, M., and Sutherland, A.: Psychological impact of cancer and its treatment, Cancer **8:**656-672, 1955.

7. Blaesing, S., and Brockhaus, J.: The development of body image in the child, Nursing Clinics of North America **7:**597-607, 1972.

8. Blues, K.: A framework for nurses providing care to laryngectomy patients, Cancer Nursing **1:**441-446, 1978.

9. Brouillette, J.N., Pryor, E., and Fox, T.A.: Evaluation of sexual dysfunction in the female following rectal resection and intestinal stoma, Diseases of the Colon and Rectum **24**(2):96-102, 1981.

10. Brown, R.S., et al.: Social and psychological adjustment following pelvic exenteration, American Journal of Obstetrics and Gynecology **114:**162-171, 1972.

11. Burnham, W.R., Lennard-Jones, J.E., and Brooke, B.N.: Sexual problems among married ileostomists, Gut **18:**673-677, 1977.

12. Carroll, R.M.: The impact of mastectomy on body image, Oncology Nursing Forum **8**(4):29-32, 1981.

13. Chapman, R.M., Sutcliffe, S.B., and Malpas, J.S.: Cytotoxic-induced ovarian failure in Hodgkin's disease. II. Effects on sexual function, Journal of the American Medical Association **242:**1882-1884, 1979.

14. Chapman, R.M., et al.: Cyclical combination chemotherapy and gonadal function: retrospective study in males, Lancet **1:**285-289, 1979.

15. Cosper, B., Fuller, S., and Robinson, G.: Characteristics of posthospitalization recovery following hysterectomy, Journal of Obstetrics, Gynecology, and Neonatal Nursing **7**(3):7-11, 1978.
16. Cunningham, C.A., and Baker, B.M.: Vocal rehabilitation of the patient with a laryngectomy. II. Assessment for vocal rehabilitation, Oncology Nursing Forum **7**(4):28-33, 1980.
17. Dempsey, M.O.: The development of body image in the adolescent, Nursing Clinics of North America **7**:609-615, 1972.
18. Dlin, B.M., and Perlman, A.: Emotional response to ileostomy and colostomy in patients over the age of 50, Geriatrics **26**:112-118, June 1971.
19. Dlin, B.M., Perlman, A., and Ringold, E.: Psychosexual response to ileostomy and colostomy, AORN Journal **10**(5):77-84, 1969.
20. Drellich, M., and Bieber, J.: The psychologic importance of a uterus and its functions: some psychoanalytic implications of hysterectomy, Journal of Nervous and Mental Diseases **126**:322-336, 1958.
21. Druss, R.G., O'Connor, J.F., and Stern, L.O.: Psychological response to colectomy. II. Adjustment to a permanent colostomy, Archives of General Psychiatry **20**:419-427, 1969.
22. Dyk, R.B., and Sutherland, A.: Adaptation of the spouse and other family members to the colostomy patient, Cancer **9**:123-138, 1956.
23. Fazio, V.W., Fletcher, J., and Montague, D.: Prospective study of the effect of resection of the rectum on male sexual function, World Journal of Surgery **4**:149-152, 1980.
24. Fedak, M.K.: Teaching the patient about sexuality. In Donovan, M.I., editor: Cancer care: a guide for patient education, New York, 1981, Appleton-Century-Crofts.
25. Gallagher, A.: Body image changes in the patient with a colostomy, Nursing Clinics of North America **7**:669-676, 1972.
26. Graf, M.S.: Sexual adjustment following mastectomy, unpublished research paper, Milwaukee, 1977, Marquette University.
27. Harrell, H.C.: To lose a breast, American Journal of Nursing **72**:676-677, 1972.
28. Kaempfer, S.H.: The effects of cancer chemotherapy on reproduction: a review of the literature, Oncology Nursing Forum **8**(1):11-18, 1981.
29. Kardiner, A.: The individual and his society, New York, 1939, Columbia University Press.
30. Kolb, L.C.: Disturbances of the body-image. In Reiser, M.F., editor: Organic disorders and psychosomatic medicine, New York, 1975, Basic Books, Inc.
31. Krant, M.J.: Psychosocial impact of gynecologic cancer, Cancer **48**:608-612, 1981.
32. Krozy, R.: Becoming comfortable with sexual assessment, American Journal of Nursing **78**:1036-1038, 1978.
33. Krumm, S.F.: Problems of sexuality in the cancer patient, Proceedings of the Second National Conference on Cancer Nursing, St. Louis, 1977, American Cancer Society.
34. Kyriakos, M., Kempson, R.L., and Perez, C.A.: Carcinoma of the cervix in young women. I. Invasive carcinoma, Obstetrics and Gynecology **38**:930-944, 1971.

35. Lamb, M.A., and Woods, N.F.: Sexuality and the cancer patient, Cancer Nursing **4:**137-144, 1981.
36. Larsen, G., Chief, Speech Pathology Section and Coordinator of Head and Neck Rehabilitation, Seattle Veterans Administration Medical Center: personal communication, Dec. 1982.
37. Larsen, G.: Rehabilitation for the patient with head and neck cancer, American Journal of Nursing **82:**119-121, 1982.
38. Lenneberg, E.S., and Sohn, N.: Modern concepts in the management of patients with intestinal and urinary stomas, Clinical Obstetrics and Gynecology **15:**542-579, 1972.
39. Lindsey, A.M., et al.: Social support and health outcomes in post mastectomy women: a review, Cancer Nursing **4:**377-384, 1981.
40. Mathis, J.L.: Psychologic aspects of surgery on female reproductive organs, Journal of Obstetric, Gynecologic, and Neonatal Nursing **2**(1):50-54, 1973.
41. McPhetridge, L.M.: Nursing history: one means to personalize care, American Journal of Nursing **68**(1):68-75, 1968.
42. Melody, G.: Depressive reactions following hysterectomy, American Journal of Obstetrics and Gynecology **83:**410-413, 1962.
43. Meyer, B.A., and Lyons, A.S.: Rectal resection: psychiatric and medical management of sequelae: report of a case, Psychosomatic Medicine **19:**152-157, 1957.
44. Meyers, A.D., et al.: Sexual behavior following laryngectomy, Ear, Nose, and Throat Journal **59:**327-329, 1980.
45. Morgan, S.: Sexuality after hysterectomy and castration, Women and Health **3**(1):5-10, 1978.
46. Murray, R.L.E.: Body image development in adulthood, Nursing Clinics of North America **7:**617-630, 1972.
47. Murray, R.L.E.: Principles of nursing interventions for the adult patient with body image changes, Nursing Clinics of North America **7:**697-707, 1972.
48. Nilsson, L.O., et al.: Sexual adjustment in ileostomy patients before and after conversion to continent ileostomy, Diseases of the Colon and Rectum **24:**287-290, 1981.
49. Orbach, C.E., and Tallent, N.: Modification of perceived body and of body concepts, Archives of General Psychiatry **12:**126-135, 1965.
50. Orifer, A.P.: Loss of sexual function in the male. In Schoenberg, B., et al., editors: Loss and grief: psychological management in medical practice, New York, 1970, Columbia University Press.
51. Owen, M.L.: Special care for the patient who has a breast biopsy or mastectomy, Nursing Clinics of North America **7:**373-382, 1972.
52. Pluchinotta, A.M., and Fabris, G.: Sexual function after abdominoperineal resection of the rectum, American Journal of Proctology, Gastroenterology and Colon and Rectal Surgery **31**(6):18-21, 1980.
53. Reach to Recovery: For women who have had breast surgery, ed. 2, New York, American Cancer Society, New York City Division, and Sloan-Kettering Memorial Cancer Center.
54. Rodriguez, D.B.: The problem for the nurse. In von Eschenbach, A.C., and Rodriguez, D.B., editors: Sexual rehabilitation of the urologic cancer patient, Boston, 1981, G.K. Hall & Co.

55. Romm, M.E.: Loss of sexual function in the female. In Schoenberg, B., et al., editors: Loss and grief: psychological management in medical practice, New York, 1970, Columbia University Press.

56. Roy, P.H., et al.: Experience with ileostomies: evaluation of long-term rehabilitation in 497 patients, American Journal of Surgery **119:**77-86, Jan. 1970.

57. Rudolph, B.J.: Lymphedema following a radical mastectomy, Oncology Nursing Forum **6**(2):13-17, 1979.

58. Sanger, C.K., and Reznikoff, M.: A comparison of the psychological effects of breast-saving procedures with the modified radical mastectomy, Cancer **48:**2341-2346, 1981.

59. Schain, W.S.: Role of the sex therapist in the care of the cancer patient. In Vaeth, J.M., editor: Frontiers of radiation therapy and oncology, vol. 15, Pharmaceutical aspects of cancer care, New York, 1981, S. Karger.

60. Schain, W.S.: Sexual problems of patients with cancer. In DeVita, V.T., Hellman, S., and Rosenberg, S.A., editors: Cancer principles and practice of oncology, Philadelphia, 1982, J.B. Lippincott Co.

61. Schilder, P.: The image and appearance of the human body, New York, 1950, International Universities Press, Inc.

62. Schoenberg, B., and Carr, A.C.: Loss of external organs: limb amputation, mastectomy and disfiguration. In Schoenberg, B., et al., editors: Loss and grief: psychological management in medical practice, New York, 1970, Columbia University Press.

63. Schoenberg, B., et al., editors: Loss and grief: psychological management in medical practice, New York, 1970, Columbia University Press.

64. Seibel, M., Freeman, M.G., and Graves, W.L.: Hysterectomy for carcinoma *in situ* and sexual function, Gynecologic Oncology **11:**195-199, 1981.

65. Silberfarb, P.M., Maurer, L.H., and Crouthamel, C.S.: Psychosocial aspects of neoplastic disease. I. Functional status of breast cancer patients during different treatment regimens, American Journal of Psychiatry **137:**450-455, 1980.

66. Stahlgren, L.H., and Ferguson, L.K.: Influence on sexual function of abdominoperineal resection for ulcerative colitis, New England Journal of Medicine **259:**873-875, 1958.

67. Stoklosa, J.M., and Bullard, D.G.: Talking about sex: suggestions for the health professional. In Vaeth, J.M., Blomberg, R.C., and Adler, L., editors: Frontiers of radiation therapy and oncology, vol. 14, Body image, self-esteem, and sexuality in cancer patients, New York, 1980, S. Karger.

68. Sutherland, A.M., et al.: The psychological impact of cancer and cancer surgery, I. Adaptation to the dry colostomy; preliminary report and summary of findings, Cancer **5:**857-872, 1952.

69. Talking together: American Journal of Nursing **72:**682, 1972.

69a. Tarpy, C.C.: Menses and related symptomatology of the premenopausal breast cancer patient treated with chemotherapy, unpublished master's thesis, Seattle, 1982, University of Washington.

70. Thomas, S.G., and Yates, M.M.: Confronting one's changed image: breast reconstruction after mastectomy, American Journal of Nursing **77:**1438-1442, 1977.

71. Wagner, L., and Bye, M.G.: Body image and patients experiencing alopecia as a result of cancer chemotherapy, Cancer Nursing **2:**365-369, 1979.

72. Wang, C., et al.: Effect of combination chemotherapy on pituitary-gonadal function in patients with lymphoma and leukemia, Cancer **45:**2030-2037, 1980.

73. Weinstein, M., and Roberts, M.: Sexual potency following surgery for rectal carcinoma: a follow-up of 44 patients, Annals of Surgery **185:**295-300, 1977.

74. Whitley, M.P., and Willingham, D.: Adding sexual assessment to the health interview, Journal of Psychiatric Nursing and Mental Health Services **16**(4):17-22, 1978.

75. Williams, J.T., and Slack, W.W.: A prospective study of sexual function after major colorectal surgery, British Journal of Surgery **67:**772-774, 1980.

76. Williams, M.A.: Cultural patterning of the feminine role: a factor in response to hysterectomy, Nursing Forum **12:**378-387, 1973.

77. Williams, M.A.: Cultural factors and hysterectomy, Paper presented at The Menstrual Cycle: an Interdisciplinary Conference, Chicago, 1977, University of Illinois.

78. Witkin, M.H.: Sex therapy and mastectomy, Journal of Sex and Marital Therapy **1:**290-304, 1975.

79. Women's attitudes regarding breast cancer: Occupational Health Nursing **22:**20-23, Feb. 1974.

80. Woods, N.F.: Human sexuality in health and illness, ed. 2, St. Louis, 1979, The C.V. Mosby Co.

81. Woods, N.F., and Earp, J.A.L.: Women with cured breast cancer: a study of mastectomy patients in North Carolina, Nursing Research **27:**279-285, 1978.

82. Yeager, E.S., and Van Heerden, J.A.: Sexual dysfunction following proctocolectomy and abdominoperineal resection, Annals of Surgery **191:**169-170, 1980.

References for clients

Binder, D.: Sex, courtship and the single ostomate, Los Angeles, 1973, United Ostomy Association, Inc.

Dickman, G.L., and Livingston, C.A.: Sex and the female ostomate, Los Angeles, 1982, United Ostomy Association, Inc.

Gambrell, E.: Sex and the male ostomate, Los Angeles, 1973, United Ostomy Association, Inc.

Reach to Recovery: For women who have had breast surgery, ed. 2, New York, American Cancer Society, New York City Division, and Sloan-Kettering Memorial Cancer Center.

20
Sexuality and disability

CINDY GATENS

Sexual health is vulnerable to both neuromuscular and musculoskeletal impairment. To assist the health care provider in delivering comprehensive services to people with a chronically disabling disease, this chapter will focus on the sexual implications for individuals with physical disability. As noted in previous chapters, illness imposes an additional dimension on adjustment in all areas. Chronic illness adds the element of time so that the effective changes last a lifetime.[24] The purposes of this chapter follow:

1. To discuss the effects of physically disabling conditions on sexuality based on current research in three disability states: arthritis, stroke, and spinal cord injury
2. To acquaint health professionals with potential sexual health problems of the physically disabled
3. To include guidelines for assessment, intervention, and evaluation to promote satisfactory sexual adjustment in neuromuscular and musculoskeletal impairment

Sex, sex acts, and sexuality

To clearly discuss issues related to sexuality and physical disability, it is essential to differentiate the terms *sex, sex acts,* and *sexuality.* Trieschmann[69] describes sex as being one of four primary drives—the others being thirst, hunger, and avoidance of pain. Originating in the subcortex, these drives are modified by learned response originating in the cortex. Thus the methods, occasions, and expressions of the primary drives are regulated by the cortex. A sex act is a specific behavior involving the genitals and secondary erogenous zones, with sexual intercourse only one kind of sex act. The relationships of the people involved and their emotions are not considered within this physical aspect of sexual expression. Sexuality includes sex drive and sex acts, with the further dimension of personality and its effect on relationships. The sexuality process can occur on many levels, such as conversation, work, socialization, and various expressions of affection, including sexual intercourse. Although a disability may impose changes on sex acts, unless there is damage to the cortex or subcenter, sex drive and sexuality remain vulnerable but intact. Thus it is important for the health professional to recognize potential sexual health problems specific for each disability.

Sexual well-being and adjustment

Much has been accomplished over the past 10 years in counseling disabled people wtih sexual problems. However, a review of the literature reveals that the needs of clients with specific disabilities, as well as individual advice for counseling, have not been fully documented. Spinal cord injury has received the largest concentration of interest in the literature, but sexual health care for the physically disabled is still an area that attracts only minimal research attention, possibly because health professionals fail to see the relationship between sexual health and optimal functioning in all activities of life.

Sexual well-being for the physically disabled cannot be treated as an isolated adjustment area. The positive correlation between sexual well-being and adjustment and satisfaction in other areas of life, such as self-esteem and vocational adjustment, is generally accepted in the literature.*

Sexual difficulties can drain clients of energy that might be used for more constructive activities. In Maslow's hierarchy of needs[46] self-esteem is given a position of central importance. A positive level of self-esteem is the final prerequisite for self-actualization; once people achieve self-esteem, they can then be free to concentrate on actualizing their potential.[65] The effects of sexual adjustment on self-esteem, social roles, marital status, and overall psychosocial adjustment and productivity have not been adequately documented, but the majority of research indicates that a positive sexual adjustment can have a significant effect on adjustment in other areas of life.[67]

Studies have indicated that clients with disabilities rated sexuality as a high priority and wanted sexual issues included with their total rehabilitation plan.[26,29,74] Health care providers must be willing to deal with the sexual aspects of disability in relation to promoting adaptation to physical disabilities in all areas of life.

Comfort[20] noted that disabled persons have two types of disabilities to deal with in the sexual field: those arising from physical problems that limit activity or response and those arising from misinformation and lack of social permission. The latter can often be the "more disabling." The young, the beautiful, and the whole comprise the sexual stereotype in American culture today. Goffman[32] notes that a physical disability is a discrediting attribute that may lead society to believe that such a person "is not quite human." Thus for some disabled men and women the effects of stigmatization may be so powerful as to impose an insurmountable obstacle for developing a relationship with another.

In assisting the disabled to attain sexual health, health professionals must address both the physical problems limiting activity and response and those problems arising from society's attitudes. Sexual assessment, subsequent discussion of concerns, and guidance and counseling can be done by any health professional who understands the problems,

---

*References 8, 14, 26, 60, 63, and 65.

is knowledgeable about the disability and potential sexual alternatives, and possesses necessary counseling skills.

Cole[15] describes the role of the health professional as that of helping disabled persons to understand their sexuality, to take responsibility for it, and to make choices based on information and on freedom from fear.

Keeping this in mind, I will consider the available research for three specific disabling conditions: arthritis, cerebrovascular accident (stroke), and spinal cord injury. There are several types of disabilities that may be likely to create sexual problems. It is hoped that these three may serve as models to assist professionals in providing appropriate sexual health counseling for the disabled.

Sexuality and arthritis

Rheumatic diseases include over 100 different conditions that have, sometimes as a major component, musculoskeletal symptoms such as pain, stiffness, loss of motion, and weakness. These diseases, collectively referred to as *arthritis,* can be localized or involve multiple body systems. Arthritic diseases are chronic in nature and have the potential of being disabling to the client.

There are more than 31 million people with arthritis severe enough to require medical care. Of these, over 20 million are women. No one knows why arthritis discriminates against women,[70] but this discrimination is likewise revealed in the literature; a majority of the existing literature about sexuality and arthritis deals with women and their sexual concerns.

Since many people with arthritis have difficulty with their usual activities of daily living because of pain, stiffness, fatigue, and limitation of joint motion, it can be presumed that the same problems may carry over to their sexuality. Sexual functioning and sexuality in general during the course of arthritis have received scant attention in the literature. Early clinical reports on the magnitude of the relationship between sexual dysfunction and arthritis are reported as being conjectural.[58]

More recently a study was done by Hill, Herstein, and Walters,[39] who studied the sexual behavior of 58 adult clients (21 men and 37 women) an average of 14.5 years after the diagnosis of juvenile rheumatoid arthritis was made. Of those clients who were sexually active, 63% reported (by interview) some limitation in sexual activity resulting from fatigue, pain, or positioning difficulty secondary to symptoms of their arthritis. In spite of these limitations these people reported that they engaged in sexual behavior comparable in both frequency and variety to their healthy peers. An exception to this were single men with juvenile arthritis who reported having coitus less regularly than their healthy peers. Of the participants, 38% expressed the need for sexual counseling as adults, and nearly all felt that sexual counseling would have been helpful during adolescence.

Currey[22] examined sexual behavior in 121 married adult arthritic clients with hip involvement. Results of the questionnaire revealed that two thirds of the respondents with osteoarthritis of the hip joint reported having sexual difficulties as a result of their arthritis. These difficulties were relatively more common in women and were attributed to stiffness and hip pain rather than to psychologic factors such as loss of libido. Although surgical procedures were successful in relieving pain in more than 90% of the clients, alleviation of sexual difficulties occurred in only 57% of the clients. This suggests the possibility that other factors also played a role in the disruption of sexual functioning. Two thirds of the clients in this study who reported sexual difficulties wanted advice with regard to their sexual problems and usually for their spouse as well.

Yoshino and Uchida[72] studied sexual activity by distribution of a questionnaire to ninety-one married women with rheumatoid arthritis. Their results indicated that half of the women experienced a decline in sexual desire and orgasm and had a lower frequency of intercourse than before their illness. The main reasons cited for this were joint pain during intercourse, fear that pain would be worse the next day, and limitation in joint mobility. Other causes were depression and anxiety about the fear of failure to please the partner.

These studies specifically define sexual dysfunction by measurement of occasion of sex acts and their frequency. There is a paucity of data available delineating the specific types of sexual dysfunction present in people with arthritis. As Richards[58] noted, this definition does not allow for voluntary flexibility in sexual behavior. Possibly, although a client's joints are in flare, a decrease in the number of sex acts is not of particular concern to the client or partner. Thus it is not truly sexual dysfunction.

Medsger and Robinson[49] analyzed marital status, considering it to be an indication of physical and emotional health and adjustment to life situations. They noted that previous studies, which also looked at marital status as an indicator of adjustment, had conflicting results: whereas the research of King and Cobb[44] supported the theory that divorce is more prevalent in people with rheumatoid arthritis, the work of Adler et al.[1] and the British Empire Rheumatology Council suggested that people with rheumatoid arthritis do not differ from the general population in frequency of divorce. All three of these studies used people without rheumatic disease as controls.

Medsger and Robinson's study[49] looked at the marital histories of 100 rheumatoid arthritis clients and 100 controls with other types of rheumatic disorders who were similar in sex, age, and race. Findings revealed a significantly greater than expected number of divorced women with rheumatoid arthritis compared to the control group. This prevalence was explained by the smaller number of remarriages in clients with rheumatoid arthritis.

Although no specific conclusions can be drawn from this research, it serves to further stress the importance of providing sexual health counseling for people with arthritis and their partners. Even though empirical data are unavailable regarding the prevalence of sexual dysfunction in people with arthritis, there is an expanding volume of clinical literature and anecdotal material that supports a correlation between sexual dysfunction and arthritis.[24,43] As with other chronic disabilities, arthritis places special stresses on the client, sexual partner, and their relationship.

Deformities of fingers and decreased range of motion in wrists, elbows, and shoulders in rheumatoid arthritis and other major forms of arthritis may prevent some modes of expressing sexuality, such as touching, mutual fondling, and foreplay. These dysfunctions may even prevent the substitution of masturbation as a potential sexual outlet. For the supine partner in the missionary position the sacroiliac joints, hips, and knees are required for intercourse. Hands, wrists, elbows, and shoulders may be needed to support the partner in the astride position. Pain in any of these joints can make sexual activities difficult.[24]

In addition to the mechanical barriers (pain, stiffness, limitation in joint movement) to sexual functioning, Katz[43] notes that pain from sources other than joints may be distracting enough to inhibit sexual responsiveness. Sjögren's syndrome is associated with many of the connective tissue diseases and may accompany rheumatoid arthritis. It alters secretions of serous and mucous glands throughout the body. Atrophic vaginitis with dryness of the vagina is common. This lack of natural lubrication often results in dyspareunia. Ehrlich[24] notes that clients with Sjögren's syndrome have marked xerostomia that, even with stimulation, will not result in increased salivary flow. This symptom, plus rapid dental caries with painful gingival involvement, often deters oral-genital activity.

Studies on the stage of sexual response in people with arthritis have not been revealed in the literature. Katz[43] commented on Masters and Johnson's description[47] of myotonia developing during the excitement phase and becoming more intense during the plateau stage of sexual response. He felt that in the person with arthritis this involuntary pelvic thrusting, carpopedal spasm, and other forms of myotonia could cause severe musculo-skeletal pain during and following sexual intercourse. He felt that this pain during sex acts might lower sexual desires. Ehrlich,[24] on the other hand, reported that his interviews with clients revealed that they achieved as much as 6 hours of relief from pain after sexual activity.

Although no empirical data were given to support his statement, Katz[43] noted that erectile impotence and orgasmic dysfunction may be present in the person with rheumatoid disease, resulting either from physical or psychogenic causes, or both. In these instances premature ejaculation (except in instances of associated prostatitis) and orgasmic dysfunction are likely to be attributable to the same causes as in the nondisabled population.

There are other factors, such as poor body image, low self-esteem, and depression, that may compound the existing physical problems and complicate sexual health in people with arthritis. Joint swelling and muscle atrophy in rheumatoid arthritis, bony overgrowth of finger joints and loss of necessary support in knee joints in osteoarthritis, butterfly rash in systemic lupus erythematosus, the drawn facial appearance in scleroderma, and stiffened spine and dorsal kyphosis in ankylosing spondylitis are visible signs of disease. Corticosteroids can cause trunkal obesity and moon facies. Appearance is a big part of self-image. If physical changes have occurred, persons are apt to see their bodies as "being different" and have a poor self-image, thus feeling less attractive sexually.

Wright[71] defined self-esteem as the more or less general self-evaluation of an individual as a worthy or unworthy person. In addition to the physical changes secondary to arthritis, the disease may also impose changes in self-care skills, family roles, employment, and recreation. Loss of the ability to work can be devastating to the person whose major source of personal identity depends on job activities. Roles such as "bread-winning" versus "homemaking" may have to be reversed. A person who was once independent may now need to ask for assistance in self-care activities. Each of these changes may lead to diminished feelings of self-worth.

Depression is a natural reaction to actual or perceived loss.[6] It may be useful as a temporary defense, allowing a person to rest and reorder life's priorities. However, prolonged depression can result in loss of energy and motivation, both of which are necessary in self-management of a chronic disease such as arthritis. Chronic pain can produce depression; similarly, depression can produce and aggravate pain.[27] All three of these emotional factors (body image, self-esteem, depression) can have a profound impact on the client's relationship with self and others and therefore sexuality. It is important to remember that achieving satisfactory adjustments regarding sexuality may be particularly complicated by the fluctuating nature of the physical and emotional states that occur with arthritis.

Assessment. An important step in assessment of sexual health for persons with arthritis is for the professional to create an atmosphere in which discussion of sexual issues can occur. A goal of intervention must be to provide recipients with information and assistance so that ultimately they can make decisions about sexuality within their own value systems.

Sexual assessment, follow-up, provision of information, and counseling can be done by any health professional who is knowledgeable about disease process, is sensitive to the problems, and possesses counseling skills. Katz[43] and Ehrlich[24] suggest that an assessment of the effects of arthritis on sexuality be included as a part of the routine aspect of the physical examination, whether or not the client initiates discussion of the subject. Ferguson and Figley[25] noted that gathering information as part of a total health assessment provides a comfortable avenue for discussion for both health professionals and clients with sexual concerns. Some carefully worded questions about sexuality and sexual functioning can reveal that the subject is open for discussion and is viewed as a health concern. A good screening question might be, ''Has your arthritis had an effect on your sexuality? Is this of concern to you?'' Further questions may include a presymptom frequency and positional variety of sexual activity evaluation, a brief evaluation of the client's value system regarding sexuality, an evaluation of present sexual activity, and the person's satisfaction with that level of activity. These questions should serve to identify areas of change or difficulty in a person's sexual health. If concerns are identified, the subsequent assessment obtained should detail the following:

1. Duration of the problem
2. How it affects the client presently
3. What, if anything, helps
4. What the client believes is the cause
5. How the client feels about dealing with the problem

With just this bit of information, professionals should be able to make a decision about their level of competence in assisting the client and determine whether the client wants help with his or her concerns at this time.

Intervention. Intervention falls within the realm of sex education and counseling. A health professional's questions with regard to sexuality often give clients permission to ask questions and discuss the topic. Allowing persons to express their feelings and letting them know that others share their concerns may often be therapeutic in itself. It is also important to remember that control and management of the disease itself may often resolve the barriers to healthy sexuality for a person with arthritis.

Essential to the management and control of the disease process is education. People with arthritis are often concerned about whether or not certain activities will be harmful.[37] Provision of basic information about arthritis, as well as the anatomy and physiology of sexual functioning, can relieve unnecessary apprehension. Health teaching should promote the understanding that the disease process of arthritis itself does not directly affect the body's capacity for sexual excitement and satisfaction. Specific difficulties secondary to arthritis can interfere with one's sexuality, but there are specific approaches that may be tried to minimize or eliminate sexual difficulties.[5]

Lack of mobility, stiffness, and deformity of skin and musculoskeleture may interfere with an otherwise healthy self-image by causing a person with arthritis to feel less feminine or masculine and less confident sexually. Counseling should promote a positive body image and acceptance of changes and enhance feelings of self-worth with emphasis on the fact that adjustment to change takes time. Open, honest communication is important to nondisabled and disabled persons but is even more essential for persons with arthritis and their partners. If possible, health professionals should talk with the partner alone and then together with the client. Questions might include, "What is the partner's perception of the dysfunction? Are there role changes within the family and society?" Both the client and partner need to be equally involved in talking through their concerns. A partner's changed sexual interest may result from the fear of causing pain. In this instance it may be helpful to have a clear, preset signal to let a partner know if one is experiencing severe pain. This signal would enable partners to continue their activities on a positive level rather than halt them abruptly because of mutual anxiety.[5]

It is a myth that good sex has to be spontaneous and unplanned. If pain and fatigue are present, preparation for sexual activities may be helpful. Perhaps a partner can help in these preparatory activities, which can serve as a type of foreplay. Timing of sexual encounters may be better in the late morning or afternoon when pain, stiffness, and fatigue are lessened. Pacing of activities before sexual encounters may avoid fatigue. Application of heat, in the form of a warm bath or shower, may have a relaxing effect and decrease pain while increasing range of motion. Range of motion exercises will relax the joints. Antiinflammatory drugs may be taken so that their effect will occur during sexual activity. Narcotics are contraindicated, since they may well decrease libido. Impotence associated with steroid treatment may be one indication for reduction of steroid treatment.[58] Suggestions regarding positioning for comfortable intercourse should be provided. Joint protection techniques apply to sexual activity as well. A side-by-side position may be preferred when there is hip involvement, upper extremity pain, and loss of strength. Hip and knee flexion contractures or limitation in hip abduction may necessitate side-lying or kneeling in a comfortable position for rear-entry intercourse.[5,24,43] Actual diagrams of positioning may be helpful in assisting clients to experiment in finding satisfactory methods of expressing themselves sexually.[4,5] Mutual pleasure giving and seeking should be stressed, including alternatives to intercourse such as hugging, kissing, talking, massaging, and oral-genital manipulation. Vibrators can be a useful aid if there is upper extremity involvement.[54] In clients with Sjögren's syndrome vaginal secretions may be diminished and cause dyspareunia. Prolonged foreplay may increase vaginal lubrication and ease penetration, thus decreasing effort and pain. A sterile surgical lubricant should also be recommended.

Fertility is not usually affected by arthritis, but some clients may be advised not to get pregnant during the active phase of the disease.[43] In rheumatoid arthritis, remissions in pregnancy are common with return of signs and symptoms after delivery. In systemic lupus erythematosus the incidence of miscarriage, premature delivery, and delivery complications is increased.[48] With pregnancy, the ligamentous structures around the pelvis become looser and thus place greater stress on affected joints. The distended womb places excessive strain on the lower back. The client with ankylosing spondylitis with diminished chest expansion may experience further difficulty with respiration because of the enlarged uterus pressing on the lungs. In scleroderma, pulmonary function is further compromised during pregnancy.[24,43] Most women with arthritis can undergo vaginal delivery. Hip flexion or adduction contractures may necessitate a cesarean section.

If contraception is desired, selection of a method must take into account the abilities of the client. A condom, diaphragm, or contraceptive foam may be difficult to use. Birth control pills may be considered if there are no contraindications. An intrauterine device (IUD) may be difficult for the health professional to insert because of lower extremity pain and limitation and may be difficult for the client to check placement.[9] An IUD may also have the potential for heavier menstrual flow affecting possible anemia of chronic disease. A vasectomy, tubal ligation, or other forms of sterilization may be considered for more permanent birth control.

Sexuality and cerebrovascular accident (stroke)

Sexual functioning following a cerebrovascular accident (CVA), or stroke, has also received only limited professional attention and investigation, although an estimated 500,000 strokes occur annually, and more than 200,000 survivors are added to the number of people who have had strokes each year.[62]

What are the effects of sexual activity on the cardiovascular system in people with hypertension? There have been no studies conducted specifically with hypertensive individuals to document the cardiovascular responses to sexual activity. Hypertension increases left ventricular work, eventually causing left ventricular hypertrophy and reduced cardiac output.[36] According to Howard,[40] the physiologic responses of hypertensive clients during coitus carry some risks. He indicated that the sustained exertion and rapid heart rate of sexual activity in the presence of decreased cardiac output may result in rapid backward pressure and acute pulmonary edema. He advocated that hypertensive persons with blood pressures of 180/110 or with target organ involvement must be cautioned to play a less aggressive role in sexual activity.

In a commentary on Howard's article Gifford[31] stressed the importance of aggressive treatment in hypertension to return blood pressure to as normal readings as possible. He stated that once this is accomplished, no restriction need be placed on physical activities, including sexual activities. Gifford also suggested resumption of sexual activity no sooner than 6 weeks after an episode of acute intracranial bleeding (subarachnoid or intracranial). Studies are needed in this area to validate these propositions.

A CVA can leave a person physically, cognitively, and emotionally disabled. Residual-free recoveries are rare; thus clients and their families must face adjustments physically, emotionally, socially, and occupationally. Sexuality is intimately involved in each of these facets of life and is therefore affected by the changes in life-style necessitated by the stroke. Renshaw[57] notes that unless the cerebral insult is severe, the actual sexual response, both anatomically and physiologically, is usually spared. Potential sexual dysfunctions resulting from the stroke depend on the extent of the cerebral damage. Partial erections, impotence, and ejaculation in men and decreased lubrication in women are all possible if there has been damage to the higher centers of the autonomic nervous system, but these are unusual occurrences.

A review of literature reveals that very little has been published concerning the specific impact of stroke on sexuality. The majority of existing studies have primarily assessed libido and frequency of coitus following stroke.[27,42,45] Kalliomaki, Markkanen, and Mustonen[42] interviewed 105 people under age 60 after stroke, and their data suggested that a CVA tends largely to diminish libido and active coitus frequency. Ford and Orfirer[27] reported on 105 stroke clients under age 60 and found that 60% said that their sexual appetite was the same or greater, 43% had decreased frequency of coitus, 22% had increased frequency of coitus, and 35% gave incomplete information. Most reported the same subjective sexual desire as before the stroke but lessened opportunity to satisfy their desire because of their partners' anxieties and revulsions. Leschner[45] interviewed 77 stroke clients after hospitalization and their partners between 50 and 70 years of age and found a decline in the frequency of intercourse as a result of their CVA, and 45% stopped having intercourse completely. The illness-specific causes for this change in sexual behavior included difficulty in maneuvering, fear of making the condition worse, and lack of sensation. This study also reported that unaffected spouses were afraid of their partners' disability or felt that their disabled spouses were physically incapable or simply sexually unattractive. Their findings indicated that male clients were more affected sexually by their strokes than female clients, with male partners being more affected regardless of whether they were the clients or the partners.

Bray, DeFrank, and Wolfe[12] investigated thirty-five persons between 33 and 80 years of age after stroke, and their findings showed no significant changes in sexual interest or desire for either men or women. They further investigated the physiologic responses associated with sexual functioning (erection and ejaculation for men). (Since the investigators did not attempt to assess vaginal lubrication in women, they concentrated on menses and orgasm as their physiologic determinant for intercourse.) Men experienced significant decreases in ability to achieve erection and to ejaculate, and all five women who were premenopausal at the time of the stroke reported major alterations in menses. Only one woman reported orgasm following stroke. In addition, 79% of the men and 73% of the women reported sexual functioning to be of importance. The results of their combined interview and questionnaire indicated that although the majority of stroke survivors maintain consistent levels of sexual desire and believe that sexual functioning is important, most will experience sexual dysfunction following stroke.

In a more recent study Allsup-Jackson[2] conducted telephone interviews with 50 stroke clients between the ages of 45 and 60. The results indicated that clients had a decrease in sexual contact with their spouses following stroke. Of the male clients, 60% reported a decrease in sexual contact, and 75% of the women reported a decrease in coitus with their spouses. Of those responding, 60% indicated that the decrease in sexual contact was upsetting, and the reduction in contact was caused by their spouses' unwillingness to participate in sexual activity. The findings were somewhat similar to Leschner's findings[45] in that a majority of the respondents indicated difficulty in adjusting to their disability and stressed that they felt the decrease in sexual contact was caused by their sexual unattractiveness, difficulty in maneuvering, and the fear of future medical problems. Allsup-Jackson summarized these problems as being overwhelming fears of inadequacy. The men appeared to be more affected by the stroke sexually, and the male partner reported more effect regardless of whether he was the client or spouse.

The fear of provoking another stroke was a concern noted by a large number of participants in the previously mentioned studies. What is the risk of having a CVA during sexual activity? There is no documented evidence that sexual activity will precipitate CVAs. However, the incidence of CVAs has been shown to increase with a corresponding increase in systolic blood pressure levels.[40] Dawber et al.[23] have analyzed the 22-year follow-up data in the Framingham study. During this time 126 men and 118 women in the study had a stroke. They concluded that classification on the basis of systolic blood pressure provided striking evidence of increasing risk of stroke with increasing blood pressure levels.

Allsup-Jackson's study[2] went beyond sexual functioning assessment and noted the importance of other outstanding factors that affect a person's sexuality after a stroke. Physical, occupational, social, and emotional adjustments all have an effect on self-image and sexuality.

Renshaw[57] delineates additional factors that affect sexuality. Hemiplegia is the most common outcome of stroke. Muscle weakness on the paralyzed side may produce mechanical difficulties and awkwardness. In addition to motor weakness, there may be an absence or excessive increase in sensation on the affected body side. Visual changes (homonymous hemianopsia) that may accompany hemiplegia of the left side will prevent recognition of objects or persons in the range of the left outer and right inner semicircle of the visual field. Loss of urinary and anal sphincter control may be present. Speech loss may occur. These physical problems, coupled with the emotional factors of disability (body image, self-esteem, and depression), are barriers to healthy sexuality in all areas of a person's existence.

Assessment. Timing for rehabilitation of a person with a stroke is important—the earlier the better, within the limits of physical tolerance. The same thing is true for sexual mobilization—the sooner the better, for the client's self-esteem and recovery.[57] Anderson and Cole's approach[3] presents sexuality activities as normal and anticipated. It is discussed within the context of the variety of losses that a person may face because of the stroke (physical, occupational, personal, and recreational). In each of these areas the client is encouraged to examine how much performance is still possible and then is shown how that performance might be improved by special training or suggestions for alternate ways of adapting. Thus the client's sexuality is approached as a natural part of life that can be expected to continue.

Some carefully worded questions about sexuality and sexual functioning can reveal that the subject is open for discussion and is viewed as a health concern. In the process of assessing the client's sexual health needs the degree of pathology must be determined. Has there been intracranial or subarachnoid bleeding within the preceding 6 weeks? What antihypertensive medications does the individual currently take? Has the client been warned against overexertion in the past? What fears might be present because of this? Other questions should assess the level of motor weakness and sensory status, as well as the level of sexual functioning before the stroke. These screening questions should give a professional an idea of potential sexual dysfunction, as well as the level of intervention needed to assist the person with a stroke and the family to attain sexual health.

Intervention. Guidelines for resumption of sexual activity after a stroke are not well established. Alterations in libido and coital frequency have been documented.[2,12,27,42,45] Clients may be encouraged to know that sexual functioning may not be altered after a CVA, but it is important to evaluate each person and situation individually. Informing clients that decreased libido and frequency are oftentimes potential problems may allow clients and their partners to express their particular concerns.

Interventions aimed at considering sexual side effects of antihypertensive medications may be very helpful for clients and their partners. If sexual dysfunction is occurring, clients and their partners should be allowed to discuss their concerns openly. Sometimes just letting clients know that others who have had a stroke have similar concerns (both in activities of daily living and sexuality) and have learned to work through them with time and practice is helpful. Renshaw[57] notes some practical suggestions for specific concerns. If muscle weakness produces mechanical difficulties and awkwardness of sexual encounters, a trapeze, pillows, or alternative coital positions may be helpful. In circumstances of absent or excessive sensation on the affected side the partner could be encouraged to use stimulating touch on the intact body side and request that the client express feelings about what is pleasurable. There may be a specific position in which the person with a stroke would be more agile and more comfortable during sexual activity. If homonymous hemianopsia exists, the partner should know this and attempt to approach the client from the intact visual field during sexual overtures, as well as daily social encounters. If bladder or bowel sphincter control is a concern, manually emptying the bowel and bladder before the sexual experience might be helpful.

A loss of speech caused by the stroke can add additional barriers to a relationship. Nonverbal cues developed by the couple may aid sexual communication.[2,27,45]

Since it has been documented that people who have had a stroke and their partners are concerned about the sexual activity provoking another stroke, it is important for health professionals to discuss this issue. Awareness of the effects of sexual activity on blood pressure may serve as an incentive for blood pressure regulation. If blood pressure is adequately controlled, there is probably no need to advise any specific coital position or precautions.[31]

Hemiparesis may make a person feel less masculine or feminine and less confident sexually. Promotion of a positive self-image is essential in assisting a person to attain sexual health. Counseling should enhance feelings of self-worth, with emphasis on the fact that adjustment to change takes time. Open and honest communication is essential for the person with a stroke and the partner. If possible, health professionals should discuss sexuality with the partner alone and then together with the client. The role of the health professional again falls within the realm of sex education and counseling. It is important to help persons with a stroke and their families to understand their sexuality, take responsibility for it, and make choices based on information free from fear.

Sexuality and spinal cord injury

The third disabling condition that will be discussed is spinal cord injury. Sexuality in the person who has experienced spinal cord injury has received more attention than other disabilities in the literature. To be energetic and independent at one moment and immobilized and dependent the next moment is a transformation affecting every aspect of a person's life and well-being. There are approximately 150,000 people with spinal cord injuries living in the United States and 7000 to 8000 traumatic injuries occurring each year as a result of automobile accidents, diving injuries, and other forms of trauma.[73] Persons with spinal cord injuries have to relearn activities in areas of mobility, skin care, bowel and bladder control, and sociosexual functioning.

After initial trauma, life-threatening situations may be present. After recovery from spinal shock, vital physiologic functions are stabilizing. Once the acute crisis is over, these persons must attempt to reevaluate and redefine their capabilities, including sociosexual activities. This is an appropriate time to discuss sexuality education and counseling with persons who have spinal cord injuries.

An understanding of the impact of spinal cord injury on the neurophysiology of the sexual response cycle is essential for the clinician who will be counseling this group of clients. Knowledge of the relationship between the level and type of cord lesion and its influence on sexual functioning and reproductive capacity will assist the client in redefining realistic goals of sexual functioning. Although this information may help predict the effects of a given lesion at a given level, clinical experiences reveal that there are many experiences to the physiologic concepts.[30] It must be stressed that sexuality involves much more than a physiologic event. The adaptations possible and necessary for sexual gratification are diverse and may be shared with the individual in the context of the practitioner-client relationship. Facilitating sexual adaptation of clients with spinal cord injuries is an integral part of the health care process.

Neurologic components of human sexual response. The human sexual response cycle depends on two main physiologic processes: vasocongestion and myotonia.[47] It is important to recall that cortical influences, as well as those of peripheral nerves, autonomic pathways, spinal cord pathways, and reflex centers, are all involved in sexual functioning.

Excitement. During the excitement phase either psychic or physical stimuli are transmitted by descending corticomotor pathways or ascending sensory pathways. Although other tissues besides the glans penis and clitoris are capable of receiving sensual stimuli, these two structures appear to be the focal neural points for tactile stimuli.[47] The glans penis in the man and the clitoris in the woman appear homologous, each being densely supplied with peripheral nerve endings. Stimuli resulting from pressure or tension in the pelvic organs or from touch applied to the external genitals excite impulses that are mediated by the afferent fibers of the pelvic and pudendal nerves. These impulses are apparently carried to the sacral cord, where synapses with parasympathetic efferent nerves to the pelvis may lead to reflex erection.[10] These pathways are illustrated in Fig. 20-1.

Erection in men appears to be under the influence of parasympathetic impulses that emanate from the sacral area of the spinal cord through the nervi splanchnici pelvini to the penis. These impulses are responsible for dilation of the arteries of the penis and to a lesser extent constriction of the penile veins. As a result, vasocongestion of the cavernous sinuses of the penis occurs.[36]

These reflex centers may be centrally activated in the brain and erection psychogenically induced. In the absence of sacral cord function, centers in the thoracolumbar segments of the cord are believed to be responsible for reflex erection.[10] Although psychic stimuli serve to enhance excitement, they are probably not essential, since appropriate genital stimulation may cause ejaculation to occur even in instances in which the cord has been severed above the lumbar regions.

In women both local and psychic stimulation may initiate the excitement phase. Local

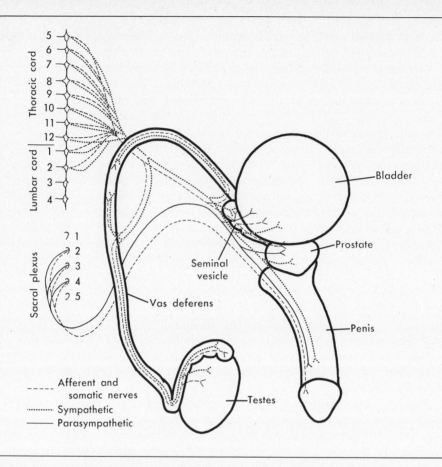

Fig. 20-1. Neurologic bases of the male sexual response.

sexual sensations are thought to be conducted to the spinal cord by way of the pudendal nerve and sacral plexus, as in men. These pathways are illustrated in Fig. 20-2. Sexual stimuli, in turn, are referred to cerebral levels. Local reflexes important in the female orgasm are thought to be integrated into the lumbar and sacral regions of the cord. The erectile tissue in the female pelvis (orgasmic platform) apparently is controlled by the parasympathetic nerves that pass through the nervi splanchnici pelvini from the sacral plexus to the genitals. During the excitement phase the parasympathetic nerves probably cause arteries in the orgasmic platform to dilate (and to a lesser extent cause congestion of veins), thus producing the vasocongestive phenomenon. This phenomenon is also responsible for lubrication of the vagina.[35]

Plateau. During the plateau phase, excitement intensifies in both sexes. The parasympathetic impulses in men cause the bulbourethral glands to secrete mucus, and in women they stimulate Bartholin's glands to secrete mucus immediately inside the vaginal introitus.[36,47]

Orgasm. As the sexual stimuli in men become intense, reflex centers of the spinal cord emit rhythmic sympathetic impulses. Propulsive contractions carrying sperm to the penile urethra (emission) are controlled by the sympathetic nerves.

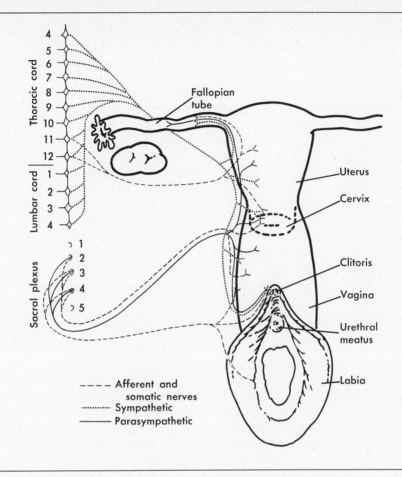

4
5
6
7
8
9
10
11
12

Thoracic cord

Lumbar cord
1
2
3
4

Sacral plexus
1
2
3
4
5

Fallopian
tube

Uterus

Cervix

Clitoris

Vagina

Urethral
meatus

Labia

– – – – Afferent and
somatic nerves
·············· Sympathetic
———— Parasympathetic

Fig. 20-2. Neurologic bases of the female sexual response.

Emission triggers afferent impulses that originate from the prostatic and membranous urethra and that flow through the pudendal and possibly pelvic nerves to the sacral cord. Here they synapse with the somatic efferent fibers of the pudendal nerve. This activity culminates in the clonic contractions of the ischiocavernosus and bulbocavernosus muscles. Synergistic innervation at the thoracolumbar and sacral levels prevents regurgitation of semen into the bladder by causing occlusion of the bladder neck during ejaculation.[36]

When afferent impulses from sympathetic pathways that synapse with efferent fibers of the hypogastric nerves stimulate the vas deferens, smooth muscles of the prostate, spermatic vessels, and bladder neck, peristalsis occurs. These impulses appear to be responsible for ejaculation. Reflex centers for ejaculation appear to be located in the sacral cord. Contraction of the perineal musculature in women is thought to be caused by neural stimuli similar to those responsible for ejaculation in men.[36]

Pathways of psychic stimuli. Central afferent stimuli may originate in many areas of the cortex, especially the temporal lobe, in parts of the limbic system, and in the hypothalamus.[10] Olfactory, visual, auditory, and somesthetic impulses may facilitate or inhibit progression of the human sexual response cycle by way of these paths.

Somatic and visceral efferents carry these impulses to the spinal cord from higher centers.

The difficulty experienced by the person with a spinal cord injury is shown in Fig. 20-3. Stimuli from areas below the cord transection are unable to descend from cortical levels to synapse with the motor neuron. However, the person may experience erection by means of the reflex arc, in which an afferent nerve synapses with an intermediate neuron, which in turn synapses with an effector neuron.

A large portion of the literature concerned with spinal cord injury deals with the mechanical and biologic aspects of sexual functioning, with primary emphasis on libido and the sex act in men.[67] A couple of factors may account for this bias. The incidence of spinal cord injury is greater in men than women, and the visible mechanics of sexual functioning are often considered easier to study in men. The lower incidence of women experiencing spinal cord injuries, as well as patterns of sexual behavior, will more likely change as women increase their participation in nontraditional occupational and social activities in environments that include higher risks of accidents. The majority of research on female sexuality and spinal cord injury deals with the reproductive aspects of menstruation and pregnancy.

Although there have been a number of studies published regarding sexual functioning of the person with a spinal cord injury,* the results are difficult to interpret and put into use clinically because of the variability in methodology. Methodological shortcomings within some of the studies include lack of documentation of the range in time from date of injury to participation in the study, documentation of the cause of injury, the terminology used in categorization of anatomic levels of injury, lack of specificity in the designation of complete verses incomplete, and documentation of current medication of participants.[38] Recognizing these limitations, practitioners can take useful generalizations from these studies to assist clients with setting expectations in the overall effect of their injury.

Male sexual functioning

Erection and ejaculation. In 1948 Munro, Horne, and Paull[53] reported the results of interviews and questionnaires administered to eighty-four men with spinal cord injuries. In their population 74% had erections, and 30% produced pregnancy. The authors concluded that a man with a spinal cord injury should be potent and fertile unless he has had a destructive lesion of the sacral cord, a transection of the cauda equina, or an injury to the cord between T6 and L3 sufficient to completely interrupt the sympathetic outflow.

Talbot[66] reviewed sexual functioning in 408 paraplegics. He found that 270 of them were able to experience erection, 186 of them in response to local stimulation (reflex) and 84 in response to psychic stimuli. Of those men who were able to have erections, one third had had intercourse. Over 50% of these men reported gratification from intercourse. Talbot also found that 76% of these men capable of erection experienced it within 1 to 6 months after injury; however, erections were regained by some subjects as long as 3½ years after injury. Comarr's findings[17] support these results.

A major difference between sexual response in persons with spinal cord injuries and nondisabled persons is that genital sexual functioning and cerebral or cognitional eroticism become separated. In those persons who have complete transections of the cord a reflex

---

*References 10, 16, 18, 19, 53, and 66.

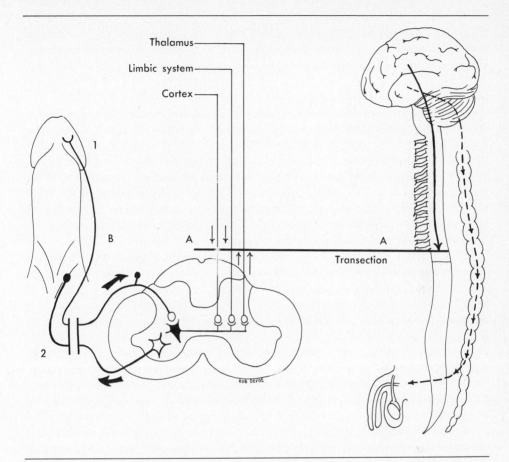

Fig. 20-3. *A,* Psychogenic erection: messages from the brain are blocked at level of lesion but may bypass lesion via the autonomic nervous system. *B,* Reflexogenic erection: sensory nerve *(1)* relays message to spinal cord and synapses with nerve that carries information to the genitals *(2)* and produces erection.

erection cannot be perceived unless the person sees it or feels it with an unaffected appendage.

        Influence of type of injury. Bors and Comarr[10] interviewed 529 men with spinal cord injuries regarding sexual functioning. Erections were more frequent in clients with complete upper motor neuron lesions than in those with complete lower motor neuron lesions. If the level of the complete lower motor neuron lesion was between T5 and T6, erection was absent and probably attributable to vascular insufficiency of the cord. Ejaculation was rare in clients with complete upper motor neuron lesions. Those who did ejaculate did not have true orgasm, but they may have derived a sense of gratification from the complete relaxation of muscle spasticity after ejaculation.

        From 90% to 100% of men with incomplete upper and lower motor neuron lesions experienced erection; ejaculation was much more frequent among those with incomplete lower motor neuron lesions. Psychogenic erections were much more frequent among clients with incomplete lesions, compared to those with complete lesions. In summary both reflexogenic and psychogenic erections were associated with incomplete lesions. Exclusively reflexogenic erections occurred with complete upper motor neuron lesions of the cervical segments, and exclusively psychogenic erections were seen in conjunction with complete lower motor neuron lesions.[10]

Comarr interviewed a series of 150 men with spinal cord injuries, 115 of whom had upper motor neuron lesions: 82% of the men were able to attain erection, 23% were able to achieve erection by means of psychic stimulation, 75% experienced spontaneous erection, and 71% had erections in response to genital stimulation. All clients with complete or incomplete lower motor neuron lesions experienced psychogenic erections only when the lesion was below T12. It also appeared that activity or hyperactivity of the sacral segments in clients with complete or incomplete upper motor neuron lesions had an inhibitory effect on ejaculation in some cases.[19] These findings reinforce the concept that the level and type of cord lesion greatly influence sexual activities.

Thus a man's sexual functioning after spinal cord injury depends on two biologic variables: the number of fibers that were severed (complete versus incomplete) and the level of injury (cervical, thoracic, lumbar, or sacral). Erections can occur in response to local stimulation that produces them reflexly or in response to psychogenic stimuli. In the latter case impulses from the brain can sometimes bypass the injured portion of the cord via the autonomic nervous system (Fig. 20-3). Usually, psychogenic erections are much less common than reflexogenic ones. Usually ejaculation cannot occur. In general the higher the lesion, the more likely the person is to be able to experience an erection.

Orgasmic experience. Clients with spinal cord injury may experience a wide variety of sensations ranging from anesthesia to orgasm. Cole[14] reported that some people with spinal cord injuries describe orgasm in spite of complete denervation of all pelvic structures and describe the experience as entirely satisfying, leading to a comfortable resolution stage of sexual excitement. Cole also reported that some adults stated that they were able to concentrate on sensation from a neurologically intact portion of their bodies and reassign that sensation to their genitals, thus experiencing it in their fantasy as orgasm. Sensory amplification is another technique that involves thinking about a physical stimulus, concentrating intensely on it, and amplifying the sensation to an intense degree.[52]

Geiger[30] noted that orgasm has been described as a cerebral event and can occur without any genital stimulation or without tactile stimulation at any level. Bors and Comarr's study[10] found that some of the male paraplegics with upper motor neuron lesions in their study reported severe flexor and extensor spasticity before and during ejaculation, followed by complete skeletal muscle relaxation. Authors have described "phantom" or "para" orgasms in persons with spinal cord injuries.[51,60] Researchers and subjects interpreted a wide variety of experiences as orgasm.[33] It is important for health practitioners to be aware of the various descriptions of sexual satisfaction and gratification experienced by people with spinal cord injuries. Provision of this information to clients and encouragement toward experimentation may be very helpful in assisting them to redefine their sexual functioning.

Female sexual functioning. Griffith and Trieschman, in a review[34] of sexual functioning in women with spinal cord injuries, revealed that only a few studies on sexual functioning refer to women, with very little descriptive data available on the physiologic and psychosocial aspects of women's sexuality. The majority of research before the 1970s with regard to female sexuality dealt with the reproductive aspects of menstruation and pregnancy. Higgins[38] notes that the counterparts to erection and ejaculation in men, including the physiologic events of genital vascular engorgement, secretions from Bartholin's glands, and vaginal lubrication, have not been directly investigated in women with spinal cord injuries, even though various authors suggest that these functions should show sparing analogous to that in men.[14,16,30]

Money's study[51] of phantom orgasm involved interviews with seven women from 21 to 65 years of age from 6 months to 14 years after injury. For the few who had the opportunity, intercourse was rare and never resulted in orgasm, but orgasm was described as being an occasional culmination of vivid fantasies or dreams in several of the subjects.

Several studies regarding the sexuality of women with spinal cord injuries have been done in recent years. Data were obtained through interviews with women with regard to their sexual behaviors and feelings. Bregman and Hadley[13] interviewed thirty-one women with spinal cord injuries, and their findings described sexual compensation and coping mechanisms of the women in areas of orgasm, bowel and bladder programs, and methods for enhancing attractiveness. All of the participants reported sexual experience after injury, and twenty-seven subjects indicated vaginal lubrication. The women who appeared to feel good about themselves psychologically also claimed to be adjusting well sexually.

A study of twenty-four women with spinal cord injuries by Fitting et al.[26] revealed an interrelationship between sexuality and self-concept in a person's adaptation to an acquired disability. The majority of their participants viewed sexual relationships as very enjoyable, although many commented that changing bowel and bladder function had inhibited sexual expression. Hindrances to sexual adjustment were noted and included the following: being treated asexually by health professionals, being given no physiologic information about their altered sexuality, having no privacy within the hospital, and being sexually rejected by a partner. Participants noted that learning how to feel good about themselves and being involved sexually after injury were evolving processes.

Thornton[68] identified and described three important aspects of concern essential in the sexuality counseling process for women with spinal cord injuries: relearning about one's altered sexual response and experimenting with this new knowledge, contraception, and social skills and realities.

My pilot study[29] involved interviews with five women with spinal cord injuries ranging in age from 21 to 25 years. Each of the women had been involved in sexual relationships before their injuries and continued to have sexual relationships after their injuries. Four of the women had experienced orgasm after their injuries. Descriptions of the orgasmic experience included a physical sensation of tingling all over, a rush of total body emotion, and a genitally centered feeling of physical release of tension. Each of the participants noted the importance of closeness and touching. Three of the women commented that sexual stimulation was primarily genitally centered before injury, and they learned to develop sensitivities in other areas above the lesion level after injury. Sexual fantasy was frequently used to enhance sexual arousal. Each of the women expressed a desire for more sexual education and counseling in areas of social issues and self-image, potential alterations in sexual response, contraception and family planning, and the physical changes that might occur in a women's body after injury.

Zwerner's study[74] of sixty-eight women with spinal cord injuries between 16 and 70 years of age examined sexual activity frequency before and after injury, including, but not limited to, intercourse. Of these women, 37% described no change in sexual activity frequency, 45% experienced a decrease, and 15% had an increase in sexual activity. Zwerner noted that only a few women commented on physical complications of sexual activities, whereas problems related to social interactions were more numerous. The need for sexual counseling information in the areas of sexual complications caused by disability, birth control and side effects, orgasm, and psychosocial issues was noted. These findings support my observations and those of Thornton.[68]

It is important to note that women with spinal cord injuries can experience orgasm if there is some residual pelvic innervation. As described previously, some women experience orgasm despite complete denervation of their pelvic structures.

Fertility

Male fertility. Munro, Horne, and Paull[53] investigated the fertility of men who had sustained traumatic injury to the spinal cord and cauda equina. A study of eighteen clients revealed no profound correlation between the level and type (complete or incomplete transection) of spinal cord injury and total sperm counts. Persons with lower spinal cord injuries involving the lumbosacral and cauda equina areas did not appear to have lower sperm counts. However, the small sample size did not permit a conclusive correlation. The investigators concluded that traumatic spinal cord injury did not, of necessity, preclude fertility.

Munro, Horne, and Paull[53] suggested that semen might be obtained by prostatic and seminal vesicle massage or electric stimulation from men with spinal cord injury who were unable to ejaculate. Electroejaculation has been used as a means of obtaining semen from men with spinal cord injuries for the artificial insemination of their wives.[7,53]

Bors et al.[11] studied fertility levels in thirty-four paraplegic men. They found that thirty of these men had regained erectile function after spinal cord injury. Microscopic examination of testicular biopsies revealed that tubular atrophy was present; however, no disturbance of Leydig's cells was found. A lesser degree of testicular pathology was found when the lesion was below the eleventh dermatome.

Sterility may be caused by loss of temperature regulation of the testes as a result of autonomic denervation or hormonal aberrations or by retrograde ejaculation.[11] Bors and Comarr[10] pointed out that reflex emission may be dribbling in nature and may lack the projectile power of true ejaculation. It is possible then that fertile men may be unable to impregnate their wives as a result of mechanical difficulties.

Female fertility and pregnancy. Again, the preponderance of research dealing with fertility and spinal cord injury has involved male samples. Early data describe the absence of menstruation in paraplegic women for 3 to 6 months after injury with a regular flow with resumption of the cycle.[21]

Twenty-five women between the ages of 18 and 50 years who had spinal cord injuries were interviewed regarding their menses.[17] Most women had a return of their menstrual periods within 6 months after injury. Half did not miss any periods, but two women had a return of menstruation after 16 and 30 months. The level and extent of the lesion and sacral sparing did not influence the return of menses. Comarr further concluded that women who had regular cycles would continue in a similar manner. Women who are in or near menopause will probably not menstruate again after their injury.

A more recent study (1982) of thirty-nine women ranging from 13 to 43 years found that 58% of the participants experienced an interruption of menses for approximately 5 months. Once menses resumed, they continued as they had in the past. Level of injury did not seem to be associated with changes in menstruation. As evidenced by available literature, there is no apparent permanent interference with the menstrual cycle in women with spinal cord injuries.

Robertson and Guttman[59] studied nine women with spinal cord injuries through eleven pregnancies. These women had lesions ranging from C4-5 to L1-2. Most of the women were able to deliver vaginally. Women with lesions above T10 had painless labor, although they had normal polarized uterine contractions. Three of the women had partially effaced and dilated cervices before the thirty-fourth week of pregnancy.

Women with lesions below T10 did experience normal pain sensations during uterine contractions. Women with spasticity experienced aggravation of muscle spasm and clonus during labor. All clients in this study were able to breast-feed successfully. They all demonstrated the normal letdown reflex during suckling. Robertson and Guttman concluded that maternal roles for women with spinal cord injuries seemed to be unlimited.

Griffith and Trieschmann[34] noted that pregnancy may be complicated by urinary tract infection, autonomic dysreflexia, and anemia. The risk of premature labor is increased as well.

Assessment. As mentioned previously, once the acute medical crisis has subsided after injury, persons with spinal cord injuries must attempt to reevaluate and redefine their capabilities, including sociosexual activities. This is an appropriate time to bring up sexuality. Cole[15] suggests discussing sexuality within the context of the total health assessment. This is a good avenue to let clients know that sexuality is normal and expected to continue and is an important part of rehabilitation.

Physiologic variables. Comarr[18] suggested that within 6 months after spinal cord injury, persons should usually know how much sexual functioning will return. The onset of erection in men usually coincides with the recovery from spinal shock and is attributable to the return of sexual autonomic reflexes. In some instances erections returned as late as 3 years after injury.[41]

To assess sexual potential, Comarr[19] recommended that a complete neurologic examination emphasizing the sacral segments be done. Since nerves emanating from S2 to S4 innervate the bladder and sexual organs, the return of bladder function seems to be a good predictor. However, this is not always the case, since sexual functioning is more vulnerable than other autonomic functions.

Presence of the bulbocavernosus reflex and rectal tone indicates that the client has an upper motor neuron lesion; their absence indicates that the lesion involves the lower motor neuron.[18] Pinprick sensation in the sacral segments when there are upper motor neuron lesions appears to be of greater prognostic significance for erection and ejaculation than preservation of light touch perception or retained voluntary motor function of the pelvic floor muscles.[18]

Psychosocial variables. The promotion of sexual health for the person with a spinal cord injury involves much more than the assessment of potential for sexual functioning. What will it be like to return to society as a disabled person? Does the person desire sexual gratification? What was sexuality like before trauma? Has the person given any thought to the subject of sexuality since injury?

Is the person married, or does the person have a current partner? What is his or her sex role in society? Do occupational requirements place constraints on the person now, necessitating a change in job or decrease in income?

What was the person's role in the family before trauma? Will the person face dramatic alterations in role performance, including sexual functioning?

Is the partner overwhelmed by what has occurred with the disability? Are there danger symptoms in the relationship? What are the expectations of the partner?

Careful consideration of the preceding questions will provide the practitioner with a data base containing information about the biopsychosocial aspects of sexuality. From this data base it is possible to infer both liabilities and strengths, learning the needs of the client and partner, and the client's concept of self as a sexual being.

Intervention. As in the majority of chronic illnesses, intervention falls within the realm of sex education and counseling. Basic to understanding sexual functioning after a traumatic spinal cord injury is comprehension of the normal human sexual response. It may be necessary to review the client's understanding of healthy sexual functioning before beginning counseling.

Counseling should be directed toward improving sexual satisfaction and enhancing self-esteem. Conjoint counseling with both the client with a spinal cord injury and the partner may be advisable. Several comprehensive programs addressing the sexual concerns of persons with spinal cord injuries have been described in the literature and summarized by the Sex and Disability Project.[63]

Formation of groups of persons with spinal cord injuries with emphasis on peer counseling in areas of sexuality has occurred during hospitalization and after discharge. The support and information engendered in the group setting are unique and often cannot be given by a professional who has not experienced a spinal cord injury.

Before proceeding with counseling, it is important to consult with the physician to get a precise determination of the level of the cord lesion and its degree of completeness. When sharing this information with clients, it is essential to stress that this determination is important in understanding sexual functioning in a broad sense but should *never* be applied to an individual.

Once the assessment of sexual functioning and concerns has been completed, particular problems should be addressed. Some clients may merely need permission to acknowledge that sexuality is important, and they should feel free to experiment and relearn new areas of sexual expression.

Atrophy of paralyzed extremities, loss of mobility, and the presence of adaptive equipment may profoundly affect a person's self-image and cause a person to feel less confident in relationships. Emphasis in education and counseling should focus on the positive aspects of one's life but at the same time allow a person time to adjust to his or her losses. Spinal cord injury has an extremely disruptive effect on the roles that a person plays in society. Teal and Athelson,[67] in reviewing Cogswell's study, reported that there appears to be a variable period of time immediately following the initial hospitalization when there is a moratorium on resocialization. It takes an individual time to adjust to the changes in life necessitated by the spinal cord injury.

Bregman and Hadley[13] found little correlation between sexual adjustment and time since injury. This finding suggests that time alone cannot ensure sexual adjustment. Education and counseling can provide information that may help a person work toward a healthy sexual adjustment. Coping with unwanted sympathy, obtaining help when needed, and handling unnecessary offers of assistance are all important social issues that should be addressed within the counseling program.[68]

Response to sexual stimulation. Specific suggestions for promoting and maintaining an erection may be helpful for men with spinal cord injuries. Manual stimulation of the penis is usually an effective method of promoting erection when psychogenic stimulation may be ineffective. A stretchable tape may be placed around the base of the penis to maintain engorgment and prevent detumescence before intromission. The tape should not be too constricting or be left in place more than 30 minutes. Vibrators for massage and stimulation may assist in inducing erection. Some men will be unable to sustain an erection long enough for coitus.[41] Sometimes stimulation of the inside surfaces of the thighs and of the lower abdomen can lead to reflex erections. Some men learn to trigger erections psychically.

The female response to sexual stimulation is not so readily observed. However, if neurologic control of vasocongestion is present, vaginal lubrication should ensue.[47] Thus one can infer that artificial lubricants would be unnecessary under these circumstances. However, it is generally good practice to inform women of the potential problem of decreased vaginal lubrication and provide suggestions that may help if it becomes a problem. Water-soluble vaginal jellies or lotions may be useful. Manual stimulation may also be helpful in activating lubrication.[68]

With an injury below T6, breasts may be sensitive to stimulation. The area around the injury may become very erogenous; some find new erogenous areas after injury (e.g., neck and shoulders) or find that areas erogenous before injury (mouth and ears) become more sensitive to stimulation.[68]

Options. Many positions for sexual activities are possible and should be limited only by inclinations and abilities.[52] Sexual options may depend on numerous factors, including the client's sexual value system, muscular strength in upper extremities, presence of hip flexors and extensors, the presence of appliances, and access to a partner. The first of these, the client's sexual value system, in conjunction with the partner's, determines what range of behaviors is acceptable. For example, oral and manual stimulation are viable means for stimulation of a partner but may be prohibited within one's value system. The muscle strength of the upper extremities will determine to what extent the person can support his or her body weight, and this influences a variety of positions that are possible. The ability to flex and extend the hips may enable the man or woman to take a more active role in intercourse by thrusting the pelvis.

Bowel and bladder control during sexual activities needs to be explored and perhaps planned for. Since many individuals with spinal cord injuries have chronic bladder infections, the potential for infecting a partner is present. For this reason, the man needs to take extra precautions, including careful cleansing of the penis and emptying of the bladder before intercourse. External catheters and leg bags can be removed before intercourse,[41] intermittent catheterization can be done, indwelling catheters can be taped in place and left in the bladder, or the urinary collection system can be positioned so that it is not likely to be clamped off. In the instance in which a man has an indwelling catheter, the female partner who is adequately lubricated usually does not have trouble accommodating the catheter.

For those men who cannot obtain a full erection, the "stuffing" technique may be a useful approach. The penis is manually tucked into the vagina. By then contracting the pubococcygeus muscle, a woman can obtain sexual sensations similar to those associated with penile thrusting.[52]

The subject of fertility should be openly discussed with both men and women after spinal cord injury. For those men unable to ejaculate, electrical stimulation of sperm for the purpose of artificial insemination may be an option. All women of childbearing age should have contraception discussed with them. One must assume that a young woman's fertility has not been altered and that the potential for normal pregnancy and delivery exists.[30] There may be an increased risk of thrombophlebitis associated with oral contraceptives.[64] An IUD may be selected, although the lack of uterine sensation may be of concern because the woman should not be aware of pain and increased cramping signaling infection or perforation of the uterus. The woman with a spinal cord injury or a partner would need to check for the IUD placement monthly. Diaphragms and contraceptive jellies and foams are reasonable methods of contraception, but a woman with poor hand function may have difficulties with their use. Tubal ligation for the woman and vasectomy for the man are ideal methods if childbearing is not a goal. This information on contraceptive alternatives should be made available to persons with spinal cord injuries so that they can make knowledgeable decisions with regard to contraceptive protection.

Predischarge planning. If weeks of hospitalization are necessary after a spinal cord injury, weekend passes and overnight visits home may allow injured persons the privacy and opportunity to attempt to resume their sexual relationships, evaluate their abilities and concerns, and find answers to their most intimate questions.

Evaluation

Evaluation of the effectiveness of teaching and counseling with persons who have experienced arthritis, a stroke, or a spinal cord injury is a difficult goal to measure, since its indices are not readily apparent. The health professional in an outpatient setting can continue to gather data over a period of time after hospitalization. Generally, asking clients specific questions with regard to sexuality is the best approach. If the subject of sexuality was openly discussed during the health teaching process, clients will probably volunteer information with regard to their concerns and progress during follow-up appointments. The practitioner should keep in mind that the goal of intervention is to provide clients with information and assistance so that ultimately they can make decisions about sexuality within their own value systems.

Summary

This chapter has focused on the sexual implications for individuals with physical disability and the practitioner's role in education and counseling. The health care process was applied to sexuality during musculoskeletal and neuromuscular impairment.

Key considerations basic to health practice include the following:
1. Knowledge of the differentiation of the terms *sex, sex acts,* and *sexuality* is essential for a discussion of issues related to sexuality.

2. Sexual well-being generally correlates with adjustment and satisfaction in other areas of life.
3. The disease process of arthritis itself does not directly affect the body's capacity for sexual excitement and satisfaction.
4. In CVA, unless the cerebral insult is very severe, the actual anatomic and physiologic sexual response is usually spared.
5. Certain components of the human sexual response cycle (such as erection and vaginal lubrication) are mediated by spinal cord reflexes, thereby precluding necessity of intact pathways from the cortex to the sex organs.
6. The level of the spinal cord lesion and the degree of interruption of nerve impulses influence the nature of sexual functioning in the person with a spinal cord injury.
7. Gratification can be experienced from feelings other than those emanating from sex organs during the human sexual response cycle.
8. Adaptation of previous sexual practices may be necessitated as a result of arthritis, stroke, and spinal cord injury.
9. Fertility and the ability to bear and nurse children are usually not compromised among women with spinal cord injuries.

The role of the health professional can be described as that of helping disabled persons to understand their sexuality, to take responsibility for it, and to make choices based on information and freedom from fear. This process is based on the assumption that the clinician possesses knowledge of the biologic, psychologic, and sociologic dimensions of sexuality, as well as acceptance of a wide variety of normal sexual behaviors.

Questions for review

1. When is the best time to initiate a discussion of sexuality and sexual functioning with a person who is disabled?
2. Mary Cannon has had rheumatoid arthritis for 16 years and is a wife and mother. She has severe deformities of her hands, which limit their mobility and dexterity. What kind of effect might this have on Mary's self-concept and feelings toward her sexuality? What other factors might you include in Mary's general assessment?
3. Marlene Hays is a 32-year-old woman who has been diagnosed as having rheumatoid arthritis. The first signs and symptoms of her disease began 6 months after the birth of her first son (now 2 years old). She and her husband are considering having another child but are concerned about the possibility of a pregnancy reactivating her disease. What information might help Marlene in making her decision?
4. Will Marlene be allowed to continue with her antiinflammatory drugs during her pregnancy? Will she be able to breast-feed her infant?
5. Ernie Brown is a 32-year-old mechanic who has rheumatoid arthritis. He has been experiencing increasing difficulty with pain, stiffness, and de-

creased strength in his hands over the past year. He told you that he is depressed about the possibility of losing his job. His wife confides in you that their relationship is deteriorating because of his fatigue and apparent lack of desire for sexual activities. What biologic variables will you need to assess? Which psychologic and sociologic variables?

6. Gloria Lund confides to you that her husband, who is in the hospital recovering from a stroke, was previously very sexually active. Now she knows (although he has not mentioned it) that he will feel "less than a man." What further data do you need for assessment purposes? What information could you share with her about the sexual aspect of his rehabilitation? Will you talk with both of them?

7. Mr. Lund has been home with his wife for 2 months now and is back for a follow-up visit. You provided counseling and education to both of them during the hospitalization. What data will you compile with regard to his sexuality at this time? Will you talk with his wife?

8. Liz Hunt, a 42-year-old woman who had a stroke 4 weeks ago, is being discharged to return home this weekend after her rehabilitation experience. She is worrying about returning to live with her husband and comments that she is concerned about their sexual activity provoking another stroke. How will you respond?

9. Steven Johnson, a 28-year-old father of two children, is admitted by ambulance to the neurologic intensive care unit after an automobile accident in which he sustained a fracture of T10, with resultant spinal cord compression. He is currently restricted to a circular electric bed, is being fed intravenously, and has a catheter for urinary drainage. He is aware that he cannot move his legs and has no feeling below his umbilicus. How can you facilitate his feeling masculine under present circumstances?

10. Two weeks later, Steven asks, "Will it ever be possible for me to have any more children?" How will you respond?

11. You find that Steven's lesion is a complete upper motor neuron transection. What implications might this have for sexual functioning?

12. What information would be important for Steven to understand before his first weekend pass home?

13. Steven asks, "How do I manage this tube (catheter) during sex?"

14. Randy Wilson, a 30-year-old woman, has been diagnosed as a T12 paraplegic after a diving accident. She is currently attending the clinic for physical therapy. Randy asks, "Will I be able to have children now that I have a spinal cord injury?" How can you respond?

15. What problems can be anticipated during Randy's labor?

16. To what extent is Randy probably able to experience sexual gratification? What techniques are available to her for enhancing her sexual pleasure?

References

1. Adler, E., Abramson, J.H., and Elkan, Z.: Rheumatoid arthritis in a Jerusalem population, American Journal of Epidemiology **85**:365-377, 1966.

2. Allsup-Jackson, G.: Sexual dysfunction of stroke patients, Sexuality and Disability **4**(3):161-168, 1981.

3. Anderson, T.P., and Cole, T.M.: Sexual counseling of the physically disabled, Postgraduate Medicine **58**(1):117-123, 1975.

4. Arthritis and sex: Rosalind Russell Arthritis Center, University of California, San Francisco, 1442 Fifth Avenue, San Francisco, Calif.

5. Arthritis: living and loving—information about sex: Atlanta, 1982, Arthritis Foundation.

6. Baum, J., and Figley, B.: Psychological and sexual heatlh in rheumatic diseases. In Kelley, W., et al.: Textbook of rheumatology, vol. II, Philadelphia, 1980, W.B. Saunders Co.

7. Bensman, A., and Kottke, F.J.: Induced emission of sperm utilizing electrical stimulation of the seminal vesicles and vas deferens, Archives of Physical Medicine and Rehabilitation **47:**436-443, 1966.

8. Berkman, A.H.: Sexuality: A human condition, Journal of Rehabilitation **41**(1):13-15, 1975.

9. Bogle, J., et al.: Family Planning Manual for Service Providers, Washington, D.C., 1980, Ebon Research Systems.

10. Bors, E., and Comarr, A.E.: Neurological disturbances of sexual function with special reference to 529 patients with spinal cord injuries, Urological Survey **10:**191-222, 1960.

11. Bors, E., et al.: Fertility in paraplegic males: a preliminary report of endocrine studies, Journal of Clinical Endocrinology **10:**381-398, 1950.

12. Bray, G.P., DeFrank, R.S., and Wolfe, T.L.: Sexual functioning in stroke survivors, Archives of Physical Medicine and Rehabilitation **62:**286, 1981.

13. Bregman, S., and Hadley, R.G.: Sexual adjustment and feminine attractiveness among spinal cord injured women, Archives of Physical Medicine and Rehabilitation **57:**448-450, 1976.

14. Cole, T.M.: Sexuality and the physically handicapped. In Green, R., editor: Human sexuality: a health practitioner text, Baltimore, 1975, Williams & Wilkins Co.

15. Cole, T.M.: Sexuality in the spinal cord injured. In Green, R., editor: Human sexuality: a health practitioner text, Baltimore, 1975, The Williams & Wilkins Co.

16. Cole, T.M.: The handicapped and sexual health. In Comfort, A., editor: Sexual consequences of disability, Philadelphia, 1978, George F. Stickley Co.

17. Comarr, A.E.: Observations on menstruation and pregnancy among female spinal cord injured patients, Paraplegia **3:**263-272, 1966.

18. Comarr, A.E.: Sexual function among patients with spinal cord injury, Urologia Internationalis **25:**134-168, 1970.

19. Comarr, A.E.: Sexual concepts in traumatic cord and equina lesions, Journal of Urology **106:**375-378, 1971.

20. Comfort, A., editor: Sexual consequences of disability, Philadelphia, 1978, George F. Stickley Co.

21. Cooper, I.S., and Hoen, T.I.: Metabolic disorders in paraplegics, Neurology **2:**322-340, 1952.

22. Currey, H.L.F.: Osteoarthritis of hip joint and sexual activity, Annals of the Rheumatic Diseases **29:**488-493, 1970.

23. Dawber, T.R., et al.: Risk factors: comparison of the biologic data in myocardial and brain infarctions. In Zulch, K.J., et al., editors: Brain and heart infarct, New York, 1971, Springer-Verlag, New York, Inc.

24. Ehrlich, G.: Sexual problems of the arthritic. In Comfort, A., editor: Sexual consequences of disability, Philadelphia, 1978, George F. Stickley Co.

25. Ferguson, K., and Figley, B.: Sexuality and rheumatic disease: a prospective study, Sexuality and Disability **2**(2):130-138, 1979.

26. Fitting, M.D., et al.: Self-concept and sexuality of spinal cord injured women, Archives of Sexual Behavior **7**(2):143-156, 1978.

27. Ford, A.B., and Orfirer, A.P.: Sexual behavior and the chronically ill patient, Medical Aspects of Human Sexuality **1**:51-61, 1967.

28. Reference deleted.

29. Gatens, C.: Sexuality and the woman with a spinal cord injury, masters thesis, Seattle, 1980, University of Washington.

30. Geiger, R.C.: Neurophysiology of sexual response in spinal cord injury, Sexuality and Disability **2**:257-266, 1979.

31. Gifford, R.W.: Commentary, Medical Aspects of Human Sexuality **7**:90-91, Oct. 1973.

32. Goffman, E.: Stigma: Notes on the management of spoiled identity, Englewood Cliffs, N.J., 1963, Prentice-Hall Inc.

33. Griffith, E.R., Tomko, M.A., and Timms, R.J.: Sexual function in spinal cord injured patients: a review, Archives of Physical Medicine and Rehabilitation **54**:539-543, 1973.

34. Griffith, E.R., and Trieschmann, R.B.: Sexual functioning in women with spinal cord injuries, Archives of Physical Medicine and Rehabilitation **56**(1):18-21, 1975.

35. Guttman, L.: The married life of paraplegics and tetraplegics, Paraplegia **2**:182-188, 1964.

36. Guyton, A.C.: Textbook of medical physiology, ed. 6, Philadelphia, 1981, W.B. Saunders Co.

37. Halstead, L.S.: Brief guide to office counseling: aiding arthritic patients to adjust sexually, Medical Aspects of Human Sexuality **2**:85-86, April 1977.

38. Higgins, G.E.: Sexual Response in spinal cord injured adults: a review of the Literature, Archives of Sexual Behavior **8**:173-196, 1979.

39. Hill, R.H., Herstein, P., and Walters, K.: JRA: follow-up into adulthood—medical, sexual, and social status, Canadian Medical Association Journal **114**:790-796, 1976.

40. Howard, E.J.: Sexual expenditure in patients with hypertensive disease, Medical Aspects of Human Sexuality **7**:82-92, Oct. 1973.

41. Jackson, R.W.: Sexual rehabilitation after cord injury, Paraplegia **10**(1):50-55, 1972.

42. Kalliomaki, J.L., Markkanen, T.K., and Mustonon, V.A.: Sexual behavior after CVA: a study on patients below the age of 60 years, Fertility and Sterility **12**:156-158, 1961.

43. Katz, W.A.: Sexuality and arthritis. In Katz, W.A., editor: Rheumatic diseases: diagnosis and management, Philadelphia, 1977, J.B. Lippincott Co.

44. King, S.H., and Cobb, S.: Psychosocial factors in the epidemiology of RA, Journal of Chronic Diseases **7**:466-475, 1958.

45. Leschner, M., Fine, H.L., and Goldman, A.: Sexual activity in older stroke patients, Archives of Physical Medicine and Rehabilitation **55**:578-579, 1974.

46. Maslow, A.H.: Motivation and personality, New York, 1954, Harper Brothers.

47. Masters, W.A., and Johnson, V.E.: Human sexual response, Boston, 1966, Little Brown & Co.

48. Medsger, A., and Chetlin, S.: Lupus and pregnancy, Wayne, Pa., 1980, Pennsylvania Lupus Foundation, Inc.

49. Medsger, A.R., and Robinson, H.: Comparative study of divorce in RA and other rheumatic diseases, Journal of Chronic Diseases **25:**269-275, 1972.

50. Mims, F.H., and Swenson, M.: Sexuality: a nursing perspective, New York, 1980, McGraw-Hill Inc.

51. Money, J.: Phantom orgasm in the dreams of paraplegic men and women, Archives of General Psychiatry **3:**373-382, 1960.

52. Mooney, T.O., Cole, T.M., and Chilgren, R.A.: Sexual options for paraplegics and quadraplegics, Boston, 1975, Little Brown & Co.

53. Munro, D., Horne, H.W., and Paull, A.P.: The effect of injury of the spinal cord and cauda equina on the sexual potency of men, New England Journal of Medicine **239:**903-911, 1948.

54. Onder, J., Lachniet, D., and Becker, M.C.: Sexual counseling—Arthritis and Women, Allied Health Professions Section Newsletter, The Arthritis Foundation **7:**1, 1973.

55. Persellin, R.H.: The effect of pregnancy on rheumatoid arthritis, Bulletin of Rheumatic Diseases **27:**922, 1977.

56. Renshaw, D.C.: Sexual problems in stroke patients, Medical Aspects of Human Sexuality **9:**1268-1274, 1975.

57. Renshaw, D.C.: Stroke and sex. In Comfort, A., editor: Sexual consequences of disability, Philadelphia, 1978, George F. Stickley Co.

58. Richards, J.S.: Sex and arthritis, Sexuality and Disability **3**(2):97-104, 1980.

59. Robertson, D.N.S., and Guttman, L.: The paraplegic patient in pregnancy and labor, Preceedings of the Royal Society of Medicine **56:**381-387, 1963.

60. Romano, M.D.: Sexuality and the disabled female, Accent on Living, Inc. **18**(3):28, 1973.

61. Reference deleted.

62. Sahs, A.L., and Hartman, E.C., editors: Fundamentals of stroke care, Washington, D.C., DHEW Pub., no. (HRA) 76-14016, 1976.

63. Sex and Disability Project: Who Cares? A handbook on sex education and counseling services for disabled people, Washington, D.C., 1979, George Washington University.

64. Shaul, S., et al.: Toward intimacy: family planning and sexuality concerns of physically disabled women, New York, 1978, Human Sciences Press.

65. Singh, S.P., and Mangner, T.: Sex and self: the spinal cord injured, Rehabilitation Literature **36**(1):2-7, 1975.

66. Talbot, H.S.: Sexual function in paraplegics, Journal of Urology **73:**91-100, Jan. 1955.

67. Teal, J.C., and Athelson, G.T.: Sexuality and spinal cord injury: some psychosocial considerations, Archives of Physical Medicine and Rehabilitation **56:**264-268, 1975.

68. Thornton, C.E.: Sexuality counseling of women with spinal cord injuries, Sexuality and Disability **2:**267-277, 1979.

69. Trieschmann, R.B.: Sexual dysfunctions associated with physical disabilities, Archives of Physical Medicine and Rehabilitation **54:**8-9, Jan. 1975.

70. Truth about arthritis and women: a case of discrimination: Atlanta, 1980, Arthritis Foundation.
71. Wright, B.: Physical disability—a psychological approach, New York, 1960, Harper & Row.
72. Yoshino, S., and Uchida, S.: Sexual problems of women with rheumatoid arthritis, Archives of Physical Medicine and Rehabilitation **62:**122-123, March 1981.
73. Young, J.S., and Northrup, N.E.: Statistical information pertaining to some of the most commonly asked questions about spinal cord injuries, part 1, Spinal Cord Injury Digest **1**(1):11-32, 1979.
74. Zwerner, J.: Yes we have troubles but nobody's listening: sexual issues of women with spinal cord injury, Sexuality and Disability **5:**158-171, 1982.

21

Sexuality and the developmentally delayed teenager

MARY BETH KNAPP and CAROL L. STADE

Nearly all of us are mentally retarded with regard to sex: and many intellectually bright people are not even educable or trainable in this respect.*

Warren R. Johnson

Most of the concerns facing developmentally disabled young persons are no different from those of their "normal" peers, but because of their handicaps and environmental restrictions stemming from their disabilities, opportunities for social interaction and development are limited and have been limited since birth. Chances to observe, develop, and practice social skills often have not and do not exist. Lacking peer reference groups and the ability to validate the accuracy of the limited sex information they may receive from others in the community only increases developmentally disabled young persons' anxieties, misperceptions, and perhaps their socially unacceptable behaviors.

Sexuality and developmental disabilities juxtapose two of the most socially unacceptable phenomena in society. "In spite of all the individual and societal preoccupation, sex has been abhorred, feared, hated, and rejected. And for all the sentimentality in our tradition, handicapping conditions including advancing age have been abhorred, rejected and even ridiculed."[8]

Generally, those with special needs have been seen as asexual, oversexed, and/or sexually menacing. It is often assumed that because they are different (e.g., cannot read, write, hear, see), they have no interest, no ability to enjoy, and no ability to assume responsibility for their actions—that they have no need for sexual expression and therefore sex is unimportant to them. The developmentally disabled, however, have the same range of sexual drives and interests as others.

As a result of the Education for All Handicapped Children Act, which was implemented in 1978, the integration of the developmentally disabled into the community is mandated in the concept of mainstreaming. The current emphasis on the sexual and human

---

*From Johnson, W.R.: Sex education and counseling of special groups, Springfield, Ill., 1975, Courtesy Charles C Thomas, Publisher.

rights of the developmentally disabled, in the ''least restrictive environment,'' is presenting new challenges to educators and health care professionals[2]:

> Today 95 percent of the retarded are living in the community and they are often the most difficult to reach with birth control services and sex education programs. Many of the teenage retarded are dropping out of school, pregnant. . . . Society expects the retarded to adopt socially acceptable behavior and to control their sexual impulses, yet society offers them almost no training to handle sex in a responsible manner. Few schools have family life sex education for the special class student, and it is particularly difficult for parents of the retarded to tell their children about ''the facts of life.''

If developmentally disabled young people in the community are misinformed or ignorant regarding sexual matters, they are vulnerable to exploitation by others and cannot be expected to make informed decisions about their own sexual needs.

Nurses working in settings providing health care services to developmentally disabled adolescents must have the information and experience necessary to be effective teachers and to initiate explanations at a level understood by their clients. For example, a 15-year-old may process information at a 5-year-old level. Other prerequisite skills for teaching effectively include (1) the ability to examine one's attitudes about sexuality in general, (2) the ability to examine one's attitudes toward the developmentally disabled and sexuality in particular, and (3) the openness to, acceptance of, and sensitivity to social and religious beliefs different from one's own.

Who are the developmentally disabled?

As defined in the new Developmental Disabilities Assistance and Bill of Rights Act of 1978,[15] a *developmental disability* is a severe, chronic disability of a person that:

1. Is attributable to a mental or physical impairment or combination of mental and physical impairments
2. Is manifested before age 22
3. Is likely to continue indefinitely
4. Results in substantial functional limitations in three or more of the following areas of major life activities:
   a. Self-care
   b. Receptive and expressive language
   c. Learning
   d. Mobility
   e. Self-direction
   f. Capacity for independent living
   g. Economic sufficiency
5. Reflects the need for a combination and sequence of special, interdisciplinary or generic care, treatment, or other services which (a) are of lifelong or extended duration and (b) are individually planned and coordinated

"The prevalence of developmental disabilities is difficult to estimate because of ambiguous definitions and conditions, uncertainties in diagnosis and difficulties in accurate casefinding due to continued ignorance, social stigmas and shame within society at large."[13] The most prevalent developmental disability in the United States is mental retardation. Approximately 3% of the population is affected, or 6 million people. It is estimated that approximately 120,000 children born annually (birth rate of 4 million per year) are or will become retarded. Of these, 89% are mildly retarded, many of whom are absorbed into the community and lead "normal" lives; 6% are classified as moderately retarded; 3.5% are severely involved; and 1.5% are profoundly so. There are 750,000 persons with cerebral palsy and an unknown number who are affected with epilepsy, sensory impairments, learning disabilities, and autism. Estimates from the U.S. Office of Education state that 7.9 million children from birth to 19 years of age are handicapped. This does not include individuals considered to be chronically ill.[13]

What are their rights?

Legal rights are, in general, drawn from two basic sources: the Constitution of the United States and state constitutions, which vary greatly. Additional legal rights are the result of statutes enacted by legislatures.

Constitutional rights of handicapped persons are the same as the constitutional rights of "normal" people. According to the Constitution, all people are created equal. Some of the constitutional rights that relate to the sociosexual development of developmentally disabled persons follow:

- The right to equal educational opportunity
- The rights to education and habilitation, which include the right to receive information about sex and contraception
- The right to be free unless proven dangerous
- The right to privacy, especially concerning one's intimate body functions, including the right to sexual expression
- The right to equal access to medical services
- The right to have relationships with one's peers, including members of the opposite sex; this includes the right to sexual expression
- The right to freely express oneself, whether it be through the choice of one's hair length, clothing styles, music, or otherwise
- The right to equal opportunities for housing
- The right to equal and fair treatment by public agencies and officials
- The right to marry, procreate, and raise children

Growing recognition of these rights by parents and professionals has resulted in judicial and legislative action. Such action has greatly enhanced acceptance of the normalization principle.

The normalization principle suggests that developmentally disabled persons should live like others to the greatest extent possible, since the deviance that justifies discrimination against developmentally disabled persons can be reduced by minimizing the degree to which they are treated differently from others. Normalization carries with it a set of

human rights given to every individual as he or she moves along the developmental continuum and is able to receive those rights. Such rights include the following:
- The right to a normal rhythm to the day (regular mealtimes, work, and playtimes)
- The right to experience the normal life cycle
- The right to grow up, to leave parents, and to move into the community
- The right to live in and experience a male-female world
- The right to the same economic standards
- The right to fail (if developmentally disabled persons are offered as much autonomy as they are capable of, this necessarily will include the possibility of failing, just as everyone else enjoys this possibility)
- The right to make choices

Nurses working as sex educators and doing sexual counseling must be prepared to discuss the ethical issues arising from these rights and their implications for developmentally disabled young persons and their families.

How can the right to choose be ensured?

"The achievement of human fulfillment, including sexual fulfillment, is a lifelong developmental process. Individual achievement of this goal is a function of the nature and quality of the interaction between life experiences and the emotional, physical, and cognitive developmental processes."[11]

The human sexual drive is second only to survival needs (food, shelter, clothing), and people must have some avenues open to them to gratify these needs. Constructive decisions about how to express one's sexuality cannot be made without knowledge of possible alternatives and consequences for choosing a particular form of expression. Without adequate education the individual has sexual drives but no goals. The most complete education possible needs to be provided given the primary nature of sexual drives and the need for personal goals.

When teenagers are developmentally disabled, one can assume that without assistance they will be unable to develop to their maximal potential in the area of sexuality as in other areas of development. Many people concerned with developmentally disabled adolescents agree that sex education is particularly crucial for these young people because of special vulnerabilities[10]:
1. They tend to be inept in social situations and often make inappropriate displays of sensuality or affection.
2. They often have difficulty putting questions into words and may be shy about asking questions at all. (Characteristically, developmentally disabled young people cannot or do not ask questions about sexuality.)
3. They tend to have a strong desire to touch, much like younger "normal" children who must touch something to "know" it or about it.
4. They are eager to please and are therefore highly suggestible.
5. They tend to be overly trusting and dependent, are not taught to problem solve and/or have a limited ability to do so, and want very much to belong to someone.
6. They are wistful about normalcy: the possibility of being married, having children, and having a sexual life. They want what others want:

    a. Friends—people to talk to and share important things with
    b. Warmth—people to touch them in ways that say "I like you"
    c. Approval—messages from others
    d. Affection—feeling and knowing they are loved
    e. Dignity—communication from others that they have worth
    f. Social outlets—avoiding loneliness
    g. Sexual satisfaction—biologic need for sex and sexual stimulation is small in comparison to other real human needs but is nonetheless a genuine need[19]

7. They are often given frightening warnings at home or in institutions about the dire consequences of sexual activity.
8. They have a realistic need to be protected against pregnancy and sexually transmitted disease.

The behaviors or attitudes that make developmentally disabled young persons particularly vulnerable can easily be explained on the basis of developmental task theory and/or current practices in socializing developmentally disabled young people. Whereas the former gives guidelines for how to best assist these young people, the latter speaks to the necessity of heightening expectations and providing more age-appropriate socialization experiences even though an individual happens to have a developmental disability.

Sex education and sexual counseling will be necessary for developmentally disabled young people to achieve social integration. Ideally sociosexual education is best taught at home by the parents on a day-to-day (informal) basis as experiences and developmental status dictate. This early and lifelong sociosexual training will allow handicapped youth to achieve social integration with minimal pain and community disruption. Unfortunately, parents are rarely prepared to approach this emotionally laden subject; they are anxious and uncomfortable and therefore avoid discussion of sexual issues. This uncomfortableness is only intensified when one's child is "not normal."

Nurses would do well to teach parents how to be sex educators of their children. More often than not, however, nurses find themselves in the role of sex educators and sexual counselors and are filled with the same discomforts and anxieties as those experienced by parents. Because nurses are the professionals most likely to become involved with developmentally disabled persons concerning the issue of sexuality, they have the professional responsibility to avail themselves of the information and experience necessary to be effective teachers and counselors.

Philosophies of sexuality counseling

    Johnson[11] has identified three philosophies concerning the sex education and counseling of special group members. Because the personal philosophy one adopts determines the direction that sex education and counseling will take, these three philosophies will be considered in brief.

    Eliminating sexuality. "This is an extension of the traditional antisexual attitude regarding sexuality in children (there is obviously no place for sexuality in children) and the confining of all legitimate sexual expression to procreative enterprise within marriage."[8] The goal of sex education or sexual counseling, according to this stance, "would be to eliminate or at least rigidly control sexual interest and expression."[8]

Tolerating sexuality (and perhaps accommodating it). This philosophy accepts the sexuality of most developmentally disabled persons and recognizes the right of each individual to experience sexual enjoyment. It views sex not as something to be eliminated but as something to be controlled within a social context. This outlook seems to suggest the following[8]:

> All right, this strong interest tends to exist in this person as it does in most members of the human race. It may be one more complicating factor in a generally difficult situation—just as it tends to be in the lives of most people. But it is there and it is real; so how might the [disabled young person] be helped to express his or her natural sexual interest safely and enjoyably within his [or her] particular social context?

Cultivating sexuality. From this perspective sexual interest is encouraged and developed for its own sake, just as other interests are cultivated. Sexual counseling and education appropriate to this philosophy would facilitate "sexual potential so that it might play the fullest possible part in the life of the individual."[8] Cultivating sexuality in developmentally disabled teenagers could ensure that they would operationalize their rights to the best of their capabilities and make informed choices concerning issues of sexuality.

Comparatively little research has been done to provide caregivers and counselors with guidelines for understanding sexuality of the developmentally disabled. However, a review of the literature does reveal some helpful facts.

1. *Developmentally disabled persons have sexual drives and interests in the opposite sex.* It is generally believed that there is a relationship between the degree of intellectual functioning, the level of social adaptive functioning, and heterosexual interest. Mildly and moderately retarded young people show as much interest in heterosexual relationships as normal adolescents.
2. *Mental age is a better predictor of self-concept and sexual knowledge than chronologic age.* For example, in looking both at the normal developmental sequence and life experiences, a 12-year-old with the mental age and adaptive functioning of a 5-year-old will have psychosexual interests more like those of a 5-year-old than those of a 12-year-old.

   One's level of cognitive functioning generally determines his or her level of psychosocial functioning. The ability to function autonomously and to form relationships with others usually corresponds closely with the level of cognitive abilities.
3. *Difficulties in motor coordination, family restriction of activities, and lack of social exposure contribute to the lag in identification with sex roles.* Gender identity is initially learned through imitation of family and friends. Therefore a child who has a limited environment because of immobility, overprotectiveness, and a paucity of social experiences has greater difficulty in discriminating sex roles. No further advancement in sociologic, psychologic, or sexual awareness can take place until one can establish gender identity, that is, until one can say with certainty, "I am a boy" or "I am a girl."
4. *The average age at which the developmentally disabled reach physiologic maturation is essentially the same as normal pubescence.* (See Chapter 3 for the normal sequence

of sexual development.) A delay in the onset and duration of pubertal changes is more frequent when the disability is genetic or prenatal in origin.

5. *Masturbation is to be anticipated as a normal expression of sexuality especially during adolescence.* It is often fostered by boredom and lack of activities. Developmentally disabled young people are more likely to masturbate at inappropriate times and in appropriate places because of the lack of social awareness and proper training.

6. *The greater the cognitive and adaptive functioning of the developmentally disabled person, the greater is his or her ability to sustain a reasonably successful marriage with no children or at most one child.* Studies have shown that the developmentally disabled adult is "capable of maintaining life in the community; able to work, maintain and manage a home and to bring up children in a manner acceptable to the community,"[5] with continued support and guidance of social agencies and/or families. The amount and type of support needed vary from couple to couple.

7. *The severity or subtlety of a young person's disability is not as relevant to a child's eventual sexuality as his or her participation in the life experiences common to the early sexual development of all people* (e.g., being held close and fed, being tickled and bounced on adult knees, being hugged and shoved by siblings, experiencing the relief of giving up body wastes at the right time and place, having curiosity about all aspects of his or her body).[12]

8. *Withholding sex knowledge will not deter the developmentally disabled from participating in sexual activity.* Knowledge of social and sexual development offers a better opportunity for appropriate behavior. Because they have more difficulty than normal persons in learning, it could be more confusing for them to be deliberately kept in ignorance.

9. *Sex education does not need to be offered on a careful time schedule.* If children are not ready to be given detailed, lengthy explanations, they will take in only the simplest aspects and become bored with the rest of the information.

10. *The developmental sequence* (social, emotional, physical) *is the same for everyone.* But the rate, pattern, and style of acquisition and the ultimate level of development attained are unique to the individual.

11. *Girls receive sex education and/or sexual information more often than boys, mainly because of concerns about the onset of menses.*

12. *Inability to move does not mean inability to please or be pleased.* The presence of deformities does not mean absence of desire. Inability to perform does not mean inability to enjoy. Loss of sensation does not mean loss of feeling.[3] Moderately and even severely developmentally disabled young people can acquire facts and attitudes that are a part of self-sufficient and responsible sociosexual behavior.

Assessment

Because the rate, pattern, and style of development are unique to the individuals involved, sex education and sexual counseling must be based on assessment of the individual needs and stage of development to guide developmentally disabled adolescents toward appropriate sociosexual expression; their sexual knowledge, level of intellectual functioning, attitudes, and biologic maturation must be considered. Present strengths and concerns, past trends, and desired future behavior must be identified in terms of their sociosexual adjustment. Assessment is a continuous process and must be organized within a developmental framework.

A developmental task is a learning experience that emerges at a certain period in the life of an individual as a result of biologic maturation, cultural pressures, personal values, and level of aspiration. Such tasks comprise the growth responsibilities individuals assume for their own development as they relate to their life situations. There exists an urge within the individual to develop in a way that will decrease the dissonance between present behavior and behavior that might be achieved. This thrust is generally intrinsic but may be evoked extrinsically; it receives direction from cultural definitions of expected behaviors at particular stages of development. Each task that is mastered becomes a tool for successfully tackling later developmental tasks. For example, young children's inclinations to explore their bodies are necessary for the successful development of gender identity, self-esteem, and self-control.

Individuals are most highly motivated to accomplish a task when they are truly ready for the next step in their development. Readiness implies that young persons have lived fully at the present stage and are not being hurried into the next stage. Individuals give readily observable clues when they want to learn new skills. Young children ready for toilet training will hold their diapers, cry, or ask to be changed when wet; children curious about reproduction will ask, "How did I get borned, Mommy?" Such clues indicate to adults in the environment that it is time to lend assistance.

There are at least four interrelated operations involved in mastering any given task: (1) perceiving new possibilities for one's behavior in what is expected of him or her, in what is available, or in the accomplishments of others in the environment who are more mature; (2) forming a new concept of self that includes the new mastery level; (3) coping effectively with conflicting demands made of him or her (perhaps most obvious in the dependence-independence struggle); and (4) desiring to achieve the next level of development enough to work toward it.

Developmental delays occur when the individual is unable to progress to the next developmental stage at the "appropriate age" for whatever reasons. Some young people continue to develop in a normal manner but at a slower rate, and some plateau at a particular level. Although these young people do not "progress" to subsequent developmental stages, they do change. They have a breadth of experience that "normal" children would not have had at the same stage in their development. Because developmental tasks are interdependent, as well as sequential, "the earlier a child's problem is recognized and treated, the more successful the treatment results will be in terms of maintaining continuity between the chronological and the functional developmental age."[1]

Table 21-1 describes the major developmental tasks and stages of sexual development, as well as the chronologic ages at which they are generally achieved.

To assess needs, the nurse may use a variety of approaches, including direct observation, verbal communication, parent interview, and administration of a variety of assessment tools.[6,7,14] Pictures depicting appropriate and inappropriate social behaviors, public and private behaviors, and the physical development and secondary sex characteristics of males and females are valuable in both assessment and teaching or counseling.

Parent interviews are helpful because they can apprise the parents of what information will be given to and obtained from their teenagers. The nurse can also deal with myths about sex education that parents may hold (e.g., sex education stimulates sexual arousal or preoccupation with sex). Parents often can share effective ways of eliciting information from their children and determine how they are currently adjusting sociosexually. Parent interviews also allow parents to discuss their own attitudes, feelings, values and beliefs toward the subject of sexuality; their expectations regarding their adolescent's adulthood; and how they deal with sexual issues and social behaviors of their children.

A comprehensive assessment will suggest the teaching and counseling approach most appropriate and determine the urgency of the particular concerns for the teenager involved. Ideally the focus of sex education could be prevention rather than a response to issues that have already become a crisis.

Some of the areas for assessment suggested by Dee[4] follow:

1. Level of intellectual functioning, including
   a. Ability to follow instructions and retain information
   b. Reading ability and comprehension
   c. Attention span
2. Physical disabilities and limitations, including
   a. Sensory status (e.g., vision, hearing)
   b. Mode of communication (through speech or gestures)
   c. Level of gross and fine motor coordination
   d. Limitations imposed by physical disability
3. Stage of biopsychosexual maturation, including
   a. State of pubertal development (menses started, secondary sex development)
   b. Curiosity about the opposite sex
   c. Special friendships with people of same sex or opposite sex
   d. Arousal of sexual feelings as a consequence of awareness of anatomic differences
   e. Ability to differentiate sexual advances from normal friendly encounters
4. Awareness of physical differences and sex roles, including
   a. Identification with same sex or opposite sex
   b. Knowledge about the anatomic differences of the sexes
   c. Opportunity to see immature or mature male or female genitals
5. Mode of sexual expression, including
   a. Expression of feeling when sad, angry, or happy
   b. Mode of displaying affection
   c. Objects of affection (family members, familiar adults, or strangers)
   d. Direction of sexual interest and expression (toward same sex, opposite sex, or self, such as masturbation)
6. Types of social experiences, including
   a. Friends (same or opposite sex)
   b. Companions available
   c. Social activities (bowling, dancing)

Table 21-1. Major tasks and stages in sexual development

| Age | Individual development | | |
	Physical	Emotional	Social
Birth to 1 year	Comfort and discomfort; physical response to sexual stimulation—erection and lubrication; masturbation	Trust and mistrust; self-centered; self-love; capacity for pleasure and discomfort	Primarily with family; some fear of strangers; likes audience
1 to 3 years	Total body exploration including genitals; toilet training (muscle control); masturbation	Begin gender identification, need to achieve, self-esteem, self-doubt or shame, and self-control	Force used to get way; sex role concepts; begin to explore with others; enjoys receiving affection and returns affection; less fear of strangers
3 to 5 years	Genital manipulation frequent: explore, pleasure, and relieve tension	Begin sense of guilt; initiative	Exploration and curiosity; basic skills for interpersonal relationships; begin same-sex parent identification; ←——— begin autonomy—assert self as individual; ←——— reinforce sexual identity—gender and roles
6 to 12 years	8 years—gradual buildup of testosterone and estrogen; 10 to 11 years—dramatic increase in hormones; menstruation (8 years and above)	Modesty; begin sexual daydreaming and fantasy	Identify with same-sex parent and peer; ambivalent feelings for opposite sex; "rehearsing" social skills; give and take in relationships

From Task Force for Sex Education for Developmentally Disabled: Personal development and sexuality: a curriculum

    d. Nature of group (mixed groups or same-sex groups)
    e. Nature of activities (supervised or unsupervised)
    f. Living condition (at home, in a foster home, or residential facility)
    g. Social behaviors adaptive to age or societal norms

Sex education and sexuality counseling

"Sex education should at all times contribute to a student's body awareness, self-image, understanding of interpersonal relationship and preparation for life in the adult world," including protection from exploitation and abuse. "Each topic should be discussed according to the (young person's) ability to understand and his or her interest in the biological, physiological and social implications."[9]

Individual development		
Intellectual	Moral and ethical	Cultural and societal
Imitating others		Primarily through parental influence
Sense of success and failure begins; language—names for body parts; begin to recognize male and female differences and similarities; reassurance regarding own genitals	Begin sense of right and wrong Nonsexual developments will provide names and judgments for later encounters with sexuality	General acceptance of limited nudity in public
Concepts of marriage and relationships; vocabulary building—"dirty words"; begin differential thinking—sex differences ————————→	Values and attitudes toward opposite sex begin to develop	General society beginning to have impact; parents still strongest
————————→		
Understand social significance of sexual behavior; vocabulary—new names; questions—more detailed and less personal	Internal urges versus demands of external world; begin decision-making independence	Influences: parents, peers, school, observing others, and media; heterosexual activity considered improper

guide for developmentally disabled, Tacoma, Wash., 1978, Planned Parenthood of Pierce County.

Teaching responsible decision making based on the concepts of public versus private behavior, individual rights and responsibilities, and appropriate versus inappropriate behavior is the key for teaching even the most severely disabled teenager acceptable community behavior.

Ideal goals for sex education include the following:

1. Sex education should remove ignorance.
2. Sex education should open communication between parents and children and ultimately between males and females.
3. Sex education should teach a person "how" to think, not "what" to think.
4. Sex education should ultimately increase the quality of interpersonal relationships.

Sex education is good—the more complete, the better. It does not occur principally in planned verbal ways but constantly in every human contact from birth onward. People do not really have the choice to provide or not to provide sexual information, but they do have an opportunity to control (influence) *how* or *what* is offered. How people conduct themselves communicates more than what they say. Parents are central to this process because children are most impressionable (experiences leave the most indelible impression) when they are young. Often adults fail to recognize the sensual and sexual nature and needs of children because their own childhood sexuality has been largely suppressed. It is important to employ every means possible to increase the ease with which males and females, and people in general, communicate and understand each other's sexuality, since human sexuality is a coeducational activity. Most people limit the concept of human sexuality to genital sex, but with education it will ideally be placed in the context of human relationships as a means (not an end) toward an expression of the most tender and closest bond between people.

Teaching strategies and curriculum

The nurse as sex educator and counselor must be flexible in using a variety of approaches in any number of learning situations to reach the aforementioned goals, objectives, and/or ideals. Good techniques are based on the educator's or counselor's ability to relate to the young person comfortably. To communicate effectively, additional techniques are often necessary because of developmentally disabled teenagers' learning handicaps. Material should be presented "more simply and repetitively . . . with use of visual aid charts, pictures, slides, movies and models."[19] Some means of clarifying and reinforcing the subject matter include behavioral demonstrations through pantomime, role play, and improvisation. Because developmentally disabled young people may or may not discuss freely and/or ask questions, it is imperative that techniques are used that will elicit what they already know so that misinformation can be corrected and new information can be presented on their individual level of understanding and interest.

For developmentally disabled young people, how they feel about themselves will be the most important factor in their adjustment. Liking and feeling good about oneself are ongoing processes. Any encounters with these young people must be handled in such a way as to honor, maintain, or increase their self-esteem. Young people with low self-esteem often continue to perform private behaviors in public and/or enter situations with high potential for sexual exploitation even after demonstrating knowledge of public versus private behavior, of appropriate versus inappropriate behaviors, and of community risks when approached by someone whom they feel is showing an interest in them.

The following outline includes specific topics and general areas of study, all of which need to be included in a complete sociosexual program*:
1. Self-esteem
   a. Liking oneself
   b. Getting along with others

---

*Based on Morrey, L.: In Task Force for Sex Education for Developmentally Disabled (Lenore Morrey, Coordinator): Personal development and sexuality: a curriculum guide for developmentally disabled, 1978, Planned Parenthood of Pierce County, 312 Broadway Terrace Bldg., Tacoma, Wash. 98402.

    c. Accepting the reality of a handicap
    d. Becoming independent
    e. Being assertive
    f. Solving problems
    g. Understanding feelings
2. Communication skills
    a. Being able to recognize and appropriately express one's emotions
    b. Being able to recognize and respond to emotions and needs of others
3. Relationships
    a. Roles and responsibilities
    b. Dating
    c. Grooming and hygiene and effect on relationships
    d. Victimless versus victimizing relationships
4. Biology and physiology
    a. Anatomy and physiology
    b. Reproduction
    c. Contraception
    d. Genetics
5. Personal hygiene and health concerns
    a. Bathing
    b. Shaving
    c. Menstrual care
    d. Clean and mended clothing
    e. Breast examination
    f. Pap smear
    g. Sexually transmitted disease
    h. Weight management
6. Sexual response and sexual expression
    a. Sexual fantasies
    b. Nocturnal emissions
    c. Special feelings in body
    d. Appropriate expression of feelings
    e. Variety of sexual expression
        (1) Abstinence
        (2) Masturbation
        (3) Homosexuality
        (4) Heterosexuality
    f. Appropriate versus inappropriate behavior
        (1) Rape
        (2) Incest

A planned outline should offer direction but should not be viewed as a set plan. Myths and misconceptions will constantly direct discussion, and flexibility will be the key to successful exchanges. One must be willing and able to deviate from planned materials to meet individual interests and needs. The more a social and sexual program is integrated into the entire learning process, the more it will meet the needs of the young people involved.

Summary

Developmentally delayed individuals are not asexual but have special needs related to the expression of their sexuality. These include learning to communicate about sexual issues, to discriminate appropriate from inappropriate displays of affection, and to protect themselves from pregnancy, sexually transmitted diseases, and sexual abuse.

There are philosophies about sexual counseling of the developmentally disabled ranging from eliminating sexuality to cultivating it. A sociosexual education and counseling program for the developmentally disabled is described dealing with self-esteem, communication skills, relationships, biology, physiology, personal hygiene and health concerns, and sexual response and expression.

Questions for review

1. Several philosophies about sexual counseling and the developmentally delayed were described. What is your personal philosophy? What factors influence your point of view?
2. How does your philosophy about counseling developmentally delayed teenagers differ from your philosophy about sexual counseling for other teenagers?
3. What are some of the major problems developmentally delayed individuals are likely to encounter as they express their sexuality? As teenagers? As adults?
4. What are some of the challenges facing parents of developmentally disabled adolescents as they express interest in sexual activity and relationships?

References

1. Banus, B., editor: The developmental therapist, Thorofare, N.J., 1972, Charles B. Black, Inc.
2. Bass, M.S.: Developing community acceptance of sex education for the mentally retarded, New York, 1970, SIECUS.
3. Cole, T.M., and Cole, S.S.: The handicapped and sexual health, Special issue on the handicapped, New York, 1976, SIECUS.
4. Dee, V.: Sex education. In de Leon Siantz, M.L., editor: The nurse and the developmentally disabled adolescent, Baltimore, 1977, University Park Press.
5. de la Cruz, F., and LaVeck, G., editors: Human sexuality and the mentally retarded, New York, 1973, Brunner-Mazel, Inc.
6. Edwards, J., and Wapnick, S.: Being me . . . a social/sexual training guide for those who work with the developmentally disabled, 1979, Ednick Communications, Box 3612, Portland, OR 97208 (slide presentation, curriculum manual, social assessment scale, and picture cards demonstrating social/sexual curriculum; includes all tools necessary for setting up a course for the handicapped).
7. Fischer, H., Krajicek, M., and Borthick, W.: Sex education for the developmentally disabled, a guide for parents, teachers and professionals, Baltimore, 1974, University Park Press.

8. Johnson, W.R.: Sex education and counseling of special groups, Springfield, Ill., 1975, Charles C Thomas, Publisher.
9. Kempton, W.: Sex education for persons with disabilities that hinder learning: a teacher's guide, North Scituate, Mass., 1975, Duxbury Press.
10. Livingston, V., and Knapp, M.B.: Human sexuality—a portfolio for the mentally retarded, Seattle, 1974, Planned Parenthood of Seattle-King County, 2211 E. Madison, Seattle, WA 98122.
11. Pattullo, A.: The socio-sexual development of the handicapped child: a preventive care approach, Nursing Clinics of North America **10:**361-372, 1975.
12. Perske, R., and Perske, M.: Sexual development. In Perske, R., and Perske, M., editors: New directions for parents of persons who are retarded, Nashville, 1973, Abingdon Press.
13. Siantz, M., editor: The nurse and the developmentally disabled adolescent, Baltimore, 1977, University Park Press.
14. Task Force for Sex Education for Developmentally Disabled (Lenore Morrey, Coordinator): Personal development and sexuality: a curriculum guide for developmentally disabled, 1978, Planned Parenthood of Pierce County, 312 Broadway Terrace Bldg., Tacoma, WA 98402.
15. Thompson, R.J., and O'Quinn, A.N.: Developmental disabilities, New York, 1979, Oxford University Press.

Suggested readings

Edgerton, R.: The cloak of competence—stigma in the lives of the mentally retarded, Berkeley, Calif., 1967, University of California Press.
Edmonson, B., McCombs, K., and Wish, J.: What retarded adults believe about sex," American Journal of Mental Deficiency **84**(1):11-18, 1979.
Edwards, J.P.: Sara and Allen—the right to choose, Portland, 1976, Ednick Communications.
Haavik, S., and Menninger, K.A.: Sexuality, law and the developmentally disabled person, Baltimore, 1981, Paul H. Brookes Publishing Co.
Hammar, S.L., and Barnard, K.E.: The mentally retarded adolescent, Pediatrics **38:**845-857, 1977.
Robinault, I.P.: Sex, society, and the disabled, New York, 1978, Harper & Row, Publishers, Inc.
SIECUS: Sexuality and the life cycle, study guide no. 8, Behavior Publications, 72 Fifth Avenue, New York, NY 10012.

Curriculum guides

Blum, G., and Blum, B.: Feeling good about yourself, 1977, Academic Therapeutic Productions, P.O. Box 899, 1539 Fourth Street, San Rafael, CA 94901.
Newton-Alricks, G.: Caring—an approach to sex education, 1979, Dan Publications, P.O. Box 333, Pringle Park Station, Salem, OR 97302 (includes picture cards).
Poulisse, L.J.: A curriculum in self-awareness and sexuality for developmentally disabled adults, Oct. 1977, Washington State Association of Group Homes, 15230 15th Ave. NE, Seattle, WA 98155.

Resource materials for teaching

Dalen, A., Dee, V., and Holmberg, N.: Menstrual self-care for the retarded girl, Seattle, 1973, University of Washington Press (Slides and teaching guide).

Social behavior; Good grooming and personal conduct; Appropriate dress for various occasions; Public and private places: Ednick Slides, Ednick Communications, Box 3612, Portland, OR 97208.

Gordon, S.: Facts about sex for exceptional youth, New York, 1969, Charles Brown.

Gordon, S.: Living fully, New York, 1975, John Day Co.

Kempton, W., Gordon, S., and Bass, M.: Love, sex and birth control for the mentally retarded—a guide for parents, Philadelphia, 1971, Planned Parenthood Association of Southeastern Pennsylvania.

Mayle, P.: Where did I come from? and What's happening to me? Lyle Stuart, Inc., 120 Interprise Avenue, Secaucus, NJ 07094.

Pattullo, A.: Puberty in the girl who is retarded, Arlington, Tex., 1969, National Association for Retarded Citizens.

22

Sexuality and alcoholism

CAROLYN A. LIVINGSTON and MARILYN C. McINTYRE

It is estimated that there are approximately 10 million adult alcoholics in the United States today.[1] Of these, 3.3 million are women and 6.7 million are men.[33] Studies agree that there is no simple explanation of the effect that alcohol has on human sexual behavior. Sexual problems may result from one or more of the following: alcohol's depressant effect on the central nervous system, disease related to alcoholism, other chemical dependency problems, or psychologic disorders in the recovering alcoholic.

Because alcohol is a powerful anesthetic that can deaden the senses, chronic alcohol abusers experience sensory and motor disturbances, diminished or absent reflexes, and a numbing of sexual feelings. Humans have various thresholds for sexual dysfunction that are related to physical and psychologic factors, as well as blood alcohol levels.[7]

Alcoholic women report sexual dissatisfactions such as lack of sexual desire, orgasmic dysfunction, dyspareunia, and vaginismus.[31] Many alcoholic men suffer from changes in their sexual desire, erectile dysfunction, and delayed orgasm or ejaculation.[7,9,21,24] Alcohol can cause irreversible sexual dysfunction for chronic abusers. Other alcoholics may recover completely from the effects of alcohol when drinking is discontinued.

To provide an understanding of the complex interaction between alcoholism and sexuality, this chapter has the following objectives:

1. To discuss the physiologic and psychologic aspects of the effects of alcohol on female and male sexual functioning
2. To explore factors that can contribute to sexual problems in relationships when one person is an alcoholic
3. To examine the role of the health care provider in treating sexual problems of the recovering alcoholic

Women, alcohol, and sex

There is relatively little research on the sexual functioning of the alcoholic woman. Most studies in the fields of both sexuality and alcoholism have focused on men. In fact, one writer shed light on the situation by pointing out that "most experts comment on human sexual behavior and alcohol as though only males drink and have sexual interests.''[10] In more recent years it has been increasingly recognized that there is a need to understand the relationship between alcoholism and sexuality in women. However, most of what clinicians are learning is still based to a large extent on clinical observation and impression rather than on research findings. There are several factors that explain this lack of data. Only a small number of the studies that have been conducted on women, alcohol, and sexuality have addressed sexual functioning per se. Instead, most studies have limited their research to questions surrounding sex-role identity, sex-role expectations, and the incidence of obstetric and gynecologic problems in alcoholic women. In addition, most of the earlier studies are technically limited, since they tend to characterize womens' sexual problems as ''frigidity,'' without differentiating between desire, arousal, and orgasm disorders. In those studies that do specify and objectively measure the physiologic effects of alcohol on the different phases of the sexual response cycle, only social drinkers have been used as subjects.[25,53] To date, it appears that alcoholic women have not been studied using objective measures. Another element of the research is that very few of the studies address sexual treatment issues for the recovering alcoholic woman. We conclude that most of the work that has been done in this field is based on clinical experience.

In any discussion of alcoholic women and sexuality it must be recognized that women in general are socialized to ignore and repress their sexual feelings, and/or to view their sexuality as a commodity. Female ignorance of sexuality from adolescence through adulthood is unfortunately the rule rather than the exception. As Potter[34] succinctly states, ''The need to be unaware of what is happening sexually is the result of how most women have been raised.'' As a result, many women tend not to deal with either the positive or negative feelings that may influence their sexuality. If and when a woman does attempt to understand or change her sexual experience, she often discovers that there are no models for her to follow, and feelings of anxiety and hopelessness may lead her back into passivity and repression. Alcohol often serves to protect her from experiencing these painful feelings. Also, alcohol, in small doses, tends to release positive feelings by dilating blood vessels and depressing control centers in the brain.[9] Female subjects in Wilsnack's study[52] said they felt ''warm, loving, considerate, expressive, open, affectionate, sexy, and feminine when drinking.'' Beckman[4] questioned alcoholic and nonalcoholic women about their sexual behavior and feelings after drinking. Her results indicated that alcoholic women report low sexual satisfaction and are more likely than nonalcoholics to believe that drinking decreases inhibition and increases sexual enjoyment, desire, spontaneity, and frequency. Other studies have revealed that these positive feelings and expectations seem to persist even when there is objective physiologic impairment of sexual functioning.[25,53]

For example, in a study by Wilson and Lawson[53] varying amounts of alcohol were administered to sixteen female social drinkers who were asked to verbally report their arousal levels while watching an erotic film. To check for physiologic arousal, a vaginal photoplethysmograph was used, which measures vaginal blood volume and pulse. The subjective reports of the subjects conflicted with the objective measures of the photoplethysmograph. As their blood alcohol levels increased, the women reported higher excitement, but according to the instrument, their arousal decreased.

Malatesta et al.[25] expanded on Wilson and Lawson's study by measuring orgasm and arousal in eighteen female social drinkers. These subjects masturbated to orgasm while watching erotic videotapes. The photoplethysmograph measured vaginal blood volumes, and questionnaires measured subjective responses to arousal and orgasm. The results showed that as the dose of alcohol increased, there was a physiologic depressant effect on orgasm. Also, the higher the blood alcohol concentration (BAC), the more the subjects reported difficulty in reaching orgasm, which when reached was less intense. However, with the higher BAC, these same women also reported increased sexual arousal and greater pleasurability of orgasm.

The consistent finding of these studies on alcohol and sexual functioning in women is that there is a discrepancy between subjective evaluations of arousal and physiologic measures of arousal. Women report enjoyment and pleasure even when there are research data indicating impairment of sexual functioning.

To explain these discrepancies, Wilson and Lawson[53] speculated that because women do not learn to recognize and identify signs of physical arousal, they are unable to report them accurately. Wilson and Lawson also suspected that the subjects may have reported their feelings based on what was expected of them by the researchers or that they were responding to the socialized belief that alcohol is supposed to be an aphrodisiac for women. It is clear that researchers do not know why this incongruity exists between the physiologic and cognitive sexual experiences in women.

Therefore, for the health care provider to fully understand the effects of alcohol on sexual functioning, it is important to be aware of the many variables that may be interacting to create a particular reaction in an individual. Although the pharmacologic action of alcohol does have physiologic effects on sexual functioning, this effect is mediated by other factors such as the dose, acute or chronic use, and the person's expectations of what the drug will do. Other factors may include the woman's relationship with her partner, her personality characteristics, and her mental state.[11]

The following sections will review in more detail some of the physiologic and psychologic effects of alcohol on sexual functioning.

Physiologic effects of alcohol on female sexual functioning.
Alcohol can influence female gynecologic and sexual functioning in several ways. Most of the earlier studies on the pathologic effects of alcohol on sexual functioning focused on liver disease and its consequences. Because of the decreased metabolism of estrogen in the liver, women with cirrhosis often experience amenorrhea and eventually atrophy of the vaginal mucosa.[39]

Because many alcoholics in earlier stages of alcoholism with normally functioning livers also experience sexual dysfunctions, researchers have begun to examine the extent to which alcohol more directly impairs the functioning of the hypothalamic-pituitary axis. Also, because data suggest that ovarian atrophy is common in alcoholic women, the role of alcohol as a direct gonadal toxin is gaining scientific interest.[47] Ovarian atrophy decreases the production of estrogen, which alters pituitary functioning, progesterone production, and ovulation. This in turn leads to sporadic growth and shedding of the endometrium, with resulting intermittent bleeding and weakening of the uterine wall. This process helps explain the high incidence of infertility and miscarriages in alcoholic women.[52]

In addition, alcohol is a depressant to the central nervous system, resulting in sensory

Table 22-1. Female sexual response cycle and effects of alcohol on each phase

Phases	Effects of alcohol		
	Early stage	Middle stage	Late stage
Desire (libido)			
Feeling vaguely sexy (''horny'')	Release of inhibitions and increased desire	Decreased desire	No desire
Interested in sex or open to sex			
Genital sensations			
Restless			
Excitement			
Vaginal lubrication—''sweating'' of vaginal walls	Increased arousal and enjoyment	Decreased lubrication and sensitivity	No lubrication or sensitivity
Expansion of inner two thirds of vaginal barrel			
Increased sensitivity of clitoris and labia			
Nipple erection			
Plateau			
Retraction of clitoris	Increased enjoyment and sensitivity	Prolonged (takes longer to reach orgasm)	Prolonged
Formation of orgasmic platform—swelling of outer one third of vagina			
Elevation of cervix and uterus—''tenting'' effect			
''Sex skin'' discoloration of labia minora			
Increase in muscle tension and breathing			

Orgasmic			
Contractions of orgasmic platform, uterus, rectal and urethral sphincters, and other muscle groups Hyperventilation and increase in heartbeat rate	Increased quality of orgasm	Fewer or no orgasms and decreased intensity of orgasm	No orgasm
Resolution			
Gradual relaxation of vaginal walls Rapid color change Sweating reaction Breathing, heartbeat, and muscle tension gradually return to normal Often during this phase, women are capable of returning to orgasm because they do not experience a refractory period, as men often do, during which sexual stimulation is unpleasant	Increased relaxation and enjoyment	Fewer orgasms	None

and motor disturbances and diminished or absent reflexes, and can thus have devastating effects on sexual functioning in both women and men. A summary of alcohol's specific physiologic effects on the phases of the female sexual response cycle is outlined in Table 22-1. Effects are listed according to the stage of alcoholism.

Sexual dysfunctions of alcoholic women. The dysfunctions that are most commonly found in alcoholic women are inhibited desire, orgasmic dysfunction, dyspareunia, and vaginismus.

Inhibited desire. Inhibited sexual desire may be the result of several complex physiologic, psychologic, and social or interactional variables. If a women is deriving little enjoyment or satisfaction from her sexual experiences or her relationship, her sexual desire is likely to diminish. Because of the many physical, social, and interpersonal problems that often accompany alcoholism, one's sexual desire is vulnerable to a partial or total shutdown. A woman may notice her lack of desire only after she has quit drinking, since it is at this time that she may begin to become aware of her sexual feelings or lack of such feelings. From a broader perspective, sexual desire may be inhibited because of the fact that the alcoholic is physically anesthetized and thus not capable of obtaining pleasurable somatic feedback.[18] Murphy et al.[31] found that of seventy-four alcoholic women interviewed early in treatment, 29.7% reported little or no sexual desire.

Orgasmic dysfunction. Primary and secondary orgasmic dysfunction may be the result of a lack of information, poor communication with one's partner, and/ or inadequate clitoral stimulation. Also, as discussed earlier, alcohol compounds the problem by depressing the central nervous system and creating sensory, motor, and reflex disturbances. Murphy et al.[31] found that 28.4% of the seventy-four alcoholic women interviewed reported orgasm less than 50% of the time during sex with a partner.

Dyspareunia. Among alcoholic women painful penetration is often an indirect result of ovarian atrophy because of drying and shrinking of the vaginal wall, which is caused by low estrogen production. Dyspareunia may also occur because of decreased or absent lubrication caused by inadequate stimulation and arousal. In their sample of seventy-four alcoholic women Murphy et al.[31] reported a relatively low incidence of dyspareunia.

Vaginismus. Any attempt at vaginal penetration causes an involuntary tightening or spasm in the outer two thirds of the vagina. Vaginismus in many instances is the result of painful intercourse, painful pelvic examinations, sexual abuse, or any unpleasant sexual experience. The women questioned by Murphy et al.[31] reported the incidence of vaginismus much less than inhibited desire and orgasmic dysfunction.

Statistical comparisons have not been made of the incidence of these dysfunctions in alcoholic women versus nonalcoholic women. Murphy et al.[31] interviewed alcoholic women regarding the incidence of specific sexual dysfunctions but did not use the questionnaire for a nonalcoholic population. Also, it was found that although the research subjects participated in a sexual enhancement group and became more comfortable and knowledgeable about sexuality, they also became more honest about their sexual dissatisfactions and revealed more sexual problems than they had reported during the initial interview. One must then question the data compiled from the interviews alone. It can only be speculated that because high doses of alcohol over a long period of time physiologically impair sexual response, and because the disease of alcoholism creates unique physical and psychologic sequelae, the incidence of dysfunctions would tend to be more prevalent among alcoholic women.

Other sexuality issues for alcoholic women. In addition to the physiologic impact that alcohol has on sexual functioning, other sexuality issues may emerge for the recovering alcoholic woman. Defense mechanisms are usually so highly developed that the woman may be out of touch with her emotions and may not even realize how she feels. The defenses protect the alcoholic from experiencing a free-floating mass of anxiety, guilt, shame, remorse, and self-hatred.[20] Evans and Schaefer[13] state that this is especially true for alcoholic women who tend to be shame based and experience high levels of guilt, low self-esteem, and a general loss of power in their lives. In most treatment programs clients are required to attend individual and group therapy sessions that are designed to help "discover ourselves and others as feeling persons, and to identify the defenses that prevent this discovery."[20] Even though little has been written or studied on how these particular feelings affect or are related to the alcoholic woman's sexuality, it is apparent that self-esteem is a crucial element in an individual's capacity for sexual fulfillment.[8]

In most treatment programs the issue of sexuality is usually not talked about, especially among women. In those programs that have addressed sexuality several findings have emerged. Surveys among Minnesota treatment centers report that 40% to 50% of the clients have been incest victims.[13] These findings are similar to those of Benward and Denson-Gerber,[5] who found that of 188 women receiving treatment, 44% had been victims of incest. Murphy et al.[31] interviewed forty-eight women receiving treatment and unexpectedly found that 54% reported being victims of rape as an adult or child. At the Chrysalis Outpatient Treatment Program in Minneapolis, Minnesota, where 50% of the women have been found to be incest victims,[13] therapy groups are offered after 1 month of sobriety. The women are given support in openly dealing with their anger, shame, and grief and are encouraged to take charge of their sexuality. The actual relationship between chemical dependency, sexual abuse, and sexual dysfunction is not clear.

One study[33] inadvertently shed some light on this area of inquiry and raised questions for further investigation. Pinhas compared sexual control and sex guilt in thirty-one alcoholic women and thirty-four nonalcoholic women. She defined sexual control as the degree to which a woman perceives that reinforcements for sexual behavior, attitudes, and feelings are contingent on herself, as opposed to external forces, and sex guilt as an expectancy for self-mediated punishment for violating standards of proper sexual conduct. The alcoholic women reported more sex guilt and less control over their sex lives. Pinhas hypothesized that alcohol is used to obtain a sense of sexual control and to minimize sex guilt and/or to avoid feelings of sexual failure. She did not examine the antecedents of sex guilt and sex control and did not control for incidence of sexual abuse and incest in her subjects. Since guilt and feelings of powerlessness are common psychological sequelae to sexual abuse and incest, one wonders what the incidence of sexual abuse was among her alcoholic population in comparison to her nonalcoholic group.

Women in recovery profess a dismal lack of knowledge about their own bodies.[13] Responsible sexual decision making and assertiveness may need to be learned, since many of the women have never taken control over preventing pregnancy, intervening in lovemaking for their own pleasure, or attracting desired sex partners.[33] Many fear their first sexual experience while sober, especially if they have never had sex without drinking.[13] This fear may be reinforced by remembering euphoria and happiness while drinking, coupled with an inability to imagine a positive sexual experience without alcohol.

Multiple problems within the woman's relationship may determine how she feels and behaves sexually and are discussed further in a subsequent section of this chapter.

Men, alcohol, and sex

The physical aspects of male sexuality are much more familiar to the general public than the psychologic aspects. Society's expectations about masculinity have become so identified with male sexual behavior that discussions of male sexual behavior are often really discussions of male role expectations. These expectations lead men to believe that they should be sexually responsive at any time, at any place, and with anyone. Male-as-initiator myths expect men to know what to do sexually and to initiate their innocent partners into the sexual arena. When the male socialization process is examined, one can see how these expectations may have developed.

Young boys are encouraged to touch and aim their penises during toilet training. Comparing penis size is part of the growing up process for adolescents. Sexual prowess is the mark of manhood for a young man.

Underneath the societal myths and role expectations for males lies a human sexual reality that is only recently coming to light. Sex therapists and researchers are making public a much different picture of male sexual behavior than the public one. First sexual experiences are often uncomfortable and anxiety arousing. Men may feel guilty or angry about sex. They may be depressed and thus not have an erection. They may ejaculate too soon or not at all. They may fear ''not getting it up'' so much that they become impotent. Most important, they may just not know how to behave sexually.[56] When alcohol is involved, all of these very real sexual issues can become heightened and compounded.

Physiologic effects of alcohol on male sexual functioning. It is difficult to make generalizations about when and if a sexual dysfunction will occur as a result of alcohol abuse. One can make generalized descriptive statements about the male sexual response cycle of chronic alcohol abusers, but it is not possible to come up with predictable physical responses that are true for all alcoholic men. For example, some alcoholic men state that they lost their erectile capacity soon after they started drinking, although for others, achieving and maintaining an erection has never been a problem. Other men will relate similar experiences about being orgasmic. Some no longer experience orgasm, although for others, having an orgasm has never been a problem.[9] The health care provider must consider each case individually because there may be marked variation.

Alcohol tends to initially remove sexual inhibitions and increase sexual libido (desire) by depressing the control centers in the brain.[9] As a result, thought and motor activities are disrupted, resulting in a loss of self-restraint. With continued drinking the blood vessels dilate, spinal reflexes slow down, and the capacity to respond sexually severely decreases.[9]

In men the brain and the genitals must be supplied with adequate levels of testosterone for good sexual functioning.[35] Alcohol abuse significantly decreases plasma testosterone levels, since alcohol inhibits testosterone production in the testes and stimulates a rapid breakdown of testosterone in the liver.[29] In a 1976 controlled laboratory study by Gordon et al.[17] eleven nonalcoholic men from 21 to 40 years of age were given alcohol for a month. The results of this study showed that at the end of 4 weeks in all of the men there was a significant reduction in both plasma testosterone levels and in the production rate of testosterone. Since normal testosterone levels are essential for the activation and maintenance of erections and sexual desire, a decrease in testosterone often provokes a failure to maintain an erection and a loss of libido.[21]

Alcohol has also been found to be a direct gonadal toxin causing atrophy of the testes, which results in decreased sperm production and possible sterility. Chronic alcohol abuse can bring about hyperestrogenemia secondary to the alcohol-induced liver damage, in which the liver converts a higher proportion of androgens to estrogens.[17,46] This may promote gynecomastia,[7] diminished body hair, and the accumulation of hypogastric and pelvic fat pads.[46]

As with the female sexual response cycle, the male sexual response cycle can be viewed as consisting of five phases. It is important to be aware of phase-specific responses in accordance with alcohol's effect on male sexuality. As an aid to the health care provider in dealing with an alcoholic client, the effects are listed according to the stage of alcoholism in Table 22-2.

Sexual dysfunctions of alcoholic men. Some of the most common sexual dysfunctions experienced by alcoholic men are inhibited sexual desire, erectile dissatisfaction, and delayed orgasm or ejaculation.

Inhibited sexual desire. Alcohol-related sexual desire seems to be situational. It is necessary to consider the interaction of the alcohol, the individual, and the environment, all of which are contingent on the amount of alcohol consumed.[9] Increased levels of sexual desire are more characteristic of the man who drinks small to moderate amounts of alcohol. With excessive prolonged alcohol consumption the testosterone level becomes markedly depressed, and sexual desire is diminished.[21]

Erectile dysfunction. Masters and Johnson[27] reported that the second most frequent cause of men failing to achieve and maintain erections could "be directly related to a specific incident of acute ingestion of alcohol or to a pattern of excessive alcohol intake." Wilson[54,55] also found decreases in erectile responses to sexual stimuli with increasing doses of alcohol in both alcoholic and nonalcoholic men. The following studies concur with these findings.

In 1976 Farkas and Rosen[14] studied sixteen men who were moderate drinkers (drank two to three times weekly). Their ages ranged from 18 to 24 years. In a laboratory setting these subjects drank alcohol while watching erotic films. Sexual arousal was measured by changes in penile diameter. It was found that large doses of alcohol depressed both penile diameter increase and the penile tumescence rate, thus suppressing the man's ability to have a hard, full erection.

Rubin and Henson[37] found in studying sixteen nonalcoholic men that small and moderate amounts of alcohol caused a marked decrease in penile tumescence. In a 1976 study of forty-eight male social drinkers Briddel and Wilson found similar results.[6]

In addition, primary and secondary erectile dysfunctions may have psychologic and

Table 22-2. Male sexual response cycle and effects of alcohol on each phase

Phases	Effects of alcohol		
	Early stage	Middle stage	Late stage
Desire (libido) Feeling vaguely sexy ("horny") Interested in sex or open to sex Genital sensations Restless	Release of inhibitions and increased desire and aggression	Decreased desire and increased aggression	Increased aggression and loss of desire
Excitement Penile erection Thickening and elevation of scrotum Moderate enlargement of testicles	Increased enjoyment and decreased penile tumescence	Increased time to erection and decreased penile tumescence	No erection
Plateau Increase in size of glans (tip) of penis Glans may become purple in color Elevation and 50% increase in size of testes Mucoid emission from Cowper's glands, possibly with sperm Increase in muscle tension and breathing	Prolonged phase and control of premature ejaculation	Decreased penile tumescence and diameter and difficulty maintaining erection	No erection or enjoyment

	Increased quality of orgasm	Uncertain orgasm	No orgasm and unpleasant ejaculation
Orgasmic			
Internal urinary sphincter closes			
Sensation of ejaculatory inevitability			
Contractions of vas deferens, seminal vesicles, prostate, and ejaculatory duct			
Relaxation of external bladder sphincter			
Contractions of urethral and rectal sphincter muscles			
Hyperventilation and increase in heartbeat rate			
Ejaculation, sperm mostly in first part			

	Increased relaxation and enjoyment	Prolonged refractory period	Loss of sexual satisfaction and no resolution phase
Resolution			
Loss of penile erection			
Refractory period when continued stimulation is uncomfortable			
Sweating reaction			
Descent of testicles			
Breathing, heartbeat rate, and muscle tension gradually return to normal			

physiologic origins. Alcohol physiologically impairs spinal reflexes, which causes both decreased sensation and decreased innervation for erection.[17] The psychologic component is that alcoholic men may typically experience the interaction of low self-esteem, fear of intimacy, and/or anxiety, which may result in erectile problems.

Men may suffer from psychologic problems because of a history of sexual dysfunction. Chronic erectile dysfunction can also be attributed to an irreversible peripheral neuropathy. In 1973 Lemere[22] reported that 8% of 17,000 chronic alcohol users complained of erectile dysfunction. Of this 8%, 50% of those who had stopped drinking had persistent erectile problems even after years of sobriety.

Delayed orgasm or ejaculation. Inhibited male orgasm or ejaculation is the persistent delay or absence of orgasm and/or ejaculation following a period of sexual excitement. Orgasm is a simple reflex. The center is located in the sacral cord, and the ejaculation reflex center is located in the cervicolumbar cord. Occasionally a man can distinguish between orgasm and ejaculation, but usually they occur almost simultaneously. "Alcohol does not seem to affect the ejaculation as distinct from orgasm."[9] Both orgasm and ejaculation relfexes may be delayed or occur with diminished quality when a man is under the influence of alcohol.[21]

In a study by Malatesta et al.[24] twenty-four men who were moderate drinkers and between the ages of 22 and 34 reported changes in their sexual response while under the influence of alcohol. After attaining a prescribed blood alcohol level and while watching erotic videotapes, the men were asked to engage in masturbation culminating in orgasm and ejaculation. The men reported increased difficulty in attaining orgasm with increased levels of alcohol consumption.

Other sexuality issues for alcoholic men. As mentioned earlier, the psychologic component of male sexuality may also suffer as a result of alcohol abuse. Good sexual functioning usually leaves one with a sense of pleasure and well-being and is the result of high sexual self-esteem, appropriate sexual assertiveness, and confident decision making. The alcoholic man is likely to be deficient in one or more of these areas and may display low sexual self-esteem, sexual aggression, and difficulty in making appropriate decisions about being sexual, such as where, when, and with whom.

Low self-esteem in alcoholic men is common.[28,45] It is accentuated by feeling physically unattractive. Chronic alcohol abuse may bring about changes in one's body, such as wrinkles, lesions, and even changes in fat distribution, all of which may contribute to feelings of unattractiveness.

Low sexual self-esteem may also be the result of achievement problems. Not only does the man experience diminished erections, but also it is not unusual that he finds he has made poor decisions about being sexual. Early into recovery he may realize that he has had very few if any sexual encounters while sober.

Many alcoholic men have developed abrasive personalities that are manifested as unreliable, disappointing, and embarrassing to their sexual partners.[43] This usually does not foster positive feelings of being sexual with anyone.

Sexual relationship issues of the alcoholic

Intimacy is the total sharing between one person and another. The feeling of trust between two people reflects a lifetime of relationship experiences. People are social animals, and without intimate relationships they tend to get lonely and become depressed.[21] When the level of intimacy becomes too close, many people will provide distance for themselves by overindulging in alcohol. Thus intimacy is avoided, and often the person's sex life suffers. A relationship can become even more stressful when understanding and companionship are not predictable and/or guaranteed. It is not unusual for the nonalcoholic partner to be turned off sexually, to be angry, and to have assumed a parenting role with the alcoholic. All of these factors are likely to result in tension, distance, and sexual disinterest.

Intimacy, trust, and open communication are often distorted or absent in these relationships, and it is not unusual for there to be a decrease in the sharing of feelings and the expressions of love and caring.[41] During recovery, intimacy and trust need to be rebuilt. The degree to which adults learn or relearn how to establish intimacy and trust depends on honest discussion of feelings, including sexual feelings, without abuse and defensiveness. An important part of the recovery process for alcoholics and their partners is to gain insight into and find resolution of their intimacy problems. This is necessary before couples can begin to enjoy loving sexual relationships.[21]

Alcoholism and sexual minorities. Alcoholism is a major health problem in the homosexual community. It is estimated that one in three homosexuals has an alcohol abuse problem.[44] This is more than three times the estimate of problem drinkers in the heterosexual population. Alcohol often plays an important part in the homosexual life-style, since gay bars and private house parties have provided a major place for meeting friends, for finding partners, and for socialization.

There is need for more research regarding homosexual and bisexual alcoholism. These women and men frequently have special needs, relating to their sexual orientation, that greatly inhibit their chances for successful recovery within heterosexual treatment models. It needs to be recognized that they are subject to a double stigma for being both homosexual and alcoholic.[38] Finnegan and McNally,[15] co-coordinators of the National Association of Alcoholism Professionals, list some of the special problems of homosexuals as fear, guilt, paranoia, rage, depression, low self-esteem, and feelings of isolation. Health care providers need to take into consideration that some homosexuals need to remain closeted. They need to feel positive about their sexual orientation in order not to use it as an excuse to drink. Finally, other important people in a homosexual's life need to be included in treatment.

Health care providers need to be aware of their own attitudes and values about sexual minorities. Many homosexuals are suspicious of traditional health and human services agencies. Self-help programs established and staffed by sexual minorities seem to be most likely to make progress in the treatment of sexual minorities who abuse alcohol. Alcoholics Anonymous now has Gay Alcoholics Anonymous in many cities, and the National Association of Gay Alcoholism Professionals is actively working to increase professional and public awareness of the specific needs of homosexual alcoholics.

There appears to be no difference between the sexual dysfunctions experienced by gay men and lesbian women and the sexual dysfunctions experienced by heterosexual men and women. What seems to be different are the feelings that homosexuals experience when seeking treatment in a heterosexual treatment agency (see Chapter 3). If a homosexual senses negative attitudes from staff members, comfort with self-disclosure and sobriety are diminished and threatened.

Role of the health care provider

Entering treatment is a stressful experience for the alcoholic and the family. Initially, the primary concern of the health care provider is to manage the client's physiologic reactions to the withdrawal of alcohol, which range from mild to severe depending on the stage of the disease. After the client is physiologically stable, a treatment plan to maintain sobriety is needed. Most counselors gather information on the client's areas of living to evaluate where and how problems are most likely to occur. Since the alcoholic suffers emotionally, mentally, and physically, major adjustments usually need to be made in all areas of living. Early assessment determines which issues require immediate intervention and which should wait until later in recovery.

Many psychosocial assessments neglect to explore current sexual functioning, as well as sexual abuse, incest, and psychologic trauma. All too often professionals who are uncomfortable with pursuing past and present issues related to sexuality will allow the area to remain unexamined. For some clients this may be a costly omission, since the area of sexuality is often fraught with anxiety and seriously threatens sobriety. Even though in-depth treatment of sexual problems may not be necessary or may not begin until 3, 6, or even 12 months into recovery, questions about sexual functioning and sexual abuse should be asked and answered early on to allow for expression of feelings and to instill hope. Hopelessness entrenches the alcoholic's low self-concept, fuels anxiety, and makes drinking more likely.[20]

A brief sexual problem history, as described in Chapter 5, is useful during assessment. Additional questions regarding alcohol use should be included to understand the client's concept of the effect that drinking has had on sexual functioning and behavior. It is also useful to ask the client how he or she thinks recovery will affect sexuality. An understanding of other pharmacologic factors that may be influencing the client's sexual functioning is paramount, since certain medications or multiple-drug abuse in combination with alcohol abuse can increase or compound sexual difficulties. Narcotics, sedatives, antianxiety drugs, and antihypertensive agents all have been reported to have negative effects on sexual response.[21] Recent studies have shown that disulfiram (Antabuse), frequently used in the treatment of alcoholism, rarely causes erectile dysfunction.[49] Van Thiel's study[48] showed that the hypothalamic-pituitary-gonadal functioning in normal men was affected in some cases when disulfiram (500 mg/day) was taken, but even with altered hormone levels, no sexual dysfunction was reported. Although it is not within the scope of this chapter to discuss the effect of these substances in detail, it should be noted that some medications, combined with alcohol, complicate the treatment of alcohol-related sexual difficulties. It is also important to consider the sociocultural background of the client, since intervention is often sabotaged when the sexual values and cultural norms of the client are overlooked. Because in-depth assessment and treatment are usually not appropriate in early recovery, a long and detailed sex history is not advised.

Once the practitioner gathers the appropriate information and understands the presenting issues, as well as the mental, emotional, and physical capabilities of the client and partner, Annon's PLISSIT model[3] may be followed as a guide to intervention. Again, the initial goal is to reduce anxiety and later to "teach them to turn themselves on as a substitute for the euphoria-producing properties of drugs, and to relax in order to replace the anxiety-reducing effects of drugs."[18] This is often a slow process and is best facilitated by a step-by-step plan that fits the specific needs of the client. Generally speaking, all interventions should include (1) permission to talk about sexuality, (2) permission to postpone sexual activity, (3) knowledge that what the client is experiencing is common for alcoholics in recovery, and (4) information about the effects of alcohol on sensory awareness and sexual functioning. The small book *Sex and Recovery*[51] is useful for the client to read, since it is written for the alcoholic and family and deals sensitively with feelings of guilt, loss of interest or ability, assertiveness, masturbation, abstinence, and emotional involvement. If the client has a partner, it is important to include that person in the counseling, since, as mentioned earlier, the sexual relationship, not just the individual, is usually dysfunctional. When and if a partner is included will depend on the presenting concern, the readiness of the client, and the willingness of the partner. Some of the common sexual concerns of recovering alcoholics and their partners and specific suggestions to help enhance sexual self-esteem are presented below.

Studies have been conducted to determine group treatment strategies for recovering alcoholics.[16,31] The enhancement group in the study by Murphy et al.[31] was divided into four stages: sex education, sexual awareness, sexual dysfunctions, and sexual assertiveness. Test scores both before and after showed significant improvements in sexual arous-

---

Sexual concerns and interventions for recovering alcoholics and their partners

Concerns	Interventions
Lack of sensory awareness	Acknowledge feelings of loss; assign Kegel exercises; suggest nongenital self-touching and looking (provide privacy and body lotion in the bathing area)
Loss of interest or ability (including inhibited desire, orgasmic dysfunction, erectile dysfunction, delayed orgasm or ejaculation, dyspareunia, and vaginismus)	Follow above suggestions; suggest sensate focus with partner (see Chapter 8); depending on counselor's skill and comfort, follow treatment guidelines for specific dysfunctions in Chapter 8 or refer client to sex therapist
Poor sexual communication and assertiveness skills	Teach basic communication skills; help client determine specific conditions for satisfying sensual and sexual contact; role play, asking for what one wants and initiating or refusing sexual activity
Resentment or guilt about past sexual experiences (including sexual abuse, incest, and rape)	Encourage expression of anger, sadness, and rage; help client gain insight and resolution

ability, sex education, and relationship satisfaction. Evans and Schaefer[13] advocate including discussions on, or even separate groups for, incest and alternative life-styles.

In many instances sexual problems improve over time with minimal intervention. If problems continue to exist after 6 months into recovery, a referral to a sex therapist may be indicated. Again, whether a person or couple is ready for intensive therapy depends on mental, emotional, and physical abilities.

Summary

This chapter has discussed the physiologic and psychologic effects of alcohol on female and male sexual functioning, as well as the interactional factors that contribute to sexual problems in alcoholic relationships.

Key considerations for health care practice include the following:

1. Whereas small amounts of alcohol may enhance a feeling of sexual desire, large amounts are usually devastating to sexual desire and performance in both women and men.
2. Alcohol is a depressant to the central nervous system, impairs the functioning of the hypothalamic-pituitary axis, and is a direct gonadal toxin.
3. The most common sexual dysfunctions of alcoholic women are inhibited desire, orgasmic dysfunction, dyspareunia, and vaginismus. The most common sexual dysfunctions of alcoholic men are inhibited desire, erectile dysfunction, and delayed orgasm or ejaculation.
4. Many recovering alcoholics are out of touch with their sensory experiences and their source of euphoria.
5. Other pharmacologic factors and medical conditions that affect sexual functioning must be stabilized before sexual counseling can begin.
6. Low self-esteem, guilt, lack of assertiveness, and lack of communication skills contribute to the sexual problems of the recovering alcoholic.
7. Sexual abuse and incest may emerge as an issue for the recovering alcoholic woman. Feelings of anger, shame, and grief are common.
8. Annon's sexual problem history and PLISSIT model are useful for assessing and responding to the sexual concerns of the recovering alcoholic.
9. Individualized treatment is necessary and is based on the mental, emotional, and physical capabilities of the client. Other considerations include the sociocultural background and sexual orientation of the client.
10. Intimacy, trust, and communication are often distorted or absent in alcoholic relationships. Whenever possible, the client's sexual partner should be included in counseling.

11. Further research is needed for a more thorough understanding of the relationship between sexuality and alcohol.

Questions for review

1. What physiologic effects does alcohol have on male and female sexual response cycles?
2. What are the most common sexual dysfunctions for the alcoholic woman?
3. What are the most common sexual dysfunctions for the alcoholic man?
4. A 35-year-old man has been in treatment 21 days and is physiologically stable. He will be leaving treatment in 1 week. He comes to you and says, "My wife and I haven't had sex for a year." How would you respond to him?
5. What issues do you need to be aware of when providing care for a lesbian or gay male alcoholic in a heterosexual treatment facility?
6. At what point would you refer a recovering alcoholic to sex therapy?
7. Discuss topics for future research in the treatment of alcoholism and sexual dysfunction.

References

1. Abel, E.L.: A review of alcohol's effects on sex and reproduction, Drug and Alcohol Dependence 5:321-332, 1980.
2. Alcohol and sex: The Bottom Line on Alcohol in Society 3(4): Aug. 1980.
3. Annon, J.S.: The behavioral treatment of sexual problems, vol. 1, Brief therapy, Honolulu, 1974, Enabling Systems, Inc.
4. Beckman, L.: Reported effects of alcohol on the sexual feelings and behavior of women alcoholics and nonalcoholics, Journal of Studies on Alcohol 40:272-282, 1979.
5. Benward, J., and Densen-Gerber, J.: Incest as a causative factor in antisocial behavior an exploratory study, Contemporary Drug Problems 4:323-340, 1975.
6. Briddell, D., and Wilson, G.T.: Effects of alcohol and expectancy set on male sexual arousal, Journal of Abnormal Psychology 85:225-234, 1976.
7. Buffum, J., et al.: Drugs and sexual function. In Lief, H., editor: Sexual problems in medical practice, Monroe, Wis., 1981, American Medical Association.
8. Burchell, R.C.: Self-esteem and sexuality, Medical Aspects of Human Sexuality 9(1):74-90, 1975.
9. Bush, P.J.: Drugs, alcohol and sex, New York, 1980, Richard Marek Publishers.
10. Carpenter, J., and Armenti, N.: Some effects of ethanol on human sexual and aggressive behavior. In Kissin, B., and Begleiter, H., editors: The biology of alcoholism, New York, 1972, Plenum Publishing Corp.
11. Dowsling, J.L.: Sex therapy for recovering alcoholics an essential part of family therapy, International Journal of Addictions 15:1179-1189, 1980.
12. Estes, N.J., and Baker, J.M.: Spouses of alcoholic women. In Estes, N.J., and Heinemann, M.E., editors: Alcoholism: development, consequences, and interventions. St. Louis, 1977, The C.V. Mosby Co.
13. Evans, S., and Schaefer, S.: Why women's sexuality is important to address

in chemical dependency treatment programs, Presented at the Chemical Abuse and Sexuality Conference, Minneapolis, Sept. 1980, unpublished.

14. Farkas, F., and Rosen, R.: Effect of alcohol on elicited male sexual response, Journal of Studies on Alcohol **37**:265-271, 1976.

15. Finnegan, D.G., and McNally, E.B.: Alcoholism recovery and health—lesbians and gay men, Oakland, N.J., 1980, unpublished.

16. Gad-Luther, I., and Dickman, D.: Psychosexual therapy with recovery alcoholics, a pilot study, Journal of Sex Education and Therapy **1**(5):11-16, 1979.

17. Gordon, G.G., et al.: Effect of alcohol (ethanol) administration on sex-hormone metabolism in normal men, New England Journal of Medicine **295**:793-797, 1976.

18. Greaves, G.: Toward an existential theory of drug dependence, Journal of Nervous and Mental Disease **159**:263-271, 1974.

19. Hugues, J.N., et al.: Hypothalamo-pituitary ovarian function in thirty-one women with chronic alcoholism, Clinical Endocrinology **12**:543-551, 1980.

20. Johnson, V.E.: I'll quit tomorrow, New York, 1973, Harper & Row, Publishers, Inc.

21. Kaplan, H.S.: Disorders of sexual desire, New York, 1979, Simon & Schuster, Inc.

22. Lemere, F., and Smith, J.W.: Alcohol induced sexual impotence, American Journal of Psychiatry **130**:212-213, 1973.

23. Levay, A.N., and Sharpe, L.: Sexual dysfunction: diagnosis and treatment. In Lief, J., editor: Sexual problems in medical practice, Monroe, Wis., 1981, American Medical Association.

24. Malatesta, V.J., et al.: Alcohol effects on the orgasmic-ejaculatory response in human males, Journal of Sex Research **15**(2):101-107, 1979.

25. Malatesta, V.J., et al.: Acute alcohol intoxication and female orgasmic response, Journal of Sex Research **18**(1):1-17, 1982.

26. Marcelle, G.: Alcoholism and the gay community: the state of knowledge today, Presented at the Third National Lesbian and Gay Health Conference, San Francisco, June 1980, unpublished.

27. Masters, W., and Johnson, V.: Human sexual inadequacy, Boston, 1970, Little, Brown & Co.

28. Matefy, R.E., et al.: Self-acceptance in alcoholics who accept and reject help, Quarterly Journal of Studies of Alcohol **32**:1088-1091, 1971.

29. Mendelson, J.H., et al.: Effects of alcohol on pituitary-gonadal hormones, sexual function and aggression in human males. In Lipton, M.A., DiMascio, A., and Killan, K.F., editors: Psychopharmacology: a generation of progress, New York, 1978, Raven Press.

30. Morin, R.A.: The alcoholic man—too much/too little, Journal of Psychedelic Drugs **12**:167-169, 1980.

31. Murphy, W., et al.: Sexual dysfunction and treatment in alcoholic women, Sexuality and Disability **3**:240-255, 1980.

32. O'Donnell, M., et al.: Lesbian health matters, Santa Cruz, Calif., 1979, Santa Cruz Women's Health Collective.

33. Pinhas, V.: Sex guilt and sexual control in women alcoholics in early sobriety, Sexuality and Disability **3**:256-272, 1980.

34. Potter, J.: Women and sex—it's enough to drive them to drink. In Burtle,

V., editor: Women who drink, Springfield, Ill., 1979, Charles C Thomas, Publisher.

35. Powell, D.J.: Sexual dysfunction and alcoholism, Journal of Sex Education and Therapy **6**(2):40-46, 1980.

36. Royce, J.: Alcohol problems and alcoholism, New York, 1981, Macmillan, Inc.

37. Rubin, H.B., and Henson, D.: Effects of alcohol on male sexual responding, Psychopharmacology **47**:123-134, 1976.

38. Sandmaien, M.: The invisible alcoholics, New York, 1980, McGraw-Hill, Inc.

39. Scheig, R.: Changes in sexual performance due to liver disease, Medical Aspects of Human Sexuality, pp. 67-79, April 1975.

40. Schuckit, M.: Sexual disturbance in the woman alcoholic, Medical Aspects of Human Sexuality, pp. 44-62, Sept. 1972.

41. Shapiro, R.J.: A family therapy approach to alcoholism, Journal of Marriage and Family Counseling, pp.71-78, Oct. 1977.

42. Smith, J.: Alcohol its effects on sexual performance, Consultant, pp. 261-264, May 1982.

43. Smith, T.M.: Specific approaches and techniques in the treatment of gay male alcohol abusers, San Francisco, March 1979, Alcoholism Evaluation and Treatment Center, unpublished.

44. Smith, T.M., and Whitney, S.: Alcohol abuse in the gay community. I. The effects of alcohol abuse, San Francisco, 1980, Bay Area Physicians.

45. Vanderpool, J.A.: Alcoholism and the self-concept, Quarterly Journal of Studies of Alcohol **30**:59-77, 1969.

46. Van Thiel, D.H., and Lester, R.: Alcoholism: its effect on hypothalamic pituitary gonadal function, Progress in Hepatology **71**:318, 1976.

47. Van Thiel, D.H., and Lester, R.: The effect of chronic alcohol abuse on sexual function, Clinics in Endocrinology and Metabolism **8**:499-510, 1979.

48. Van Thiel, D.H., et al.: Disulfiram-induced disturbances in hypothalamic-pituitary function, Alcoholism: Clinical Experimental Research **3**:230-234, 1979.

49. Wagner, G., and Jensen, S.B.: Alcohol and erectile failure. In Wagner, G., and Green, R., editors: Impotence: physiological, psychological, surgical diagnosis and treatment, New York, 1981, Plenum Publishing Corp.

50. Watts, R.J.: The physiological interrelationship between depression, drugs, and sexuality, Nursing Forum **17**:168-183, 1978.

51. Weinberg, J.R.: Sex and recovery, Minneapolis, 1977, Recovery Press.

52. Wilsnack, S.C.: Femininity by the bottle, Psychology Today, pp. 39-85, April 1973.

53. Wilson, G.T., and Lawson, D.: Effects of alcohol on sexual arousal in women, Journal of Abnormal Psychology **5**:489-497, 1976.

54. Wilson, G.T., and Lawson, D.M.: Expectancies, alcohol, and sexual arousal in male social drinkers, Journal of Abnormal Psychology **85**:587-594, 1976.

55. Wilson, G.T., et al.: Effects of alcohol on sexual arousal in male alcoholics, Journal of Abnormal Psychology **87**:609-616, 1978.

56. Zilbergeld, B.: Male sexuality, New York, 1978, Bantam Books.

23

Drug effects on human sexual behavior

JAMES S. WOODS

The past few decades have seen a tremendous alteration in traditional attitudes regarding many aspects of the human experience. Prevalent among these changes are new approaches to sexual behavior and drug use. Recent advances in social technology and biomedical research have permitted and encouraged both a higher level of understanding and deeper experimentation into many heretofore unanswered questions about human sexuality. In a society characterized by an increased awareness of sexual functioning and the widespread availability, use, and even abuse of drugs that modify every facet of human behavior, it is important to consider the effects of drugs on human sexual functioning and activity. The purpose of this chapter is to consider recent developments from biomedical and clinical research, as well as some of the more traditional concepts and misconceptions regarding the effects of drugs on sexual behavior in humans.

Oral contraceptives

The oral contraceptives stand alone as a class of drugs that has had a primary influence on the shaping of contemporary attitudes regarding sexual behavior. The ready availability of oral contraceptives to millions of women over the past 20 to 25 years not only has meant a welcome approach to family planning but also has made possible a separation of sexual activity from concern about conception and reproduction. Thus "the pill" has played a major role in creating a pervasive sense of sexual freedom in contemporary society.

For the most part the oral contraceptives available today are primarily for use by women. Modern preparations consist of a combination of progestational and estrogenic steroids and require once-a-day use throughout the pill cycle. Progestational steroids, such as dimethisterone, norethindrone, or norethynodrel, and estrogenic steroids, such as ethinyl estradiol or mestranol, are commonly used. Estrogenic steroids suppress secretion of follicle-stimulating hormone, blocking follicle development and ovulation. Progestational steroids suppress luteinizing hormone so ovulation cannot occur even if the follicle develops. Progestins also thicken the cervical mucus, which interferes with sperm migration and causes endometrial changes that prevent implantation of the fertilized ovum. Combination contraceptive preparations require precoital administration, and, if used conscientiously, are considered to have a failure rate of not greater than 1%.

In addition to oral contraceptives containing a combination of steroidal compounds, preparations containing only a progestogen, norethindrone or norgestrel, at a very low dose level, have also become available.[6] The dosage is one tablet daily without interruption. These "minipill" preparations (Micronor, Ovrette, Nor-Q.D.) exert their contraceptive action by reducing the penetrability of the sperm in the cervical mucus, by interfering with luteal function by suppressing the secretion of gonadotropins, and by interfering with the implantation of the ovum. The minipill does not prevent ovulation and is therefore believed to be somewhat less effective as a contraceptive than preparations that contain both progestogens and estrogen.

Postcoital "morning-after" preparations that prevent implantation of the fertilized ovum by blocking or incapacitating the corpus luteum subsequent to ovulation[15] are also available. These preparations are composed of estrogenic steroids such as diethylstilbestrol (DES) or conjugated estrogens (Premarin), which, in large doses, shorten transit time for the fertilized ovum into the uterine cavity, accounting for their postcoital activity.[18] The use of DES for this purpose is controversial because of the development of vaginal cancer in daughters[35] of some women who have taken DES during pregnancy. It has been shown that the progestogen d-norgestrel, taken within 3 hours of sexual intercourse, is also effective in preventing pregnancy.[43]

Several attempts have been made toward developing continuous action drugs that are effective in providing contraceptive protection for women for prolonged periods. Recently an experimental birth control capsule that can be implanted under the arm has been shown to be highly effective in preventing pregnancy in up to 99% of women tested. The capsules contain the progestin levonorgestrel, which is slowly released into the blood, providing continuous protection against pregnancy for up to 7 years. The capsule can be easily removed if pregnancy is desired. Although still in the experimental stage in the United States, capsule contraceptives are currently available in Egypt, Thailand, and other countries and should be approved for use in the United States by the end of the 1980s.

Work is also in progress on a once-a-month birth control pill that may be ready for use by women by 1984 or 1985. This pill employs a newly discovered drug, antiprogesterone, which acts by selectively blocking the effects of progesterone on cells of the uterus, thereby allowing the fertilized ovum to be expelled along with the normal shedding of the uterine lining during menstruation. The once-a-month pill is expected to have none of the potentially deleterious side effects associated with once-a-day combination preparations. Another once-a-month contraceptive device, the ring, may also be available for use by women by the mid-1980s. The ring is designed to be worn in the vagina for 3-week periods during the ovulatory cycle, during which a combination of d-norgestrel and estradiol is released to provide continuous contraceptive protection.

Although the chemical contraceptives available today are for use only by women, research continues into the development of oral contraceptive agents for men. Unfortunately, this area is plagued with problems, most of which bear either on male sexuality or on male reproductive physiology. Foremost is the presumption that men will not use chemical contraceptives because of fear of psychologic and clinical effects on libido and masculinity. These fears are not completely unfounded, since adverse effects on sexual physiology have been observed with spermatogenic agents. Thus the pharmaceutics industry has been slow to institute research programs in this area. Another problem lies in the complexity of the male reproductive system. Experimental drugs that block spermatogenesis, such as nitrofurans, thiophenes, hydrazines, and sex steroids, require approximately 2 months between drug action and contraceptive effectiveness. In addition, the disulfiram-like effect of some of these agents, which produce acute toxic effects in persons taking them in combination with alcohol, limits their use in contemporary society, where alcohol consumption is often associated with sexual activity.

A more effective approach to controlling fertility in men has been proposed to lie in the use of agents that will interfere with the fertilizing capacity of spermatozoa in the epididymis.[5] Cyproterone acetate, an antiandrogen, has been shown to produce spermatogenic arrest in rats[54] and to interfere with androgen-dependent maturation of epididymal spermatozoa.[56] In clinical trials cyproterone acetate, administered orally, has induced infertility in men, but pronounced depression of both sperm count and sperm motility occurs as well. These observations suggest that the drug affects spermatogenesis, as well as epididymal maturation.[31] Whether this property of cyproterone will affect its eventual utility as an effective contraceptive drug in men remains to be determined. Another class of potential male contraceptive drugs, the α-chlorhydrins, appears to act on the epididymal phase of sperm maturation almost immediately after administration. These effects are reversible with cessation of therapy and, apparently, neither alter libido nor interfere with genetic material.[40] Unfortunately, α-chlorhydrins are toxic to other organ systems and are therefore unlikely to have practical application as a male contraceptive.[4] Nevertheless, many laboratories are currently studying the utility of this class of compounds as a model of a posttesticular contraceptive agent that may eventually lead to the development of a successful male birth control drug.

Drugs that decrease sexual activity and functioning

Drugs that have an adverse effect on sexual functioning and activity may do so either through an overall depressive effect on the central nervous system or through a somewhat more specific action on a portion of the autonomic nervous system that affects sexual functioning, or both. Male potency, in particular, seems to be susceptible to the effects of drugs that interact with the autonomic nervous system. This section describes some of these drugs, which comprise a surprisingly large variety of over-the-counter and clinically prescribed agents in use today.

The autonomic nervous system consists of nerves, ganglia, and plexuses that are distributed throughout the body to provide innervation for the automatic functioning of various body organs. Included under the control of this system are the sex organs and associated glands and blood vessels. The two main anatomic divisions of the autonomic nervous system, the sympathetic (adrenergic) outflow and the parasympathetic (cholinergic) outflow, are viewed as physiologic antagonists. Often, however, these systems function cooperatively, as in their synergistic effect on sexual functioning.

In men, adrenergic impulses produce ejaculation by causing contraction of the prostate and seminal vesicles in association with an effect on the bulbocavernosus and ischiocavernosus muscles. Drugs that block adrenergic impulses may affect ejaculatory function as a result of sympathetic blockade.

On the other hand, parasympathetic stimulation controls penile erection. This response is secondary to congestion of the vascular sinuses in the corpora resulting from parasympathetic nerve action in the venous channels. Drugs that interfere with parasympathetic nerve transmission will block this function.

Ganglionic blocking agents, which may simultaneously block both sympathetic and parasympathetic nerve function, may result in complete impotence and therefore sexual dysfunction.

Antihypertensive drugs. Drugs used in the treatment of hypertension can be classified into three principal categories: vasodilators, sympatholytics, and diuretics. The latter two categories have been reported to impair sexual functioning in humans.

Sympatholytic agents are those substances that exert their effects by blocking sympathetic nervous system function. Such agents can be grouped into several categories according to their primary site(s) of action. These include centrally acting agents, ganglionic blocking agents, sympathetic receptor blockers, and agents that alter the release of neurotransmitter from sympathetic nerve terminals.

Among the centrally acting agents, the most commonly employed in the clinical control of hypertension are clonidine (Catapres), methyldopa (Aldomet), and reserpine (Serpasil). Clonidine is a relatively new drug that acts to reduce blood pressure by decreasing the sympathetic outflow from the medulla.[11] This drug has been reported to also have peripheral anticholinergic effects, including urinary retention and gynecomastia in men. The incidence of erectile failure and other adverse effects on sexual functioning in men has been reported to be as high as 24%.[51] No adverse effects of clonidine on female sexual functioning have been reported.

Methyldopa acts centrally to reduce blood pressure. This effect is brought about when the drug is converted in the central nervous system to α-methylnorepinephrine through the action of two enzymes, dopa decarboxylase and dopamine β-hydroxylase.[34] α-Methylnorepinephrine then acts as a weak "false transmitter," replacing the more potent norepinephrine in central sympathetic nerve transmission. Adverse sexual effects of methyldopa that have been reported include erectile and ejaculatory failure and decreased libido in men and decreased libido and galactorrhea in women.[57,67] Adverse effects of methyldopa disappear within about 2 weeks after drug use is discontinued.

Reserpine acts as a hypotensive agent both centrally and peripherally by stimulating the release of neurotransmitters from cellular binding sites and by preventing their reaccumulation in nerve endings. This action leads to numerous sympatholytic side effects, including sexual dysfunction. Reported effects include erectile difficulties, decreased emission, and delayed ejaculation in men and decreased libido in women.[37,51] Reserpine has also been shown to block ovulation, cause infertility and pseudopregnancy, and induce lactation in women. Because mental depression may also be precipitated by reserpine, as well as its numerous other side effects, this drug is no longer recommended for routine use as an antihypertensive medication.

Of the ganglionic blocking agents that are available for hypertension therapy, only trimethaphan (Arfonad) is currently employed for this purpose. Drugs of this class may block both sympathetic and parasympathetic innervation of the sex organs. Hence both erectile capability and ejaculatory function may be adversely affected as a consequence of these effects.

Sympathetic receptor blocking agents exert their effects by selective blockade of α- or β-adrenergic receptors. Only those that specifically act as β-receptor blockers are commonly used for controlling hypertension. Two drugs of this class that are available in the United States are propranolol (Inderal) and metoprolol. Since these agents alter blood pressure principally through direct effects on the heart and by inhibition of renal renin secretion, adverse effects on sexual functioning are minimal. In a few cases, however, loss of libido and decreased potency in men have been reported.[36,77] α-Adrenergic receptor blocking agents such as phenoxybenzamine (Dibenzyline) and phentolamine (Regitine) are not commonly used in hypertension therapy because of severe adverse side effects, including nausea. The potential effects of these drugs on sexual functioning, therefore, are of little clinical importance. A new drug, prazosin (Minipress), has recently been introduced as an antihypertensive agent and appears to have the properties of an α-blocker. Current literature on the clinical effects of this drug does not document a significant incidence of sexual dysfunction in association with its use in hypertension treatment.

Guanethidine (Ismelin) is the only drug used in the United States in the control of hypertension that acts solely by depleting neurotransmitter from sympathetic nerve endings and preventing its reuptake. This action produces impotence in a number of men using the drug, since the nervous mechanisms responsible for sexual functioning are essentially inactivated by the drug's action. Experiments with guanethidine have shown that erectile potency, ability to ejaculate, and intensity of climax are all reduced significantly during drug use.[52] Retrograde ejaculation resulting from incompetence of the urethral sphincter caused by inadequacy of sympathetic transmitter release has also been reported. The incidence of these effects is as high as 60% among guanethidine users and appears to be directly related to the dose of the drug taken.[76]

Diuretics comprise the second principal category of antihypertensive drugs that impair sexual functioning in humans. Thiazide diuretics, such as bendroflumethiazide (Naturetin) and chlorothiazide (Diuril), are commonly used as part of a combination drug therapy program in treatment of hypertension. These agents act principally by increasing renal excretion of sodium and chloride, which is accompanied by osmotic diuresis of water. Clinical studies indicate that about 5% of men who use thiazide diuretics on a regular basis experience disturbances in potency that are attributable to the drug. The mechanisms of impotence associated with the use of thiazides are not known but may be associated in part with potassium depletion accompanying drug use.

Another diuretic employed in the treatment of hypertension is the steroid analog spironolactone (Aldactone). This agent acts by displacement of aldosterone in the kidneys, thereby interfering with the normal reabsorption of calcium ions. Sexual dysfunction in both men and women has been reported in association with spironolactone use,[30] although the mechanism by which this effect occurs is not known. Among the manifestations of sexual dysfunction reported are decreased libido, impotence, and gynecomastia in men and menstrual irregularities, including amenorrhea, and breast tenderness in women.

An important question that arises regarding the effects of drugs used in hypertension on sexual functioning is to what extent the person taking antihypertensive medication should be informed of the potential for sexual dysfunction associated with such therapy. This question has major implications with respect to client compliance, since side effects that result in impairment of sexual functioning may lead to reduction or discontinuation of medication. In this regard it would seem that an informed understanding on behalf of the client with respect to the potential for adverse sexual side effects of the medicine taken would be desirable, so that an assessment of the willingness of the client to tolerate such effects could be made. Adjustments in the antihypertensive drug regimen resulting from such counseling may thereby improve both client compliance and sexual functioning while providing for effective blood pressure control.

   Antidepressants. Depression is considered to include emotional disorders ranging from mild despondency without somatic manifestations to severely retarded states and suicidal risks. In an increasingly complex society, characterized by increased demands on both time and ability as a way of life, depression and its manifestations are becoming more and more common. Depression is usually accompanied by decreased sexual drive, interest, and activity.

   Treatment of depression by either psychologic support or relief from stressful conditions often results in a return of normal sexual interest and behavior. Often, however, the use of antidepressant drug therapy is recommended. Some agents, unfortunately, have the inherent capacity to promote the development of impotence and to adversely affect other aspects of sexual behavior. Thus the positive aspects of these drugs resulting from mood elevation may be counterbalanced by their negative effects on sexual functioning.

   Two principal categories of antidepressant drugs are currently in use. The first group consists of chemicals known as tricyclic compounds and includes imipramine (Tofranil), desipramine (Norpramin, Pertofrane), amitriptyline (Elavil), nortriptyline (Aventyl), and protriptyline (Vivactil). Although the antidepressant effect of these drugs is not clearly understood, their peripheral anticholinergic effects are similar to those produced by many antihypertensive agents. It is primarily the anticholinergic actions to which the untoward effects of these drugs on sexual functioning are attributed. Thus tricyclic compounds are most often associated with the development of male impotence. Inhibition of ejaculation in a small percentage of men being treated with these drugs has been reported, with the effects subsiding when the dosage is reduced.

   The second group of drugs used as antidepressants are the monoamine oxidase (MAO) inhibitors. These drugs are also used as antihypertensive agents. Their primary mechanism of action is blockade of the enzyme monoamine oxidase in the brain and in adrenergic nerve terminals. Substances normally oxidized by MAO, especially serotonin and norepinephrine, therefore accumulate and in some way produce stimulation of mood.

   Two types of MAO inhibitors are currently available for clinical or therapeutic use: hydrazine derivatives, which include phenelzine sulfate (Nardil), and nonhydrazine compounds, including tranylcypromine sulfate (Parnate) and pargyline (Eutonyl). Impotence may result from the use of these drugs because of their tendency to block peripheral ganglionic nerve transmission. Delayed or impaired ejaculation has also been reported in 25% to 30% of men using MAO inhibitors. These effects are usually reversible within 2 to 3 weeks after discontinuation of the drug.

   Lithium carbonate is a third class of drug that has been introduced in recent years for treatment of depression primarily associated with manic-depressive illness. Disturbed sexual functioning in clients treated with lithium carbonate has been reported,[37] although specific effects on sexual behavior or functioning have not been defined. A variety of endocrine changes induced by lithium compounds, including interference with antidiuretic hormone action[4,65] and suppression of serum testosterone levels in men,[59] may contribute to the adverse effects on sexual functioning that have been observed.

Antihistamines. Histamine is a naturally produced substance that possesses a variety of physiologic properties, including smooth muscle stimulation, mediation of the inflammatory response, and cardiovascular effects. Antihistaminic drugs act as competitive inhibitors of histamine at physiologic receptor sites and prevent its action. Well-known examples of such drugs include diphenhydramine (Benadryl), promethazine (Phenergan), and chlorpheniramine (Chlor-Trimeton). These drugs are annually consumed by millions of people for use as antiemetics, as mild sedatives, and for the control of allergy and cold symptoms. Most antihistamines display anticholinergic effects, such as dryness of the mouth, urinary retention, and constipation. Continuous use of these drugs may result in interference with sexual activity. This effect is presumably mediated by means of the blockade of parasympathetic nerve impulses to the sex glands and organs.

Antispasmodics. For the most part antispasmodic drugs are quaternary ammonium compounds. Their primary effect is relaxation of the smooth muscle of the gastrointestinal tract, biliary tract, ureter, and uterus. Because these drugs may act as ganglionic blocking agents, postural hypotension and impotence may result from their use. Drugs in this category include methantheline (Banthine), glycopyrrolate methobromide (Robinul), hexocyclium (Tral), and poldine (Nacton).

Sedatives and tranquilizers. A wide variety of sedatives and tranquilizers have become available in recent years. Many of these drugs have both direct and indirect effects on sexual interest and capability. Two of the most frequently used classes of tranquilizers include phenothiazines and benzodiazepine compounds. In addition, several minor categories of sedative drugs are also available, and these may also affect sexual functioning.

Phenothiazines comprise one of the most widely used classes of drugs in medical practice today. Over thirty phenothiazines with a broad spectrum of action are currently available. Known as the major tranquilizers, phenothiazines are primarily used in the treatment of psychosis, but they have additional use as preanesthetic medications, in the treatment of parkinsonism, and as antiemetics and analgesics. Chlorpromazine (Thorazine, Megaphen) is the best-known example. Others include prochlorperazine (Compazine), thioridazine (Mellaril), and mesoridazine (Serentil). Although the details of the mechanism of the sedative effect of phenothiazines are not fully understood, these drugs are thought to act by modifying sensory input into the reticular formation of the brainstem. The sedative effect they produce may partially account for a decrease in interest in sexual activity of persons receiving phenothiazine therapy.

In addition to their central effects, these drugs exert a variety of peripheral actions that may also contribute to inhibition of sexual functioning. Phenothiazines decrease skeletal muscle tone and block cholinergic synapses at both muscarinic and nicotinic receptor sites. Inhibition of various adrenergic impulses may occur as well. Impotence, decreased libido, and ejaculation disorders have been reported in clients taking phenothiazines. Singh[66] reported the failure of ejaculation in men treated with thioridazine, although erection and orgasm were not affected. Ejaculation problems have also been reported in association with the use of chlorprothixene (Taractan)[17] and mesoridazine (Serentil).[63]

Chlorpromazine may also influence sexual functioning by affecting the endocrine glands, possibly through acting on the hypothalamus. In animal studies phenothiazine derivatives have been shown to cause a suppression of hypothalamic and pituitary function, resulting in decreased secretion of hormones affecting the function of sex organs in both males and females.[64] Chlorpromazine has been shown to be spermicidal in dogs[20] and to reduce the copulation rate of male rats.[27] Regressive and atrophic changes in the testes of experimental animals receiving phenothiazines have also been reported.[62] Chlorpromazine has been shown to reduce urinary levels of gonadotropins, estrogens, and progestins. As with reserpine, chloropromazine blocks ovulation, suppresses estrus cycles in animals, induces lactation, and maintains a decidual reaction. The release of pituitary gonadotropins by relatively small doses of chlorpromazine has been shown to delay ovulation and menstruation in women. Prolonged amenorrhea, galactorrhea, and gynecomastia have been reported to accompany treatment with certain phenothiazine derivatives.[39,67,68]

Benzodiazepine compounds comprise the second most widely used class of tranquilizing drugs. The two best known are chlordiazepoxide (Librium) and diazepam (Valium). As mild tranquilizers, both drugs are used in the treatment of anxiety, as skeletal muscle relaxants, and in the treatment of alcoholism. Impairment of sexual functioning has been associated with the effects of chlordiazepoxide and diazepam on the activity of both cholinergic and adrenergic facets of the autonomic nervous system. As with the phenothiazine derivatives, ejaculation problems have been reported for men using chlordiazepoxide.[38] Aspermia, the absence of ejaculation during coitus or masturbation, has also been reported in association with the use of chlordiazepoxide.[38] The definitive sedative and relaxing activity of these drugs may also account for the decreased interest in sexual activity observed in clients using them. Alternatively, the efficacious use of these tranquilizers has been considered to be of value in the treatment of sexual impotence and other problems involving sexual performance.[1]

Several other types of drugs used in the treatment of psychologic problems have been shown to depress sexual activity in humans. Benperidol, a sedative and mild tranquilizer, has been shown to have antilibidinous effects on men. In a study of sex offenders benperidol was effective in abolishing sexual desire and the ability to maintain an erection.[19] Failure of ejaculation without concomitant alteration of erection or orgasm has been reported in clients treated with phenoxybenzamine (Dibenzyline), an α-adrenergic blocking agent once used as an adjunct to psychiatric therapy. The potent sympatholytic effects of this drug have been advanced to account for the adverse effects on sexual functioning.[29] Methaqualone (Quaalude), another commonly used sedative, is a mild, nonbarbiturate hypnotic agent that has achieved wide popularity for the euphoric effects that sometimes accompany its abuse. Although some have attributed aphrodisiac properties to methaqualone, such effects have never been identified in relation to medical use of the drug. In fact, adverse sexual effects, including impotence, have been reported in association with its use.[24] Similarly, meprobamate (Miltown, Equanil), one of the most commonly used sedative drugs during the 1960s, may also impair sexual functioning, principally as a result of its action as a depressant of the central nervous system during continued use.

Ethyl alcohol. Ethyl alcohol deserves to be considered for its effects on human sexual functioning and behavior as a drug of individual and unique notoriety.

Revered for centuries as a sexual stimulant and cure-all, alcohol is in fact a depressant and is recognized today to have far greater social than therapeutic value. Its use as a social amenity has become widely accepted in contemporary society. Although it is a sedative, alcohol in moderate amounts may help to enhance sexual activity by relieving anxieties and loosening the inhibitions that often shroud sexual behavior. Beyond a certain limit, however, neither desire nor virility will overcome the depression of physical capability that occurs under its influence.

Studies on the pharmacologic action of alcohol have shown that the central nervous system is more markedly affected by alcohol than is any other system of the body. Electrophysiologic studies indicate that alcohol exerts its first depressant effect on the reticular activating system, a part of the brain responsible for the integration of activity in various parts of the nervous system.[41] The cortex is thus released from integrating control, with the result that various processes related to thought and motor activities become disrupted. The first mental processes affected are those related to sobriety and self-restraint. The result is a less inhibited and less restrained approach to sexual behavior and other activities that are normally inhibited by previous training or experience. Subsequent to the continued consumption of alcohol, however, the brain becomes narcotized, reflexes become retarded, blood vessels are dilated, and the capacity for sexual functioning is diminished. In addition, alcohol produces a severe diuretic effect, which also interferes with sexual functioning.

Chronic alcoholism frequently is associated with impotence and, in fact, is considered the most common cause of nonfunctional male impotence and sterility in the United States.[71] Feminization is commonly seen in chronic male alcoholics and is associated with testicular atrophy, gynecomastia, diminished body hair,[72] and decreased plasma testosterone levels.[28] These effects are probably related to disruption of the maintenance of normal sex hormone balance by the liver, the organ most severely damaged by prolonged alcohol intake. These effects, if continued, can lead to irreversible liver and testicular damage, resulting in permanent alteration of a person's ability to function sexually. The effects of chronic alcoholism on sexual functioning in women have not yet been clearly characterized, although many female alcoholics complain of diminished sexual interest and orgasmic dysfunction, similar to that experienced by men.

Alcohol may also precipitate a negative social orientation with regard to sexual behavior. Overindulgence in alcohol by men has been shown to be a frequent cause of forcible sexual assault on women. In a study in which various types of sex offenders were assessed for frequency of offense, drunk persons were involved in 12% to 16% of reported incidents.[25] In these cases alcoholic consumption had not reached the point of physical incapacitation but rather a stage characterized by confusion, belligerence, and misinterpretation, resulting in violent, antisocial acts. Thus, although initially permitting a less inhibited approach to sexual behavior, alcohol eventually decreases the capability and enjoyment of sexual activity through both physical incapacitation and depression of a rational approach to sexual behavior.

Barbiturates. Barbiturates, such as amobarbital (Amytal), pentobarbital (Nembutal), secobarbital (Seconal), and thiopental (Pentothal), are sedative-hypnotic drugs that produce a wide range of general depressant effects on all nervous tissues. As with alcohol, these drugs, when taken in prescribed dosages, produce relaxation, hypnosis, and sleep with concomitant depression of a wide range of body functions, including sexual performance and ability. With prolonged use or overdose, barbiturates can lead to respiratory failure and death. Withdrawal following continued heavy consumption of barbiturates may precipitate convulsions. There is no rationale for their use in altering sexual behavior in humans.

      Sex hormone preparations. In recent years it has been observed that sex hormones may act on parts of the central nervous system and other organs of the body to influence sexual and aggressive behavior, as well as mood and emotional outlook. Thus variations in female hormones may produce anxiety, irritability, and depression, whereas male hormones are associated with aggression and increased sexual interest.[47] Currently there is growing evidence that the sexual drives of both men and women may be influenced by treatment with sex hormones. In one study male hormones prescribed to women were shown to increase sexual interest and enjoyment, whereas male subjects treated with the female hormone estrogen almost always experienced a decrease or cessation of libido.[53]

      These observations have now been extended to the production of synthetic sex hormone preparations, many of which have been shown to influence sexual behavior. The antiandrogen steroid cyproterone acetate decreases libido and potency and has been successfully used in the treatment of hypersexuality in men.[9] Synthetic estrogens and progesterones have, of course, found wide acceptance as oral contraceptive agents. Another class of synthetic sex hormones are the anabolic steroids, which are derivatives of the male sex hormone testosterone. These drugs, which include methandrostenolone (Dianabol), nandrolone phenpropionate (Durabolin), and norethandrolone (Nilevar), are used clinically to promote nitrogen retention and weight gain in elderly or undernourished clients. In recent years considerable controversy has arisen over the use and misuse of these drugs by athletes and other postpubertal boys to promote muscle growth and endurance.[21,22,73] When these drugs are used by normally developed, well-nourished individuals, the anabolic effects on strength and development are questionable.[73] There is considerable evidence, in fact, that sexual activity may be adversely affected by these drugs because of their antigonadotropic effects on sexual functioning. These effects have been dramatically demonstrated in human studies in which men treated with norethandrolone for 8 to 25 weeks all showed loss of libido, decreased potency, diminished testicular size, and azoospermia.[21] Although recovery from most of these effects occurred in most clients within 6 months after treatment was stopped, testicular morphology remained abnormal, and it was questionable as to whether normal sexual functioning would ever be regained.

      Saltpeter. Saltpeter (potassium nitrate) has long been claimed to be an effective means of decreasing sexual appetite and is often rumored to constitute a substantial portion of the diet at boarding schools, prisons, and other institutions where sexual activity is discouraged. In actuality, saltpeter does not decrease sexual drive but, as a fairly effective diuretic, may act as a sexual deterrent by increasing urine flow. Otherwise, it has no known effects on sexual interest or potency.

Drugs that enhance sexual behavior (aphrodisiacs)

      The search for substances that increase potency or drive has existed almost as long as civilization itself. Inscriptions found in the ruins of ancient cultures have described the preparation of "erotic potions," and an endless number of "aphrodisiacs" have been described since then to modern times.[42] In contemporary society the continuous proliferation of drugs and chemicals that modify mood and behavior has enhanced the claim that many such drugs have aphrodisiac properties, and more and more substances are considered by some to fulfill this purpose.

In reality there are no known drugs that specifically increase libido or sexual performance, and every chemical taken for this purpose, without medical advice, especially in combination with other drugs, poses the danger of drug interaction or overdose to the user. Still, a number of pharmacologically active agents are capable of temporarily modifying both physiologic responsiveness and subjective perception in such a manner as to enhance the enjoyment, if not the fulfillment, of the sex act. Some of these agents are considered in this section.

Cantharis. Cantharis (cantharidin, Spanish fly), a legendary sexual stimulant, is in reality a powerful irritant and potent systemic poison. A powder made from dried beetles *(Cantharis vesicatoria)* found in southern Europe, cantharis is capable of producing severe illness characterized by vomiting, diarrhea, abdominal pain, and shock. When taken orally, it causes irritation and inflammation of the genitourinary tract and dilation of the blood vessels of the penis, producing, in some instances, prolonged erections, usually without an increase in sexual desire. Deaths have been reported from the frequent use of cantharis as an aphrodisiac.[13] It is currently recognized that cantharis is not an effective sexual stimulant, and it is seldom used in modern medical practice.

Yohimbine. Another natural substance with supposed aphrodisiac properties is yohimbine, an alkaloid derived from the West African tree *Corynanthe yohimbi.* Yohimbine produces a competitive α-adrenergic blockage of limited duration and antidiuresis, probably caused by the release of antidiuretic hormone. Although yohimbine stimulates the lower spinal nerve centers controlling erection, there is no convincing evidence that it acts as a sexual stimulant. It currently has no therapeutic uses.

Strychnine. Strychnine, the active ingredient in the extract of seeds from *Strychnos nux-vomica,* has long been used as an aphrodisiac and as an attempted treatment for impotence. As an extremely powerful stimulant of the whole neuraxis, especially the spinal cord, strychnine may produce priapism and has been used along with yohimbine as a remedy for impotence. In reality strychnine has no known selective effects on sexual performance, and there is no scientific rationale for its use in altering sexual behavior in humans.

Narcotics and psychoactive agents. The use of drugs such as morphine, heroin, cocaine, marijuana, LSD, and amphetamines as aphrodisiacs has become somewhat prevalent in contemporary society, and there is little doubt that these agents can, under certain circumstances, seem to enhance the enjoyment of the sexual experience for some who try them. The reason for such variation in responsiveness is that these agents have no particular properties that specifically increase sexual potency, but rather they tend to affect the user according to the particular circumstances under which they are used. Thus the state of mind of the individual user and the amount consumed contribute considerably to the effect achieved. Like alcohol, these drugs act on the central nervous system to release inhibitions, which are often the cause of problems involving sexual behavior. Taken in excess or too often, however, these drugs, like alcohol, will have the opposite response and will inhibit sexual drive and functioning.

Recent studies have shown that both morphine and heroin in sufficient doses produce marked reduction in sexual activity in male and female users. In male addicts nonemissive erections and impotence can result,[14] and female addicts report a high incidence of amenorrhea, infertility, reduced libido, and spontaneous abortions.[49] The reduction in sexual potency and capability is complicated in narcotics users who are concomitantly taking other types of drug therapy. These complications are of special importance when one considers the potent addicting powers of the narcotic agents. The sexual problems of heroin users are rapidly reversible with cessation of drug use or with replacement by methadone therapy. Unfortunately, however, methadone itself has also been found to produce both serious fertility problems and impaired sexual performance in male users of the drug.[10] Infertility is associated with a pronounced reduction in the size and secretory activity of the secondary sex organs, resulting in extremely low ejaculate volume and low sperm motility in methadone users. Whether this condition is reversible after withdrawal from the drug is not yet known, although animal studies suggest that normal secondary sex organ function will return after discontinuation of methadone treatment.

Cocaine abuse has endured since antiquity but has become particularly widespread in recent years in contemporary society because of its central stimulant properties. As with other psychoactive drugs, cocaine is reported to increase sex drive and to intensify the quality of the total erotic experience. Reported effects are variable, ranging from multiorgasmic capacity to spontaneous erections and painful priapism.[74] Although occasional use does appear to facilitate the sexual experience for some persons, chronic use of cocaine, as with alcohol, invariably leads to a decline in sexual functioning and interest.

Marijuana (cannabis), an extract of the *Cannabis sativa* plant, is considered by many to be a sexual stimulant. However, like alcohol, its effect results indirectly from relaxation and release of inhibitions surrounding sexual activity. The main active ingredient in marijuana is tetrahydrocannabinol, to which its pharmacologic effects are attributed. As with other psychoactive drugs, the subjective effects resulting from smoking marijuana depend on the personality of the user, the dose, and the circumstances under which it is smoked. Most commonly, the effect of marijuana is a distortion of time and an enhanced suggestibility, producing the illusion that sexual climax is somewhat prolonged. Thus the subjective consideration of the user of marijuana as an aphrodisiac may enhance his or her enjoyment of the sex act. Studies on the properties of marijuana for a specific effect on sexual behavior, however, have shown that it has no such properties.[10] On the contrary, there is evidence that marijuana smokers have a higher incidence of decreased libido and impaired potency than nonusers.[44] In addition, chronic intensive use of marijuana has been shown to depress plasma testosterone levels in healthy men[44] and has produced gynecomastia in some users.[33] Decreased sperm counts and changes in sperm motility have also been observed.[50] One recent report[9] indicates that tetrahydrocannabinol interferes with the normal functioning of the male reproductive organs by reducing the activities of various enzymatic processes in the testis, prostate, and epididymis. Young persons who smoke marijuana may be at particularly high risk of adverse effects on sexual functioning and fertility because of the effects of the drug on developing sex organs.[50] Although studies to determine the potential for marijuana to cause birth defects in humans have not yet been conducted, tetrahydrocannabinol has been shown to block ovulation in female rhesus monkeys and is known to cross the placenta and cause birth defects in some animal species.[50] The evidence for the potential adverse effects of marijuana and its active ingredients on sexual functioning and reproductive capability would therefore seem to strongly militate against the use of marijuana during the reproductive years and especially during pregnancy.

Lysergic acid diethylamide (LSD) is another drug that, although considered an aphrodisiac by some, has potentially untoward effects on sexual functioning and behavior. As with other psychoactive drugs, any alteration of sexual performance produced by LSD is principally subjective, the effects of this drug being almost entirely on the central nervous system. Little response, if any, has been seen in other organ systems that can be attributed to a direct effect of LSD, and there is no biochemical or pharmacologic evidence to support the contention that LSD or similar drugs contain any sex-stimulating properties.[23] On the other hand, the repeated use of LSD may produce serious psychologic problems, which could have an overall adverse effect on sexual interest or activity. The use of LSD during pregnancy may cause a higher rate of malformed babies or stillbirths than is observed in nonusers.[61]

Amphetamines (Benzedrine, Dexedrine, Methedrine) have also been used for the purpose of stimulating sexual functioning. These drugs have a powerful central stimulant action in addition to peripheral α- and β-sympathomimetic effects. The main results of an oral dose of 10 to 30 mg are wakefulness and alertness, mood elevation, increased motor and speech activity, and often elation and euphoria. Physical performance is usually improved, and fatigue can be prevented or reversed. The effects of amphetamines on sexual performance, however, are inconsistent. At moderate dosage levels there is seldom any effect on sexual behavior, aside from that accompanying elevation of mood or reversal of fatigue. Doses in the range of 20 to 50 mg have been reported to alter sensations to enhance the orgasmic feeling. However, higher doses, such as 1 g taken intravenously, will produce loss of interest and withdrawal from sexual activity.[14] Amphetamines, along with the other psychoactive agents, will do little to promote the enjoyment of sexual activity and may produce, in the long run, adverse psychologic and physical effects that may reduce sexual interest and capability.

Ethyl alcohol. One final word about the powers of alcohol as an aphrodisiac should be included in this section. A study of 20,000 well-educated men and women of high socioeconomic status revealed that for almost 60% of them alcohol heightened the enjoyment of sex. It was concluded that the removal of inhibitions through consumption of alcohol more than counterbalances the loss of physical ability that accompanies its use.[3] This fact suggests that at least for wealthier, better-educated, and more inhibited persons, alcohol in moderation can actually increase sexual functioning despite depressed physical reactions.

Other drugs that may affect sexual behavior

A number of clinically used or experimental drugs have been shown to positively affect sexual interest or potency in both clients and laboratory animals. This effect seems to occur independent of their prescribed intention or use. Several of these drugs are described in this section.

L-Dopa. Levodihydroxyphenylalanine (L-dopa) is a natural interme-diate in the biosynthesis of catecholamines in the brain and peripheral adrenergic nerve terminals. In the biologic sequence of events it is converted to dopamine, which in turn serves as a substrate of the neurotransmitter norepinephrine. L-Dopa has been used with gratifying success in the treatment of Parkinson's disease, a disease of the basal ganglia characterized by dopamine deficiency. When L-dopa is administered to a client with Parkinson's disease, amelioration of the symptoms is observed, presumably because of the conversion of the drug to dopamine. It has been observed that clients, especially older men, who are treated with L-dopa experience a sexual rejuvenation. It is to this effect that the sexual stimulating powers of L-dopa have been attributed. Consequently, studies with younger men complaining of decreased erectile ability have similarly shown that L-dopa increases libido and incidence of penile erections. Overall, however, these effects were short lived and did not promote satisfactory sexual functioning and potency. Thus it is conceded that L-dopa is not a true aphrodisiac but that increased sexual activity experienced by clients with Parkinson's disease treated with L-dopa reflects an improve-ment of well-being, along with partial recovery of normal sexual functions that were impaired by the disease.[48]

PCPA. p-Chlorophenylalanine (PCPA), a drug chemically related to L-dopa, has been claimed to have potent aphrodisiac properties in laboratory animals.[69] Considerable controversy has characterized the potential sex-stimulating powers of this drug,[26] which has been used experimentally as a selective blocker of serotonin biosynthesis in the brain. In one report[16] PCPA, when used with the MAO inhibitor phenelzine, significantly increased sexual activity in men suffering from debilitating essential head-aches and sexual deficiency. The sexual improvement paralleled the amelioration of headaches and mood. Because PCPA has not come into clinical use, it is not known what direct effects it may have on human libido or sexual ability.

Amyl nitrite. Amyl nitrite, a drug used in the treatment of angina pectoris, is alleged to enhance sexual activity in humans. As a potent peripheral vasodilator and smooth muscle stimulant, amyl nitrite has been reported to intensify the orgasmic experience if inhaled at the moment of orgasm. This effect is probably the result of relaxation of smooth muscles and consequent vasodilation of the genitourinary tract. No effects of amyl nitrite on libido or sexual functioning have been reported.

Caffeine. Caffeine is the principal central nervous system stimulant in coffee, tea, and certain other widely consumed beverages and over-the-counter drug preparations. In the past caffeine has been misrepresented by some as possessing properties that stimulate sexual behavior.[45] Although the stimulant effect of caffeine may be beneficial for enhancing sexual performance in persons who are otherwise disinterested because of fatigue, no specific effect of caffeine on sexual functioning has been demonstrated in amounts normally consumed. Higher doses, however, might tend to mimic, to some extent, some of the effects of amphetamines.

Vitamin E. Much has been said in recent years about the positive effects of vitamin E (α-tocopherol) on sexual performance and ability in humans. Un-fortunately, there is little scientific rationale to substantiate such claims. The primary reasons for attributing a positive role in sexual performance to vitamin E come mainly from experiments on vitamin E deficiency in laboratory animals. In such experiments the principal manifestation of this deficiency is infertility, although the reasons for this condition differ in males and females. In female rats there is no loss in ability to produce apparently healthy ova, and no defect in the placenta or uterus exists. However, fetal death occurs shortly after the first week of embryonic life, and fetuses are reabsorbed. This situation can be prevented if vitamin E is administered any time up to the fifth or sixth day of embryonic life. In male rats the earliest observable effect of vitamin E deficiency is immobility of spermatozoa, with subsequent degeneration of the germinal epithelium. However, there is no alteration in the secondary sex organs or diminution of sexual vigor, although the latter may occur with continued vitamin E deficiency. Because of experimental results such as these, it has been thought that vitamin E could restore or preserve virility, fertility, sexual interest, potency, and endurance in humans. There is no evidence to support any of these contentions, but since sexual performance is often influenced by mental attitude, a person who believes vitamin E may improve sexual prowess may actually find such improvement.

Selenium. Selenium is a trace element that appears to have a nutritional requirement in peroxide-destroying processes in certain tissues. Although excess levels of selenium in the diet are highly toxic, selenium deficiency in animals has been associated with low sperm counts and decreased fertility in males and sterility in females. Little is known of the effects of selenium or selenium deficiency on sexual ability or fertility in humans, although persons given selenium supplements have reported enhancement of sexual urge and an increase in frequency of sexual activity. As in the case of vitamin E, however, it is likely that the improvement of sexual ability associated with use of selenium is principally the result of psychologic expectation of such improvement associated with its use.

Clomiphene citrate (Clomid). Clomiphene citrate, an antiestrogen, has been widely used in the treatment of infertility in women who fail to ovulate. The drug acts by stimulating the anovulatory ovary to secrete estrogen and the hypothalamus to stimulate production and release of gonadotropins that stimulate follicle maturation and ovulation. In men clomiphene citrate increases depressed testosterone levels and enhances low sperm count. Several studies[12,46] have indicated that an increase in sexual potency and libido occurs in clients during clomiphene citrate therapy. These effects most likely occur as a result of enhanced expectations on behalf of the users of achieving ovulation and/or conception rather than because of specific properties of the drug itself.

Bromocriptine mesylate (Parlodel). Bromocriptine is an ergot alkaloid derivative used in the treatment of amenorrhea and galactorrhea associated with hyperprolactinemia. Although sometimes used in the treatment of infertility in women, it is not recommended for this purpose because its safety during pregnancy has not been established. Bromocriptine has been reported to restore gonadal function in men with galactorrhea and hyperprolactinemia, and in preliminary trials in infertile men it has been shown to produce a rapid rise in depressed testosterone associated with elevated serum prolactin levels.[58] No alterations in sexual behavior or performance in either men or women who have taken bromocriptine have been reported.

Cimetidine (Tagamet). Cimetidine acts to antagonize the effect of histamine on gastric acid secretion in the stomach by competitively inhibiting the action of histamine on the so-called H_2 receptor. Its principal use is in the treatment of peptic and duodenal ulcers. Recently a number of reports have appeared citing a loss of libido and sexual potency in men who had been using cimetidine for this purpose. Effects ranging from breast soreness and gynecomastia[32] to complete impotence[55,75] have been reported. Although the reason for these effects is not clear, cimetidine has been shown to produce an antiandrogenic effect in animals[55] and to cause a substantial drop in sperm count in men,[70] suggesting an inhibitory effect of the drug on testosterone production. This action, however, remains to be established. The consequences of prolonged cimetidine therapy on fertility and sexual activity in either men or women are not as yet known.

Clofibrate (Atromid S). Clofibrate, a monochlorophenoxy acid derivative, has been widely used in the treatment of hypertriglyceridemia and hypercholesterolemia and is under clinical trial in atherosclerosis when there is evidence of coronary disease. Although the precise mechanism of its blood lipid-lowering effect is not clear, clofibrate apparently acts by interfering with cholesterol synthesis in the liver. Although there is no obvious rationale for an adverse effect of this drug on sexual capability, one report has appeared describing erectile impotence in men who were receiving clofibrate therapy.[60] This circumstance was reversed within 4 weeks after drug treatment was stopped but reoccurred when therapy was resumed. Further studies are required to determine the cause of this effect. No alteration of sexual functioning in women who have taken clofibrate has been reported.

Disulfiram (Antabuse). Disulfiram (tetraethylthiuram disulfide) is an antioxidant that, when taken with ethyl alcohol, blocks the intermediary metabolism of alcohol at the aldehyde stage. Subsequent accumulation of aldehyde in the system leads to intense and dramatic illness (aldehyde syndrome) characterized by flushing, nausea, pulsating headache, hypotension, blurred vision, and vertigo. As little as 7 ml of alcohol can precipitate symptoms in sensitive persons. This property of disulfiram accounts for its therapeutic usefulness in the treatment of chronic alcoholism, not as a cure but as a strong deterrent to further alcohol consumption. Disulfiram, given by itself, is relatively nontoxic, and few untoward side effects are observed. However, reduced sexual potency and temporary impotence[67,68] have been reported in some users. Since disulfiram has no therapeutic uses except in the treatment of chronic alcoholism, it is likely that these effects are associated with past chronic alcohol abuse rather than with the drug itself.

Summary

It may be said that whereas many drugs have an adverse effect on sexual functioning and performance, few actually enhance sexual behavior (Table 23-1). Drugs that decrease sexual drive and potency often act directly on the mechanisms controlling physical performance. In addition, they may decrease interest through a depressant effect on the central nervous system. Drugs that seem to enhance sexual behavior do so indirectly through a transient relaxation of tensions, alleviation of discomfort, or release of inhibitions. Ultimately the effect of any drug on sexual performance is likely to be diminution of interest and capability, a fact that should always be taken into account when there is reduction of sexual functioning in association with prolonged drug therapy or in cases of drug abuse.

Table 23-1. Drug effects on human sexual behavior

Drug or drug category	Effect	Probable mechanism of action
Oral contraceptives	Positive	Permits separation of sexual activity from concern about conception
Antihypertensives Clonidine (Catapres) Guanethidine (Ismelin) Methyldopa (Aldomet) Propranolol (Inderal) Reserpine (Serpasil) Trimethaphan (Arfonad)	Negative	Peripheral blockade of nervous innervation of sex glands
Antidepressants Amitriptyline (Elavil) Desipramine (Norpramin, Pertofrane) Imipramine (Tofranil) Nortriptyline (Aventyl) Pargyline (Eutonyl) Phenelzine sulfate (Nardil) Protriptyline (Vivactil) Tranylcypromine sulfate (Parnate)	Negative	Central depression; peripheral blockade of nervous innervation of sex glands
Antihistamines Chlorpheniramine (Chlor-Trimeton) Diphenhydramine (Benadryl) Promethazine (Phenergan)	Negative	Blockade of parasympathetic nervous innervation of sex glands
Antispasmodics Glycopyrrolate methobromide (Robinul) Hexocyclium (Tral) Methantheline (Banthine) Poldine (Nacton)	Negative	Ganglionic blockade of nervous innervation of sex glands
Sedatives and tranquilizers Benperidol Chlordiazepoxide (Librium) Chlorpromazine (Thorazine, Megaphen) Chlorprothixene (Taractan) Diazepam (Valium) Mesoridazine (Serentil) Methaqualone (Quaalude) Phenoxybenzamine (Dibenzyline) Prochlorperazine (Compazine) Thioridazine (Mellaril)	Negative and positive	Central sedation; blockade of autonomic innervation of sex glands; suppression of hypothalamic and pituitary function Tranquilization and relaxation
Ethyl alcohol	Negative	Central depression; suppression of motor activity; diuresis
	Transiently positive	Release of inhibitions; relaxation
Barbiturates	Negative	Central depression; suppression of motor activity; hypnosis
Diuretics Bendroflumethiazide (Naturetin) Chlorthiazide (Diuril) Spironolactone (Aldactone)	Negative	Diuresis

Table 23-1. Drug effects on human sexual behavior—cont'd

Drug or drug category	Effect	Probable mechanism of action
Sex hormone preparations Cyproterone acetate Methandrostenolone (Dianabol) Nandrolane phenpropionate (Durabolin) Norethandrolone (Nilevar)	Negative	Antiandrogenic effects on sexual function; loss of libido; decreased potency
Methadone	Negative	Suppresses secondary sex organ function in men
Potassium nitrate (saltpeter)	Questionable	Diuresis
Cantharis (Spanish fly)	Negative	Irritation and inflammation of genitourinary tract; systemic poisoning
Yohimbine	Questionable	Stimulation of lower spinal nerve centers
Strychnine	Questionable	Stimulation of neuraxis; priapism
Narcotics and psychoactive drugs Amphetamines Cocaine	Negative	Central depression; decreased libido and impaired potency
Heroin LSD Marijuana Methadone Morphine	Transiently positive	Release of inhibitions; increased suggestibility; relaxation
L-Dopa and *p*-chlorophenylalanine (PCPA)	Questionable	Improvement of well-being
Amyl nitrite	Questionable	Vasodilation of genitourinary tract; smooth muscle relaxation
Caffeine	Questionable	Central nervous system stimulant
Vitamin E	Questionable	Supports fertility in laboratory animals
Selenium	Questionable	Supports fertility in laboratory animals
Lithium carbonate	Questionable	Produces broad endocrine changes; diuresis
Clomiphene citrate (Clomid)	Questionable	Stimulates gonadotropic hormones; enhances expectations of achieving pregnancy
Bromocriptine (Parlodel)	Questionable	Stimulates gonadotropic hormones
Cimetidine (Tagamet)	Negative	Unknown
Clofibrate (Atromid S)	Questionable	Unknown
Disulfiram (Antabuse)	None by itself; negative with alcohol	Blocks alcohol metabolism; produces aldehyde syndrome

Perhaps the best individual approach to a healthy and enjoyable sexual experience lies not in the use of drugs to stimulate or otherwise modify sexual performance but, rather, in an understanding and appreciation of the many facets of human behavior that constitute sexuality.

Questions for review

1. Consider your area of clinical practice. Which types of drugs are most frequently prescribed for your clients? Of these drugs, which are most likely to interfere with sexual functioning?
2. Of the drugs listed in Table 23-1, what pharmacologic action is most frequently responsible for sexual dysfunction?
3. Which drugs, when used in combination, are likely to potentiate one another in their negative effects on sexual functioning?
4. Which drugs tend to have both positive and negative effects on sexuality?
5. To what extent do you believe it is helpful to explain the effects of drugs to clients? What might be some positive and negative effects of telling a client his drug therapy may lead to impotence?

References

1. American Medical Association Committee on Human Sexuality: Problems of male sexual response: human sexuality, Chicago, 1972, AMA.
2. Athanasiou, R., Shaver, P., and Travis, C.: Sex, Psychology Today **4**(2):39-52, 1970.
3. Baldessarini, R.J., and Lipinski, J.F.: Lithium salts:1970-1975, Annals of Internal Medicine **85**:527-533, 1975.
4. Barwin, B.N.: Recent advances in the pharmacologic regulation of fertility in men, CMA Journal **119**:757-759, 1978.
5. Bennett, J.P.: Chemical contraception in the male. In Bennett, J.P., editor: Chemical contraception, New York, 1974, Columbia University Press.
6. Bennett, J.P.: The second generation of hormonal contraceptives: continuous low-dose progestin (minipill) and depot contraceptive methods. In Bennett, J.P., editor: Chemical contraception, New York, 1974, Columbia University Press.
7. Brotherton, J., and Harcus, A.W.: Effects of oral cyproterone acetate on urinary FSH and LH levels in adult males being treated for hypersexuality, Journal of Reproduction and Fertility **33**:356-357, 1973.
8. Chakravarty, I.: Enzymatic changes in the male reproductive organs by δ-9-tetrahydrocannabinol, Biochemical Pharmacology **31**:415-418, 1982.
9. Churchill, W.: Do drugs increase sexual drive? Sexology, pp. 164-167, Oct. 1968.
10. Cicero, T.J., et al.: Function of the male sex organs in heroin and methadone users, New England Journal of Medicine **292**:882-887, 1975.
11. Clonidine (Catapres) and other drugs causing sexual dysfunction: Medical Letter **19**:81-82, 1977.
12. Cooper, A.J., et al.: Effects of clomiphene in impotence: a clinical and endocrine study, British Journal of Psychiatry **120**:327-330, 1972.
13. Craven, J.D., and Polak, A.: Cantharidine poisoning, British Medical Journal **2**:1386-1388, 1954.

14. Cross, R.R.: Management of sexual dysfunction in family practice, Paper presented for Interstate Post-Graduate Medical Association of North America, Chicago, Nov. 1973.
15. Dierassi, C.: Birth control after 1984, Science **169:**941-957, 1970.
16. Del Bene, E., and Sicuteri, F.: Drug interaction on the human sexual behavior, International Journal of Clinical Pharmacology and Biopharmacy **14:**231, 1976.
17. Ditman, K.: Inhibition of ejaculation of chlorprothixene, American Journal of Psychiatry **120:**1004-1005, 1964.
18. Emmens, C.W.: Postcoital contraception, British Medical Bulletin **26:**45-51, Jan. 1970.
19. Field, L.H.: Benperidol in the treatment of sexual offenders, Medicine, Science and the Law **13:**195-196, 1973.
20. Foote, R.H., and Gray, L.C.: Effects of tranquilizers on libido, sperm production and in vitro sperm survival in dogs, Proceedings of the Society of Experimental Biology and Medicine **114:**396-398, 1963.
21. Frasier, S.D.: Androgens and athletes, American Journal of Diseases of Children **125:**479-480, 1973.
22. Freed, D., Banks, A.J., and Longson, D.: Anabolic steroids in athletes, British Medical Journal **3:**761, 1972.
23. Freedman, A.M.: Drugs and sexual behavior, Medical Aspects of Human Sexuality **1:**25-31, 1967.
24. Gay, G.R., et al.: Drug-sex practice in the Haight-Ashbury or "The Sensuous Hippie." In Sandler, M., and Gessa, G.L., editors: Sexual behavior: pharmacology and biochemistry, New York, 1975, Raven Press.
25. Gebhard, P.H., et al.: Sex offenders, New York, 1965, Harper & Row, Publishers.
26. Gessa, G.L., Tagliamonte, A., and Tagliamonte, P.: Aphrodisiac effect of p-chlorophenylalanine, Science **171:**706, 1971.
27. Gillette, E.: Effects of chlorpromazine and D-lysergic acid diethylamide on sex behavior of male rats, Proceedings of the Society of Experimental Biology and Medicine **103:**392-394, 1960.
28. Gordon, G.G., et al.: Effect of alcohol (ethanol) administration on sex-hormone metabolism in normal men, New England Journal of Medicine **295:**793-798, 1976.
29. Green, M.: Inhibition of ejaculation as a side-effect of Mellaril, American Journal of Psychiatry **118:**173-174, 1961.
30. Greenblatt, D.J., and Koch-Webster, J.: Gynecomastia and impotence complications of spironolactone therapy, Journal of the American Medical Association **223:**82, Jan. 1973.
31. Greep, R.O., Koblinsky, M.A., and Jaffe, F.S.: Reproduction and human welfare: a challenge to research, Bioscience **26:**677-684, 1976.
32. Hall, W.H.: Breast changes in males on cimetidine, New England Journal of Medicine **295:**841, 1976.
33. Harmon, J., and Aliapoulis, M.A.: Gynecomastia in marijuana users, New England Journal of Medicine **287:**936, 1972.
34. Henning, M., and Rubenson, A.: Evidence that the hypertensive action of alpha-methyldopa is mediated by central actions of alpha-methyl noradrenaline, Journal of Pharmacy and Pharmacology **23:**407-414, 1971.

35. Herbst, A.L., Ulfelder, H., and Poskanzer, D.C.: Adenocarcinoma of the vagina: association of maternal stilbestrol therapy with tumor appearance in young women, New England Journal of Medicine **284:**878-881, 1971.

36. Hollifield, J.W., et al.: Proposed mechanism of propranolol's antihypertensive effect in essential hypertension, New England Journal of Medicine **295:**68-71, 1976.

37. Hollister, L.E.: Drugs and sexual behavior in man, Life Sciences **17:**661-668, 1975.

38. Hughes, J.M.: Failure to ejaculate with chlordiazepoxide, American Journal of Psychiatry **121:**610-611, 1964.

39. Jarvik, M.E.: Drugs used in the treatment of psychiatric disorders. In Goodman, L.S., and Gilman, A., editors: The pharmacological basis of therapeutics, ed. 4, New York, 1970, The Macmillan Co.

40. Jones, A.R.: The antifertility actions of alpha-chlorhydrin in the male, Life Sciences **23:**1625-1646, 1978.

41. Kalant, H.: Some recent physiological and biochemical investigations on alcohol and alcoholism, Quarterly Journal of Studies on Alcohol **23:**52-93, 1962.

42. Katchadourian, H.A., and Lunde, D.T.: Fundamentals of human sexuality, New York, 1972, Holt, Rinehart & Winston, Inc.

43. Kesseru, E., Larranaja, A., and Parada, J.: Postcoital contraception with D-norgestrel, Contraception **7:**367-379, 1973.

44. Kolodny, R.C., et al.: Depression of plasma testosterone levels after chronic intensive marijuana use, New England Journal of Medicine **290:**872-874, 1974.

45. Lewin, L.: Phantastic: narcotics and stimulating drugs, their use and abuse, New York, 1964, E.P. Dutton & Co., Inc.

46. Lim, V.S., and Fang, V.S.: Restoration of plasma testosterone levels in uremic men with clomiphene citrate, Journal of Clinical Endocrinology and Metabolism **43:**1370-1377, 1976.

47. Lunde, D.T., and Hamberg, D.A.: Techniques for assessing the effects of sex hormones on affect, arousal and aggression in humans, Recent Progress in Hormone Research **28:**627-663, 1972.

48. Maliz, S.: L-Dopa and behavior, New York, 1972, Raven Press.

49. Mathis, J.L.: Sexual aspects of heroin addiction, Medical Aspects of Human Sexuality **4**(9):98-109, 1970.

50. Marijuana and health: 1982, Committee to Study the Health-Related Effects of Cannabis and its Derivatives, Washington, D.C., 1982, Institute of Medicine, National Academy of Sciences, National Academy Press.

51. Mills, L.C.: Drug-induced impotence, American Family Physician **12:**104-106, 1975.

52. Money, J., and Yankowitz, R.: The sympathetic-inhibiting effects of the drug Ismelin on human male eroticism, with a note on Mellaril, Journal of Sexual Research **3:**69-82, 1967.

53. Neiger, S.: Sex potions, Sexology, pp. 730-733, June 1968.

54. Neumann, F., et al.: Aspects of androgen-dependent events as studied by antiandrogens, Recent Progress in Hormone Research **26:**337-410, 1970.

55. Pedan, N.R., et al.: Male sexual dysfunction during treatment with cimetidine, British Medical Journal **1:**659, 1979.

56. Prasad, M.R.N., Singh, S.P., and Rajalakshmi, M.: Fertility control in male rats by continuous release of microquantities of cyproterone acetate from subcutaneous Silastic capsules, Contraception **2:**165-178, 1970.

57. Riddinough, M.A.: Presenting, detecting and managing adverse reactions of antihypertensive agents in the ambulant patient with essential hypertension, American Journal of Hospital Pharmacy **34:**465-479, 1977.

58. Saidi, K., Wenn, R.V., and Sharif, F.: Bromocriptine for male infertility, Lancet **1:**250-251, 1977.

59. Sanchez, R.S., et al.: Pituitary-testicular axis in patients on lithium therapy, Fertility and Sterility **27:**667-669, 1976.

60. Schneider, J., and Kaffarnik, H.: Impotence in patients treated with clofibrate, Atherosclerosis **21:**455-457, 1977.

61. Sex in the news: Sexology, p. 25, Sept. 1971.

62. Shader, R.I.: Male sexual function. In Shader, R.I., and DiMascio, A., editors: Psychotrophic drug side-effects, Boston, 1970, The Williams & Wilkins Co.

63. Shader, R.I.: Sexual dysfunction associated with mesoridazine besylate (Serentil), Psychopharmacologia **27:**293-294, 1972.

64. Shader, R.I., and Grinspoon, G.I.: Schizophrenia, oligospermia, and the phenothiazines, Diseases of the Nervous System **28:**240-244, 1967.

65. Singer, I., and Rotenberg, D.: Physiology in medicine: mechanisms of lithium action, New England Journal of Medicine **298:**254-260, 1973.

66. Singh, H.: Case of inhibition of ejaculation as side-effect of Mellaril, American Journal of Psychiatry **117:**1041-1042, 1961.

67. Story, N.L.: Sexual dysfunction resulting from drug side effects, Journal of Sexual Research **10:**132-149, 1974.

68. Stohs, S.J.: Drugs and sexual effects, U.S. Pharmacist **3:**51-68, 1978.

69. Tagliamonte, A., et al.: Compulsive sexual activity induced by *p*-chlorophenylalanine in normal and pinealectomized male rats, Science **166:**1433, 1969.

70. Van Thiel, D.H., et al.: Hypothalamic-pituitary-gonadal dysfunction in men using cimetidine, New England Journal of Medicine **300:**1012-1015, 1979.

71. Van Thiel, D.H., and Lester, R.: Sex and alcohol, New England Journal of Medicine **291:**251-253, 1974.

72. Van Thiel, D.H., Sherins, R.J., and Lester, R.: Mechanisms of hypogonadism in alcohol liver disease, Gastroenterology **65:**574-582, 1973.

73. Wade, N.: Anabolic steroids: doctors denounce them, but athletes aren't listening, Science **176:**1399-1403, 1972.

74. Watts, R.J.: The physiological interrelationships between depression, drugs, and sexuality, Nursing Forum **17:**169-183, 1978.

75. Wolfe, M.M.: Impotence on cimetidine treatment, New England Journal of Medicine **300**(2):94, 1979.

76. Woosley, R.L., and Nies, A.S.: Guanethidine, New England Journal of Medicine **295:**1053-1057, 1976.

77. Zacharias, F.J.: Patient acceptability of propranolol and the occurrence of side effects, Postgraduate Medical Journal **52**(Suppl. 4):87-89, 1976.

Suggested readings

Csaky, T.Z.: Cutting's handbook of pharmacology, ed. 6, New York, 1979, Appleton-Century-Crofts.

Goodman, L.S., and Gilman, A., editors: The pharmacological basis of therapeutics, ed. 6, New York, 1980, The Macmillan Co.

References for clients

Graedon, J.: The people's pharmacy, ed. 1, New York, 1977, Avon Books.

Graedon, J.: The people's pharmacy, ed. 2, New York, 1980, Avon Books.

Index

A

Abdominal pain, lower, in sexually transmitted diseases, 272

Abortion
  antecedents of, 183-190
    biologic, 184-185
    contraceptive use as, 185-187
    psychologic, 187
    sexual decisions as, 183-184
    sociologic, 187-190
  availability of, 189
  health care process in, 196-197
  health practitioner's role in, 194-196
  legal availability of, 188-189
  for pregnancy from rape, 251, 253
  public attitudes toward, 189-190
  sequelae of, 190-194
    biologic, 190-192
    psychologic, 192-194
    sexual, 194
  spontaneous, age and, 185

Abstinence for contraception, sexual behavior and, 215*t*

Abuse, sexual, sexual dysfunction and, 134

Acting out, sexual, 287-288

Acyclovir for genital herpes, 277

Adjustment, sexual well-being and, 371-372

Adolescence
  sexual problems and concerns in, 56-59
  sexuality in, 53-59

Adrenogenital syndrome, 48

Adulthood
  sexuality in, 65-66
  young, sexuality in, 63-65

Age
  abortion and, 184-185
  fertility and, 207-208, 223
  psychologic response to rape and, 239
  refractory time and, 10

Aging ostomate, 353, 358

Aggravated assault, definition of, 232

Air embolism from oral-genital sex in pregnancy, 175

Alcohol
  physiologic effects of, on sexual functioning in female, 417-420

Page numbers in *italic* indicate illustrations.
Page numbers followed by *t* indicate tables.

Alcohol—cont'd
  physiologic effects of, on sexual functioning in male, 422-423

Alcoholism
  in men
    delayed orgasm or ejaculation and, 426
    erectile dysfunction and, 423-426
    inhibited sexual desire and, 423
    physiologic effects of, on sexual functioning, 422-423
    sexual dysfunctions and, 423
    sexuality and, 422-426
    sexuality issues and, 426
  recovery from, sexual concerns in, 429
  and sexual minorities, 427
  sexual relationship issues in, 426-427
  sexuality and, 415-431
    health care provider and, 428-430
  in women
    dyspareunia and, 420
    inhibited desire and, 420
    orgasmic dysfunction and, 420
    physiologic effects of, on sexual functioning, 417-420
    sexual dysfunctions and, 420
    sexuality and, 415-422
    sexuality issues and, 421-422
    vaginismus and, 420-421

Aldactone, sexual behavior and, 438, 450*t*

Aldomet, sexual behavior and, 437, 450*t*

Amebiasis, sexually transmitted, 279

Amitriptyline, sexual behavior and, 439, 450*t*

Amniotic fluid infections, coitus and, 174

Amobarbital, sexual behavior and, 442-443

Amphetamines, sexual behavior and, 446, 451*t*

Ampicillin, oral
  for *Gardnerella* vaginalis vaginitis, 279
  for gonorrhea, 274

Amyl nitrite, sexual behavior and, 447, 451*t*

Amytal, sexual behavior and, 442-443

Anabolic steroids, sexual behavior and, 443, 451*t*

Anal intercourse, effects of, on cardiovascular system, 297

Androgen-insensitivity syndrome, 47-48

Androgens, levels of, diminished, in male climacteric, *67*, 68

Androgyny, sexual behavior and, 21-22

Disseminated gonococcal infection (DGI), 274-275

Disulfiram, sexual behavior and, 449, 451*t*

Diuretics, sexual behavior and, 438, 450*t*

Diuril, sexual behavior and, 438, 450*t*

Donovanosis, 277

L-Dopa, sexual behavior and, 447, 451*t*

Double standard in sexual behavior in United States, 19-20

Drug(s)

   antidepressant, sexual behavior and, 439-440, 450*t*

   antihistamine, sexual behavior and, 440, 450*t*

   antihypertensive, sexual behavior and, 437-439, 450*t*

   antispasmodic, sexual behavior and, 440, 450*t*

   barbiturate, sexual behavioral and, 442-443, 450*t*

   decreasing sexual activity and functioning, 436

   effects of, on sexual behavior, 434-452

   enhancing sexual behavior, 443-446

   ethyl alcohol as, sexual behavior and, 441-442, 446, 450*t*; *see also* Alcohol; Alcoholism

   narcotic, sexual behavior and, 444-446

   oral contraceptive

      sexual behavior and, 215*t*, 434-436, 450*t*

      sexually transmitted diseases and, 267-268

   psychoactive, sexual behavior and, 444-446

   saltpeter as, sexual behavior and, 443, 451*t*

   sedative, sexual behavior and, 440, 450*t*

   sex hormone preparations as, sexual behavior and, 443, 451*t*

   tranquilizing, sexual behavior and, 440-441, 450*t*

Durabolin, sexual behavior and, 443, 451*t*

Dysfunction

   erectile, 138-141; *see also* Erectile dysfunction

   orgasmic, in female, 144-145

   sexual, 132-148

      of alcoholic men, 423

      of alcoholic women, 420

      from cerebrovascular accident, 377-379

      in chronic renal disease, 314, 316-320, 321-324

Dysfunction—cont'd

   sexual—cont'd

      of diabetic men, 328-332; *see also* Erectile dysfunction in diabetic men

      of diabetic women, 332-337

      etiology of, 132-134

      female, 143-147; *see also* Female sexual dysfunction

      hormonal factors in, 133

      male, 137-143; *see also* Male sexual dysfunction

      neural factors in, 133

      in ostomate, 352-358

      physiologic influences on, 132-133

      psychologic influences on, 133-134

      sexual health care and, 126-127

      treatment modalities for, 134-137

         Annon's, 135

         group, 137

         Kaplan's, 136-137

         Masters and Johnson's, 135-136

      vascular factors in, 133

Dyspareunia, 127, 147

   in alcoholic women, 420

   rape and, 232

E

Educating clients, nurse's role in, 121-122

Education, sex, 103-113

   for alcoholic, 429

   approaches to, 106

   for arthritis client, 375-376

   for developmentally delayed teenager, 408-410

   evaluation of program for, 111

   for myocardial infarction client, 300, 303

   need for, 104-105

   objectives of, 105-106

   preparation of health professional for, 106-111; *see also* Health professional as sex educator, preparation of

   resources for, 112-113

   scope of, 104-106

   for spinal cord injury client, 390-391

Educational skills for sex educator, 109-111

Ejaculation

   dysfunctional, in diabetes, 329

   inhibited, 127, 143